Canine Anatomy

A SYSTEMIC STUDY

Canine Anatomy

A SYSTEMIC STUDY

DONALD R. ADAMS

Department of Veterinary Anatomy
College of Veterinary Medicine
Iowa State University

THE IOWA STATE UNIVERSITY PRESS / AMES

Authorization to photocopy items for internal or personal use,
or the internal or personal use of specific clients, is granted by
Iowa State University Press, provided that the base fee of $.10
per copy is paid directly to the Copyright Clearance Center, 27
Congress Street, Salem, MA 01970. For those organizations
that have been granted a photocopy license by CCC, a separate
system of payments has been arranged. The fee code for users
of the Transactional Reporting Service is 0-8138-0281-4/86 $.10.

♾ Printed on acid-free paper in the United States of America

First edition, 1986
Second printing, 1988
Third printing, 1992
Fourth printing, 1994

Library of Congress Cataloging in Publication Data

Adams, Donald R. (Donald Robert)
    Canine anatomy.

    1. Dogs — Anatomy.   I. Title.
SF767.D6A33   1986   636.7'0891   85–23114
ISBN 0-8138-0281-4

CONTENTS

PREFACE

This text is written to provide introductory anatomical information on the dog and cat for the first year veterinary student. Since this text was prepared as an adjunct to the very fine reference textbook <u>Miller's Anatomy of the Dog</u>, specific details and references have been omitted. Terminology generally conforms to that of <u>Nomina Anatomica Veterinaria</u>, 3rd edition, 1983.

This text has been used as a guide to the systemic dissection of nonembalmed canine carcasses. To achieve diversity in student dissection and to enhance learning, specific dissection instructions have been omitted. An effort has been made to present directional and structural terminology gradually and sequentially. Anatomical terms introduced for the first time in the text, or emphasized in a particular chapter, are typed in capital letters. Information about some words known to cause students difficulty has for clarification been included in parentheses after they first appear. Information on these words may include their singular and plural spellings, pronunciation, and/or meaning. It is hoped that students will be motivated by this additional information to make regular use of a medical dictionary.

I am indebted to Neal Cholvin, former chairman of Veterinary Anatomy, Pharmacology, and Physiology, Iowa State University, for his support of instructional innovation; Ron Flatt, the late director of Laboratory Animal Resources, Iowa State University, for his assistance in procuring sufficient animals for laboratory dissection; the Iowa State University Research Foundation for providing partial support for the illustrative work; and to Dean Biechler, April Damaska, Suzie

Rayne, Frank Schneider, and Chari Wessel for their many excellent anatomical drawings. The illustrations, most which were drawn from prosected specimens, are original contributions to the discipline. I also wish to thank the many students, faculty, and staff who contributed to this book and to the course for which it was prepared. The numerous revisions of this text, prepared prior to the availability of word processing, were achieved through the very capable secretarial assistance of Glenda Burkheimer.

Introduction

FIG. 1.1. Long axis.

LONG AXIS

FIG. 1.2. Proximal—distal.

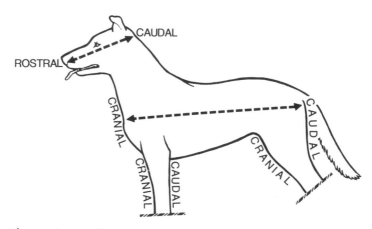

FIG. 1.3. Cranial/rostral—caudal.

1 DIRECTIONAL TERMINOLOGY

A number of adjectives are used to describe the position of structures in the body. Descriptive terms are also used to name many anatomical structures. The terms described in this chapter are utilized throughout the remainder of the text.

An imaginary line through the center of the length of an organ or structure of the body forms the LONG AXIS (pl. axes) of that organ or structure (Fig. 1.1). The weight of the organ is almost symmetrically distributed around its long axis. Proximal and distal are used to describe position along the long axis of a structure relative to the main body mass. PROXIMAL implies a position near or toward the main mass of a structure; DISTAL implies a position away from the main mass (Fig. 1.2).

CRANIAL and CAUDAL are directional terms meaning toward or relatively near the cranium (brain case) and tail, respectively (Fig. 1.3). Cranial and caudal, when used in describing structures of the trunk (neck, thorax, abdomen, and pelvis), refer to position along the long axis of the trunk. Cranial and caudal, when used in reference to forelimb and hind limb structures of a standing dog, refer to the surfaces toward the head and tail, respectively; only the portions of the limbs proximal to the carpus (wrist) and tarsus (ankle) are said to have cranial and caudal surfaces. ROSTRAL, rather than cranial, is used to describe the positions of most structures along the long axis of the head; the word rostral refers to a position facing the apex of the nose. In the head the opposite direction to rostral is caudal.

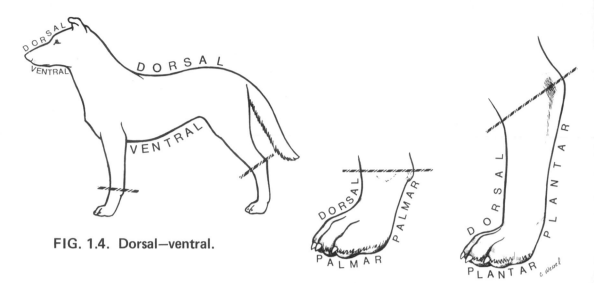

FIG. 1.4. Dorsal—ventral.

FIG. 1.5. Dorsal—palmar/plantar.

FIG. 1.6. Anterior - posterior/superior - inferior.

FIG. 1.7. Median plane.

FIG. 1.8. Sagittal plane.

DORSAL and VENTRAL are directional terms meaning toward or relatively near the back and belly, respectively (Fig. 1.4). Dorsal and ventral, when used in describing structures of the head, trunk, and tail, refer to opposing positions along the long axis. Distal to the carpus and tarsus, dorsal refers to the surface opposite that of the footpads (Fig. 1.5). The dorsal surfaces of the distal portions of the thoracic and pelvic limbs are continuous proximally with the cranial surfaces of the respective limb. The surface of the thoracic limb distal to the carpus, which bears footpads, is the PALMAR surface; the surface of the pelvic limb distal to the tarsus, which bears footpads, is the PLANTAR surface (Fig. 1.5). The palmar and plantar surfaces of the distal portion of the limbs are continuous with the caudal surfaces of the proximal portion of the limbs.

When describing certain structures of the head (eye, eyelids, lips, inner ear, pituitary gland), the terms cranial, caudal, dorsal, and ventral are replaced by ANTERIOR, POSTERIOR, SUPERIOR, and INFERIOR, respectively (Fig. 1.6).

An organ or structure may be divided into two nearly identical halves by a MEDIAN PLANE (Fig. 1.7). A median plane passing longitudinally through the dog's body divides it into right and left halves. The DORSAL MEDIAN LINE and VENTRAL MEDIAN LINE are imaginary lines through which the median plane passes on the dorsal and ventral surfaces, respectively, of the dog. A SAGITTAL (PARAMEDIAN) PLANE (Fig. 1.8) is parallel to the median plane. MEDIAL and LATERAL refer to positions toward and away from the median plane, respectively (Fig. 1.9). Some structures, such as blood vessels of the external ear, occur in groups of three and are described as MEDIAL, INTERMEDIATE, and LATERAL.

FIG. 1.9. Medial—intermediate—lateral.

FIG. 1.10.   Dorsal and transverse planes.

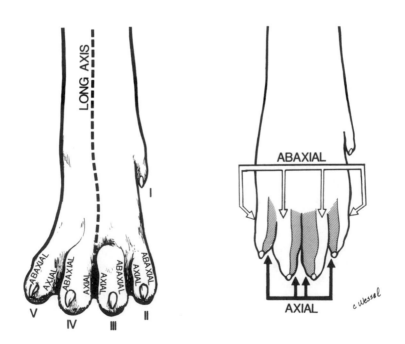

FIG. 1.11.   Axial versus abaxial.

A TRANSVERSE PLANE passes through a structure perpendicular to its long axis; a DORSAL PLANE, perpendicular to both the median and transverse planes, divides the body longitudinally into dorsal and ventral portions (Fig. 1.10).

Axial and abaxial are directional terms used in reference to the digits and relate to the long axis of the limb. The long axis of the thoracic and pelvic limbs of the dog passes between the third and fourth digits. Digits are named I, II, III, IV, and V according to position from medial to lateral. If an animal species has less than five digits the remaining digits are usually designated II, III, IV, and V (as in the hind feet of many dogs); II, III, and IV; III and IV; or III. The AXIAL surface of digits I-V is the surface of each digit nearest the axis; the ABAXIAL surface of digits I-V is the surface of each digit away from the axis (Fig. 1.11).

Superficial and deep are terms used in reference to position in the body or in a solid organ (Fig. 1.12). SUPERFICIAL means near the surface and DEEP refers to near the center of the body or solid organ.

FIG. 1.12. Superficial - deep.

Internal and external describe the position of a structure in the body or in a hollow organ (Fig. 1.13). INTERNAL implies that a structure is near the lumen of an organ; EXTERNAL implies that the structure is away from the center of a hollow organ.

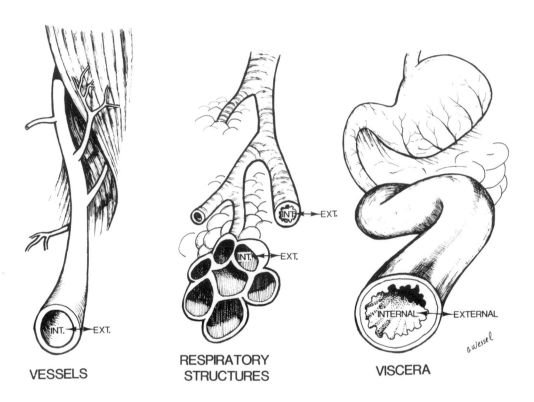

VESSELS

RESPIRATORY STRUCTURES

VISCERA

FIG. 1.13. External—internal.

Superficial Morphology

FIG. 2.1. Nasal plane.

NASAL ALA

NASAL SULCUS

LATERAL VIEW

NASAL ALA   NASAL ALA

NASAL   NASAL
SULCUS   SULCUS

ROSTRAL VIEW

SUPERIOR PALPEBRA

CILIA

LATERAL PALPEBRAL
COMMISSURE

INFERIOR PALPEBRA

SUPERIOR LACRIMAL
PUNCTUM

MEDIAL PALPEBRAL
COMMISSURE

INFERIOR LACRIMAL PUNCTUM

SEMILUNAR CONJUNCTIVAL
FOLD

FIG. 2.2. Palpebrae.

PALPEBRAL CONJUNCTIVA

CONJUNCTIVAL
SAC

CORNEA

BULBAR
CONJUNCTIVA

CONJUNCTIVAL FORNIX

FIG. 2.3. Conjunctiva and cornea.

2 THE COMMON INTEGUMENT

The term COMMON INTEGUMENT, or common covering, includes the skin, hair, skin glands, mammary glands, pads, and claws. The SKIN, which covers the external surface of the body, is variously modified over the surface of the external nose, eye, and ear. The NASAL PLANE is the nonhaired tip of the nose that is divided by small fissures into numerous polygons (Fig. 2.1). Each external NARIS (pl. nares; nostril) is bounded laterally by a movable wing, or NASAL ALA (a'lah, pl. alae). The grooves ventral to the nasal alae are the NASAL SULCI (sul'kee, sing. sulcus).

The PALPEBRAE (sing. palprebra; eyelids) are modified integumentary structures that protect the anterior surface of the eye (Fig. 2.2). Both SUPERIOR and INFERIOR PALPEBRAE have a haired superficial surface, but CILIA (sil'e-ah, sing. cilium; eyelashes) are present only on the superior palpebra. The lateral and medial angles formed by the junctions of the superior and inferior palpebrae are termed LATERAL and MEDIAL PALPEBRAL COMMISSURES (CANTHI) (can'thie, sing. canthus), respectively. A third eyelid, the SEMILUNAR CONJUNCTIVAL FOLD (NICTITATING MEMBRANE), projects laterally from the medial commissure of the eye.

The skin of the superficial surface of the palpebrae is continuous with the mucous membrane of the deep surface. This mucous membrane is the CONJUNCTIVA (Fig. 2.3), a delicate lining that covers the deep surface of the palpebrae (PALPEBRAL CONJUNCTIVA) and the anterior surface of the eyeball (BULBAR CONJUNCTIVA). The bulbar conjunctiva is continuous with the most superficial layer of the CORNEA, the anterior corneal epithelium. The angle formed by the reflection of the conjunctiva from the palpebral surface to

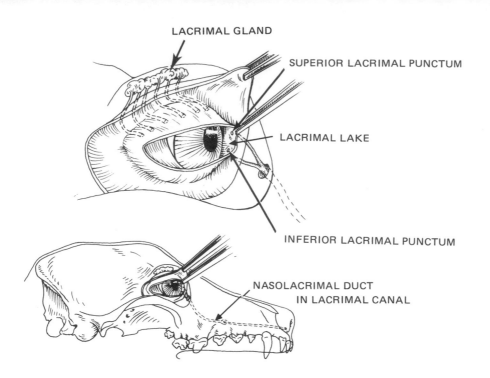

FIG. 2.4. Lacrimal apparatus.

LACRIMAL GLAND

SUPERIOR LACRIMAL PUNCTUM

LACRIMAL LAKE

INFERIOR LACRIMAL PUNCTUM

NASOLACRIMAL DUCT
IN LACRIMAL CANAL

FIG. 2.5. Lymph nodules on the deep surface of the semilunar conjunctival fold.

FIG. 2.6. External ear.

APEX

ANTITRAGIC MARGIN

TRAGIC MARGIN

AURICLE

SCAPHA

SPINE OF HELIX

CUTANEOUS
MARGINAL SAC

ANTIHELIX

ANTITRAGUS

CRURA OF THE HELIX

INTERTRAGIC
INCISURE

TRAGUS

PRETRAGIC INCISURE

ANNULAR CARTILAGE

the bulbar surface is termed the CONJUNCTIVAL FORNIX (for⁄niks, pl. fornices).

The fluid-filled space between the palpebrae and bulbar conjunctiva is the CONJUNCTIVAL SAC. At the medial palpebral commissure there is a larger fluid-filled space, the LACRIMAL LAKE (Fig. 2.4). A small orifice, difficult to see with the unaided eye, is present in both the superior and inferior palpebrae. These orifices, termed LACRIMAL PUNCTA (punk⁄tah, sing. punctum), are situated near the medial palpebral commissure. LACRIMAL FLUID (tears) is produced primarily by LACRIMAL GLANDS (70%), located dorsal to the eyeball, and by the superficial gland of the third eyelid (30%). Fluid collects in the lacrimal lake and passes away from the surface of the eye through the lacrimal puncta; it is then discharged into the rostral part of the nasal cavity by the NASOLACRIMAL DUCT.

The posterior (deep) surface of the semilunar conjunctival fold bears prominent LYMPH NODULES (Fig. 2.5). These nodules when inflamed and swollen may block flow through the secretory ducts of the superficial glands of the third eyelid.

The external ear (Fig. 2.6) consists of a canal, the EXTERNAL ACOUSTIC MEATUS (me-a⁄tus; passage), and the PINNA (pin⁄nah, pl. pinnae). The pinna is that portion of the ear that is readily seen; it is fundamentally the same in the various breeds of dogs. The rostral margin of the pinna is the TRAGIC MARGIN and the lateral margin is the ANTITRAGIC MARGIN. The tip of the ear is termed the APEX. The SCAPHA is that portion of the pinna situated between tragic and antitragic margins. The cartilaginous skeleton of the ear is formed by two cartilages: auricular and annular. The AURICULAR CARTILAGE, which provides shape to the external ear, is thin and pliable over most of its distal portion. The proximal portion of the auricular cartilage is rolled, forming a tubelike wall around much of the external acoustic eatus. A number of folds, or wrinkles, formed in the auricular cartilage present structural landmarks for treatment of the ear. The most prominent is a transverse fold on the concave surface of the external ear. The free end of this fold, the ANTIHELIX (he⁄liks, pl. helices; coil), is directed caudolaterally. At the base of the ear a thickened structure, the TRAGUS (tra⁄gus, pl. tragi), forms the superficial wall of the cartilaginous external acoustic meatus. The tragic margin separates proximally into two CRURA (kru⁄ra, sing. crus) between which is positioned the

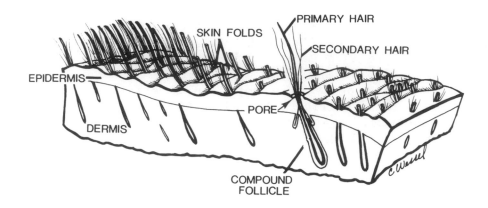

FIG. 2.7. Diagram of an excised block of skin.

FIG. 2.8. Specialized hair types.

rostral margin of the tragus. The groove between these crura and the tragus is named the PRETRAGIC INCISURE. Caudal to the antihelix on the caudal part of the concave surface of the pinna, several longitudinal ridges may be observed, two of which are the lateral and medial processes of the ANTITRAGUS. The fissure between the antitragus and tragus is called the INTERTRAGIC INCISURE. The tragus and the pretragic and intertragic incisures are important landmarks for surgery to drain the external acoustic meatus. A CUTANEOUS MARGINAL SAC of unknown significance occurs in the antitragic margin. The ANNULAR CARTILAGE is a short, cartilaginous tube that extends from the osseous external acoustic meatus of the skull to the auricular cartilage; thus it encloses the proximal portion of the membranous external acoustic meatus.

Microscopically the skin may be divided into two major parts, the EPIDERMIS and DERMIS (Fig. 2.7), each of which is subdivided into various layers. The deepest layer of the epidermis is a layer of living cells, which, by mitosis, produces cells of the more superficial epidermal layers and of hair and claws. The dermis is a layer of connective tissue deep to the epidermis; it contains blood vessels, nerves, nerve endings, and glands. Macroscopic examination of the dermal layer of the dog reveals the basal portion of hair embedded in it; the layer of living cells of the epidermis folds down into the dermis, forming a sheath or follicle around the base of the hair shaft. Each hair is a nonliving structure produced by an epidermal HAIR FOLLICLE. A number of individual hairs (a larger PRIMARY HAIR plus several smaller SECONDARY HAIRS), each with its own follicle, project from the surface of the skin through a common opening, or PORE. Small muscle fibers attach to the hair follicle deeply and to the dermis superficially. Contraction of these smooth muscle fibers straightens the hair.

Some examples of specialized types of hair present over the surface of the body (Fig. 2.8) are: CILIA, TRAGI (hair at the opening of the external ear), and the large TACTILE HAIRS present over much of the face. Types of tactile hairs include SUPRAORBITAL, ZYGOMATIC, BUCCAL (buk'al), SUPERIOR and INFERIOR LABIAL, MENTAL, and INTRAMANDIBULAR. Tactile hairs are termed "vibrissae" by many comparative anatomists. In Veterinary Anatomy the term vibrissae is restricted to specialized hairs present in the nasal vestibule; such vibrissae are not present in the dog. Tactile hairs are large single hairs, each of which is produced by a large follicle. The tactile hair follicle is surrounded by a blood

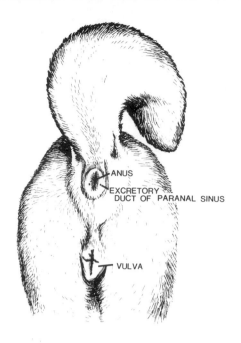

FIG. 2.9. Duct orifices of paranal sinuses, anal sphincters relaxed.

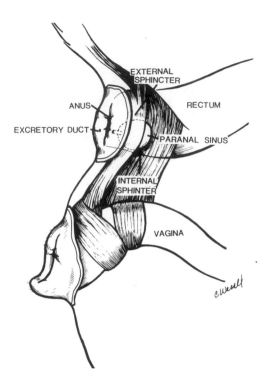

FIG. 2.10. Paranal sinus—anal sphincter relationship.

FIG. 2.11. Caudal gland.

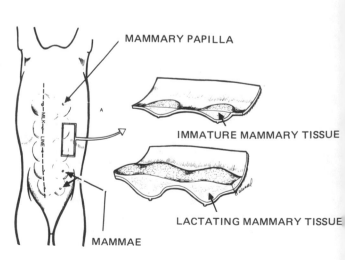

FIG. 2.12. Mammary glands.

sinus composed of a superficial ring and a deeper spongy portion. Abundant nerve fiber terminals in the connective tissue walls of the blood sinuses are responsive to tactile sensation. Both the blood pressure in the sinus and the skeletal muscle attaching to the dermal sheath of the follicle may modify the responsiveness of the hair to stimulation. (In the cat, tactile hairs with blood sinuses are also present in the skin of the distal portion of the thoracic limb).

Microscopic glands occurring in the dermis are sebaceous, odoriferous, or sudoriferous in character. The SEBACEOUS GLANDS secrete a fatty material and are usually associated with hair follicles. ODORIFEROUS (APOCRINE SUDORIFEROUS) GLANDS, located over most of the dog's surface area, are also associated with hair follicles; these glands, which secrete odorous substances, may function in olfactory communication between animals. SUDORIFEROUS (MEROCRINE SUDORIFEROUS) GLANDS, or true sweat glands, are restricted in location to the footpads, where their watery secretions may have a function in gripping the surface. Some larger specialized glands are the CERUMINOUS GLANDS of the external auditory meatus, TARSAL GLANDS of the palpebrae, CIRCUMANAL GLANDS of the anal region, paranal sinus glands (glands of the anal sacs), caudal glands, and mammary glands.

The PARANAL SINUSES (anal sacs) are paired cutaneous sacs located one to each side of the anus; a duct from each sinus opens onto the surface of the skin at the lateral margin of the anus (Figs. 2.9, 2.10). The paranal sinuses are covered by skeletal muscle that encircles the anal canal.

The CAUDAL GLAND is a densely grouped collection of microscopic glands on the dorsal surface of the proximal portion of the tail (Fig. 2.11).

The MAMMARY (milk producing) GLANDS develop in a row on each side of the ventral median line; this row, or line, is termed the "milk line" (Fig. 2.12). The mammary glands (MAMMAE) of the bitch are usually present as four to six pairs. Five pairs of mammae are the most common, although there may be four mammae on one side and five on the other. The mammae are described as being thoracic, cranial abdominal, middle abdominal, or caudal abdominal according to their regional placement. Each functional mammary gland (MAMMA) produces milk, which passes to the surface of the skin via 7-16 ducts in a MAMMARY PAPILLA (pah-pil'ah, pl. papillae), or nipple (Fig. 2.13). Both male and young female

FIG. 2.13. Mammary papilla.

PAPILLARY OSTIA

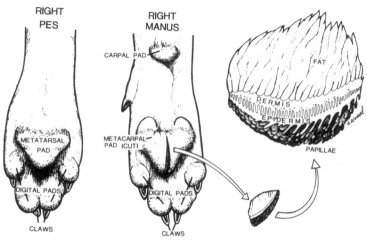

RIGHT PES

RIGHT MANUS

CARPAL PAD

METACARPAL PAD (CUT)

METATARSAL PAD

DIGITAL PADS

DIGITAL PADS

CLAWS

CLAWS

FAT

DERMIS

EPIDERMIS

PAPILLAE

FIG. 2.14. Footpads.

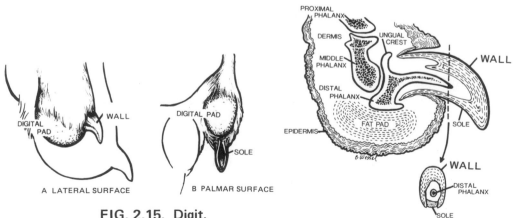

WALL

DIGITAL PAD

DIGITAL PAD

WALL

SOLE

A LATERAL SURFACE

B PALMAR SURFACE

FIG. 2.15. Digit.

PROXIMAL PHALANX

DERMIS

UNGUAL CREST

WALL

MIDDLE PHALANX

DISTAL PHALANX

EPIDERMIS

FAT PAD

SOLE

WALL

DISTAL PHALANX

SOLE

TRANSVERSE SECTION THROUGH THE DISTAL PHALANX AND CLAW

FIG. 2.16. Digit, sectioned sagittaly.

mammae consist of papillae and small primary ducts. Beginning with the onset of the first estrus the mammary duct system and glandular elements of the bitch develop. After conception the mammae continue developing until tissue of adjacent glands crowd each other.

PADS, roughened by small projecting papillae, are present on the palmar and plantar surfaces of the limbs. These papillae provide traction as they come into contact with the ground. Each pad consists of thickened epidermal and dermal parts plus a deeper fat pad (Fig. 2.14) that is highly vascular. The pads are named according to their location. The DIGITAL PADS are small pads located in the distal interphalangeal region of digits II–V. The large pads in the metacarpophalangeal and metatarsophalangeal regions are the METACARPAL and METATARSAL PADS, respectively. A small pad on the palmar surface of the carpal region is the CARPAL PAD.

A CLAW is a cutaneous structure, the proximal portion of which wraps around the distal portion of the digital skeleton (Figs. 2.15, 2.16). The dorsal and lateral epidermal portion of the claw (WALL) is stronger than the ventral portion (SOLE). The proximal portion, or coronary border, of the wall is situated in the osseous depression formed by the ungual crest of the distal phalanx. The dermis of the claw is continuous with connective tissue lining the bone of the distal phalanx. When the claw is clipped too close, the nerves and blood vessels of the dermis respond by producing pain and bleeding.

A DEWCLAW is not a claw but rather a relatively functionless digit. The dewclaw (first digit of the hind foot), if present, may possess one, two, or all three phalanges. For show, the Briard and Great Pyrenees breeds are required to have double dewclaws.

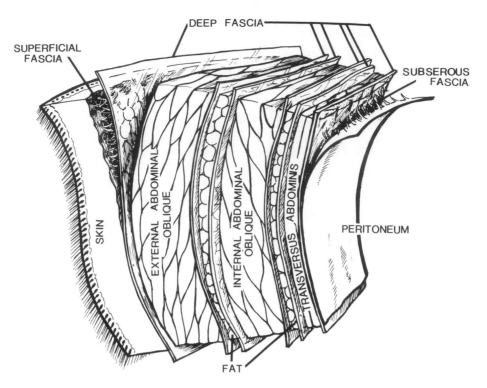

FIG. 3.1. Diagram of an excised block of abdominal wall.

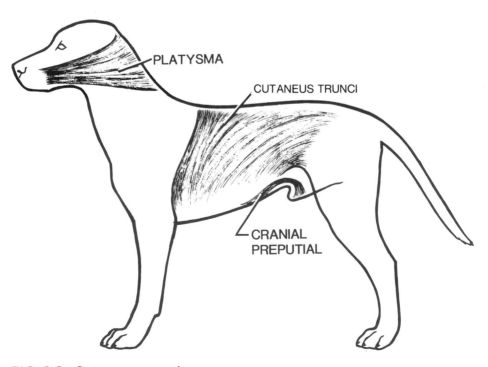

FIG. 3.2. Cutaneous muscle.

3 FASCIA

FASCIA (fash'e-ah, pl. fasciae; band) is composed of connective tissue bands or sheets that bind skin to deeper structures and ensheath structures deep to the skin.

For descriptive purposes, fascia may be subdivided into three major types: superficial, deep, and subserous (Fig. 3.1); the superficial and deep fascial sheets are named according to the anatomical regions where they are located.

The SUPERFICIAL FASCIA (TELA SUBCUTANEA) (te'lah, pl. telae) is an elastic layer that connects the dermis of the skin to deeper structures. (Many authors consider this layer to be part of the dermis of the skin.) In some locations there is little superficial fascia and the skin is held tightly to underlying structures; in other places the skin is quite loose.

A thin layer of cutaneous muscle, which functions to move or shake the skin, lies within the superficial fascia (Fig. 3.2). The portion of cutaneous muscle that attaches most of the skin of the trunk to the axillary region is the CUTANEUS TRUNCI MUSCLE. Other cutaneous muscles include that of the head (the PLATYSMA) and the ventrally situated CRANIAL PREPUTIAL MUSCLE of the dog, which, as part of the cutaneus trunci muscle, attaches to the cutaneous sheath of the penis. The mammary glands are located primarily in the superficial fascial layer (the female homolog of the cranial preputial muscle is the CRANIAL SUPRAMAMMARY MUSCLE). In well-fed animals the superficial fascia is often densely infiltrated with fatty deposits; the term PANNICULUS ADIPOSUS refers to a fatty superficial fascia. Injections into the superficial fascia are rapidly absorbed by the abundant small blood and

FIG. 3.3. Deep lumbar and abdominal fascia.

SKIN
SUPERFICIAL FASCIA
SUPRASPINOUS LIGAMENT
FAT
DEEP FASCIA
LUMBAR VERTEBRA
EPAXIAL MUSCLES
LAYERS OF DEEP FASCIA
TRANSVERSUS ABDOMINIS
INTERNAL ABDOMINAL OBLIQUE
EXTERNAL ABDOMINAL OBLIQUE
PERITONEUM

FIG. 3.4. Regional thickenings of the superficial layer of deep fascia.

CRURAL FASCIA
CRURAL EXTENSOR RETINACULUM
TARSAL EXTENSOR RETINACULUM
FLEXOR RETINACULUM

FIG. 3.6. Retinacula of the pelvic limb.

ANTEBRACHIAL FASCIA
EXTENSOR RETINACULUM
FLEXOR RETINACULUM

FIG. 3.5. Retinacula of the thoracic limb.

lymph vessels present there. Some larger veins course near the surface of the body within the superficial fascia.

DEEP FASCIA, a stronger and denser layer than superficial fascia, encases individual muscles and groups of muscles (Fig. 3.3); intermuscular connective tissue SEPTA extend between individual muscles, providing a slippery medium in which muscles may shorten during contraction against little resistance. Each layer of fascia splits into other layers that invest muscles, tendons, and bones in a continuous system. Deep fascia may be arbitrarily described in three levels according to position: (1) a superficial layer that covers the body immediately deep to the superficial fascia; (2) a number of intermediate layers that invest the various muscles and other structures of the body wall; and (3) a deep layer that surfaces the major cavities of the trunk. The intermediate layers interconnect the superficial and deep layers by means of numerous intermuscular septa.

The superficial layer of deep fascia is very well developed in certain anatomical regions (Fig. 3.4) and thus will be given special attention. The THORACOLUMBAR FASCIA (1) is present in the thoracic vertebral and lumbar regions; it is continuous caudally with the GLUTEAL (2) and CAUDAL (3) FASCIA. The fascia of the lateral and cranial femoral regions, the FASCIA LATA (la'tah; wide) (4), is a very strong connective tissue sheet. The superficial layer of the deep fascia invests the distal portions of the thoracic and pelvic limbs, where it is termed the ANTEBRACHIAL (5) and CRURAL (6) FASCIA. It forms a tight sheath around the limbs that under normal physiological conditions prevents the limbs from accumulating blood and lymph.

The deep fascia forms retaining bands around tendons in the carpal and tarsal regions of the thoracic and pelvic limbs, respectively. The retaining band of dorsal carpal fascia is named the EXTENSOR RETINACULUM (ret"i-nak'u-lum, pl. retinacula; rope); it acts to maintain certain tendons in place (Fig. 3.5). The retaining band of palmar carpal fascia is named the FLEXOR RETINACULUM. There are two dorsal retaining bands of thickened fascia in the pelvic limb, named the CRURAL and TARSAL EXTENSOR RETINACULA, and one plantar band, the flexor retinaculum (Fig. 3.6).

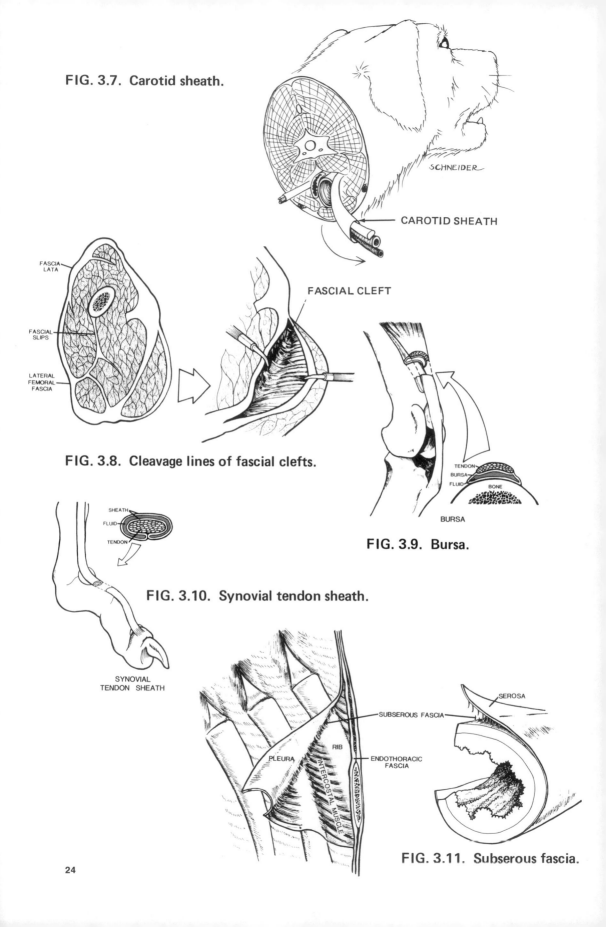

FIG. 3.7. Carotid sheath.

CAROTID SHEATH

SCHNEIDER

FASCIA LATA

FASCIAL SLIPS

LATERAL FEMORAL FASCIA

FASCIAL CLEFT

FIG. 3.8. Cleavage lines of fascial clefts.

TENDON
BURSA
FLUID
BONE

BURSA

FIG. 3.9. Bursa.

SHEATH
FLUID
TENDON

FIG. 3.10. Synovial tendon sheath.

SYNOVIAL TENDON SHEATH

SEROSA

SUBSEROUS FASCIA

PLEURA
RIB
INTERCOSTAL MUSCLE
ENDOTHORACIC FASCIA

FIG. 3.11. Subserous fascia.

24

The deep fascia that forms a sheath around the common carotid artery and vagosympathetic trunk is called the CAROTID SHEATH (Fig. 3.7). The compartments between layers of fascia that enclose muscles, vessels, and lymph nodes may contain an infection and delay its spread. The greater the freedom needed by muscles for contraction, the greater is the degree of fascial separation from muscle surfaces. As muscles are dissected out, these FASCIAL CLEFTS become evident (Fig. 3.8); they are places of cleavage between adjacent muscles.

Fluid-filled connective tissue sacs, or SYNOVIAL BURSAE (ber'sah, pl. bursae), are located in many parts of the body between muscle tendons and underlying bone (Fig. 3.9); bursae reduce friction that otherwise would be produced during muscular activity by tendons sliding on bone. SYNOVIAL TENDON SHEATHS (Fig. 3.10) occur in the manus and pes as specializations of deep fascia forming elongated sacs that wrap around tendons; the deepest portion of the fascial sac adheres to the tendon. The fluid-filled sheaths permit a degree of movement while reducing friction.

The deep layer of deep fascia that forms part of the deep surface of the thoracic wall is termed ENDOTHORACIC FASCIA (Fig. 3.11). The deep layer of deep fascia in the abdominal and pelvic regions is the TRANSVERSALIS FASCIA. SUBSEROUS FASCIA is situated deep to the deep layer of deep fascia and immediately superficial to the serous membrane that surfaces the body wall of the thoracic, abdominal, and pelvic cavities. The subserous fascia is grossly indistinguishable from the deep layer of the deep fascia. Subserous fascia is continuous from the thoracic and abdominal walls to the various internal organs, where it is internal to the external glistening wet (serous) membrane. The fat deposits around the kidney are located primarily within the subserous fascia.

Musculoskeletal System

FIG. 4.1. Regions of the thoracic limb.

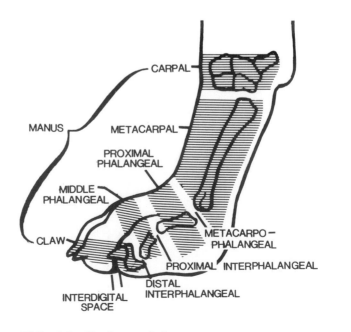

FIG. 4.2. Regions of the manus.

4 THORACIC LIMB

The thoracic limb has scapular, humeral articulation, axillary, brachial, cubital, antebrachial, carpal, metacarpal and phalangeal regions (Fig. 4.1). The SCAPULAR REGION is subdivided longitudinally by the spine of the scapula into the SUPRASPINOUS REGION (craniodorsally) and the INFRASPINOUS REGION (caudoventrally). The region of the HUMERAL ARTICULATION is superficial to the shoulder joint; the POINT OF THE SHOULDER is the most cranial osseous prominence of the bones forming the shoulder joint. The AXILLARY REGION is the area superficial to the AXILLA, a space or tissue compartment medial to the proximal portion of the arm and lateral to the cranial portion of the thorax. The BRACHIAL REGION is superficial to the arm to which it refers. The CUBITAL REGION is superficial to the elbow joint. The POINT OF THE ELBOW is the most caudal osseous projection at the elbow joint; the specific area of the cubital region over the point of the elbow is the OLECRANON (o-lek'rah-non) REGION. The ANTEBRACHIAL REGION is the surface of the forearm. The area of the wrist is the CARPAL REGION. The METACARPAL REGION is distal to the carpal region and proximal to the digits. The area superficial to the digits is the PHALANGEAL REGION.

The MANUS (ma'nus, pl. manus) is the portion of the thoracic limb that includes the carpal, metacarpal, and phalangeal regions (Fig. 4.2). The area superficial to the junction of the digits with the remainder of the foot of the thoracic limb is the METACARPOPHALANGEAL REGION. The regions superficial to the bones of the proximal and middle segments of the digits are termed PROXIMAL and MIDDLE PHALANGEAL; the distal area of each digit is termed the CLAW REGION. Regions superficial to the joints between osseous elements of the digit are termed PROXIMAL and DISTAL INTERPHALANGEAL. The area between individual digits is the INTERDIGITAL SPACE.

FIG. 4.3. Appendicular structures.

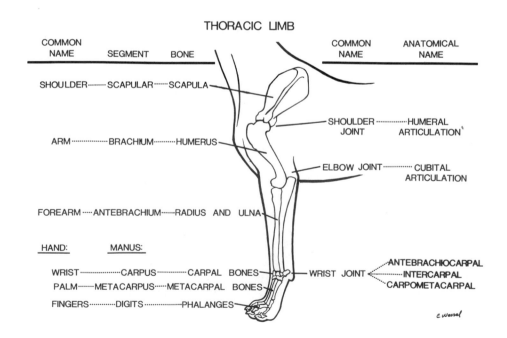

FIG. 4.4. Anatomical segments of the thoracic limb.

The bones and muscles of the major appendages of the body, the thoracic and pelvic limbs, form the APPENDICULAR SKELETON and MUSCLES (Fig. 4.3). The thoracic limb is arbitrarily divided into a number of anatomical segments, which correspond to the names of regions that overlay them (Fig. 4.4).

BONES

Bones are classified according to their shape as long, short, flat, or pneumatic (Fig. 4.5). LONG BONES generally are longer than they are wide ʹor thick. SHORT BONES are of various shapes and are usually nearly as wide as they are long. FLAT BONES are those laterally compressed bones that provide protection for soft structures. PNEUMATIC BONES are those with air-filled cavities or sinuses. The various bones of the thoracic limb are long, short, or flat.

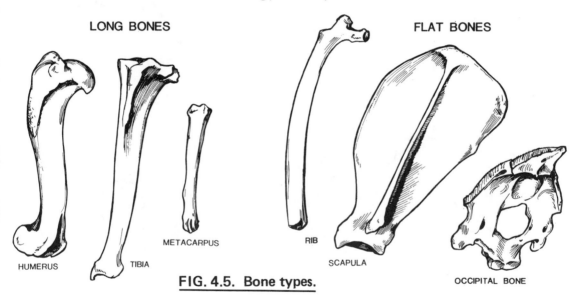

LONG BONES

HUMERUS   TIBIA   METACARPUS

FLAT BONES

RIB   SCAPULA   OCCIPITAL BONE

FIG. 4.5. Bone types.

SHORT BONES

VERTEBRAE   CARPAL BONES

PNEUMATIC BONES

FRONTAL BONE

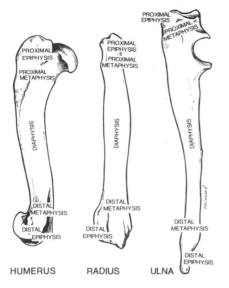

FIG. 4.6. Portions of long bone.

FIG. 4.7. Centers of ossification in long bone.

FIG. 4.8. Physes of long bone.

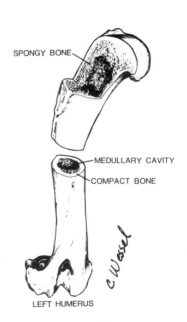

FIG. 4.9. Spongy and compact bone.

A long bone (Fig. 4.6) is composed of a shaft (DIAPHYSIS) and two extremities (EPIPHYSES). The epiphyses usually have a larger diameter than does the diaphysis. The thickened portions of the diaphysis adjacent to the epiphyses are termed METAPHYSES.

With few exceptions, all bones of the neck, trunk, and appendages develop from CARTILAGE. Cartilaginous models of long bone undergo ossification in DIAPHYSEAL CENTERS present in the middle of the models and in EPIPHYSEAL CENTERS at the extremities; in addition, ossification occurs in tissue around the perimeter of the model (Fig. 4.7). The first appearance of ossification centers occurs in the dog embryo about half way through the gestation period. The diaphyseal (primary) ossification centers are present in the diaphyses prior to birth; short bones and the epiphyses of long bones are without ossification centers at the time of birth. In the dog, short bones develop centers of ossification between the ages of 2 weeks and 10 months; all epiphyses of long bones possess epiphyseal (secondary) centers of ossification at 4 months. Many long bones have accessory centers of ossification.

Prior to a dog achieving full growth, cartilage is present in long bones over the surface of the epiphyses and as a plate between the diaphysis and the epiphyses (Fig. 4.8). Bone growth is achieved by proliferation of cartilaginous cells concurrent with ossification of some of the cartilage tissue. The EPIPHYSEAL PLATE (PHYSIS) (fi′sis, pl. physes; growth) consists of a zone of resting cartilage adjacent to the epiphysis, a zone of proliferating cartilage, a zone of hypertrophy and maturation, and a zone of calcification adjacent to the metaphysis. When cartilaginous cells of the physis (which are under the influence of growth hormone) cease to proliferate, the plate becomes ossified and growth in length of the long bone ceases. Growth in diameter occurs by deposition of calcium around the outside of the diaphysis coincident with reabsorption of bone from the inside of the diaphysis.

Bones of the skeleton are described as being spongy or compact (Fig. 4.9) depending upon the ratio of osseous to nonosseous material present. SPONGY BONE is composed of numerous interlacing OSSEOUS TRABECULAE (trah-bek′ u-lee, sing. trabecula) or fibers, the direction of which indicates the various lines of stress imposed on the bone. COMPACT BONE appears visually as a solid substance. Compact bone, with a compressive strength four times that of concrete and a

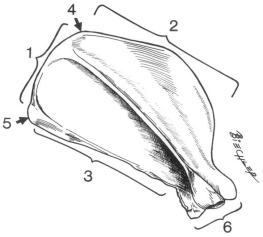

FIG. 4.10. Right scapula, lateral surface.

FIG. 4.11. Right scapula, medial surface.

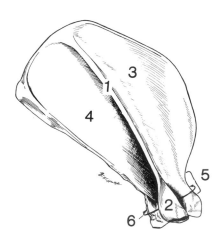

FIG. 4.12. Right scapula, lateral surface.

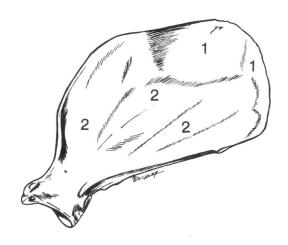

FIG. 4.13. Right scapula, medial surface.

tensile strength half that of steel, forms the superficial layer of the entire osseous skeleton, the diaphysis of long bones, and much of the pectoral and pelvic girdles. Spongy bone is present in the deeper portions of short and flat bones and in the epiphyses and metaphyses of long bones.

Bones of the Thoracic Limb

The SCAPULA (pl. scapulae) (Fig. 4.10) is the most proximal bone of the thoracic limb. Its borders are the DORSAL (1), CRANIAL (2), and CAUDAL (3) MARGINS and the CRANIAL (4), CAUDAL (5), and VENTRAL (6) ANGLES.

The ventral angle of the scapula (Fig. 4.11) is that portion articulating with the humerus; it is characterized by a shallow concavity, the GLENOID (socket shape) CAVITY (1), and a cranial enlargement, the SUPRAGLENOID TUBERCLE (2). The CORACOID PROCESS (3) is a small medial projection from the supraglenoid tubercle. Located near the caudal edge of the ventral angle is another enlargement, the INFRAGLENOID TUBERCLE (4).

On the lateral surface of the scapula (Fig. 4.12), an elongated projection, the SCAPULAR SPINE (1), protrudes distally as the ACROMION (2). Two spaces, one on either side of the scapular spine, are termed from cranial to caudal, SUPRASPINOUS (3) and INFRASPINOUS (4) FOSSAE (fos'ee, sing. fossa; channel). The cranial margin forms the SCAPULAR NOTCH (5) just proximal to the supraglenoid tubercle. The NECK OF THE SCAPULA (6) is the constricted portion of the scapula at the transverse plane of the acromion and scapular notch.

The deep surface of the scapula (Fig. 4.13) is divided into a proximal SERRATED FACE (1) and a distal SUBSCAPULAR FOSSA (2).

(DIFFERENCES TO BE NOTED IN THE CAT: The cat possesses an osseous CLAVICLE. This radiographically observable bone, embedded in the brachiocephalicus muscle, does not articulate with other bones. The feline acromion is composed of HAMATE (ham'ate; hooked) and SUPRAHAMATE PROCESSES. The suprahamate process is a caudally projecting prominence near the distal end of the scapular spine; the hamate process is a distal extension of the acromion that reaches the level of the humeral articulation.)

FIG. 4.14. Right humerus, medial surface of proximal portion.

FIG. 4.15. Right humerus, lateral surface of proximal portion.

FIG. 4.16. Right humerus, caudal surface.

FIG. 4.17. Right humerus, caudal surface of distal portion.

The scapula articulates with the HUMERUS (pl. humeri). The proximal portion of the humerus (Fig. 4.14) consists of a caudal articular projection, or HEAD (1); a large semicircular prominence, or MAJOR TUBERCLE (2), cranial to the head; and a smaller MINOR TUBERCLE (3), located medial to the head. The depression between the minor and major tubercles on the proximal craniomedial surface of the humerus is the INTERTUBERCULAR GROOVE (4). The major tubercle of the humerus forms the point of the shoulder.

The linear elevation on the lateral surface of the proximal part of the humerus (Fig. 4.15) is termed the TRICIPITAL MUSCLE LINE (1). It terminates distally at a roughened prominence, the DELTOID TUBEROSITY (2).

The TERES (te′reez; round and long) MAJOR TUBEROSITY (1, Fig. 4.16) is a small, roughened eminence on the medial surface of the humerus opposite and just proximal to the deltoid tuberosity (2). The NUTRIENT FORAMEN (pl. foramina) (3) of the diaphysis is on the caudal surface of the distal half of the humerus. There are a number of nutrient foramina on the medial and lateral surfaces of the major and minor tubercles. The distal end of the humerus is composed of a CONDYLE (kon′dil; knuckle) (4) and LATERAL and MEDIAL EPICONDYLES (5). (Many clinicians consider the distal end of the humerus to be composed of both medial and lateral condyles.)

The HUMERAL CONDYLE includes the HUMERAL TROCHLEA (trok′le-ah; pulley) (1, Fig. 4.17) and several depressions formed proximal to the trochlea by the radius and ulna. The trochlea forms most of the humeral surface that articulates with the ulna. The OLECRANON FOSSA (2) is the large depression on the distal caudal surface of the humerus. It is continuous with a depression on the cranial surface of the humerus via the SUPRATROCHLEAR FORAMEN. The depression on the distal cranial surface of the humerus (RADIAL FOSSA) is formed by articulations with the radius. The epicondyles are the laterally and medially projecting prominences on the distal end of the humerus. The medial epicondyle (3) is larger than the lateral epicondyle (4). The ridge of bone proximal to the lateral epicondyle on the caudolateral surface of the humerus is the LATERAL EPICONDYLAR CREST (5).

(DIFFERENCES TO BE NOTED IN THE CAT: The supratrochlear foramen is usually absent; however, a SUPRACONDYLAR FORAMEN is present in the distal medial portion of the feline humerus, forming an osseous passageway for the median nerve and brachial artery.)

FIG. 4.18. Right ulna.

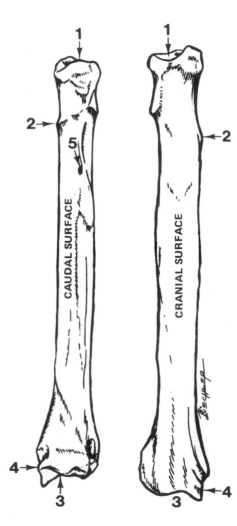

FIG. 4.19. Right radius.

The ULNA (pl. ulnae) (Fig. 4.18), the longest bone of the dog's body, extends from the point of the elbow to the carpus.   The OLECRANON (1), or proximal extremity of the ulna, projects caudally past the cubital articulation forming the point of the elbow. A relatively long olecranon provides strength in extending the cubital articulation, whereas a relatively short olecranon provides for rapid extension. A large TROCHLEAR NOTCH (2), present on the proximal cranial surface of the ulna, articulates with the humeral trochlea. The two projections forming the proximal and distal margins of the trochlear notch are the ANCONEAL (ang-ko′ne-al) (3) and CORONOID (crownlike) (4) PROCESSES, respectively. When the cubital articulation is extended, the anconeal process is positioned within the olecranon fossa of the humerus. There are two coronoid processes; the RADIAL NOTCH (5) of the ulna is present between the large medial and small lateral coronoid processes.   When rotator muscles contract, the proximal portion of the radius rotates against the radial notch of the ulna.   The ULNAR TUBEROSITY (6) is a small prominence just distal to the medial coronoid process.   The roughened cranial surface of the body of the ulna is the border facing the radius. Note the nutrient foramen (7) in the proximal portion of this rough surface. The distal pointed portion of the ulna is termed the LATERAL STYLOID (pillarlike) PROCESS (8).

In the prone position, the RADIUS (pl. radii) (Fig. 4.19) is positioned craniolaterally to the ulna at the cubital articulation and craniomedially at the carpal articulation.   The concave FOVEA (fo′ve-ah, pl. foveae) CAPITIS (1) of the head of the radius articulates with the lateral portion of the condyle of the humerus.   The RADIAL TUBEROSITY (2) is a small eminence on the medial surface of the radius near the transverse level of the ulnar tuberosity. The tendons of insertion of the brachialis and biceps brachii muscles, which attach to the ulna, also attach to the radial tuberosity.   The RADIAL TROCHLEA (3) is the distal articular surface by which the radius articulates with carpal bones. The elongated medial projection of the distal end of the radius is the MEDIAL STYLOID PROCESS (4).   The rough caudal surface of the radius is the border facing the ulna; this interosseous surface has a nutrient foramen (5) near the proximal end of the radius.

FIG. 4.20. Right carpus and proximal portion of the metacarpus, dorsal surface.

FIG. 4.21. Right carpus and metacarpus, dorsal surface.

II - V

FIG. 4.22. Digits, lateral surface.

FIG. 4.23. Distal phalanx, lateral surface.

Seven bones form the skeleton of the dog CARPUS; the carpal bones are arranged in two rows, a proximal row of three bones and a distal row of four bones (Fig. 4.20). The medial bone of the proximal row articulates with the radius; it is the largest of the carpal bones and is termed the RADIAL CARPAL BONE (1). The lateral bone of the proximal row, which articulates with the ulna and the radius, is the ULNAR CARPAL BONE (2). The ACCESSORY CARPAL BONE (3) is caudal to the ulnar carpal bone on the lateral surface of the carpus. The distal row of four carpal bones are named from medial to lateral as CARPAL BONES I, II, III, and IV.

The METACARPUS, which is distal to the carpus and proximal to the digits, contains five METACARPAL BONES numbered I through V (Fig. 4.21). Each metacarpal bone has a proximal BASE (1), a BODY (2), and a distal HEAD (3). Metacarpus I is quite small.

DIGITS II, III, IV, and V (Fig. 4.22) have three PHALANGES (fa′lan-jez, sing. phalanx) each; digit I usually has two. The proximal phalanx of digit I and the proximal and middle phalanges of digits II, III, IV, and V have a proximal base (1), a body (2), and a distal head (3).

The distal phalanx (Fig. 4.23) of digits I through V has a dorsal prominence, the EXTENSOR PROCESS (1); a palmar FLEXOR TUBERCLE (2); a distal CREST OF THE CLAW (3); and a PROCESS OF THE CLAW (4). The crest of the distal phalanx projects distally superficial to the dorsal and lateral proximal surfaces of the cutaneous claw; the base of the crest of the distal phalanx is the extensor process. A pair of elastic ligaments attach the crest of the distal phalanx to the middle phalanx, resulting in overextension of the distal interphalangeal joint (see p. 95). The process of the claw is the bony extension of the distal phalanx into the cutaneous claw.

MOVEMENT

OPPOSING GRAVITY

TENSION

SHORTENED

TENSION

TENSION

NOT SHORTENED

TENSION

FIG. 4.24. Results of
tension in appendicular muscle.

FOOT OFF THE GROUND

FOOT ON THE GROUND

POINT OF ORIGIN

BICEPS BRACHII

FIG. 4.25. Skeletal muscle, its
regions and points of attachment.

BELLY

POINT OF INSERTION

MEDIAL VIEW

TENDON

CONNECTIVE
TISSUE FIBERS

TENDON

BONE

APONEUROSIS

TENDON

FIG. 4.26. Skeletal muscle,
types of attachment.

MUSCLES

Microscopically, skeletal muscle is composed of fibers (cells) that function by creating tension along their long axes. This tension may result in shortening of a muscle, which effects movement of osseous structures to which the muscle is attached, or it may prevent movement by either acting against opposing gravitational forces or countering contraction of other muscles (Fig. 4.24).

A skeletal muscle (Fig. 4.25) is composed of a main portion and two extremities; the major portion, or BELLY, of a muscle contains the greatest number of muscle fibers. The muscle extremities attach to bone or fascia. If contraction of a muscle results in movement, the most mobile end of the muscle is termed the INSERTION (TERMINATION); the extremity with least movement is called the ORIGIN. the portion of a muscle adjacent to the origin is the HEAD. Usually the origin of an appendicular muscle is the attachment closest to the body. Many muscles produce movement at both points of attachment, while other muscles produce movement at one end one time and at the other end another time, depending on the position of the body and its functional state. In these cases it is not necessary to describe points of origin and insertion, only points of attachment.

Among the muscle fibers in the belly of a muscle are numerous connective tissue fibers; these fibers coalesce at the extremities of most muscles, forming tough cords called TENDONS or flat sheets termed APONEUROSES (ap"o-nu-ro'ses, sing. aponeurosis) (Fig. 4.26). Aponeuroses are often continuous with deep fascia. Some muscles attach directly to bone by means of their investing fascia and by connective tissue fibers within the muscle rather than by means of tendons or aponeuroses. Connective tissue fibers of tendons, by merging into the intercellular substance of bone, are strongly attached. Muscle fibers are more likely to tear under stress than are the tendons of attachment.

FLEXION   EXTENSION

FIG. 4.27. Action of muscles, flexion versus extension.

ABDUCTION   ADDUCTION

FIG. 4.28. Action of muscles, abduction versus adduction.

Descriptive terms indicate the action of groups of muscles on the structures to which they attach. FIXATION MUSCLES are those that fix or stabilize bones of a joint against movement in one direction, while other muscles act to effect movement of the joint in another direction. Muscles that span a joint, attaching to two different bones, may either increase the angle of the joint, EXTENSION, or decrease it, FLEXION (Fig. 4.27). Muscles that move a structure toward the median plane are said to be ADDUCTORS; those that move the limbs away from the median plane are ABDUCTORS (Fig. 4.28). A muscle that raises a structure dorsally is a LEVATOR. The antagonistic muscle to a levator is a DEPRESSOR (Fig. 4.29). A muscle responsible for rotating the cranial surface of a limb medially is a PRONATOR, while the opposing muscle, which rotates the cranial surface of the limb laterally, is a SUPINATOR (su″pi-na′tor) (Fig. 4.30).

LEFT LIMB, CRANIAL VIEW

FIG. 4.29. Action of muscles, elevation versus depression.

RIGHT LIMB, CRANIAL VIEW

FIG. 4.30. Action of muscles, supination versus pronation.

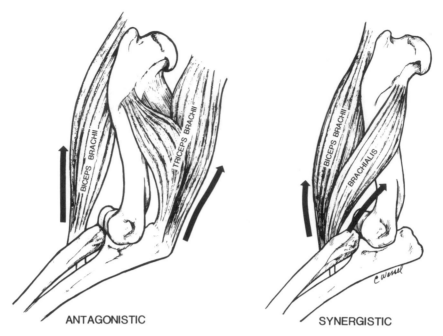

FIG. 4.31. Action of muscles, antagonistic versus synergistic.

MUSCLE TYPES:

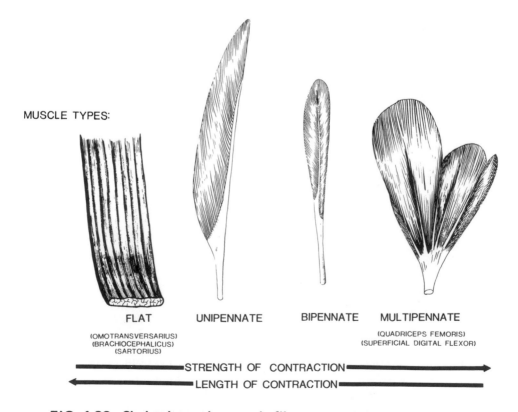

| FLAT | UNIPENNATE | BIPENNATE | MULTIPENNATE |

(OMOTRANSVERSARIUS)
(BRACHIOCEPHALICUS)
(SARTORIUS)

(QUADRICEPS FEMORIS)
(SUPERFICIAL DIGITAL FLEXOR)

STRENGTH OF CONTRACTION

LENGTH OF CONTRACTION

FIG. 4.32. Skeletal muscle, muscle fiber arrangement.

The function of one muscle is usually opposed by another; e.g., if a muscle functions to straighten a joint, another one, an ANTAGONISTIC MUSCLE, will have the function of bending the joint. If two or more muscles work together to perform a function, they are said to be SYNERGISTIC (Fig. 4.31).

The pattern of muscle fibers within a muscle and the number of motor units activated (a motor unit is one motor nerve fiber and all the muscle fibers it activates) determine the amount of change in length and the force that a contracting muscle may produce (Fig. 4.32). The longer a muscle is and the more parallel its fibers are to the long axis, the greater will be the length of contraction. FLAT (STRAPLIKE) MUSCLES have long fibers parallel to the long axis of the muscle. PENNATE MUSCLES have fibers that are oriented at an angle to the long axis of the muscle; the fibers are shorter and more numerous in pennate than in straplike muscles. Various types of pennate muscles are classified by the complexity of fiber arrangement: unipennate, bipennate, and multipennate. A UNIPENNATE MUSCLE has a row of fibers parallel to each other but at an angle to the long axis of the muscle. A BIPENNATE MUSCLE has two rows of fibers converging on the long axis of the muscle. The most powerful is the MULTIPENNATE MUSCLE, which is characterized by more than two rows of parallel fibers, each attaching to longitudinally oriented tendinous tissue within the muscle itself.

Muscles are usually named according to their action, shape, or attachment. A muscle with the name common digital extensor produces extension of the digits. The pronator teres muscle is a round muscle that produces pronation. The trapezius muscle is shaped like a trapezoid. However, the name of a muscle may be misleading for a particular species; e.g., the triceps brachii muscle has three heads in the human and four in the dog. The names of some muscles provide information on both origin and insertion; e.g., the spinodeltoideus arises on the spinous process of the scapula and inserts on the deltoid tuberosity of the humerus.

FIG. 4.33. Magnification of limb displacement.

OMOTRANSVERSARIUS

FIG. 4.34. Extrinsic muscles of the thoracic limb that attach to the scapula.

FIG. 4.35. Schematic of thoracic limb muscles: craniolateral view of muscles that attach to the scapula.

48

Muscles of the Thoracic Limb

More than 53 muscles act upon the thoracic limb. The actions of individual muscles or muscle groups may be readily estimated by mentally visualizing relative positions of bone, muscle, and muscle attachments. By shortening the length of a muscle or part of a muscle, the function or action of that muscle (whether a flexor, extensor, abductor, adductor, levator, depressor, pronator, supinator, sphincter, dilatator, or other) is determined. However, a muscle acts in conjunction with a number of other muscles, and the direction of pull on the skeletal part is due to the sum of the forces applied by individual muscles.

Eight of the thoracic limb muscles are EXTRINSIC, i.e., these muscles are related or attach to bones that are not a part of the thoracic limb skeleton. Extrinsic muscles of the limbs produce differential movement of axial and appendicular structures. The extrinsic muscles of the thoracic limb are responsible for movement of the shoulder and upper arm; a small movement of the limb proximally may result in a much larger displacement of the distal end of the limb (Fig. 4.33).

Four extrinsic muscles of the thoracic limb that attach the scapula to the axial skeleton are the trapezius (trah-pe′ ze-us), rhomboideus, omotransversarius (omo; shoulder), and serratus ventralis. Three of these may be observed from a lateral view (Figs. 4.34, 4.35); two superficially, the trapezius (1) and omotransversarius muscles (2), and one more deeply, the rhomboideus muscle (3). The fourth extrinsic muscle of the scapular region, the serratus ventralis (4), requires considerable dissection for visualization.

FIG. 4.36. Trapezius muscle, dorsal view of cervical and thoracic portions.

FIG. 4.37. Omotransversarius muscle.

The TRAPEZIUS MUSCLE of each side attaches the spine of a scapula to a ligament positioned longitudinally along the dorsal median line of the body (Fig. 4.36). Each trapezius is divided cranially into a cervical portion (1) and caudally into a thoracic portion (2), named according to region of origin. The two trapezii span the interscapular region, forming the shape for which they are named.

The OMOTRANSVERSARIUS (1, Fig. 4.37) is a strap-shaped muscle that connects the distal end of the scapular spine (acromion) to the transverse process of the 1st (most cranial) cervical vertebra. Another extrinsic muscle of the thoracic limb, the brachiocephalicus, is superficial to the omotransversarius muscle in the lateral cervical region.

Deep to the trapezius muscles, a pair of muscles arise from the dorsal median line and insert on the proximal end of each scapula near the dorsal border (Fig. 4.38). This paired muscle has a rhomboid (diamond) shape, hence its name, RHOMBOIDEUS. The rhomboideus muscle is divided into a capital portion (1), a cervical portion (2), and a thoracic portion (3). The RHOMBOIDEUS CAPITIS MUSCLE is a slender straplike portion that separates proximally from the RHOMBOIDEUS CERVICIS MUSCLE to attach to the skull.

FIG. 4.38. Left rhomboideus muscle: dorsal view of capital, cervical, and thoracic portions.

FIG. 4.39. Left serratus ventralis muscle: lateral view of cervical and thoracic portions.

FIG. 4.40. Schematic of left serratus ventralis muscle, dorsolateral view.

The remaining extrinsic muscle that inserts on the scapula, the SERRATUS VENTRALIS, is situated deep to the scapula (Figs. 4.39, 4.40). The long axis of the serratus ventralis muscle is in a dorsolateral direction from the trunk to the scapula. The serratus ventralis muscles suspend the thorax from the deep proximal surfaces (serrated faces) of the scapulae. Each serratus ventralis arises from the neck and from the thorax; the serrated origins give the muscle its name. The SERRATUS VENTRALIS CERVICIS MUSCLE (1) arises from the transverse processes of the caudal five cervical vertebrae (note that at the base of the neck the cervical vertebrae are situated quite far ventrally). The muscular slips of the SERRATUS VENTRALIS THORACIS MUSCLE (2) arise ventral to the midlength of the first seven or eight ribs.

Four extrinsic muscles of the thoracic limb that attach the humerus to the axial skeleton (Fig. 4.41) are the brachiocephalicus (1), latissimus dorsi (2), superficial pectoral (3), and deep pectoral (4).

FIG. 4.41. Extrinsic muscles of the thoracic limb, humeral attachment.

FIG. 4.42. Right brachiocephalicus muscle, ventral view.

The BRACHIOCEPHALICUS (brak″e-o-se-fal′i-kus; arm and head) MUSCLE attaches by one end to the skull and median dorsal line of the neck and by the other to the distal cranial surface of the humerus (Fig. 4.42). A transverse tendinous line is present in the brachiocephalicus dorsal to the level of the point of the shoulder. The vestige of the clavicle may be palpable at this CLAVICULAR INTERSECTION (arrow) as a small piece of cartilage or bone. Considering the clavicular intersection as the least movable point within this muscle (which is several separate muscles in animals with functional clavicles), the part of the brachiocephalicus that inserts on the humerus is the CLEIDOBRACHIALIS MUSCLE (1); the other two portions, which insert on the neck and skull, are the cervical (2) and mastoid (3) parts of the CLEIDOCEPHALICUS MUSCLE, respectively. The STERNOCEPHALICUS (4), a trunk muscle (see p. 155), is located immediately cranioventral to the cleidocephalicus and adjacent to the external jugular vein.

The LATISSIMUS (lah-tis′i-mus) DORSI (1, Fig. 4.43) is a broad, flat muscle caudal to the thoracic limb region and deep to the cutaneus trunci muscle. It is wide at its aponeurotic origin from the dorsal median line and relatively narrow and thick near its insertion on the proximal medial surface of the humerus (teres major tuberosity). The caudal portion of the trapezius muscle is superficial to the craniodorsal portion of the latissimus dorsi muscle.

FIG. 4.43. Left latissimus dorsi muscle, lateral view.

SCHEMATIC OF THE CRANIAL VIEW

FIG. 4.44. Pectoral muscles.

VENTRAL SURFACE

FIG. 4.45. Jugular fossae.

The SUPERFICIAL PECTORAL MUSCLE (Fig. 4.44) arises from the ventral median line and inserts on the cranial proximal surface of the humerus. It is subdivided into two parts, a smaller, superficial descending portion and a deeper, broader transverse portion. The fibers of the DESCENDING PECTORAL (1) are oriented in a caudolateral direction; those of the TRANSVERSE PECTORAL (2) are oriented transversely. The DEEP (ASCENDING) PECTORAL (3) arises from the ventral median line and inserts on the proximal medial surface of the humerus. It may be divided by fascial clefts into several smaller muscles. The muscle fibers of the cranial portion of the deep pectoral are deep to the superficial pectoral and are oriented transversely. The caudal portion of the deep pectoral is superficial and is oriented craniolaterally.

A depression, the JUGULAR (jug´u-lar; neck) FOSSA (arrow, Fig. 4.45), is present on each side of the ventral median line, cranial to the superficial pectoral (1,2), medial to the cleidobrachialis (3) and the clavicular intersection (4), and lateral to the straplike sternocephalicus (5), which attaches the sternum to the skull. The superficially situated external jugular vein passes deeply from the neck at the jugular fossa into the thoracic cavity.

(DIFFERENCES TO BE NOTED IN THE CAT: The descending portion of the superficial pectoral muscle arises more caudally on the sternum and is thus more transversely oriented than that of the dog. Extrinsic muscles such as the brachiocephalicus and superficial pectoral insert distally on the proximal portion of the antebrachium.)

INTRINSIC muscles of the thoracic limb are those that both arise from and insert upon bone or fascia of the thoracic limb. Nine intrinsic muscles of the thoracic limb that span the surfaces of the humeral articulation are: laterally--the deltoideus, infraspinatus, teres minor, and supraspinatus; caudally--the teres major and triceps brachii; cranially--the biceps brachii; and medially--the subscapularis and coracobrachialis.

FIG. 4.46. Intrinsic muscles of the right shoulder, lateral view.

LATERAL VIEW

MEDIAL VIEW

FIG. 4.47. Left teres minor and triceps brachii muscles.

The DELTOIDEUS MUSCLE (1,2, Fig. 4.46) is the most superficial of four intrinsic muscles that cross the lateral surface of the shoulder joint. It has two origins, two bellies, and one insertion. The most distal portion of the deltoideus (1), which arises from the acromion, is situated across the humeral articulation, caudal to the major tubercle. Both the acromial portion and a second more proximal portion (2), which arises by an aponeurosis from the scapular spine, insert in common on the deltoid tuberosity, deep to the cleidobrachialis muscle. The portion of the deltoideus that arises from the scapular spine is easily confused with a deeper muscle, the INFRASPINATUS (3), which arises from the infraspinous fossa. The tendon of the infraspinatus muscle is situated lengthwise across the lateral surface of the humeral articulation and inserts on the lateral surface of the major tubercle. The SUPRASPINATUS MUSCLE (4) arises from the supraspinous fossa of the scapula, deep to the trapezius and omotransversarius muscles, and inserts on the major tubercle of the humerus.

The small TERES MINOR MUSCLE (1, Fig. 4.47) arises from the caudal border of the scapula and inserts distally on the lateral surface of the proximal portion of the humerus. The teres minor is deep to the deltoideus muscle and caudal to the distal portion of the infraspinatus muscle.

The TRICEPS (three heads) BRACHII MUSCLE has four heads of origin, three of which are from the proximal portion of the humerus and one is from the caudal border of the scapula. The head of the triceps brachii, which has a muscular origin from the caudal margin of the scapula, appears to have two or three bellies; these muscle masses are the LONG HEAD OF THE TRICEPS BRACHII (2, 3, 4), which forms the major portion of the muscle. The other three heads of the triceps brachii muscle are named lateral, medial, and accessory according to their positions around the caudal surface of the humerus. The common point of insertion of the triceps brachii muscle is on the olecranon of the ulna (point of the elbow); the caudal margin of the triceps brachii muscle mass along the caudal surface of the arm, formed mostly by the long head, is termed the TRICIPITAL MARGIN (5). The LATERAL HEAD (6) arises from the tricipital line of the humerus; this part of the triceps brachii forms the major muscular mass on the lateral surface of the arm. The MEDIAL HEAD (7) arises from the proximal medial surface of the humeral diaphysis and by position forms the medial portion of the four-part triceps. The ACCESSORY HEAD (8), which is positioned between the medial, lateral, and long heads, arises from the proximal surface of the humerus.

FIG. 4.48. Intrinsic muscles of the right shoulder, medial view.

FIG. 4.49. Left biceps brachii and coracobrachialis muscles, medial view.

The SUBSCAPULARIS (1, Fig. 4.48) is a muscle situated on the deep surface or subscapular fossa of the scapula from which it arises. It crosses the medial surface of the humeral articulation and inserts on the minor tubercle of the humerus. A portion of the belly of the supraspinatus muscle (2), which overlaps the cranial border of the scapula onto its medial surface, is often mistaken for the subscapularis muscle. On the medial surface of the thoracic limb the proximal portion of the TERES MAJOR MUSCLE (3) may be observed between the more craniodorsally located subscapularis muscle and the more caudally positioned latissimus dorsi muscle (4). The teres major muscle arises from the caudal angle of the scapula and inserts, in common with the latissimus dorsi and cutaneus trunci muscles, on the teres major tuberosity of the humerus.

The BICEPS (two heads) BRACHII MUSCLE (1, Fig. 4.49) arises from the supraglenoid tubercle of the scapula and inserts on the proximal cranial surface of the radius and ulna in the ANTEBRACHIUM. The tendon of origin of the biceps brachii muscle passes through the intertubercular groove of the craniomedial surface of the humerus, where the tendon is held in place by the TRANSVERSE HUMERAL LIGAMENT (2). The transverse humeral ligament attaches to the major and minor tubercles of the humerus. The CORACOBRACHIALIS MUSCLE (3) arises from the coracoid process of the scapula, crosses the minor tubercle, and inserts on the medial surface of the proximal half of the humerus.

Fifteen intrinsic muscles of the thoracic limb span the cubital articulation; seven of these directly effect movement of the antebrachium. The other muscles arise from the humerus and effect movement of the carpus and/or digits. The intrinsic muscles of the BRACHIUM that act upon the antebrachium may be grouped into muscles that are caudal to the long axis of the limb--the triceps brachii, tensor fasciae antebrachii, and anconeus; craniolateral to the cubital articulation--the brachialis and supinator; and craniomedial to the cubital articulation--the biceps brachii and pronator teres.

FIG. 4.50. Right tensor fasciae antebrachii and anconeus muscles, caudal view.

FIG. 4.51. Muscles adjacent to the cranial surface of the cubital articulation, craniolateral view.

The TENSOR FASCIAE ANTEBRACHII (1, Fig. 4.50) is a thin, strap-shaped muscle located on the caudomedial surface of the arm, superficial to the long head of the triceps (2). It arises from the latissimus dorsi muscle (3), near its attachment on the teres major tuberosity, and inserts on fascia of the olecranon. The ANCONEUS (4) is a short muscle that arises on the distal caudal surface of the humerus and inserts on the proximal lateral surface of the ulna.

(DIFFERENCES TO BE NOTED IN THE CAT: Both the cleidobrachialis and the superficial pectoral muscles of the cat insert on the proximal portion of the antebrachium. A small EPITROCHLEOANCONEUS MUSCLE, present on the proximomedial surface of the feline cubital articulation, arises from the medial epicondylar crest and inserts on the olecranon.)

The BRACHIALIS MUSCLE (1, Fig. 4.51) arises from the proximal caudolateral surface of the humerus and inserts craniomedially on the ulna and radius, just distal to the cubital articulation. It forms a half spiral around the humerus in its course from origin to insertion. The SUPINATOR (2) is a short muscle that arises from the lateral epicondyle of the humerus and inserts on the cranial surface of the radius. This rotator muscle of the antebrachium is situated craniolateral to the cubital articulation, deep to other antebrachial muscles. The biceps brachii muscle (3) stretches from the scapula (proximally) through the intertubercular groove of the humerus to its dual insertion on the radius and ulna, distal to the cubital articulation (see Fig. 4.49). The biceps brachii muscle is situated along the craniomedial surface of the humerus, superficial and cranial to the medial head of the triceps muscle. Much of the proximal portion of the biceps brachii muscle is covered by the superficial and deep pectoral muscles. The PRONATOR TERES (4) is a small muscle that arises from the medial humeral epicondyle and inserts on the medial border of the radius.

The intrinsic muscles of the thoracic limb that arise, at least in part, from the humerus and insert on bones of the manus may be grouped into extensors of the carpus, extensors of the carpus and digits, flexors of the carpus, and flexors of the carpus and digits. They arise, at least in part, from an epicondyle of the humerus and cross two or more joints. Those muscles originating from the lateral epicondyle are EXTENSOR MUSCLES OF THE MANUS; those arising from the medial epicondyle are FLEXOR MUSCLES OF THE MANUS.

FIG. 4.52. Extensor muscles of the right manus, lateral view.

The extensor group of muscles, located on the craniolateral surface of the antebrachium, includes the extensor carpi radialis, common digital extensor, lateral digital extensor, and extensor carpi ulnaris (ulnaris lateralis).

The EXTENSOR CARPI RADIALIS (1, Fig. 4.52) is the large muscle palpable through the skin on the cranial surface of the radius. The craniomedial border of the extensor carpi radialis muscle is a commonly used site for injections into the cephalic vein. A rudimentary thin strip of muscle, the BRACHIORADIALIS, may be present medial to and parallel with the cephalic vein. The extensor carpi radialis muscle originates from the lateral epicondylar crest and inserts on the proximal dorsal surface of metacarpal bones II and III. A transversely oriented thick band of carpal fascia, the EXTENSOR RETINACULUM (2), binds the two extensor carpi radialis tendons in place against the carpus (dorsally).

(DIFFERENCE TO BE NOTED IN THE CAT: The brachioradialis muscle is well developed.)

The COMMON DIGITAL EXTENSOR MUSCLE (3) is lateral and partially deep to the extensor carpi radialis. It arises from the lateral epicondyle and inserts by four tendons on the proximal surface (extensor process) of the distal phalanx of digits II, III, IV, and V. The extensor retinaculum (2) on the dorsal surface of the carpus also retains the four common digital extensor tendons in position. The LATERAL DIGITAL EXTENSOR MUSCLE (4) is caudolateral and partially deep to the common digital extensor muscle. It arises from the lateral epicondyle of the humerus and inserts by three tendons, which join with tendons of the common digital extensor muscle on the proximal dorsal surface of the distal phalanx of digits III, IV, and V. The three tendons of insertion of the lateral digital extensor are also held in place on the dorsal surface of the carpus by the extensor retinaculum (2). The EXTENSOR CARPI ULNARIS (5), which is considered to be a flexor muscle in the dog, is situated along the lateral surface of the antebrachium, where it arises from the lateral epicondyle of the humerus and inserts via two tendons on the accessory carpal bone and proximal lateral surface of metacarpal V. The LONG ABDUCTOR MUSCLE OF DIGIT I (6), which is oriented distomedially, arises from the craniolateral surface of the ulna and inserts on the proximal end of metacarpus I. A SESAMOID (ses′ ah-moid; sesame-seed-like) BONE, frequently observed in radiographs of the carpal joint, is present in the tendon of insertion.

SUPERFICIAL DISSECTION

SUPERFICIAL DIGITAL FLEXOR REMOVED

S. RAYNE

FIG. 4.53. Flexor muscles of the left manus, medial view.

The flexor group of muscles (Fig. 4.53), located on the caudomedial surface of the antebrachium, includes the flexor carpi radialis, superficial digital flexor, flexor carpi ulnaris, and deep digital flexor. The short belly of the FLEXOR CARPI RADIALIS MUSCLE (1), present on the medial surface of the proximal portion of the antebrachium, is caudal and partially deep to the pronator teres. The flexor carpi radialis muscle arises from the medial epicondyle of the humerus and inserts on the proximal palmar surface of metacarpals II and III. The SUPERFICIAL DIGITAL FLEXOR MUSCLE (2) is caudal to the flexor carpi radialis and forms the caudomedial surface of the antebrachium. It arises from the medial epicondyle of the humerus and inserts by means of four tendons on the proximal palmar surfaces of the middle phalanx of digits II, III, IV, and V. A thickening of deep fascia, the FLEXOR RETINACULUM, binds the insertion tendon of the superficial digital flexor into a hollow in the palmar surface of the carpus. The CARPAL CANAL is a space formed by the flexor retinaculum and the accessory, ulnar, and radial carpal bones. The flexor retinaculum is divided into two parts, one superficial and the other deep to the superficial digital flexor tendon.

The FLEXOR CARPI ULNARIS (3) consists of two parts that appear as separate muscles, an ulnar (3a) and a humeral (3b) head. The short bellied ulnar head arises from the caudal surface of the olecranon and inserts distally as a tendon on the accessory carpal bone. The humeral head originates proximally from the medial epicondyle, deep to the ulnar head, and also inserts on the accessory carpal bone. The DEEP DIGITAL FLEXOR MUSCLE (4) has three points of origin: the medial epicondyle of the humerus, the proximal caudal border of the ulna, and the medial border of the radius. The two portions that arise from the ulna and radius are small and combine with the tendon of the humeral head at the level of the carpus. All three heads of the deep digital flexor have one common tendon of insertion, which, after passing through the carpal canal, divides into five tendons. The five tendons insert on the proximal palmar surface (flexor tubercle) of the distal phalanx of digits I, II, III, IV, and V. The flexor retinaculum maintains the deep digital flexor tendon in the carpal canal.

FIG. 4.54. Left pronator quadratus muscle, caudomedial view.

TABLE 4.1. Classification of articulations

General type	Class of joint
Synarthroses (little movement)	
A. One bone directly fused to another bone	Synostosis
B. Bone attached to bone by cartilage (cartilaginous articulations)	
1. Hyaline cartilage	Synchondrosis
2. Fibrocartilage	Symphysis
C. Bone attached to bone by dense connective tissue (fibrous articulations)	
1. Broad zone of dense connective tissue	Syndesmosis
2. Narrow zone of dense connective tissue between flat bones	Suture
3. Tooth anchored in an alveolus of the jaw by dense connective tissue	Gomphosis
Synovial articulations (movable)	
A. Shape (of opposing articular surfaces)	
1. Flat surface with a flat surface	Plane
2. Convex surface with a concave surface	Spheroidal
3. Elongated convex surface with an elongated concave surface	Ellipsoidal
4. Knuckle-shaped surface fitting into a reciprocal depression	Condylar
5. Circular surface rotating in a concave or ring-shaped surface	Trochoid
6. Concavoconvex surface with a reciprocal convexoconcave surface	Saddle (sellar)
B. Plane of movement — one plane only	Ginglymus
C. Number of bones involved	
1. Two opposing surfaces	Simple
2. More than two articular surfaces	Composite

A muscle in the interosseous space between the ulna and radius (Fig. 4.54), deep to the deep digital flexor, is the PRONATOR QUADRATUS (four sided) (1). This muscle attaches to the rough surfaces of the radius (2) and ulna (3).

JOINTS

There are a number of osseous joint types in the body (Table 4.1), but the articulations of greatest importance in veterinary medicine are the cartilaginous and synovial joints. CARTILAGINOUS JOINTS permit limited movement; SYNOVIAL JOINTS, with lubricating fluid between opposing bones, are characterized by greater freedom in movement.

Cartilaginous joints are composed of two bones united by either hyaline cartilage or fibrocartilage; these two types of joints are termed SYNCHONDROSES and SYMPHYSES (sim'fi-ses, sing. symphysis). An osseous epiphysis joined to the diaphysis of a long bone by epiphyseal cartilage is an example of a synchondrosis (Fig. 4.55); most synchondroses are lost through ossification during the maturation process. Junctions between right and left pelvic bones and between individual vertebrae are examples of symphyses.

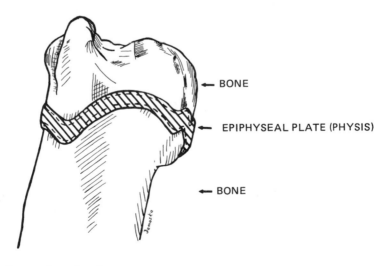

BONE

EPIPHYSEAL PLATE (PHYSIS)

BONE

FIG. 4.55. A synchondrosis.

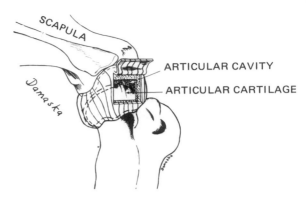

FIG. 4.56. Contents of a synovial joint.

FIG. 4.57. Collateral ligaments of a synovial joint.

FIG. 4.58. Synovial joint, simple articulation.

FIG. 4.59. Synovial joint, composite articulation.

Synovial joints are characterized by the presence of an ARTICULAR CAVITY between the articular cartilages surfacing opposing bones (Fig. 4.56).   The ARTICULAR CAPSULE of a synovial joint passes from the superficial layer of one bone to the superficial layer of the opposing bone, forming a sheath around the articular cavity; thus the articular cavity is completed by walls of articular cartilage and the articular capsule. The articular capsule is composed of two connective tissue layers: a deep SYNOVIAL STRATUM and superficial FIBROUS STRATUM. The thin synovial membrane produces the lubricating fluid, SYNOVIA, which fills the articular cavity. Fat deposits are often present between the synovial and fibrous membranes. Such deposits may protrude into the space between the opposing bones of a joint; however, the synovial membrane folds around the deep surface of the fat.

Thickenings of the fibrous membrane, called EXTRACAPSULAR LIGAMENTS, aid in maintaining the integrity of synovial joints. A pair of extracapsular ligaments, termed COLLATERAL LIGAMENTS (Fig. 4.57) are associated with the fibrous membrane of the articular capsule of a number of articulations; these articulations are characterized by bending in only one plane. Collateral ligaments that cross the joint to each side of the plane of movement help prevent lateral movement and overextension.

Synovial joints are described in subtypes according to the shape of their articular surfaces, the direction of movement they permit, and the number of articular surfaces within the same capsule. A SIMPLE ARTICULATION (Fig. 4.58) is a synovial joint formed by only two opposing articular surfaces within the same connective tissue sheath or joint capsule; many of the synovial joints classed according to shape are also simple articulations. A COMPOSITE ARTICULATION (Fig. 4.59) is a synovial joint having more than one pair of opposing articular surfaces within the same articular capsule. The GINGLYMUS (jing′gli-mus; hinge) ARTICULATION is a type of synovial joint that permits movement in one plane only.

B. SPHEROIDAL ARTICULATION:
RIGHT COXAL JOINT, VENTRAL VIEW

A. PLANE ARTICULATION:
COSTOTRANSVERSE JOINT,
CRANIAL VIEW

C. ELLIPSOIDAL ARTICULATION: RIGHT
RADIOCARPAL JOINT, PALMAR VIEW

FIG. 4.60. Synovial joints, classed according to the shape of the articular surface.

Synovial joints are described according to shape (Fig. 4.60) as: PLANE ARTICULATIONS (A), opposing bones with flat surfaces; SPHEROIDAL ARTICULATIONS (B), opposing convex surface fitting into a reciprocally concave surface; ELLIPSOIDAL ARTICULATIONS (C), similar to spheroidal but elongated; CONDYLAR ARTICULATIONS (D), surface with knuckle-shaped prominences fitting into opposing surface with reciprocal depressions; TROCHOID ARTICULATIONS (E), shaped like a wheel, with a circular surface turning or pivoting within an opposing ring-shaped surface or on an opposing circular surface; and SADDLE ARTICULATIONS (F), opposing bones with concavoconvex surfaces.

E. TROCHOID ARTICULATION: RIGHT PROXIMAL RADIOULNAR JOINT, LATERAL VIEW

D. CONDYLAR ARTICULATION: RIGHT FEMOROTIBIAL JOINT, CRANIAL VIEW

F. SADDLE ARTICULATION: PROXIMAL INTERPHALANGEAL JOINT, DORSAL VIEW

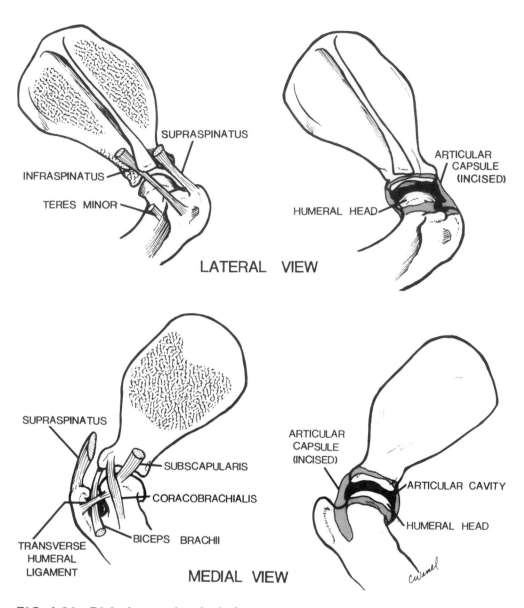

FIG. 4.61. Right humeral articulation.

Joints of the Thoracic Limb

The HUMERAL ARTICULATION (Fig. 4.61) is a spheroidal type of synovial joint. It is characterized by a small amount of movement in any direction. The fibrous membrane of the articular capsule blends with the transverse humeral ligament and the tendons of insertion of the subscapularis, infraspinatus, and supraspinatus muscles. The articular capsule, with synovial fluid, extends distally through the intertubercular groove between the humerus and tendon of the biceps brachii. The tendons of the subscapularis, infraspinatus, and supraspinatus, which act as muscular (active) collateral ligaments, are quite efficient; dislocations of the humeral articulation are rare. The tendons of the biceps brachii and coracobrachialis muscles also strengthen the humeral articulation.

When radiographing the humeral articulation of dogs younger than 7 months, a separate accessory epiphyseal center of ossification may be noted in the region of the supraglenoid tubercle, which has not yet undergone fusion to the remainder of the scapula (Fig. 4.62). The proximal epiphysis of the humerus may be separated from the diaphysis by a cartilaginous plate in dogs younger than 1 year.

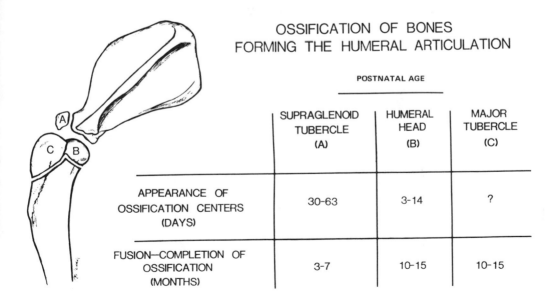

OSSIFICATION OF BONES FORMING THE HUMERAL ARTICULATION

POSTNATAL AGE

	SUPRAGLENOID TUBERCLE (A)	HUMERAL HEAD (B)	MAJOR TUBERCLE (C)
APPEARANCE OF OSSIFICATION CENTERS (DAYS)	30-63	3-14	?
FUSION—COMPLETION OF OSSIFICATION (MONTHS)	3-7	10-15	10-15

FIG. 4.62. Ossification of bones forming the left humeral articulation.

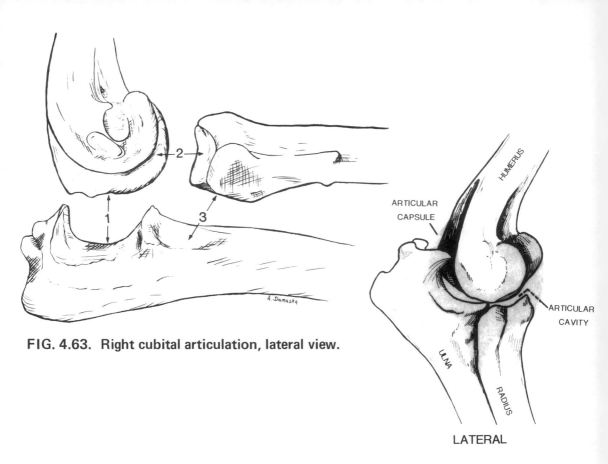

FIG. 4.63. Right cubital articulation, lateral view.

ARTICULAR
CAPSULE

HUMERUS

ARTICULAR
CAVITY

ULNA

RADIUS

LATERAL

FIG. 4.64. Articular capsule of
the right cubital articulation,
lateral view.

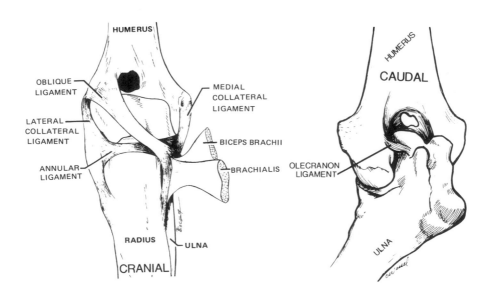

HUMERUS

OBLIQUE
LIGAMENT

MEDIAL
COLLATERAL
LIGAMENT

LATERAL
COLLATERAL
LIGAMENT

BICEPS BRACHII

ANNULAR
LIGAMENT

BRACHIALIS

RADIUS   ULNA

CRANIAL

HUMERUS

CAUDAL

OLECRANON
LIGAMENT

ULNA

FIG. 4.65. Extracapsular ligaments of the right cubital articulation.

The CUBITAL ARTICULATION (Fig. 4.63), an example of a ginglymus, is composed of three articulations: HUMEROULNAR (1), HUMERORADIAL (2), and PROXIMAL RADIOULNAR (3). A single articular capsule and articular cavity filled with synovial fluid serve all three articulations of the cubital region (Fig. 4.64). Thus the cubital articulation is a composite articulation. All ligaments associated with the cubital articulation are extracapsular (Fig. 4.65). Thickenings of the fibrous membrane of the articular capsule form the LATERAL and MEDIAL COLLATERAL LIGAMENTS, which attach the lateral and medial epicondyles of the humerus, respectively, to the radius and ulna. The ANNULAR LIGAMENT OF THE RADIUS is a connective tissue band, deep to the collateral ligaments, that partially encircles the head of the radius; the annular ligament and radial notch of the ulna form a ring in which the radius rotates. The OBLIQUE LIGAMENT crosses the flexor angle of the cubital articulation; attaching to the humerus and ulna, it aids in preventing overextension. The OLECRANON LIGAMENT attaches the anconeal process of the ulna to the caudal surface of the medial epicondylar crest.

Dislocations (luxations) of the cubital articulation are infrequent; however, the condyle is prone to fracture because of the presence of the olecranon fossa and supratrochlear foramen. These fractures result in a separation of either one or both of the medial and lateral portions of the condyle from the diaphysis. The main axis of stress in the thoracic limb during locomotion is through radial carpal bone, radius, and lateral portion of the humeral condyle.

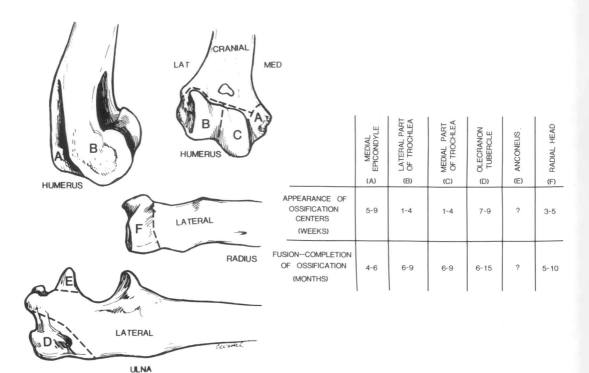

	MEDIAL EPICONDYLE	LATERAL PART OF TROCHLEA	MEDIAL PART OF TROCHLEA	OLECRANON TUBERCLE	ANCONEUS	RADIAL HEAD
	(A)	(B)	(C)	(D)	(E)	(F)
APPEARANCE OF OSSIFICATION CENTERS (WEEKS)	5-9	1-4	1-4	7-9	?	3-5
FUSION—COMPLETION OF OSSIFICATION (MONTHS)	4-6	6-9	6-9	6-15	?	5-10

FIG. 4.66. Ossification of bones forming the right cubital articulation.

FIBROUS MEMBRANE

SYNOVIAL MEMBRANE

FIG. 4.67. Left carpal articulation.

The distal portion of the humerus develops three ossification centers by 9 weeks of age; the distal centers fuse with the diaphysis and each other by 9 months (Fig. 4.66). The radius and ulna each have one proximal ossification center, which is present by 7 weeks and is fused by 10 months of age; in addition, a center of ossification may be present in the anconeal process of the ulna. Elbow dysplasia, which is characterized by the partial or complete failure of the anconeal process to fuse with the olecranon, is most frequent in large dogs such as the German Shepherd.

The CARPAL ARTICULATION (Fig. 4.67) includes the ANTEBRACHIOCARPAL (1), MIDDLE CARPAL (2), other INTERCARPAL (3), and CARPOMETACARPAL (4) ARTICULATIONS. Opposing articular surfaces of individual carpal bones constitute the various intercarpal articulations. The middle carpal articulation, a joint between proximal and distal rows of carpal bones, includes several intercarpal articulations. The combined action of individual portions of the carpal articulation is described as a ginglymus.

The fibrous membrane portion of the carpal articulation capsule extends as a sleeve from the distal end of the radius and ulna, over the carpal bones, to the proximal end of the metacarpal bones. The synovial membrane is present as two separate entities, forming two articular cavities, each containing synovia: one between the antebrachium and the proximal row of carpal bones, the other between the proximal and distal rows of carpal bones and between the distal carpal and metacarpal bones. The antebrachiocarpal articulation is a composite articulation since a common articular cavity extends between the DISTAL RADIOULNAR ARTICULATION and the RADIOCARPAL and ULNOCARPAL ARTICULATIONS.

APPROXIMATE AGE OF APPEARANCE OF:

		Ossification center (in weeks)	Fusion (in months)
1	Distal radial epiphysis	3	10
2	Distal ulnar epiphysis	8	10
PROXIMAL ROW			
3	Accessory carpal bone	2	
4	Accessory carpal bone (2° center)	7	5
5	Radial carpal	3	
6	Intermediate carpal	3	
7	Central carpal	6	4
8	Ulnar carpal	6	
DISTAL ROW			
I	Carpal bone I of distal row	3	
II	Carpal bone II of distal row	4	
III	Carpal bone III of distal row	4	
IV	Carpal bone IV of distal row	3	

FIG. 4.68. Ossification of bones forming the left carpal articulation.

Ossification centers appear in the carpal bones and in the distal epiphyses of the radius and ulna postnatally; ossification is completed with loss of cartilaginous epiphyseal plates by the age of 12 months (Fig. 4.68). Fracture of the accessory carpal bone occurs frequently in Greyhounds. The sesamoid bone of the long abductor of digit I is present on the medial surface of the carpus.

The articulations between proximal and middle phalanges and between the middle and distal phalanges are termed the PROXIMAL (1) and DISTAL (2) INTERPHALANGEAL ARTICULATIONS, respectively (Fig. 4.69). The digital pads are located on the palmar surfaces of the distal interphalangeal articulations. A small sesamoid bone, present dorsally in the joint capsule of each metacarpophalangeal joint, is positioned between the common digital extensor tendon and joint. Larger, paired sesamoid bones on the palmar surface of each metacarpophalangeal joint are positioned between superficial digital flexor tendons and each joint.

FIG. 4.69. Interphalangeal articulations.

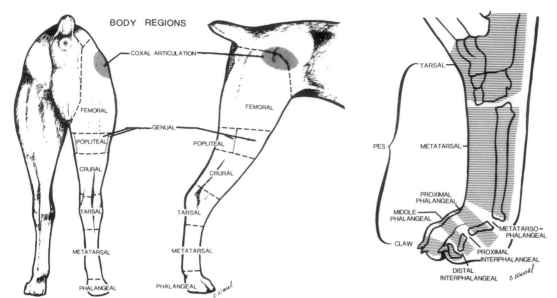

BODY REGIONS

COXAL ARTICULATION

FEMORAL

FEMORAL

GENUAL

POPLITEAL

POPLITEAL

CRURAL

CRURAL

TARSAL

TARSAL

METATARSAL

METATARSAL

PHALANGEAL

PHALANGEAL

FIG. 5.1. Subregions of the pelvic limb.

TARSAL

PES

METATARSAL

PROXIMAL PHALANGEAL

MIDDLE PHALANGEAL

METATARSO-PHALANGEAL

CLAW

PROXIMAL INTERPHALANGEAL

DISTAL INTERPHALANGEAL

FIG. 5.2. Regions of the pes.

COMMON NAME	SEGMENT	BONE		COMMON NAME	ANATOMICAL NAME
			HIP JOINT		COXAL ARTICULATION
THIGH	FEMORAL	FEMUR			
			KNEE (STIFLE) JOINT		GENUAL ARTICULATION
SHANK	CRUS	TIBIA AND FIBULA			
FOOT:	PES:				
ANKLE	TARSUS	TARSAL BONES	HOCK	ANKLE JOINT	TARSAL JOINT
ARCH	METATARSUS	METATARSAL BONES			TARSOCRURAL
					INTERTARSAL
TOES	DIGITS	PHALANGES			tarsometatarsal

FIG. 5.3. Anatomical segments of the pelvic limb.

5 PELVIC LIMB

The pelvic limb is divided into coxal articulation, femoral, genual, crural, tarsal, metatarsal, and phalangeal regions (Fig. 5.1). COXAL ARTICULATION refers to the hip joint, FEMORAL to the thigh, GENUAL to the knee, CRURAL to the leg, and TARSAL to the ankle. The PATELLAR REGION is the subregion of the genual region that overlies the patella (knee cap). The POPLITEAL (pop-lit'e-al) REGION is the area caudal to the knee.

The METATARSUS is that portion of the foot (PES) (pes, pl. pedes) between the ankle and the digits (Fig. 5.2). The term pes signifies the TARSAL, METATARSAL, and PHALANGEAL REGIONS. The surface area superficial to the joint between the skeleton of the metatarsus and the proximal segment of the digit is the METATARSOPHALANGEAL REGION. The other regions distal to the metatarsus are named the same as corresponding areas of the thoracic limb (see Fig. 4.2)

BONES OF THE PELVIC LIMB

The bones of the pelvic limb include those of the pelvic girdle and the femoral, genual, crural, tarsal, metatarsal, and phalangeal regions (Fig. 5.3).

FIG. 5.4. Bony pelvis, cranial view.

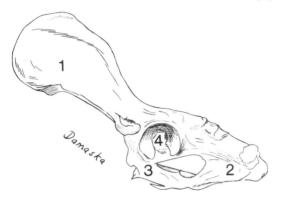

FIG. 5.5. Bones forming the left os coxae, lateral view.

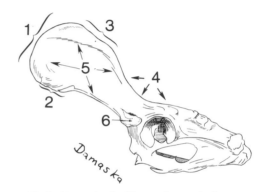

FIG. 5.6. Left ilium, lateral view.

FIG. 5.7. Left ischium: lateral view (A); caudodorsal view (B).

The PELVIS (Fig. 5.4) consists of the PELVIC GIRDLE (1) and the SACRUM (2). The pelvic girdle (OSSA COXARUM) consists of right and left OS (pl. ossa) COXAE (kok′see, sing. coxa).

The three bones forming the mature os coxae (Fig. 5.5)-- ILIUM (1), ISCHIUM (is′ke-um, pl. ischia) (2), and PUBIS (3)--are united to each other around the ACETABULUM (4), a concave articular surface. The ilium forms the craniodorsal portion, the pubis the cranioventral portion, and the ischium the caudoventral portion of the os coxae. Dogs younger than 7 months have a separate acetabular bone, which may be apparent on radiographs.

The dorsocranial marginal ridge of the ilium is the ILIAC CREST (1, Fig. 5.6), which includes a cranioventral prominence, the TUBER COXAE (2), and a long dorsal prominence, the TUBER SACRAL (3). The MAJOR ISCHIATIC NOTCH (4) is the elongated concavity on the dorsal surface of the ilium, caudal to the tuber sacral. The smooth, shallow depression in the lateral surface of the thin wing of the ilium is named the GLUTEAL (gloo′te-al) SURFACE (5). A smooth prominence on the lateral surface of the body of the ilium, cranial to the acetabulum, is the RECTUS FEMORIS AREA (6), the point of origin of a muscle of similar name.

The TUBER ISCHIADICUM (1, Fig. 5.7) is the broad, caudally projecting margin of the ischium and its lateral projection. A space present on the dorsal margin of the ischium between the ISCHIATIC SPINE (2) and the tuber ischiadicum is termed the MINOR ISCHIATIC NOTCH (3).

The ILIOPUBIC EMINENCE (1, Fig. 5.8) is a small prominence on the cranial margin of the pubic bone, lateral to the PELVIC SYMPHYSIS (2).

FIG. 5.8. Ossa coxarum, caudoventral view.

FIG. 5.9. Bony pelvis and sacrotuberous ligament, caudodorsal view.

FIG. 5.10. Left acetabular fossa and notch.

The two halves of the ossa coxarum articulate ventrally at the pelvic symphysis (1, Fig. 5.9); this articulation is composed of two parts, the PUBIC and ISCHIATIC SYMPHYSES. The pelvic symphysis becomes ossified in dogs older than 5 years. The ISCHIATIC ARCH (2), on the caudoventral margin of the two ischia, extends from one tuber ischiadicum to the other. The two large OBTURATOR FORAMINA (3), one on each side, are enclosed by the ischiatic and pubic bones. A smooth surface on the craniodorsal margin of the obturator foramen is the OBTURATOR GROOVE (4). A cordlike structure, the SACROTUBEROUS LIGAMENT (5), attaches the lateral portion of the tuber ischiadicum to the sacrum and 1st caudal vertebra.

(DIFFERENCES TO BE NOTED IN THE CAT: A sacrotuberous ligament is not present in the cat.)

The ACETABULAR FOSSA (1, Fig. 5.10) is incomplete ventromedially due to the presence of the ACETABULAR NOTCH (2).

The proximal portion of the FEMORAL BONE (Fig. 5.11) bears an articular HEAD (1), which is directed medially; a small FOVEA (fo′ve-ah, pl. foveae) OF THE FEMORAL HEAD (2) is present on the caudomedial surface. A distinct constriction, the NECK OF THE FEMORAL BONE (3), is present between the head and the remainder of the proximal extremity. The large, dorsally projecting MAJOR TROCHANTER (4) is separated from the head and neck by the large, cavernous TROCHANTERIC FOSSA (5) on the caudal surface of the proximal extremity. The MINOR TROCHANTER (6) is present on the caudomedial surface of the femoral bone, distal to the neck.

FIG. 5.11. Proximal portion of the left femoral bone, caudal view.

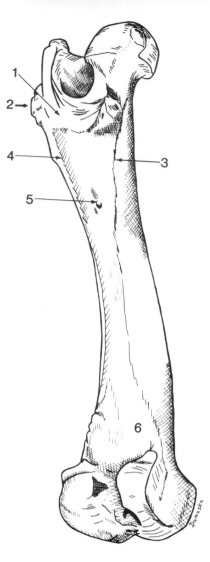

FIG. 5.12. Left femoral bone,
caudomedial view.

FIG. 5.13. Distal portion of the
left femoral bone, caudolateral view.

FIG. 5.14. Distal portion of the
left femoral bone, caudal view.

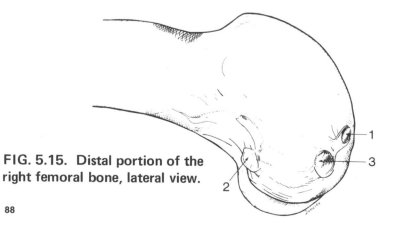

FIG. 5.15. Distal portion of the
right femoral bone, lateral view.

The ridge of bone that extends from the minor to the major trochanter is the INTERTROCHANTERIC CREST (1, Fig. 5.12). The area of the THIRD TROCHANTER (2) occurs on the caudolateral surface of the femoral bone, near the same transverse plane as the minor trochanter. A ROUGH SURFACE extends longitudinally along the caudal surface of the femoral bone; the edges of the rough surface are termed the MEDIAL (3) and LATERAL (4) LIPS of the rough surface. The NUTRIENT FORAMEN is present in the rough surface (5). The distal caudal surface of the femoral diaphysis is named the POPLITEAL SURFACE (6).

The distal end of the femoral bone (Fig. 5.13) is characterized by a TROCHLEA (1) and two caudally projecting CONDYLES (2). The trochlea is a smoothly grooved surface with lateral and medial lips (3); each lip is continuous distally with a condyle. The trochlear groove of the femoral bone is continuous distally with the INTERCONDYLAR FOSSA (4), a large concavity between the condyles.

Smooth, circular, articular surfaces (1, Fig. 5.14) are present proximally on the caudally projecting condyles. These are the articular surfaces of the medial and lateral sesamoid bones of the gastrocnemius muscle. Two small prominences, the LATERAL (2) and MEDIAL (3) EPICONDYLES, are on the caudolateral and caudomedial surfaces, respectively, of the distal extremity; each epicondyle is adjacent to an articular surface of a sesamoid bone. Proximal to the epicondyles are two large prominences on the caudal surface of the diaphysis; these SUPRACONDYLAR TUBEROSITIES, MEDIAL (4) and LATERAL (5), are continuous with the lips of the rough surface of the femoral bone.

A small concave depression, the EXTENSOR FOSSA (1, Fig. 5.15), is present on the distal end of the femoral bone at the junction of the lateral lip of the trochlea and the lateral condyle. Between the articular surface (2) of the lateral sesamoid bone and the extensor fossa, a third smooth articular surface may be noted, the FOSSA OF THE POPLITEAL MUSCLE (3).

FIG. 5.16. Right tibia and fibula, cranial view.

CRANIAL VIEW   CAUDAL VIEW

FIG. 5.17. Proximal portion of the right tibia.

FIG. 5.18. Distal portion of the right tibia, caudal view.

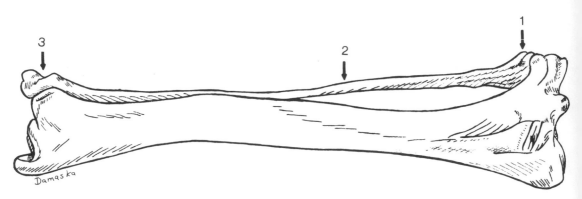

FIG. 5.19. Right tibia and fibula, cranial view.

The crural region is nearly the same length as the femoral region; two bones (Fig. 5.16), a large TIBIA (1) and a slender FIBULA (2) are present in the CRUS (krus, pl. crura; leg).

The proximal end of the tibia (Fig. 5.17) bears three large prominences: a caudomedial prominence, the MEDIAL CONDYLE (1); a caudolateral prominence, the LATERAL CONDYLE (2); and a cranial longitudinal crest, the CRANIAL MARGIN (3). The proximal portion of the cranial margin, the TIBIAL TUBEROSITY (4), provides for insertion of the primary extensor muscle mass of the knee joint. Two small eminences on the proximal tibial articular surface project proximally into the intercondylar fossa of the femoral bone; these medial and lateral intercondylar tubercles are collectively termed the INTERCONDYLAR EMINENCE (5). Depressions cranial and caudal to the intercondylar eminence are the CRANIAL (6) and CAUDAL (7) INTERCONDYLAR AREAS, respectively. The groove in the caudal surface of the tibial epiphysis, distal to the caudal intercondylar area, is the POPLITEAL NOTCH (8). The EXTENSOR GROOVE (9) is a furrow in the proximolateral surface between the lateral tibial condyle and the tibial tuberosity.

The medial portion of the distal end of the tibia (Fig. 5.18) projects distally as the MEDIAL MALLEOLUS (mal-le'o-lus, pl. malleoli) (1). The distal articular surface of the tibia is the TIBIAL COCHLEA (2).

The fibula (Fig. 5.19), which is lateral to the tibia, is characterized by a proximally enlarged HEAD (1), a long, slender BODY (2), and an enlarged distal extremity, the LATERAL MALLEOLUS (3).

FIG. 5.20. Bones of the right tarsus, dorsal view.

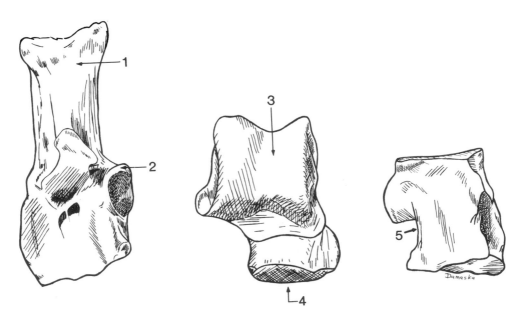

FIG. 5.21. Right calcaneus, talus, and fourth tarsal bones, dorsal view.

The bones of the TARSUS (Fig. 5.20) are arranged in three rows: a proximal row of two bones, the CALCANEUS (kal-ka'ne-us) (1) and TALUS (2); a middle row formed by a single bone, the CENTRAL TARSAL BONE (3); and a distal row of four bones, TARSAL BONES I, II, III, and IV. The laterally positioned calcaneus is the largest bone of the tarsus.

The TUBER CALCANEI (1, Fig. 5.21) is the large, proximally projecting prominence of the calcaneus on which the common calcanean tendon inserts. A medial projection near the distal end of the calcaneus, the SUSTENTACULUM (sus″ten-tak'u-lum; support) TALI (2), articulates with the medial plantar surface of the talus. The talus articulates with the dorsal surface of the calcaneus and with the distal extremity of the tibia. The proximal dorsal surface of the talus is in the form of a trochlea (3), which matches, in a reciprocal manner, the cochlear surface of the tibia. The head (4), or distal end, of the talus articulates with the central tarsal bone, which in turn articulates with tarsal bones I, II, and III. The distal articular surface of the calcaneus contacts the proximal articular surface of tarsal bone IV. A groove (5) in the lateral surface of tarsal bone IV indicates the site where the fibularis longus tendon crosses to the plantar surface of the pes.

FIG. 5.22. Right metatarsal bones and distal two rows of tarsal bones, dorsal view.

FIG. 5.23. Bones of a digit (II-V), lateral view.

There are four main METATARSAL BONES, II–V (Fig. 5.22); in most breeds a small metatarsal I is also present. Each metatarsal bone has a proximal BASE (1), a BODY (2), and a distal HEAD (3). The metatarsus is longer than the metacarpus of the same dog.

DIGITS II–V have PROXIMAL (1), MIDDLE (2), and DISTAL (3) PHALANGES (Fig. 5.23). Digit I may be absent; if present, it will usually contain one or two phalanges.

(DIFFERENCES TO BE NOTED IN THE CAT: Retractile claws (Fig. 5.24) are characteristic of the Felidae (cat family). The articular surfaces of the distal interphalangeal articulation are shaped such that during hyperextension, the distal phalanx (1) swivels past the lateral surface of the middle phalanx (2). Two elastic ligaments (3), tautly stretched between the middle and distal phalanges, maintain the claw in retraction. Protrusion of the claw requires contraction of the digital extensors (4) for fixation of the proximal interphalangeal articulation and of the deep digital flexor muscle (5) for flexion of the distal interphalangeal articulation.)

LATERAL VIEW   CRANIAL VIEW

FIG. 5.24. Retractile claw mechanism of the cat. (Modified from Gonyea and Ashworth 1975. *J. Morphol.* 145(2): 229-38.)

FIG. 5.25. Gluteal muscles, dorsal view.

BICEPS FEMORIS BISECTED
AND PARTIALLY REFLECTED

FIG. 5.26. Caudal femoral muscles, lateral view.

MUSCLES OF THE PELVIC LIMB

The proximal portion of the pelvic limb contains gluteal, caudal femoral, medial femoral, cranial femoral, and coxal articulation muscles.

The GLUTEAL MUSCLES (Fig. 5.25) include the small, caudal superficial gluteus (1), the large middle gluteus (2), and the deeply situated deep gluteus (3). The SUPERFICIAL GLUTEUS (1), which arises from gluteal fascia (the sacrum) and the sacrotuberous ligament, inserts on the third trochanter of the proximal caudolateral surface of the femoral bone. The MIDDLE GLUTEUS (2), the fibers of which are oriented caudodistally, is the major superficial muscle of the gluteal region. It arises from the iliac crest and the gluteal surface of the ilium; its tendon inserts on the major trochanter of the proximal surface of the femoral bone. A caudal portion of the middle gluteus, the PIRIFORMIS (pear shape) MUSCLE, situated deep to the superficial gluteus, arises from the caudal vertebrae and is easily confused with a small deep slip (4) of the superficial gluteus. Fibers of the DEEP GLUTEUS MUSCLE (3) are oriented caudodistally from the ilium to the major trochanter on the proximal lateral surface of the femoral bone. The origin of the deep gluteus muscle is from the ilium at the dorsal level of the major ischiatic notch.

Caudal femoral muscles (Fig. 5.26) are the biceps femoris (1), semitendinosus (2), semimembranosus (3), and the slender caudal crural abductor (4). The BICEPS FEMORIS (1) forms the major muscle mass on the caudolateral surface of the femoral region; it arises from the tuber ischiadicum and the sacrotuberous ligament, passes over the insertion of the superficial gluteus muscle (5), and inserts by means of aponeuroses at various points distally. The SEMITENDINOSUS (sem″e-tend″i-no′sus) MUSCLE (2) arises from the tuber ischiadicum and inserts distally on the medial surface of the tibia; it also inserts by means of a fascial attachment on the tuber calcanei. The SEMIMEMBRANOSUS MUSCLE (3) arises from the tuber ischiadicum, at which level it is visible superficially. Distally, the muscle fibers are covered laterally by the semitendinosus muscle and medially by the gracilis muscle (6). The semimembranosus muscle attaches by means of two tendons of insertion, one to the distal medial lip of the femoral rough surface and one to the proximal medial surface of the tibia (medial tibial condyle). The long, thin, straplike CAUDAL CRURAL ABDUCTOR MUSCLE (4) is situated along the caudal deep margin of the biceps femoris;

SUPERFICIAL DISSECTION   SCHEMATIC, DEEP MUSCLES REMOVED

FIG. 5.27. Medial femoral muscles, medial view.

GRACILIS

FIG. 5.29. Medial femoral muscles, medial view.

FIG. 5.28. Right pelvic limb, caudal view.

it arises from the sacrotuberous ligament and inserts by a fascial attachment on the lateral surface of the crus.

(DIFFERENCES TO BE NOTED IN THE CAT: The GLUTEOFEMORALIS, an elongate muscle adjacent to the cranial margin of the biceps femoris muscle, arises from the 2nd and 3rd caudal vertebrae and inserts on the patella.)

Medial femoral muscles (Fig. 5.27) are the sartorius (1), pectineus (pek-tin'e-us) (2), gracilis (gras'il-is; slender) (3), and adductor (4). The SARTORIUS MUSCLE (1) forms the craniomedial surface of the femoral region. This muscle is divided longitudinally into two straplike muscles, one caudal to the other. The cranial part of the sartorius muscle arises from the iliac crest and inserts on the patella; the caudal part arises from the tuber coxae and inserts on the cranial margin of the tibia. The PECTINEUS (2) is a spindle-shaped muscle that is palpable in the abducted limb on the proximal medial surface of the femoral region. It arises from the iliopubic eminence and inserts deep to the sartorius muscle on the distal rough surface of the femoral bone (caudomedially). A triangular "space," formed by the converging sartorius and pectineus muscles, is termed the FEMORAL TRIANGLE (5). The GRACILIS (3) is a broad, flat muscle that forms the caudomedial surface of the femoral region. The fibers of the ADDUCTOR MUSCLE (4), deep to the gracilis muscle and caudal to the femur, are directed distolaterally from the pelvic symphysis to the caudal surface of the femoral bone.

Viewed from the caudal aspect (Fig. 5.28), the gracilis is the most medial of the four superficial muscles observed: biceps femoris (1), semitendinosus (2), semimembranosus (3), and gracilis (4). The gracilis muscle arises from the pelvic symphysis and inserts by an aponeurosis on the proximal craniomedial surface of the tibia; a caudal portion of the aponeurosis inserts on the tuber calcanei.

The adductor muscle (Fig. 5.29) may be subdivided into two parts: adductor magnus et brevis (1) and adductor longus (2). The adductor muscle is deep and caudal to the pectineus muscle (3) and cranial to the semimembranosus muscle (4). The ADDUCTOR MAGNUS ET BREVIS (large and short) MUSCLE (1) arises from the pelvic symphysis and inserts on the lateral lip of the rough surface of the femoral bone. The ADDUCTOR LONGUS MUSCLE (2) arises from the pubic bone and inserts on the caudal surface of the femoral bone near the intertrochanteric crest. Both the gracilis and adductor

FIG. 5.30. Schematic of prepubic and symphyseal tendons, ventral view.

FIG. 5.31. Schematic of cranial femoral muscles, lateral view.

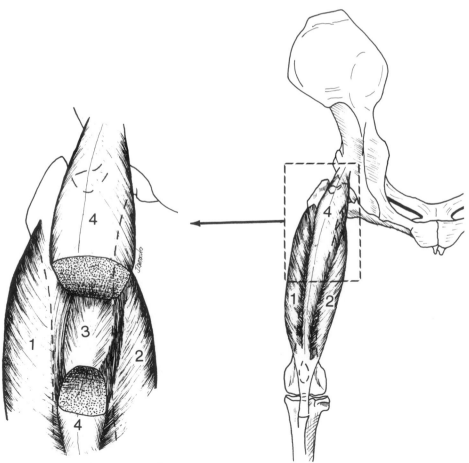

FIG. 5.32. Schematic of quadriceps femoris muscle, cranial view.

muscles arise from the pelvic symphysis via strong connective
tissue termed the symphyseal tendon.

The SYMPHYSEAL TENDON (1, Fig. 5.30) is situated along
the ventral median line superficial to the pelvic symphysis.
The transversely oriented CRANIAL PUBIC LIGAMENT (2) attaches
one iliopubic eminence to the other at right angles to the
symphyseal tendon. Abdominal muscles attach to the cranial
pubic ligament via a strong PREPUBIC TENDON (3).

The cranial femoral muscles (Fig. 5.31) include the
tensor fasciae latae and quadriceps femoris. The TENSOR
FASCIAE LATAE (1) is a short, double-bellied muscle situated
on the proximal lateral surface of the femoral region between
the sartorius muscle (2) craniomedially, the middle gluteus
muscle (3) proximally, and the biceps femoris muscle (4)
caudally. The tensor fasciae latae muscle arises from the
tuber coxae and inserts on the FASCIA LATA (5).

The large QUADRICEPS (four heads) FEMORIS MUSCLE (Fig.
5.32) arises from four points, three from the proximal end of
the femoral diaphysis and one from the ilium. The three
heads, which arise from the femoral bone, are partially
separable and are named according to their position as VASTUS
LATERALIS (1), VASTUS MEDIALIS (2), and VASTUS INTERMEDIUS
(3) MUSCLES. The vastus intermedius muscle is positioned
directly against the cranial surface of the femoral bone.
The RECTUS (straight) FEMORIS MUSCLE (4), the fourth and most
cranial portion of the quadriceps femoris, arises from an
attachment area on the lateral surface of the ilium, cranial
to the acetabulum. All four bellies of the quadriceps muscle
form one common tendon of insertion that extends distally
around the patella to insert on the tibial tuberosity.

FIG. 5.33. Deep muscles associated with the coxal articulation.

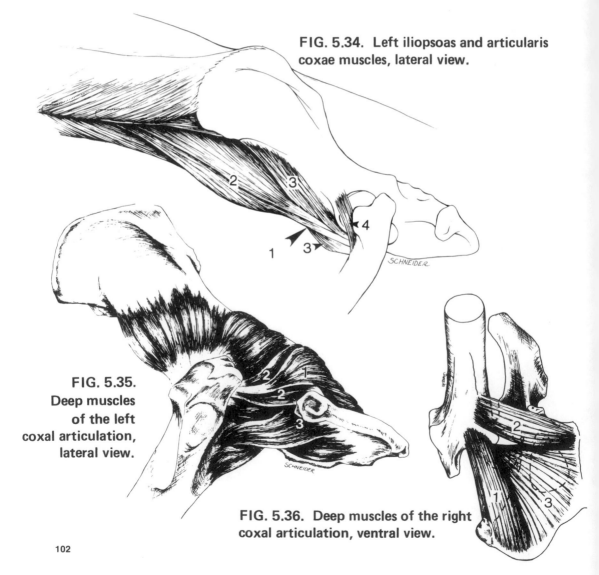

FIG. 5.34. Left iliopsoas and articularis coxae muscles, lateral view.

FIG. 5.35. Deep muscles of the left coxal articulation, lateral view.

FIG. 5.36. Deep muscles of the right coxal articulation, ventral view.

Deep muscles closely associated with the coxal articulation (Fig. 5.33) are the iliopsoas (il"e-o-so'as) (1), articularis coxae (2), internal obturator (3), gemelli (jem'el-li) (4), quadratus femoris (5), and external obturator (6).

The ILIOPSOAS MUSCLE (1, Fig. 5.34), which will be described later with the trunk (see p. 163), is formed by two muscles, the PSOAS (so as) MAJOR (2) and ILIACUS (3). The iliacus muscle arises from the ventral concave surface of the ilium, caudal to the tuber coxae, and extends caudally past the proximal medial surface of the femoral bone to attach to the minor trochanter. The ARTICULARIS COXAE (4) is a short, straplike muscle that arises from the ilium caudal to the origin of the rectus femoris and inserts on the proximal cranial surface of the femoral diaphysis. The articularis coxae muscle is in contact with the more deeply situated articular capsule.

The INTERNAL OBTURATOR MUSCLE (1, Fig. 5.35) arises from the dorsal marginal surface of the obturator foramen. This obturator muscle is considered internal since it arises from within the canal formed by the pelvic bones. The tendon of the internal obturator muscle crosses the dorsal surface of the minor ischiatic notch, ventral to the sacrotuberous ligament, and inserts on the trochanteric fossa of the femoral bone. The GEMELLI (2) are small muscular masses arising from the dorsolateral surface of the minor ischiatic notch, deep to the tendon of the internal obturator muscle. The tendon of the gemelli muscles inserts on the trochanteric fossa. The QUADRATUS FEMORIS (3) is a short, strong muscle arising from the ventral surface of the ischium, medial to the tuber ischiadicum, and inserting on the intertrochanteric crest of the femoral bone.

The quadratus femoris (1, Fig. 5.36) and adductor longus (2) muscles together form a V shape; they have a common area of insertion and one arises from the ischium (caudally) and the other from the pelvic symphysis (cranially). The broad, flat EXTERNAL OBTURATOR MUSCLE (3) arises from the ventral surface of bones forming the obturator foramen and inserts on the proximal caudal surface of the femoral bone in the trochanteric fossa. The external obturator muscle is covered cranially by the more superficial long adductor muscle and caudally by the quadratus femoris muscle.

FIG. 5.37. Action of crural muscles on the pes.

FIG. 5.38. Muscles of the right crus, lateral view.

The muscles that arise from the femoral bone or proximal portion of the crus and insert on bones of the pes (Fig. 5.37) may be grouped into flexors of the tarsus (1), flexors of the tarsus and extensors of the digits (2), extensors of the tarsus (3), and the extensors of the tarsus and flexors of the digits (4).

The flexors of the tarsus and extensors of the digits form the craniolateral muscles of the crus (Fig. 5.38). The CRANIAL TIBIAL (1), LONG DIGITAL EXTENSOR (2), FIBULARIS (peroneus) LONGUS (3), LATERAL DIGITAL EXTENSOR (4), and FIBULARIS BREVIS (5) form the craniolateral muscular mass. The tendons of insertion of the cranial tibial and long digital extensor muscles pass deep to a thickening of the deep fascia, the CRURAL EXTENSOR RETINACULUM (6), on the distal cranial surface of the crus. A second fascial band on the dorsal surface of the tarsus, the TARSAL EXTENSOR RETINACULUM (7), binds down the long digital extensor tendon. The large cranial tibial muscle, which is the most cranial of the craniolateral muscle group, arises from the lateral surface of the tibial tuberosity; the tendon of insertion passes deep to the crural extensor retinaculum, arches around the medial surface of the tarsus, and inserts on the proximal plantar surface of metatarsals I and II. The long digital extensor muscle (2) is caudolateral and partially deep to the cranial tibial muscle. It crosses the genual articulation and all joints distal to the stifle, arising from the extensor fossa of the femoral bone and inserting by means of four tendons on the proximal dorsal surfaces of the distal phalanx of digits II, III, IV, and V. Both crural and tarsal extensor retinacula retain the tendon of insertion in place, proximal to where the tendon separates into its four cords.

The extensors of the tarsus and flexors of the digits form the caudal muscles of the crus; this caudal muscle mass is formed by the gastrocnemius (8), superficial digital flexor (9), deep digital flexor (10), caudal tibial, and popliteus (pop-lit′e-us) muscles.

(DIFFERENCES TO BE NOTED IN THE CAT: A muscle in the proximal lateral portion of the feline crus is the SOLEUS (sole′us). It arises from the fibular head and inserts as part of the common calcanean tendon on the calcanean tuberosity. The soleus and gastrocnemius muscles are collectively named the TRICEPS SURAE (su′rye, sing. sura; calf.)

FIG. 5.39. Deep muscles of the crus, lateral view of proximal portion.

FIBULARIS BREVIS

LONG EXTENSO
OF DIGIT I

SCHNEIDER

Fig. 5.40. Fibularis brevis and extensor muscle of digit I, lateral view.

GRACILIS

SEMITENDINOSUS

BICEPS FEMORIS

FIG. 5.41. Caudal muscles of the right crus, caudal view.

FIG. 5.42. Plantar surface of the left pes.

The short-bellied fibularis longus muscle (1, Fig. 5.39) is caudal and superficial to the long digital extensor muscle (2). The fibularis longus arises from the lateral collateral ligament (3), lateral tibial condyle, and head of the fibula; the distal tendon of the fibularis longus muscle crosses the lateral surface of the tarsocrural articulation and divides into two tendons at the level of tarsal bone IV. One tendon inserts on the proximal dorsolateral surface of metatarsal bone IV; the other passes to the plantar surface of the pes through a groove in tarsal bone IV and inserts on the proximal plantar surface of one or more metatarsal bones. The slender lateral digital extensor muscle (4), which is deep and caudal to the fibularis longus muscle, arises from the fibula proximally and inserts either on the proximal dorsal surface of the proximal phalanx of digit V or in common with the lateral tendon of the long digital extensor muscle.

The fibularis brevis muscle arises from the lateral surface of the fibula and tibia, near their midlength, and inserts on the proximal dorsolateral surface of metatarsal V (Fig. 5.40). A small LONG EXTENSOR MUSCLE OF DIGIT I may be observed deep against the tibia; it arises from the fibula and passes distally through the crural extensor retinaculum, deep to the long digital extensor muscle.

The MEDIAL (1) and LATERAL (2) HEADS OF THE GASTROCNEMIUS MUSCLE (Fig. 5.41) arise from the medial and lateral supracondylar tuberosities of the femoral bone, respectively. The common tendon of insertion attaches to the tuber calcanei. The SUPERFICIAL DIGITAL FLEXOR MUSCLE (3) arises from the lateral supracondylar tuberosity of the femoral bone, deep to the gastrocnemius. The superficial digital flexor muscle and lateral head of the gastrocnemius muscle are difficult to separate proximally; distally, the tendon of insertion of the superficial digital flexor (4) crosses the medial surface of the gastrocnemius tendon (5) to become superficial near the tuber calcanei.

The superficial digital flexor tendons insert on the tuber calcanei and on the proximal plantar surface of the middle phalanx of digits II, III, IV, and V (arrows, Fig. 5.42).

FIG. 5.43. Popliteus and deep digital flexor muscles, caudal view of right pes (A); deep digital flexor tendons in the left pes, plantar surface (B).

FIG. 5.44. Tarsal canal, transverse section through the left pes.

TALUS

FIG. 5.45. Relationship of superficial and deep digital flexor tendons in the digits.

FIG. 5.46. Common calcanean tendon, caudomedial view.

The POPLITEUS MUSCLE (1, Fig. 5.43A) arises from the popliteal muscle fossa of the lateral femoral condyle. The belly of the popliteus is oriented distomedially across the caudal surface of the articular capsule to insert on the proximal caudal surface of the tibial diaphysis. The deep digital flexor is composed of LATERAL (2) and MEDIAL (3) DIGITAL FLEXOR MUSCLES. The larger lateral head arises from the caudal surface of the fibula and tibia; the smaller medial head arises from the caudal border of the tibia between the popliteus and lateral head of the deep digital flexor muscles. The lateral deep digital flexor tendon passes through the TARSAL CANAL, medial to the tuber calcanei; distal to the tarsal canal, the two digital flexor tendons unite on the plantar surface of the tarsus to form a common tendon (4). This tendon is separated distally into four units (Fig. 5.43B).

The osseous tarsal canal (Fig. 5.44), through which the tendons of the deep digital flexor (1) pass, is a space medial to the calcaneus (2) on the plantar surface of the tarsus. Vessels, nerves, and tendons within the tarsal canal are held in place by the flexor retinaculum (superficially) and the fibrous membrane of the articular capsule (deeply).

The individual tendons of the deep digital flexor muscle (1, Fig. 5.45) pass through the superficial digital flexor tendons (2) at the level of the metatarsophalangeal articulation. Each deep digital flexor tendon inserts on the proximal plantar surface of each distal phalanx (of digit II, III, IV, or V). Strong deep fascial thickenings retain the tendons in position.

The common tendon (Fig. 5.46) of the gastrocnemius (1), superficial digital flexor (2), biceps femoris (3), semitendinosus (4), and gracilis (5) muscles, which inserts on the tuber calcanei, is termed the COMMON CALCANEAN TENDON (6).

The CAUDAL TIBIAL MUSCLE, with a small body and a long, thin tendon, is positioned between the medial digital flexor and popliteus muscles. It arises from the fibula and inserts on the medial surface of the tarsus.

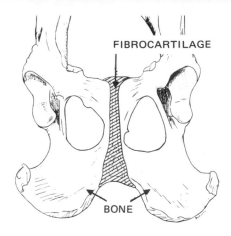

FIBROCARTILAGE

BONE

FIG. 5.47. Pelvic symphysis, ventral view.

FIBROUS MEMBRANE   SYNOVIAL MEMBRANE

SYNOVIA

LIGAMENT
OF THE
FEMORAL
HEAD

ARTICULAR CAPSULE

FIG. 5.48. Coxal articulation.

B   A

C

D

SCHNEIDER

	OSSEOUS ELEMENT			
	ACETABULUM	FEMORAL BONE		
	A			
POSTNATAL STATUS		HEAD	MAJOR TROCHANTER	MINOR TROCHANTER
		B	C	D
OSSIFICATION CENTER FIRST DISCERNED (weeks)	11–12	3	10-12	12-16
FUSION/CLOSURE OF PHYSIS (months)	7	10-12	12	13

FIG. 5.49. Ossification of bones in the proximal femoral region.

JOINTS OF THE PELVIC LIMB

The fibrocartilaginous junction formed midventrally between bones of the pelvis midventrally is an example of a symphysis (Fig. 5.47; see Table 4.1).

The COXAL ARTICULATION (hip joint) is a spheroidal type of synovial joint (Fig. 5.48). An intracapsular ligament, the LIGAMENT OF THE FEMORAL HEAD, attaches the fossa of the femoral head to the acetabular fossa. INTRACAPSULAR LIGAMENTS pass between two bones of a joint within an articular cavity, deep to the fibrous portion of the articular capsule. Such ligaments are not in the synovial fluid since they are surrounded by a synovial membrane sheath. Intracapsular ligaments assist in maintaining alignment of bones of a joint and provide a pathway across the articular cavity for vessels and nerves. An extracapsular TRANSVERSE ACETABULAR LIGAMENT completes the ACETABULAR LIP (ventromedially) by spanning the acetabular notch. The articular capsule is relatively large, attaching from the peripheral margins of the acetabular lips to the neck of the femoral bone.

Radiographic examination of the coxal articulation may reveal a slipped proximal femoral epiphysis (common in smaller breeds), fractures of the femoral head, and/or dislocations.

The acetabulum is completely ossified in a 7-month-old dog (Fig. 5.49). The head of the femoral bone develops a center of ossification by 3 weeks and is fused to the diaphysis by 12 months. Both major and minor trochanters begin ossifying by 4 months and are fused to the diaphysis by 13 months postnatally.

FIG. 5.50. Left genual articulation, lateral view.

FIG. 5.51. Patellar attachments.

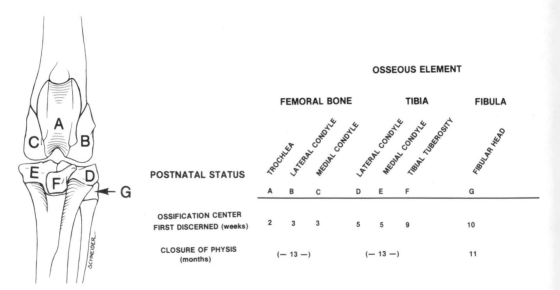

	OSSEOUS ELEMENT						
	FEMORAL BONE			TIBIA			FIBULA
POSTNATAL STATUS	TROCHLEA	LATERAL CONDYLE	MEDIAL CONDYLE	LATERAL CONDYLE	MEDIAL CONDYLE	TIBIAL TUBEROSITY	FIBULAR HEAD
	A	B	C	D	E	F	G
OSSIFICATION CENTER FIRST DISCERNED (weeks)	2	3	3	5	5	9	10
CLOSURE OF PHYSIS (months)		(— 13 —)			(— 13 —)		11

FIG. 5.52. Ossification of bones forming the genual articulation.

The STIFLE (sti′fl) JOINT, or GENUAL ARTICULATION (Fig. 5.50) includes the FEMOROPATELLAR (1), FEMOROTIBIAL (2), and PROXIMAL TIBIOFIBULAR (3) ARTICULATIONS; since the articular surfaces of the three bones are present within a single interconnecting articular capsule, the GENU (je′nu; knee) is a composite articulation. Movement of the genual articulation occurs primarily in one plane, characteristic of a ginglymus; however, rotation of 5-6 degrees laterally or medially does occur. Freedom for medial rotation increases to 19 degrees during flexion.

Four sesamoids are present in the genual region (Fig. 5.50): the PATELLA (4) in the tendon of insertion of the quadriceps femoris, the LATERAL (5) and MEDIAL (6) FABELLAE (fah-bel′lee; sing. fabella; little bean) in the tendons of origin of the heads of the gastrocnemius, and a SESAMOID (7) in the TENDON OF THE POPLITEUS MUSCLE.

The osseous patella bears lateral and medial extensions, the PARAPATELLAR FIBROCARTILAGES (1, Fig. 5.51) that articulate with the lateral and medial trochlear lips of the femoral bone. MEDIAL and LATERAL PATELLAR RETINACULA (2) connect the parapatellar fibrocartilages to the medial and lateral fabellae, respectively.

During radiographic examination of the genual articulation, the appearance of normal structures must be differentiated from incidences of distal femoral epiphyseal separation, dislocation of the patella, proximal tibial epiphyseal separation (relatively common), and separation of the tibial tuberosity. The distal epiphysis of the femoral bone has three centers of ossification (medial and lateral condyles and trochlea), which are present by 3 weeks of age (Fig. 5.52). By the age of 4 months the trochlea fuses with the condyles, and by 13 months the distal epiphysis is fused with the diaphysis. The proximal epiphysis of the tibia develops three centers of ossification by 11 weeks of age: the medial and lateral condyles and the tibial tuberosity. The condyles are fused to the tuberosity by 8 months of age and to the diaphysis by 13 months. The head of the fibula is fused to the diaphysis by 11 months of age.

FIG. 5.53. Ligaments and menisci
of the left genual articulation,
craniolateral "exploded" view.

Two intracapsular ligaments attach the tibia to the femoral bone (Fig. 5.53). These cruciate ligaments, which cross each other, are named according to their distal attachment on the tibia. The CRANIAL CRUCIATE (kroo'she-ate; cross shape) (1) stretches between the caudolateral surface of the intercondylar fossa of the femoral bone and the cranial intercondylar area of the tibia. The CAUDAL CRUCIATE (2) stretches from the craniomedial surface of the femoral intercondylar fossa, past the medial surface of the cranial cruciate, to the caudolateral surface of the tibial medial condyle. The cruciate ligaments are ensheathed by synovial membrane. The lateral and medial femoral condyles do not articulate directly with the lateral and medial tibial condyles; instead, a pair of fibrocartilaginous pads, termed MENISCI (sing. meniscus) (3, 4), separate the two bones. The peripheral margin of the MEDIAL MENISCUS (3) is attached to the articular capsule. A MENISCOFEMORAL LIGAMENT (5) attaches the caudal surface of the LATERAL MENISCUS (4) to the intercondylar fossa of the femoral bone. Medial and lateral menisci are attached to each other cranially and to the cranial and caudal intercondylar areas of the tibia. The articular capsule encloses a large articular cavity that separates the patella from the femoral bone, the femoral condyles from the tibial condyles, and the lateral tibial condyle from the fibular head. Cranial to the articular cavity, the two layers of the articular capsule, fibrous and synovial, are separated by an INFRAPATELLAR FAT BODY (6). Thickenings in the fibrous membrane portion of the articular capsule (laterally and medially) form the lateral and medial collateral ligaments. The LATERAL COLLATERAL LIGAMENT (7) attaches to the lateral femoral epicondyle (proximally) and to the head of the fibula and lateral tibial condyle (distally). The tendon of origin of the popliteus muscle is deep to the lateral collateral ligament. The MEDIAL COLLATERAL LIGAMENT (8) attaches to the medial femoral epicondyle (proximally) and to the medial surface of the medial tibial condyle (distally). Injuries to the genual articulation frequently involve the cranial cruciate, medial collateral ligament, and medial meniscus. The femoral attachment of both cranial and caudal cruciate ligaments is caudal to the joint axis during flexion. The cranial cruciate, the tibial attachment of which is cranial to the axis, is taut during extension of the genual articulation and also partially taut during flexion. The cranial cruciate ligament assists in preventing both hyperextension (148 degrees +) and hyperflexion of the stifle. If the cranial cruciate is completely ruptured, cranial movement of the tibia relative to the femur (slight during extension, 2 mm)

FIG. 5.54. Right tarsal articulation, lateral view.

FIG. 5.55. Ossification of bones forming the pes.

OSSEOUS ELEMENT

POSTNATAL STATUS	TIBIA DISTAL EPIPHYSIS	FIBULA DISTAL EPIPHYSIS	TALUS	CALCANEUS	TUBER CALCANEUS	CENTRAL TARSAL	TARSAL I–IV	METATARSUS HEADS	PHALANGES BASES
	A	B	C	D	E	F	G	H	I
OSSIFICATION CENTER FIRST DISCERNED (weeks)	3	6	1	1	8	5	3-7	4	6
CLOSURE OF PHYSIS (months)	11	9	—	—	7	—	—	9	7

is marked during flexion (9.5 mm). Cranial displacement of
the tibia on the femur is known clinically as "cranial drawer
movement." When the entire caudal cruciate is ruptured, a
caudal movement of the tibia (slight during extension, 2 mm)
is marked during flexion of the genual articulation (8 mm).
Caudal displacement of the tibia is termed "caudal drawer
movement." Medial rotation of the tibia is prevented
primarily by both cranial and caudal cruciates as they twist
against each other. Lateral rotation of the tibia is
prevented primarily by the collateral ligaments.

The TARSAL ARTICULATION (Fig. 5.54) includes the
TARSOCRURAL (1), TARSOMETATARSAL (2), and various intertarsal
articulations. The fibrous membrane of the articular capsule
extends distally from the distal end of the tibia and fibula
to the proximal end of the metatarsal bones; between its
proximal and distal extent, the fibrous tissue is fused to
the superficial surface of the tarsal bones. Synovial
membranes, attaching to the peripheral margins of articular
cartilage, span the distance from one osseous element of the
tarsal articulation to another. The synovial sac of the
tarsocrural joint is continuous with that of the proximal
intertarsal articulations forming a single articular cavity.
The synovial cavities of the distal intertarsal and
tarsometatarsal articulations also interconnect.

The distal epiphyses of the tibia and fibula are fused
to their respective diaphyses in dogs 11 months of age (Fig.
5.55). Most of the tarsal bones develop ossification centers
postnatally; a secondary ossification center develops in the
tuber calcanei. Ossification is complete in the calcaneus by
7 months of age. The diaphyses of the metatarsal and
phalangeal bones are ossified at birth. The distal ends of
the metatarsal bones (heads) and the proximal ends of the
phalanges (bases) develop ossification centers by 6 weeks and
ossify to the diaphyses by the time the dog is 9 months old.
Trauma of the tarsal bones frequently includes fracture of
the talus and central tarsal bone and epiphyseal separation
of the tuber calcanei. Fracture of the central tarsal bone
often occurs in racing Greyhounds.

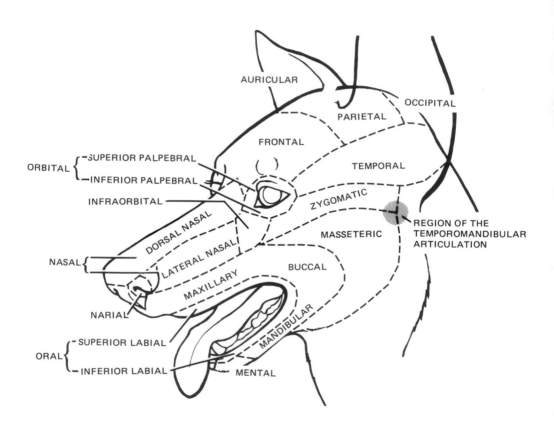

FIG. 6.1. Regions of the face and cranium.

6 HEAD

The FACIAL REGION, which overlies the bones that make up the face, is subdivided into 13 regions (Fig. 6.1): nasal, oral, mental, buccal, orbital, infraorbital, temporomandibular articulation, masseteric, maxillary, mandibular, zygomatic, intermandibular, and subhyoid. The NASAL REGION overlies the nasal cavity and is subdivided into NARIAL and DORSAL and LATERAL NASAL REGIONS. The region of the NARIS is the surface area around the external opening into the nasal cavity. The ORAL REGION is subdivided into SUPERIOR and INFERIOR LABIAL REGIONS. The MENTAL REGION is the surface over the chin. The BUCCAL REGION refers to the cheek, which it overlies. The ORBITAL REGION is the area superficial to the bony socket that protects the eye; the SUPERIOR and INFERIOR PALPEBRAL REGIONS are subdivisions of the orbital region. Beneath and rostral to the orbit is the INFRAORBITAL REGION, named after the bony canal and foramen deep to the surface. The joint between the lower jaw and the skull lies deep to the REGION OF THE TEMPOROMANDIBULAR ARTICULATION. The MASSETERIC (mass″e-ter′ik) REGION is superficial to the masseter muscle, a muscle of mastication. The MAXILLARY and MANDIBULAR REGIONS are superficial to facial bones with the same names. The ZYGOMATIC REGION overlies the zygomatic bone and zygomatic salivary gland. The ventral facial subregion, between right and left mandibles, is the INTERMANDIBULAR REGION. The SUBHYOID REGION, situated between intermandibular and laryngeal regions, is superficial to the hyoid apparatus and root of the tongue.

The CRANIAL REGION, superficial to the cranial bones that encase the brain, is subdivided into OCCIPITAL, PARIETAL, TEMPORAL, AURICULAR, and FRONTAL REGIONS. The

FIG. 6.2. Right cranial bones, lateral view.

FIG. 6.3. Fontanelle of a mature chihuahua.

HYPOGLOSSAL CANAL

FIG. 6.4. Occipital bone, caudoventral view

FORAMEN OF THE DORSAL SAGITTAL SINUS

GROOVE OF THE TRANSVERSE SINUS

CONDYLOID CANAL

FORAMEN MAGNUM

FIG. 6.5. Internal surface of occipital bone, rostral view.

SUPRAORBITAL FOSSA is a depression in the temporal region above and behind the eye; this fossa is not as pronounced in dogs as it is in larger domestic mammals.

BONES OF THE HEAD

The SKULL, a bony case, houses the brain, inner ear, and the upper respiratory and digestive systems. It also partially encloses and protects the eye and larynx. The skull will be described prior to considering the soft structures of the head. Dentition is discussed with the remainder of the digestive system (pp. 224-29); foramina of the skull are described more fully in the chapters on the vessels and nerves of the head (see Chaps. 20, 26). The skull may be divided into cranial and facial bones, which provide support and protection for the brain and face, respectively.

The CRANIUM (Fig. 6.2) is composed of the following bones: occipital (1), parietal (2), frontal (3), temporal (4), pterygoid (ter'i-goid; winglike) (5), basisphenoid (6), presphenoid (7), ethmoid (8), and vomer.

The ossification of frontal and parietal bones may not yet be completed in a young puppy, thus this area may be soft and nonradiopaque. Such osseous gaps between bones of the cranium are called FONTANELLES (fon"tah-nelz'). A fontanelle (1, Fig. 6.3) will also normally be observed in the adult Chihuahua where ossification of these bones is not complete.

The following external openings and prominences should be identified in the OCCIPITAL BONE (Fig. 6.4): the FORAMEN MAGNUM (1), the osseous border of which encircles the spinal cord; the paired OCCIPITAL CONDYLES (2), which articulate with the 1st cervical vertebra; the NUCHAL (nu'kal) CREST (3), which provides for attachment of certain neck muscles; the EXTERNAL OCCIPITAL PROTUBERANCE (4), which is the dorsocaudal prominence with which right and left nuchal crests merge; the INTERPARIETAL PROCESS (5), positioned dorsomedially, which arises as a separate bone and fuses prenatally with the occipital bone; and the bilateral JUGULAR PROCESSES (6), which provide for attachment of several muscles, one of which (the digastricus) functions to open the jaw. On the internal surface of the occipital bone, the TENTORIUM PROCESS (1, Fig. 6.5) projects rostroventrally into the cranial cavity from the dorsocaudal osseous wall.

FIG. 6.7. Frontal bones.

SUPRAORBITAL FORAMEN

ETHMOIDAL FORAMINA

FIG. 6.6. Parietal bones.

FIG. 6.8. Left temporal bone, lateral view.

RETROARTICULAR FORAMEN

HYPOGLOSSAL CANAL

TYMPANOOCCIPITAL FISSURE

STYLOMASTOID FORAMEN

FIG. 6.9. Right temporal bone, ventral view.

The PARIETAL BONE forms much of the dorsal and lateral walls of the cranium (Fig. 6.6). The EXTERNAL SAGITTAL CREST (1), as a dorsal median spine, is continuous in many dogs from the external occipital protuberance (caudally) to the frontal bones (rostrally). Brachycephalic breeds, dogs with dome-shaped cranial vaults, and young dogs with weakly developed jaw muscles may have paired TEMPORAL LINES (2) in place of the external sagittal crest. The TEMPORAL SURFACE (3) is a convex surface that serves as the area of origin for the temporalis muscle; the temporal and frontal bones (to be described later) also provide a portion of the temporal surface and temporal line. Intracranially, the parietal bone forms a portion of the bony tentorium process, which projects rostroventrally between the cerebrum and cerebellum.

Much of the FRONTAL BONE (FIG. 6.7) is separated into a superficial (1) and a deep (2) bony layer by an air space termed the FRONTAL SINUS (3). The air-filled cavity of the frontal sinus, like all paranasal sinuses, opens into that of the nasal cavity. The ZYGOMATIC PROCESS OF THE FRONTAL BONE (4) is a ventrolaterally projecting process from the external surface of the frontal bone.

The TEMPORAL BONE forms much of the caudolateral portion of the skull (Figs. 6.8, 6.9). The ZYGOMATIC PROCESS OF THE TEMPORAL BONE (1) forms a protective cover for more deeply situated nerves and vessels and provides an area of origin for the masseter muscle. The ventral proximal portion of the zygomatic process of the temporal bone has a concave MANDIBULAR FOSSA (2), a surface that articulates with the mandible. The large, rostroventrally directed RETROARTICULAR PROCESS OF THE TEMPORAL BONE (3) forms much of the articular surface. The EXTERNAL ACOUSTIC MEATUS (4) is the large opening immediately caudal to the retroarticular process; sound waves are transmitted through the external acoustic meatus to the middle ear. The TYMPANIC BULLA (bul′ah, pl. bullae) (5), a rounded prominence situated between the retroarticular and jugular processes, contains the middle ear cavity.

The MUSCULOTUBAL CANAL (6, Fig. 6.9) is separated from the larger, more medial CAROTID CANAL (7) by a slender, bony septum. The musculotubal canal contains the tendon of a tensor muscle and the AUDITORY (Eustachian) TUBE, which functions to allow air to pass between the pharynx and middle ear equalizing air pressure on each side of the ear drum. The MASTOID PROCESS (8) is a blunt eminence dorsolateral to the tympanic bulla and rostrodorsal to the jugular process.

INTERNAL ACOUSTIC MEATUS

FIG. 6.10. Right petrous temporal bone, deep surface.

ORBITAL FISSURE

OPTIC CANAL

SMALL ALAR FORAMEN

ROSTRAL ALAR FORAMEN

OVAL FORAMEN

CAUDAL ALAR FORAMEN

ROUND FORAMEN

FIG. 6.11. Basisphenoid and presphenoid.

OPTIC CANAL
ORBITAL FISSURE
ROUND FORAMEN

OVAL FORAMEN

FIG. 6.12. Deep surface of the sphenoid bone.

It provides a point of attachment for the hyoid apparatus and the sternomastoideus, cleidomastoideus, and splenius muscles.

On the internal surface of the skull (Fig. 6.10) the PETROUS (pet'rus; rocklike) PORTION OF THE TEMPORAL BONE (1) projects into the cranial cavity, partially separating the cerebrum from the cerebellum. The PETROSAL CREST (2) is continuous with the tentorium process of the occipital and parietal bones.

The BASISPHENOID and PRESPHENOID BONES (Fig. 6.11) each consist of a body and two wings (alae). The body of the basisphenoid (1) and the body of the presphenoid (2) form much of the ventral floor of the cranium. The external surface of the wings of the sphenoid bones (3) contain a number of important foramina through which nerves and vessels pass.

The SELLA TURCICA (sel'ah tur'sik-ah; Turkish saddle) (1, Fig. 6.12) is on the internal surface of the basisphenoid; it forms an osseous cradle for the hypophysis (pituitary). The DORSUM SELLAE (2) is a bony projection forming the caudal part of the cradle; the HYPOPHYSEAL FOSSA (3) is the depression that supports the hypophysis.

The ETHMOID BONE (Fig. 6.13) is a complex structure situated deep within the skull between the nasal and cranial cavities. It is discussed with the respiratory system.

ROSTRAL VIEW   LATERAL VIEW   CAUDAL VIEW

FIG. 6.13. Ethmoid bone.

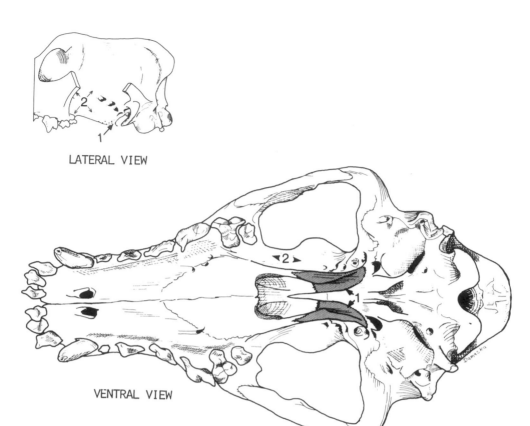

LATERAL VIEW

VENTRAL VIEW

FIG. 6.14. Pterygoid bone.

FIG. 6.15. Vomer, ventral view.

The PTERYGOID BONE (1, Fig. 6.14), which forms part of the lateral wall of the air passageway dorsal to the soft palate, also serves as a point of origin for the medial pterygoid muscle, a muscle of mastication. Portions of a number of important nerves and vessels are present laterally, adjacent to the palatine bone; this area containing muscle, nerves, and vessels is termed the PTERYGOPALATINE FOSSA (2).

The VOMER (1, Fig. 6.15) may be observed on the ventral surface of the skull, where it forms part of the dorsal wall of the nasopharyngeal meatus, and within the nasal cavity (dotted lines), where it forms a median U-shaped trough. A ventral extension from the vomer partially divides the air passage near the caudal portion of the hard palate.

Bones of the face (Fig. 6.16) are nasal (1), maxilla (2), incisive (3), ventral nasal concha (kong'kah, pl. conchae; shell) (4), palatine (5), lacrimal (6), zygomatic (7), mandibles (8), and the hyoid apparatus (9). The zygomatic bone and zygomatic process of the temporal bone form much of the ZYGOMATIC ARCH. Nasal, ventral nasal concha, lacrimal, and zygomatic bones will not be discussed further.

FIG. 6.16. Left facial bones, lateral view.

MINOR PALATINE FORAMEN
MAJOR PALATINE FORAMEN

FIG. 6.17. Incisive, maxillary, and palatine bones, ventral view.

INFRAORBITAL FORAMEN
INFRAORBITAL CANAL
MAXILLARY FORAMEN
SUPERIOR ALVEOLAR FORAMINA
SPHENOPALATINE FORAMEN
CAUDAL PALATINE FORAMEN

FIG. 6.18. Incisive, maxillary, and palatine bones, caudolateral view.

FIG. 6.19. Mandibles, dorsolateral view.

BONE
BONE
BONE
FIBROCARTILAGE

FIG. 6.20. Intermandibular articulation.

TYMPANOHYOID

FIG. 6.21. Hyoid apparatus, lateral view.

The MAXILLA (1, Figs. 6.17, 6.18) forms a major part of the hard palate and osseous lateral walls of the nasal cavity. The LACRIMAL CANAL is a tunnel through the maxillary bone extending from the FOSSA OF THE LACRIMAL SAC (in the lacrimal bone) to the nasal cavity; the nasolacrimal duct, which conveys lacrimal fluid or tears from the surface of the eye to the nose, is partially situated within the lacrimal canal (see p. 13).

The INCISIVE BONE (2, Figs. 6.17, 6.18) supports the six upper incisors and contributes to the formation of the PALATINE FISSURE (3, Fig. 6.17). The PALATINE BONE (4, Fig. 6.17; 3, Fig. 6.18) forms part of the hard palate and pterygopalatine fossa.

Each MANDIBLE (Fig. 6.19) bears three processes on its proximal part: the coronoid process (1), the condylar process (2), and the angular process (3). The CONDYLAR PROCESS articulates with the mandibular fossa of the temporal bone at the TEMPOROMANDIBULAR ARTICULATION (4). The CORONOID PROCESS of the mandible, positioned between the zygomatic arch and the medial osseous wall of the orbit, provides a surface area for insertion by the powerful temporalis muscle. The ANGULAR PROCESS forming the caudoventral portion of the mandible provides a point of insertion for another muscle of mastication, the masseter. The depression on the lateral surface of the mandible near the base of the coronoid process is the MASSETERIC FOSSA (5), which serves as an area of insertion for the masseteric muscle. The INTERMANDIBULAR ARTICULATION (Fig. 6.20), between right and left mandibles, is formed by cartilaginous and fibrous connective tissue.

The HYOID APPARATUS (Fig. 6.21) is composed of a number of bones that articulate at one point with the mastoid process of the skull, at another point with the larynx, and third by means of connective tissue with the tongue. The individual bones of the hyoid apparatus are a single BASIHYOID (1) and on each side a THYROHYOID (2), a CERATOHYOID (ser″ah-to-hi′oid) (3), an EPIHYOID (4), and a STYLOHYOID (5). The TYMPANOHYOID is usually cartilaginous, as may be a number of the other hyoid components in young animals.

FIG. 6.22. Superficial facial muscles, right lateral view.

FIG. 6.23. Facial muscles, right lateral view.

MUSCLES OF THE HEAD

The muscles of facial expression function to move the lips, nasal alae, and the ears. Muscles of the face include the platysma; zygomaticus; orbicularis oris; buccinator; levator nasolabialis; orbicularis oculi; and rostral, dorsal, caudal, and ventral groups of auricular muscles.

The PLATYSMA (plah-tiz'mah) (1, Fig. 6.22) is a cutaneous muscle that passes from the middorsal RAPHE (ra'fe; seam) of the neck, across the parotid and masseteric regions, to the angle of the mouth, where it radiates into the ORBICULARIS ORIS MUSCLE (2). The platysma, which acts to pull the commissure of the lips caudally, is a superficial muscle covering the ventrolateral surface of the head.

The ZYGOMATICUS MUSCLE (1, Fig. 6.23) extends cranioventrally from the SCUTIFORM (sku ti-form; shield) CARTILAGE (2) of the ear to the caudal edge of the superior lip, where its fibers radiate into the orbicularis oris muscle (3). The scutiform cartilage is a small, flat cartilage interposed in the rostral auricular muscle group, rostromedial to and separate from the cartilage of the external ear. The orbicularis oris is a superficial muscle, the fibers of which are situated between the skin of the outer surface of the lips and the mucous membrane of the inner surface of the lips. As the orbicularis oris extends from the superior lip to the inferior lip around the ANGLE OF THE MOUTH, its pursestring action results in a closing of the lips. Fibers of the obicularis oris muscle intermingle with the larger and more deeply situated BUCCINATOR MUSCLE (4). The buccinator muscle lies deep to the zygomaticus muscle and between the rostral margin of the masseter muscle and the caudal margin of the orbicularis oris muscle. It functions to make the cheek taut. The LEVATOR NASOLABIALIS (5) is a flat muscle that arises from the frontal region between the eyes and inserts on the superior lip and nasal ala; it elevates the superior lip and dilates the nostril. The ORBICULARIS OCULI (6) is composed of a group of muscle fibers that encircle the eye, situated partially within the eyelids. Contraction of the orbicularis oculi closes the PALPEBRAL FISSURE (space between the free margins of the eyelids).

FIG. 6.24. Auricular muscles.

FIG. 6.25. Muscles of mastication, right lateral view.

The muscles that move the external ear (Fig. 6.24) are divided into four groups: rostral, dorsal, caudal, and ventral auricular. The ROSTRAL AURICULAR MUSCLES (1) arise from the forehead, rostromedial to the ear, and insert on the cartilaginous skeleton of the external ear. The DORSAL AURICULAR MUSCLES (2) extend from the medial raphe of the caudal half of the head to insert on the cartilaginous skeleton of the external ear. The CAUDAL AURICULAR MUSCLES (3) are a group of muscles that extend from the dorsum of the neck to the cartilaginous skeleton of the ear. The small PAROTIDOAURICULAR MUSCLE (4) is the larger of two VENTRAL AURICULAR MUSCLES.

Muscles of mastication (Fig. 6.25) include the orbicularis oris, buccinator, masseter (mas-se'ter) (1), temporalis (2), medial pterygoid, lateral pterygoid, and digastricus (di-gas"trik'us; two bellies) (3). The orbiculars oris and buccinator muscles keep food within the oral cavity by means of their purse-string action. The MASSETER MUSCLE--a large muscular mass located ventral to the zygomatic arch, rostral to the parotid salivary gland, and caudal to the facial vein--arises from the zygomatic arch and inserts in the masseteric fossa on the lateral surface of the mandible. The TEMPORALIS is a thick muscle located between the sagittal crest of the skull (dorsally) and the zygomatic process of the frontal bone (rostrally). Deep to the rostral, dorsal, and caudal auricular muscles, the temporalis muscle arises from the temporal fossa of the skull and inserts on the medial surface of the coronoid process of the mandible. Both the temporalis and the masseter muscles, the fibers of which intermingle at the zygomatic arch, act to close the mouth by elevating the lower jaw.

FIG. 6.26. Deep muscles of mastication, right lateral view.

FIG. 6.27. Extrinsic hyoid muscles, ventral view.

Deep to the zygomatic arch and the coronoid process of the mandible, the MEDIAL PTERYGOID MUSCLE (1, Fig. 6.26), covered with glistening deep fascia, is observed deep and medial to a number of vessels and nerves that course through the pterygopalatine fossa. The medial pterygoid muscle arises from the pterygopalatine fossa and inserts on the medial surface of the mandible, ventral to the area of insertion by the temporalis muscle. The LATERAL PTERYGOID MUSCLE (2), which is smaller than the medial pterygoid, arises from the sphenoid bone and passes caudolaterally to insert on the medial surface of the mandibular condyle. Both the medial and lateral pterygoid muscles aid the masseter and temporalis muscles in closing the jaw. The DIGASTRICUS MUSCLE (3), which is located along the caudoventral surface of the mandible, arises from the jugular process of the occipital bone and inserts on the caudoventral portion of the body of the mandible. The digastricus functions to open the jaw.

Deglutition (swallowing) is a complex action involving the tongue, soft palate, larynx, hyoid bones, pharynx, and esophagus. These structures are discussed in chapters covering the upper respiratory and digestive organs.

Extrinsic muscles of the hyoid apparatus (Fig. 6.27) include the sternohyoideus (1), thyrohyoideus (2), mylohyoideus (3), and geniohyoideus. The sternohyoideus and sternothyroideus muscles are also described with the muscles of the neck. The MYLOHYOIDEUS MUSCLE is a thin sheet of transversely directed fibers situated superficially between the body of the right and left mandibles. The fibers of the mylohyoideus muscle arise from the medial surface of the body of the mandible and insert on the contralateral muscle in the midline between the mandibles; the paired muscle thus forms a sling ventral to the tongue. A small vein (submental) courses rostrally from the venous hyoid arch along the raphe of the mylohyoideus muscle.

FIG. 6.28. Extrinsic hyoid muscles, with the right mandible removed, right lateral view.

RIGHT GENIOHYOIDEUS

RIGHT MYLOHYOIDEUS

FIG. 6.29. Extrinsic tongue muscles, with the right mandible removed, right lateral view.

The STERNOHYOIDEUS (1, Fig. 6.28) and THYROHYOIDEUS (2) MUSCLES exert a caudally directed force on the hyoid apparatus. The paired GENIOHYOIDEUS (3) is a straplike muscle, deep (dorsal) to the mylohyoideus (4), that extends from the hyoid bone to the mandibular symphysis.

The extrinsic muscles of the tongue (Fig. 6.29) include the styloglossus (1), the hyoglossus (2), and the genioglossus (3). The fibers of the paired GENIOGLOSSUS (glossa: glos'ah; tongue) MUSCLE pass from the medial surface of the mandible (caudodorsally) into the body and root of the tongue, forming an inverted V-shaped mass dorsal to the geniohyoideus. The HYOGLOSSUS MUSCLE passes from the hyoid bone into the body of the tongue, lateral to the caudodorsal extent of the genioglossus and dorsal to the mylohyoideus. The STYLOGLOSSUS is a straplike muscle extending from the stylohyoid bone to the body of the tongue; it is located lateral to the distal end of the hyoglossus muscle and medial to the body of the mandible.

FIG. 7.1. Regions of the body.

FIG. 7.2. Cervical subregions.

FIG. 7.3. Pectoral subregions.

138

7 TRUNK

The trunk is a general term for that portion of the body not including the head or limbs. The surface of the trunk is divided into cervical, pectoral, abdominal, dorsal, and pelvic regions (Fig. 7.1).

The CERVICAL REGION is subdivided into parotid, dorsal cervical, lateral cervical, and ventral cervical regions (Fig. 7.2). The PAROTID REGION is the area ventral to the base of the ear that is superficial to the parotid salivary gland. The DORSAL CERVICAL REGION is dorsal to the cervical vertebrae. The LATERAL CERVICAL REGIONS form the lateral surfaces of the neck. The VENTRAL CERVICAL REGION is again subdivided into LARYNGEAL and TRACHEAL REGIONS. The external jugular vein separates the lateral and ventral cervical regions. The JUGULAR FOSSAE are depressions on each side of the base of the neck where right and left external jugular veins course deep to enter the thorax.

The PECTORAL REGION is composed of PRESTERNAL, STERNAL, and COSTAL REGIONS (Fig. 7.3). The sternal and costal regions are named according to location of the underlying sternum and ribs, respectively. The CARDIAC REGION is a subregion superficial to the heart. The COSTAL ARCHES, one on each side of the animal, are arches formed by cartilage of three of the most caudal four pairs of ribs.

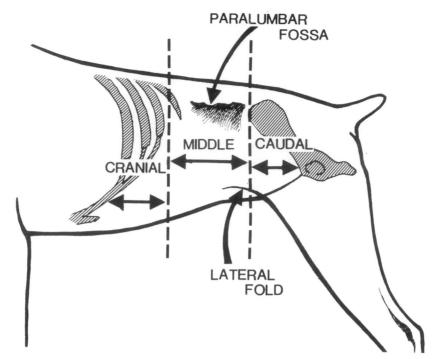

FIG. 7.4. Three major abdominal subregions.

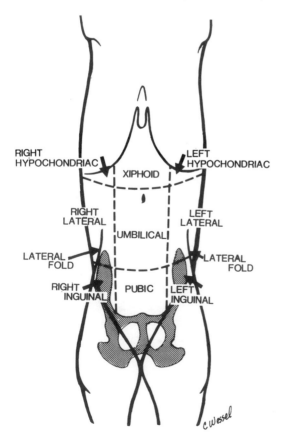

FIG. 7.5. Nine abdominal subregions.

FIG. 7.6. Dorsal subregions.

The ABDOMINAL REGION is divided into nine regions by two transverse and two sagittal lines on the surface of the abdomen as a result of imaginary planes passed through the abdomen. CRANIAL, MIDDLE, and CAUDAL ABDOMINAL REGIONS are formed by two transverse planes passing through the trunk; one transverse plane passes through the caudal border of the costal arch and the other passes through the cranial border of the hip bones (Fig. 7.4).

The cranial, middle, and caudal abdominal regions are each subdivided into three smaller regions by passing two sagittal planes through the trunk (Fig. 7.5); the sagittal planes, one on each side of the ventral median line, are located approximately half way between the median plane and the lateral surface of the animal. The cranial abdominal region is thus divided into RIGHT and LEFT HYPOCHONDRIAC (under cartilage) REGIONS and a XIPHOID (zif'oid; swordlike) REGION. The middle abdominal region is subdivided into RIGHT and LEFT LATERAL ABDOMINAL REGIONS and a midventral UMBILICAL REGION. In thin animals, a depression may be observed in the dorsal portion of the lateral regions termed the PARALUMBAR FOSSA. A fold of skin connects the thigh (cranially) with the abdomen; this LATERAL FOLD occurs in each lateral abdominal region. The caudal abdominal region is subdivided by the sagittal planes into RIGHT and LEFT INGUINAL REGIONS and a midventral PUBIC REGION. The PREPUTIAL REGION, or area of the sheath of the penis, is a subregion of the male pubic region.

The DORSAL REGION is the area dorsal and superficial to the trunk vertebrae; it is subdivided into a THORACIC VERTEBRAL REGION and a LUMBAR (loin) REGION (Fig. 7.6). The portion of the thoracic vertebral region between the dorsal borders of the scapulae is the INTERSCAPULAR REGION; it is the most dorsal portion of the back.

FIG. 7.7. Pelvic subregions.

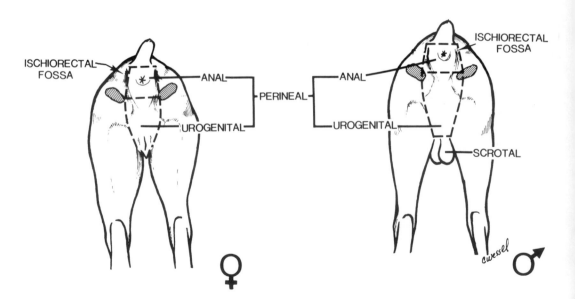

FIG. 7.8. Perineal subregions.

The PELVIC REGION is subdivided into sacral, caudal, gluteal, clunial, tuber coxae, tuber ischiadicum, perineal, and scrotal or supramammary entities (Figs. 7.7, 7.8). The SACRAL, CAUDAL, and GLUTEAL REGIONS overlie the sacral and caudal vertebrae and gluteal muscle groups, respectively. The CLUNIAL (kloo'ne-al; buttocks) REGION is the area dorsal to the caudal extent of the pelvis. A depression in the clunial region, the ISCHIORECTAL (is″ke-o-rek'tal) FOSSA, may be observed in gaunt animals. The regions of the TUBER COXAE and TUBER ISCHIADICUM, which are superficial to osseous enlargements of the bony pelvis, are located cranial and caudal to the hip joint, respectively. The PERINEAL (per″i-ne'al) REGION extends ventrally from the base of the tail to the caudal attachment of the scrotum in the dog or to the ventral margin of the external genitalia in the bitch. The perineal region is subdivided into ANAL (dorsally) and UROGENITAL (ventrally) REGIONS by a transverse line connecting the ischiatic tuber of each side. In the dog the SCROTAL REGION extends from the urogenital region (dorsally) to the pubic region (cranially); the corresponding region in the bitch is the SUPRAMAMMARY REGION.

The head, trunk, and tail are positioned along the long axis of the body; the bones providing support and protection for these parts are collectively termed the AXIAL SKELETON (Fig. 7.9). Skeletal muscles associated with the axial skeleton are termed AXIAL MUSCLES.

FIG. 7.9. Axial musculoskeletal system.

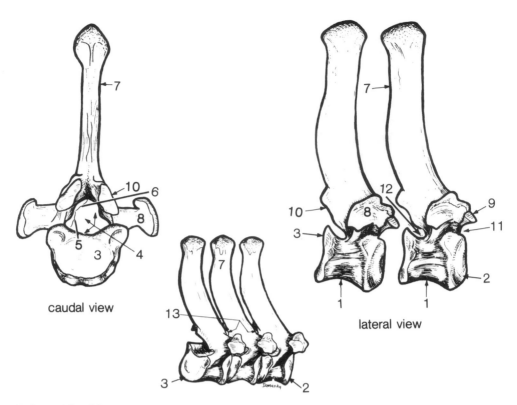

caudal view

lateral view

FIG. 7.10. Vertebrae, structures in common.

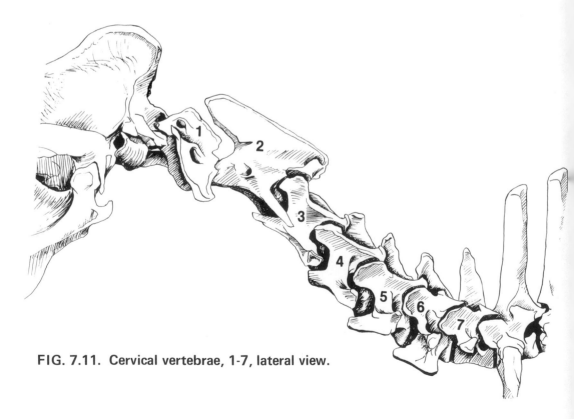

FIG. 7.11. Cervical vertebrae, 1-7, lateral view.

BONES OF THE TRUNK

A VERTEBRA (pl. vertebrae) (Fig. 7.10) typically is characterized by having a BODY (1); a CRANIAL (2) and a CAUDAL (3) EXTREMITY; a VERTEBRAL FORAMEN (4), which forms one unit of the VERTEBRAL CANAL; a VERTEBRAL ARCH, consisting of ventral PEDICLES (5) and dorsal LAMINAE (sing. lamina) (6); a SPINOUS PROCESS (7); a pair of TRANSVERSE PROCESSES (8); paired CRANIAL (9) and CAUDAL (10) ARTICULAR PROCESSES; CRANIAL (11) and CAUDAL (12) VERTEBRAL NOTCHES (each forms half of an INTERVERTEBRAL FORAMEN when articulated with adjacent vertebrae); and an INTERARCUATE SPACE (13). Cranial and caudal extremities begin to ossify 2 months postnatally and fuse with the body between 7 and 10 months. Nutrient foramina are usually present in the dorsal and ventral surfaces of the vertebral bodies.

The presence of 7 CERVICAL VERTEBRAE (Fig. 7.11) is characteristic of most mammalian species. The 1st (most cranial) cervical vertebra is the ATLAS (1), which articulates cranially with the occipital condyles and caudally with the AXIS (2), or 2nd cervical vertebra. The 7th cervical vertebra articulates with the first (most cranial) thoracic vertebra and with the head of the 1st pair of ribs.

TRANSVERSE FORAMINA (1, Fig. 7.12) are present in the transverse processes of the cranial six cervical vertebrae; blood vessels and nerve fibers course along the vertebral column through the transverse foramina.

FIG. 7.12. Transverse foramina of cervical vertebrae 1-6.

CRANIAL VIEW

FIG. 7.13. Atlas.

CRANIAL VIEW

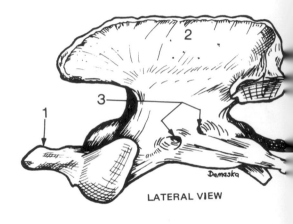

LATERAL VIEW

FIG. 7.14. Axis.

CAUDAL VIEW

LATERAL VIEW

FIG. 7.15. Cervical vertebrae 3-5.

The atlas (Fig. 7.13), lacking both a body and spinous process, may be identified as a cervical vertebra by the presence of transverse foramina (1). The transverse processes (2) are large lateral projections, which may be palpated in the live animal. A second pair of foramina, the LATERAL VERTEBRAL FORAMINA (3), are present in the cranial portion of the dorsal vertebral arch; the first pair of spinal nerves pass out from the spinal cord through the lateral vertebral foramina (blood vessels pass through these foramina also). The typical vertebral body and extremities are not present in the atlas; instead, a VENTRAL ARCH (4) is present. The thickest portion of the atlas is its LATERAL MASS (5), which includes the transverse process, and the CRANIAL (6) and CAUDAL (7) ARTICULAR FOVEAE. The cranial margin of the transverse process is notched, owing to the presence of blood vessels and a branch of the 1st spinal nerve; this notch is the ALAR INCISURE (8). Small processes that project into the vertebral foramen provide attachment for a transverse ligament that divides the vertebral foramen into a dorsal and a ventral portion. The spinal cord occupies the dorsal portion; the ventral portion contains a tooth-shaped process of the 2nd cervical vertebra.

The axis (Fig. 7.14), the 2nd cervical vertebra, is also highly modified from the shape of a typical vertebra. The two most pronounced identifying features are the cranially extending DENS (1) and the well-developed elongated SPINOUS PROCESS (2). The spinous process serves as a point of attachment for a number of neck muscles and for a strong ligament, the LIGAMENTUM NUCHAE. A transverse foramen (3) is located in the base of each slender transverse process (4).

Cervical vertebrae 3-5 are similar morphologically (Fig. 7.15). Each is characterized by the presence of transverse foramina (1), bifurcated transverse processes (2), and relatively small spinous processes (3).

CRANIAL VIEW

LATERAL VIEW

FIG. 7.16. Sixth cervical vertebra.

CAUDAL VIEW   LATERAL VIEW

FIG. 7.17. Seventh cervical vertebra.

FIG. 7.18. Thoracic vertebrae 1-13, lateral view.

The 6th cervical vertebra (Fig. 7.16) appears similar to cervical vertebrae 3-5 except for a pronounced extension of the bifurcated transverse processes (1). The 7th cervical vertebra (Fig. 7.17) has an elongated spinous process (1); bears CAUDAL COSTAL FOVEAE (2); and lacks transverse foramina. The caudal costal fovea provides part of the articular surface with the head of the 1st rib.

Thirteen THORACIC VERTEBRAE (Fig. 7.18) are present in the dog. The first (cranial) 10 thoracic vertebrae have spinous processes (1) directed caudodorsally. The thoracic vertebra with spinous process perpendicular to the long axis of the vertebral column, the ANTICLINAL (an"ti-klie'nal) VERTEBRA (2), is usually the 11th; spinous processes of the 12th and 13th thoracic vertebrae are directed craniodorsally. Each side of the first 10 thoracic vertebrae bears two surfaces for articulating with the heads and one surface for articulating with the tubercles of ribs. The articular surfaces for the costal head are the CRANIAL COSTAL FOVEA (3) and the caudal costal fovea (4), present on the vertebral bodies. The articular surface for each costal tubercle is the COSTAL FOVEA OF THE TRANSVERSE PROCESS (5), present on the lateral surface of each transverse process. The 11th, 12th, and 13th thoracic vertebrae usually have only two costal articular surfaces per side, the transverse (5) and cranial costal fovea (each rib, 11-13, articulates with only one vertebra). Each of the 11th, 12th, and 13th thoracic vertebrae has an ACCESSORY PROCESS (6).

FIG. 7.19. Lumbar vertebrae 1-7, lateral view.

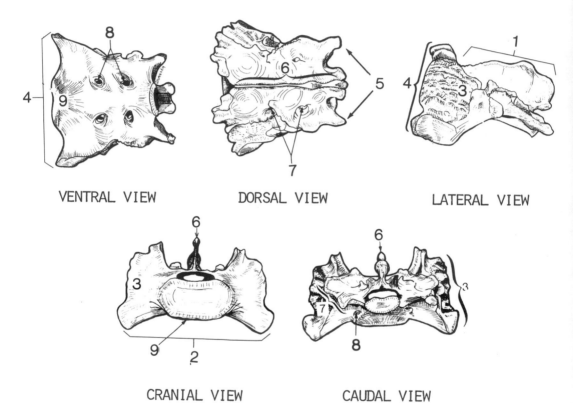

VENTRAL VIEW   DORSAL VIEW   LATERAL VIEW

CRANIAL VIEW   CAUDAL VIEW

FIG. 7.20. Sacrum.

FIG. 7.21. Caudal vertebrae.

The vertebral column of the dog contains seven LUMBAR VERTEBRAE (Fig. 7.19). A lumbar vertebra has a large body (1), long, cranioventrally directed transverse processes (2), and small MAMILLARY PROCESSES (3). Mamillary processes are also present on a number of thoracic vertebrae. Accessory processes (4) are also present on a number of lumbar vertebrae.

The SACRAL BONE (Fig. 7.20) is composed of three SACRAL VERTEBRAE, which fuse together within a few months postnatally. The sacrum has DORSAL (1) and PELVIC (2) SURFACES, a LATERAL PART (3), a BASE (4), and an APEX (5). The dorsal surface bears a MEDIAN SACRAL CREST (6) of fused spinous processes and DORSAL SACRAL FORAMINA (7). The pelvic surface bears VENTRAL SACRAL FORAMINA (8) and a PROMONTORY (9). The promontory, present on the pelvic (ventral) surface of the sacral base, may create difficulties during parturition, particularly in dogs with dome-shaped crania.

CAUDAL VERTEBRAE (Fig. 7.21) vary in number and shape. A vertebral arch (and therefore a vertebral foramen and canal) is not present caudally past the 6th or 7th caudal vertebra.

Eight bones, or STERNEBRAE, and seven INTERSTERNEBRAL CARTILAGE segments form the STERNUM (Fig. 7.22). The sternebra situated farthest cranially is the MANUBRIUM (1); the following six sternebrae are termed the BODY, and the last sternebra is the XIPHOID PROCESS (2). XIPHOID CARTILAGE projects caudally from the xiphoid process.

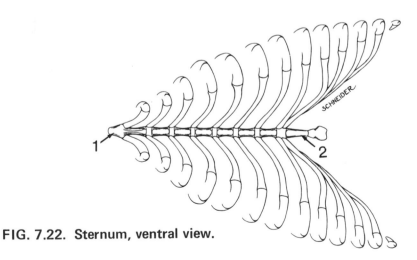

FIG. 7.22. Sternum, ventral view.

FIG. 7.23. Ribs 1-13, lateral view.

FIG. 7.24. Costal bone, cranial view.

There are 13 pairs of RIBS in the thorax (Fig. 7.23). The first (most cranial) 9 pairs of ribs are termed STERNAL RIBS (1) since they each attach directly to the sternum. The last 4 pairs of ribs are named ASTERNAL RIBS (2), although the ventral tips of the 10th, 11th, and 12th pairs of ribs attach to preceding ribs and thus to the sternum. Each rib is composed of COSTAL BONE (3) and COSTAL CARTILAGE (4). The costal cartilages of the 9th, 10th, 11th and 12th ribs form the COSTAL ARCH (5). The ventral portion of the 13th rib is not attached to the preceding rib or sternum; thus it is often described as "floating."

The 1st costal cartilage articulates with the 1st sternal segment; the following eight costal cartilages articulate with cartilage between sternal segments, with the 8th and 9th costal cartilages sharing an intersternebral point of attachment.

Each costal bone (Fig. 7.24) consists of a HEAD (1), NECK (2), COSTAL TUBERCLE (3), and BODY (4). The costal tubercles of all 13 pairs of ribs articulate with the transverse processes of thoracic vertebrae of corresponding number. The heads of the first 10 or 11 ribs articulate with surfaces on the caudal edge of the body of each preceding vertebra and on the cranial edge of the body of each correspondingly numbered vertebra.

MUSCLES OF THE TRUNK

Trunk muscles may be described as belonging in one of two major groups: epaxial or hypaxial muscles. EPAXIAL MUSCLES are those muscles dorsal to the long axis of the vertebral column; bilateral contraction of epaxial muscles results in extension of the vertebral column. HYPAXIAL MUSCLES, those muscles ventral to the long axis of the vertebral column, have a number of functions; however, most hypaxial muscles contribute to flexion of the vertebral column. Specialized muscles concerned with respiration, digestion, urination, and copulation are discussed later with the specific body systems concerned.

FIG. 7.25. Sternocephalicus, ventral view.

FIG. 7.26. Muscles overlying the cranial portion of the epaxial muscle system.

The epaxial (extensor) group is composed of a number of complex muscles that are difficult to separate and identify. The epaxial muscles may be divided into the following divisions: splenius, erector spinae, transversospinalis, interspinalis, and intertransversarius muscles. To observe the epaxial muscles in the cervical and thoracic regions, the STERNOCEPHALICUS MUSCLE (1, Fig. 7.25), the pectoral limb, and the serratus dorsalis muscle need to be removed. The sternocephalicus muscle has two parts both of which arise from the manubrium of the sternum. A cranioventral part of the sternocephalicus muscle inserts on the mastoid process of the skull and a caudodorsal part inserts on the nuchal crest of the skull.

The SERRATUS DORSALIS CRANIALIS MUSCLE (1, Fig. 7.26), which is deep to the serratus ventralis (2) and rhomboideus (3) muscles, arises from the dorsal cervical raphe and the spinous processes of thoracic vertebrae; its fibers are directed caudoventrally to insert on ribs 2-10. The very small SERRATUS DORSALIS CAUDALIS MUSCLE (4) is oriented in a cranioventral direction from the thoracolumbar fascia to the last several ribs.

FIG. 7.27 Superficial epaxial muscles, with extrinsic limb muscles and serratus dorsalis removed (A); epaxial skeleton for visual comparison (B), lateral view.

The SPLENIUS CERVICIS (1, Fig. 7.27) is a flat muscle that attaches caudally to the dorsal midline from the 1st cervical to the 3rd thoracic vertebrae and cranially to the nuchal crest. The three subdivisions that form the ERECTOR SPINAE MUSCLE are the iliocostalis, longissimus, and spinalis muscles, from ventrolateral to dorsomedial in position. The ILIOCOSTALIS MUSCLE is present as a series of short muscle fascicles occurring in the lumbar and thoracic regions as the ILIOCOSTALIS LUMBORUM (2) and ILIOCOSTALIS THORACIS (3) MUSCLES. The iliocostalis lumborum muscle attaches caudally to the wing of the ilium and cranially to the last ribs. The iliocostalis thoracis muscle attaches ribs to ribs and to the transverse process of the last cervical vertebra.

The LONGISSIMUS (lon-jis'i-mus) MUSCLE (Fig. 7.27) is present as a series of short muscle fascicles, located dorsal to the iliocostalis system, that occur in the lumbar, thoracic, and cervical regions. The LONGISSIMUS LUMBORUM MUSCLE (4) extends from iliac crest and spinous processes of lumbar vertebrae (caudally) to the vertebral arch and accessory processes of lumbar vertebrae (cranially). The LONGISSIMUS THORACIS MUSCLE (5) is a thoracic continuation of the longissimus that inserts on accessory and transverse vertebral processes and on ribs adjacent to the costal tubercles. The LONGISSIMUS CERVICIS MUSCLE (6), as a cervical continuation, inserts on the transverse processes of the last four cervical vertebrae. The LONGISSIMUS CAPITIS MUSCLE (7) is that portion of longissimus, dorsomedial to the longissimus cervicis muscle and deep to the splenius muscle, that extends from the transverse processes of the first three thoracic vertebrae and the caudal articular processes of the last five cervical vertebrae to the mastoid process of the temporal bone. A caudal continuation of the longissimus muscle into the tail is named, descriptively, the SACROCAUDALIS DORSALIS LATERALIS MUSCLE (8).

The SPINALIS MUSCLE is composed of thoracic and cervical portions, with the thoracic portion fused to fibers of the semispinalis thoracis. The fused muscle, SPINALIS AND SEMISPINALIS THORACIS (9, Fig. 7.27), arises from the thoracolumbar fascia and the dorsomedial surface of the longissimus thoracis muscle. The spinalis and semispinalis thoracis muscle inserts on the spinous processes of the last two cervical and first six thoracic vertebrae. The SPINALIS CERVICIS MUSCLE (1, Fig. 7.28) arises from the spinous process of the 1st thoracic vertebra and inserts cranially on spinous processes of the 2nd to 5th cervical vertebrae.

FIG. 7.28. Deep epaxial muscles of the cervical region, lateral view: splenius, longissimus cervicis, and longissimus capitis muscles removed (A); semispinalis muscle also removed (B); all muscles removed (C).

The TRANSVERSOSPINALIS MUSCLE division is a series of deep epaxial muscles and includes the semispinalis, multifidi, and rotator muscles. The SEMISPINALIS MUSCLES consists of thoracic, cervical, and capital portions. The thoracic portion of the semispinalis muscle, fused with the spinalis, has been described (9, Fig. 7.27). Another segment of the semispinalis muscle, the SEMISPINALIS CAPITIS, composed of biventer cervicis and complexus, is superficial to the spinalis cervicis muscle (Fig. 7.28). The BIVENTER (two bellies) CERVICIS MUSCLE (2) arises medial to the longissimus muscle from the transverse processes of the 2nd to 4th thoracic vertebrae and inserts on the skull near the external occipital protuberance. The COMPLEXUS MUSCLE (3), ventrolateral to the biventer cervicis, arises from the caudal articular processes of the last 5 cervical and 1st thoracic vertebrae; the complexus muscle inserts on the nuchal crest of the skull.

The MULTIFIDI (mul-tif'i-die, sing. multifidus) MUSCLES (4, Fig. 7.28; 1, Fig. 7.29) are a series of short muscles that attach caudoventrally to mamillary, transverse, or articular processes, pass craniodorsally over two vertebrae, and usually attach to spinous processes of other vertebrae. Muscles belonging to the multifidi subdivision are present from the caudal vertebrae to the skull. The multifidus series is continued cranially in the region of the first two cervical vertebrae (Fig. 7.28) as the caudal and cranial capital oblique muscles. The CAUDAL CAPITAL OBLIQUE MUSCLE (5) arises from the spinous process of the axis and inserts craniolaterally on the transverse process of the atlas. The CRANIAL CAPITAL OBLIQUE MUSCLE (6) arises on the transverse process of the atlas and inserts craniodorsally on the nuchal crest of the skull. The multifidi continue caudally into the tail as the SACROCAUDALIS DORSALIS MEDIALIS.

FIG. 7.29. Deep epaxial muscles of the thoracic and abdominal regions, lateral view, with iliocostalis and longissimus muscles removed (A); skeleton deep to the deep cranial muscles of the thoracic and abdominal regions (B).

In the cranial thoracic region, short muscle groups are present that act to pivot or rotate the thoracic vertebrae around their long axes. These ROTATOR MUSCLES (2, Fig. 7.29) occur as short and long fascicles. The short rotator muscles pass between the transverse process of one thoracic vertebra to the spinous process of the next preceding (cranial) vertebra; long rotator muscles pass by one vertebra from their origin to their point of insertion.

INTERSPINALIS muscles (3, Fig. 7.29) are segmental muscles that attach to the spinous processes of adjacent vertebrae. Muscles that may be considered modified interspinalis muscles are the RECTUS CAPITIS MUSCLES, which arise on the dorsal surface of the axis or atlas and insert on the skull near the nuchal crest. The RECTUS CAPITIS DORSALIS MAJOR MUSCLE (7, Fig. 7.28; 1, 2, Fig. 7.30) arises on the spinous process of the axis and inserts on the occipital bone. This major dorsal straight muscle of the head is comprised of two parts, a more superficial part (1, Fig. 7.30) which arises from the caudal portion of the spinous process and a deeper part (2, Fig. 7.30) which arises from the cranial portion of the spinous process. The RECTUS CAPITIS DORSALIS MINOR MUSCLE (3) arises from the dorsal arch of the atlas and inserts on the occipital bone directly dorsal to the foramen magnum. INTERTRANSVERSE MUSCLES, occurring from head to tail, are best developed in the cervical (8, Fig. 7.28) and caudal vertebral regions. These muscles arise from mamillary, articular, accessory, or transverse processes, pass over one or more vertebrae, and insert on transverse processes of other vertebrae.

FIG. 7.30. Rectus capitis dorsalis muscles, dorsal view.

FIG. 7.31. Ventral vertebral muscles: deep flexor muscles of the head and neck, ventrolateral view (A); deep flexor muscles of the trunk, ventral view (B); deep flexor muscles of the lumbar, sacral, and caudal vertebrae, ventral view (C).

For consideration of muscles ventral to the long axis of the vertebral column, these hypaxial muscles may be divided into three groups: deep flexors of the vertebral column, lateral thoracic and abdominal muscles, and ventral trunk muscles.

The deep vertebral (subvertebral) muscles (Fig. 7.31) include the rectus capitis ventralis, rectus capitis lateralis, longus capitis, longus colli, psoas minor, quadratus lumborum, psoas major, sacrocaudalis ventralis lateralis, and sacrocaudalis ventralis medialis. The RECTUS CAPITIS VENTRALIS MUSCLE (1) attaches from the ventral arch of the atlas to the ventral surface of the occipital bone. Lateral to the rectus capitis ventralis, the RECTUS CAPITIS LATERALIS MUSCLE (2) attaches the transverse process of the atlas to the jugular process of the skull.   The LONGUS CAPITIS MUSCLE (3) arises from transverse processes of cervical vertebrae and inserts on the ventral surface of the occipital bone. The LONGUS COLLI MUSCLE (4) in the thorax arises from the ventral surfaces of the first six thoracic vertebrae and inserts on the transverse processes of the last two cervical vertebrae; in the neck, the longus colli muscle arises from the transverse process of one vertebra and inserts on the ventral surface of the preceding (cranial) vertebral body. The longus colli muscle is situated medial to the longus capitis muscle.

The PSOAS MINOR MUSCLE (5, Fig. 7.31) arises from the ventral surfaces of the last thoracic and first four or five lumbar vertebrae and inserts as a cordlike tendon on the ilium adjacent to the iliopubic eminence. The QUADRATUS LUMBORUM MUSCLE (6) arises dorsal to the psoas minor muscle from the ventral surfaces of the bodies of the last three thoracic vertebrae; it inserts on the transverse processes of the lumbar vertebrae and the medial surface of the wing of the ilium. The PSOAS MAJOR MUSCLE (7) arises from the last six lumbar vertebrae and inserts, in common with the ILIACUS MUSCLE as the ILIOPSOAS, on the minor trochanter of the femoral bone (see p. 107).

The ventral tail muscles are the SACROCAUDALIS VENTRALIS LATERALIS (8, Fig. 7.31) and MEDIALIS (9). The major artery to the tail is situated in a depression between right and left sacrocaudalis ventralis medialis muscles.

FIG. 7.32. Superficial layer of hypaxial muscles, lateral view.

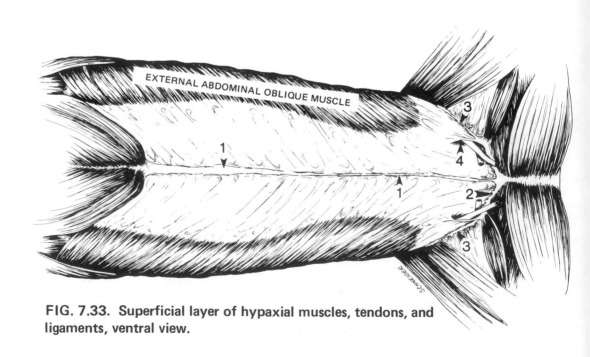

FIG. 7.33. Superficial layer of hypaxial muscles, tendons, and ligaments, ventral view.

The lateral thoracic and abdominal muscles occur in three layers from superficial to deep. The superficial muscle layer of the lateral thorax (Fig. 7.32) includes the scalenus, external intercostals, levator costarum and external abdominal oblique. The superficial muscle of the abdomen is the external abdominal oblique. The muscle fibers of all four muscles are oriented in a caudoventral direction. The scalenus has superficial and deep parts that form the DORSAL (1) and MIDDLE (2) SCALENUS MUSCLES; the fascicles of the scalenus muscle attach the 1st, 3rd, 4th, and 8th or 9th ribs to the last five cervical vertebrae. The EXTERNAL INTERCOSTAL MUSCLES (3) arise from the caudal surface of a rib and insert on the cranial surface of the next rib (caudally). The short, fusiform-shaped LEVATOR COSTARUM MUSCLES (4) are deep to the longissimus thoracis muscle; 12 levator muscles attach the transverse processes of thoracic vertebrae to cranial borders of adjacent ribs. The EXTERNAL ABDOMINAL OBLIQUE MUSCLE (5) arises from the superficial surfaces of ribs 4–13 and from the thoracolumbar fascia; it inserts by means of a wide aponeurosis on the linea alba and the prepubic tendon.

The LINEA ALBA (al'bah; white) (1, Fig. 7.33), or white line, is the combined aponeuroses of the abdominal muscles that extends along the ventral median line from the xiphoid process of the sternum to the pelvic symphysis. The cranial pubic ligament (2) is a thickening of connective tissue that attaches the iliopubic eminence of one side to the pubic symphysis on the ventral median line and then to the iliopubic eminence of the other side. A thickening in the dorsocaudal portion of the external abdominal oblique muscle's aponeurosis forms a part of the INGUINAL ARCH (3), which spans the distance from the tuber coxae to the iliopubic eminence. The SUPERFICIAL INGUINAL RING (4) is a slitlike opening in the aponeurosis of the external abdominal oblique muscle. The peritoneal outpocketing, vessels, and reproductive structures that pass through the superficial inguinal ring are described on pages 271–75, 317, and 479.

EXTERNAL ABDOMINAL OBLIQUE MUSCLE

2

3

1

EXTERNAL INTERCOSTAL MUSCLES,
INTACT ON THE LEFT SIDE, ARE
REMOVED FROM THE RIGHT SIDE

FIG. 7.34. Middle layer of hypaxial muscles, ventral view.

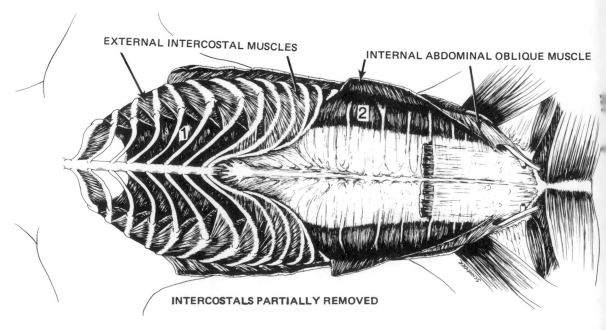

EXTERNAL INTERCOSTAL MUSCLES

INTERNAL ABDOMINAL OBLIQUE MUSCLE

2

1

INTERCOSTALS PARTIALLY REMOVED

FIG. 7.35. Deep layer of hypaxial muscles, ventral view.

The middle layer of lateral thoracic and abdominal muscles (Fig. 7.34) includes the INTERNAL INTERCOSTAL (1), INTERNAL ABDOMINAL OBLIQUE (2), and CREMASTER (to suspend) (3) muscles. The muscle fibers of both the internal intercostals and internal abdominal oblique muscles are oriented cranioventrally at right angles and deep to the superficial layer of muscles. The internal intercostal muscles attach the cranial surface of individual ribs to the caudal surface of adjacent ribs. The internal abdominal oblique muscle arises from the thoracolumbar fascia, the tuber coxae, and the inguinal arch; it inserts on the 12th and 13th ribs and by an aponeurosis on the linea alba. The cremaster muscle, which is derived from the internal abdominal oblique, is described with the male reproductive system (see p. 271).

The deep layer of lateral thoracic and abdominal muscles (Fig. 7.35) includes the transversus thoracis and transversus abdominis muscles. These two muscle groups are characterized by having muscle fibers oriented transversely to the long axis of the axial skeleton. Deep to the ribcage, the TRANSVERSUS THORACIS MUSCLE (1) arises from the sternum and inserts on the deep surfaces of the 2nd to 7th costal cartilages. The TRANSVERSUS ABDOMINIS MUSCLE (2) arises from the medial surfaces of the last five ribs, the transverse processes of the lumbar vertebrae, and the tuber coxae; it inserts by an aponeurosis on the linea alba.

The ventral trunk muscles include the rectus thoracis; the rectus abdominis; and the rectus cervicis complex, formed by the sternohyoideus, sternothyroideus, thyrohyoideus, and geniohyoideus muscles (see pp. 135-37). The STERNOHYOIDEUS is a straplike muscle that arises from the manubrium of the sternum and the 1st costal cartilage and inserts on the basihyoid. The STERNOTHYROIDEUS MUSCLE arises with the sternohyoideus from the 1st costal cartilage and inserts on the lateral surface of the thyroid cartilage of the larynx. The sternothyroideus muscle is immediately deep to the sternohyoideus muscle. To approach the trachea along the ventral median line, an incision would be made between the sternohyoideus and the sternothyroideus of one side and the same muscles of the other side. The THYROHYOIDEUS is a short muscle that attaches the thyroid cartilage to the thyrohyoid bone. The RECTUS THORACIS MUSCLE, the fibers of which are oriented caudoventrally, attaches the costal cartilage of the 2nd to 4th ribs to the 1st rib. The RECTUS ABDOMINIS MUSCLE is a long, straplike muscle that arises cranially by an aponeurosis from the sternum and 1st rib and inserts caudally

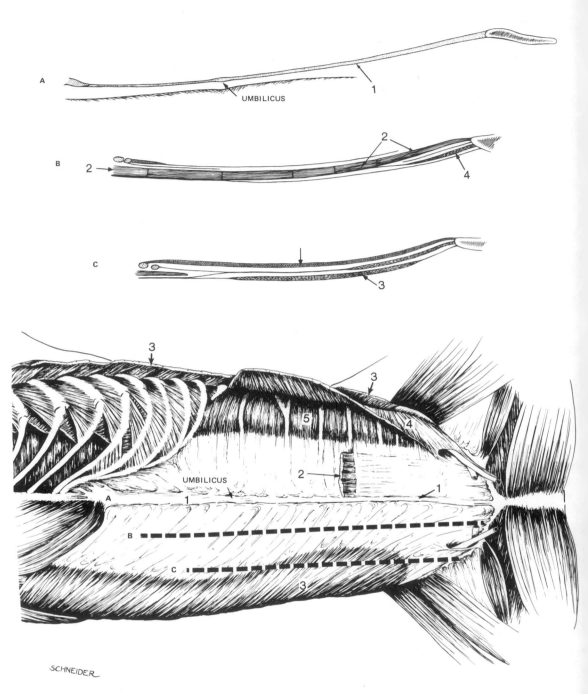

A

UMBILICUS

1

B

2

2

4

C

3

3

3

5

4

UMBILICUS

A

1

2

1

B

C

3

SCHNEIDER

FIG. 7.36. Change in position of rectus abdominis muscle in the abdominal wall, from cranial to caudal.

on the cranial pubic ligament via the prepubic tendon.   The
paired recti abdomini muscles are separated at the ventral
median line by the linea alba.

Depending upon location of an incision in the abdominal
wall, different layers of tissue will be encountered.   In the
cranial part of the abdominal wall, the aponeuroses of the
two oblique muscles of each side come together to form a
sheath that surrounds each rectus abdominis muscle (Fig.
7.36).   Caudally, in the inguinal region, the rectus
abdominis muscle is deep, next to the peritoneum, with the
aponeuroses of the other three abdominal muscles superficial
to it.   The linea alba (1), situated along the ventral median
line between right and left rectus abdominis muscles (2),
demarcates a line at which right and left sheathes are fused;
at this point of fusion (A) an incision needs to pass through
only one fused layer of deep fascia to reach the peritoneum.
A sagittal incision a few centimeters to one side of the
linea alba (B) would pass progressively through 3-5 layers
depending upon whether the site of incision is cranial or
caudal to the UMBILICUS.   A more lateral sagittal incision
(C) would involve both oblique muscles, or their separate
aponeuroses, and the transversus abdominis muscle (5).

FIG. 7.37. Atlantooccipital articulation, dorsolateral view.

FIG. 7.38. Atlantoaxial articulation, dorsal view. Dorsal arch of the atlas removed (A); muscles and articular capsule removed (B).

JOINTS OF THE TRUNK

Synovial joints in the vertebral column are present between articular processes (cranial and caudal) of adjacent vertebrae and between vertebrae and ribs.

The ATLANTOOCCIPITAL ARTICULATION (Fig. 7.37) is a site commonly used for puncturing membranes to remove (tap) cerebrospinal fluid. An articular capsule (1), enclosing a synovia-filled cavity, passes from the circumference of the articular surface of the occipital bone to the circumference of the cranial articular surface of the atlas. Thus the U-shaped articular capsule is lateral and ventral to the spinal cord. The thin VENTRAL ATLANTOOCCIPITAL MEMBRANE (a part of the fibrous articular capsule) passes from the ventral arch of the atlas to the ventral edge of the foramen magnum. The DORSAL ATLANTOOCCIPITAL MEMBRANE (2) attaches from the dorsal arch of the atlas to the dorsal edge of the foramen magnum.

The articular cavity of the ATLANTOAXIAL ARTICULATION (Fig. 7.38) is continuous with the cavity of the atlantooccipital articulation. As in the atlantooccipital articulation, the articular cavity is lateral and ventral to the spinal cord, but not dorsal to it. The dens of the axis (1) is bound in the ventral part of the vertebral foramen of the atlas by the TRANSVERSE ATLANTAL LIGAMENT (2).

A

B

FIG. 7.39. Intervertebral and costovertebral articulations. Lateral view of several intervertebral symphyses and thoracic and lumbar vertebrae (A); cranial view of a thoracic vertebra and proximal portions of associated ribs (B).

The INTERVERTEBRAL SYMPHYSES (Fig. 7.39) are fibrocartilaginous joints between adjacent bodies of vertebrae. Each such symphysis contains a layer of fibers connecting the periphery of one vertebral body to the next; these crisscrossing fibers pass obliquely relative to the long axis of the vertebral column. A ring of fibrous tissue is thus formed around the space between adjacent vertebral bodies. This ring, termed the ANULUS FIBROSUS (1), forms the outer portion of the INTERVERTEBRAL DISC. Deep to the thick layers of the anulus fibrosus, a soft, gelatinous, glistening white material maintains separation of adjacent vertebral articular cartilage; termed the NUCLEUS PULPOSUS (2), it forms the center of the intervertebral disc. Degenerative changes in the anulus fibrosus and/or a traumatic compression of the intervertebral disc may result in a herniation of the nucleus pulposus. If such a herniation occurs dorsally, a compression of the spinal cord and/or spinal nerves may result. Most intervertebral disc problems of the cervical region occur between C2 and C3; disc problems of the thoracolumbar region usually occur between T11 and L2. An intervertebral disc does not occur between C1 (atlas) and C2 (axis).

Ribs articulate with vertebrae at two synovial joints (Fig. 7.39): the COSTAL HEAD ARTICULATION (3), and the COSTOTRANSVERSE ARTICULATION (4). The head of each rib (1-10) articulates with costal articular surfaces on the bodies of two adjacent vertebrae and with an intervening intervertebral disc. The heads of each pair of ribs (2-10) are held tightly against their articular surfaces on the various vertebrae by an INTERCAPITAL LIGAMENT (5). Each intercapital ligament is a connective tissue band that is situated transversely across the dorsal surface of an intervertebral disc and attaches to the heads of right and left ribs. The synovial membrane of the articular capsule on one side is continuous across the vertebral column, between the intercapital ligament and the intervertebral disc, with that of the articular capsule of the other side. The RADIATE LIGAMENT OF THE COSTAL HEAD (6) attaches each rib head to the lateral surfaces of the bodies of two adjacent vertebrae (except for the last two or three pairs of ribs) and to the anulus fibrosus between them. The costotransverse articulations are synovial joints between articular surfaces of costal tubercles and vertebral transverse processes. Peripheral to the synovial membrane, each costal tubercle is bound to a transverse process by a COSTOTRANSVERSE LIGAMENT (7).

CRANIAL VIEW

LATERAL VIEW

SAGITTAL SECTION THROUGH THE LEFT PORTION OF VERTEBRAE T$_9$ - T$_{11}$

FIG. 7.40. Intervertebral ligaments.

A number of other articulations occur within the trunk. the SACROILIAC ARTICULATION (which craniodorsally is fibrocartilage and caudoventrally contains a synovial joint), the STERNOCOSTAL ARTICULATIONS (which are synovial joints), the STERNAL SYNCHONDROSES (joints between sternebrae without synovia), and the COSTOCHONDRAL ARTICULATIONS (joints between costal bone and costal cartilage without synovia).

Each vertebra is united to adjacent vertebrae by various ligaments (Fig. 7.40). A dorsal longitudinal band, the SUPRASPINOUS LIGAMENT (1) attaches to each spinous process between the 1st thoracic and 3rd caudal vertebrae. The NUCHAL LIGAMENT is a cranial extension of the supraspinous ligament; it attaches to the spinous process of the 1st thoracic vertebra (caudally) and to the spinous process of the axis (cranially). Two other longitudinal bands of connective tissue in the vertebral column are the ventral and dorsal longitudinal ligaments. The VENTRAL LONGITUDINAL LIGAMENT (2) is a slender band on the ventral surfaces of the vertebral bodies and intervertebral discs from the axis to the sacrum. The DORSAL LONGITUDINAL LIGAMENT (3) is present on the dorsal surfaces of vertebral bodies and intervertebral discs from the axis to the caudal termination of the vertebral canal. The intercapital ligaments of the ribs pass between the dorsal longitudinal ligament and the intervertebral discs. The LIGAMENTA FLAVA (flav'ah; yellow) spans the distance between individual vertebrae, attaching vertebral arch to vertebral arch. This yellow ligament should not be confused with the more deeply situated dura mater, the outermost layer of the meninges. Other connective tissue bands that may be encountered are INTERSPINOUS and INTERTRANSVERSE LIGAMENTS.

(DIFFERENCE TO BE NOTED IN THE CAT: A nuchal ligament is not present.)

MANDIBLE   RIB

FIG. 8.1. Contribution of stress to the production of flat bone.

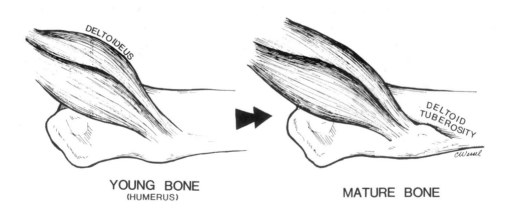

YOUNG BONE   MATURE BONE
(HUMERUS)

FIG. 8.2. Contribution of stress to osseous projections.

8 BIOMECHANICS

STRESS

The musculoskeletal system is designed for support and movement; its component parts are bone, cartilage, muscle, ligament, tendon, and fascia. Immobility results in a decrease in size of a muscle and loss of calcium from bones. This decrease in size of a structure is termed ATROPHY. HYPERTROPHY is the opposite of atrophy and describes an enlargement resulting from exercise. Exercise places stress on bone through muscular activity. Muscles that attach on two opposite surfaces of a bone create stress in only one plane. This unidirectional stress, which stimulates the development of osseous tissue in one plane, contributes to the production of flat bone (Fig. 8.1). The pull of muscles on their points of attachment on bone results in development of osseous projections that enlarge as the animal ages (Fig. 8.2). There is much variation in size and shape of osseous enlargements in various species since the same muscle in different species may perform different levels of activity and provide different degrees of tension on bone.

The weight of every part of the standing or moving dog is supported by the limbs. Most weight loads applied to long bones place stresses on them that are parallel (COMPRESSION) and perpendicular (SHEAR) to their long axes. These stresses are greatly increased during running, when the pelvic limbs push against the ground or when the thoracic limbs catch and cushion the fall of the forward moving body after each pelvic thrust.

A series of bones placed end to end would be capable of carrying more weight than if they were placed at angles to each other because bone can withstand a greater compressive force than shear force. Bone that is slightly and temporarily deformed by stress develops STRESS LINES parallel to the weight load.

Stress is progressively less toward the central axis of a cylinder. The compact bone in the diaphyses of long bones is also strengthened by having a minimum of cavities, grooves, and notches that would weaken its structure. Thus, by being hollow and cylindrical, long bones have a greater strength (per unit weight) for resisting compression than solid or rectangular bones.

Due to the attachment of muscles to the epiphyses and metaphyses, the ends of long bones are subjected to bending forces; to resist bending, the ends of long bones are often oval in cross section, with thicker walls toward and away from the points of muscle attachment.

Forces transmitted by one bone to another across a partially flexed joint are carried through trabeculae in the epiphyses and metaphyses of each bone; the trabeculae are oriented linearly along the lines of stress. An injury to bone or disuse of a muscle will result in an alteration of force and hence in a change in the direction and quantity of trabeculae.

Synovial joints (see pp. 69-73) permit long bones to move while under relatively little shearing stress. The synovia, which lubricates the articular cavity, reduces friction and wear by molecular shearing that occurs within the fluid itself. The reciprocal surfaces of the articulating epiphyses are so morphologically incongruous that the film of lubricant between them is shaped like a wedge. Stress during movement forces the wedge of synovia between newly developing contiguous surfaces.

MOVEMENT

A Whippet is able to travel 55 km/hr (35 miles/hr); the coyote and red fox run at 69 and 72 km/hr (43.9 and 45.8 miles/hr), respectively. Mammals with rapid cursorial locomotion are characterized by having elongated distal limb segments and points of muscular insertion close to the joints. This lengthening of the limb in relation to body size results in a longer stride; stride is a full cycle of limb movement or the total distance covered after all limbs have moved. Speed in movement is equal to length of stride times the rate of stride. Muscles of various mammals do not vary greatly in speed of contraction. The rate of stride is dependent upon proximity of the points of muscle insertion to limb joints (Fig. 8.3). When a tendon is inserted close to the joint, a larger stride is achieved in a shorter time, since a shorter distance of contraction is required to produce the same movement than an insertion farther from the joint would necessitate. Insertion by a tendon farther from the joint provides greater strength.

FIG. 8.3. Strength/speed versus relative proximity of muscle insertion to the center of a joint.

FIG. 8.4. Vertical movement and
the sequence of limb movements
in the walk type of gait.

The dog initiates movement with a thoracic limb; as movement occurs, the metacarpal and metatarsal pads make contact with the ground before the digital pads do. The shock of the limbs striking the ground is cushioned by overextension of the carpal joints and flexion of the tarsal joints. The tendons of superficial and deep digital flexors, flexors carpi ulnaris and radialis, and the common calcanean tendon take on the stress of impact, cushioning and dampening the shock. The ulnar and genual articulations have limited movement or cushioning function. The digital flexor muscles of both manus and pes increasingly contract, resulting in greater flexion such that the body weight is transferred to the digital pads.

Muscles of a limb that are active during that portion of movement when the limb is supporting weight usually have a pennate fiber pattern and are thus powerful and contract a short distance. Limb muscles that are active during the period of the stride when the limb is swinging and not in ground contact usually have parallel fibers, are relatively weak, and shorten a greater distance.

A GAIT is a regularly repeated sequence of leg movements; the walk, trot, pace, and gallop are each characterized by a unique sequence of movements.

The WALK (Fig. 8.4) is a gait in which each foot is in contact with the ground more than 50% of the time. Each foot moves independently (out of synchrony), and two or three feet provide support at all times. The sequence of limb movements in one stride occurs as follows: right manus, left pes, left manus, right pes (or left manus, right pes, right manus, left pes). The angle formed by the ground with a line passing through the acetabulum and supporting pad of a walking Greyhound is approximately 66 degrees both at the beginning and at the end of the support phase.

FIG. 8.5. Vertical movement and the sequence of limb movements in the trot type of gait.

The TROT (Fig. 8.5) is a gait in which a thoracic limb and the opposite pelvic limb move nearly in unison (one diagonal followed by the other). The trot may produce a rise and fall of the shoulders, which evidences a jolting gait; much of the shock will be absorbed by the thoracic limb if the scapula and long axis of the trunk are positioned at an angle of approximately 45 degrees to each other. Some dogs, such as the German Shepherd, are able to trot rapidly enough to utilize their momentum for forward motion while all four feet are off the ground (SUSPENSION); the "flying trot" is characterized by suspension in two phases: one following movement of one diagonal and the other following movement of the other diagonal.

Animals are often moved at a trot while diagnosing lamenesses as abnormal movement becomes more apparent during this gait. The degree of flexion and extension is decreased and the swing and support phases of limb movement are shortened in an injured limb such that the affected limb bears weight for a shorter period of time. Verticle movement of the head and neck in animals with limb lameness may be utilized to determine whether the right or left limb is affected; the head is lowered during the supportive phase of the sound thoracic limb and raised during the supportive phase of the lame limb. An animal with a lameness in a pelvic limb will carry its pelvis tilted such that less weight is applied to the injured limb.

The PACE, or amble, is a gait in which first one lateral (thoracic and pelvic) and then the other lateral move in unison. This gait is faster than the trot and is often utilized by a tired or unsound dog.

FIG. 8.6. Vertical movement and the sequence of limb movements in the gallop type of gait.

In the GALLOP (Fig. 8.6), the two pelvic limbs make contact with the ground out of synchrony and then the two thoracic limbs do likewise. There are various forms of galloping (sustained, normal, and leaping). The sustained gallop (CANTER) is a sequence of three supports per stride: one pes, the opposite pes with its diagonal, and the opposite manus. The portion of the stride with the single support by the manus provides a catapultlike action; the body is propelled forward like that of a polevaulter by the extended thoracic limb. A scapula-thoracic angle of 45 degrees will permit optimum propulsion by this single support. The normal gallop is characterized by four distinct supports sequenced as follows: left pes, right pes, left manus, right manus. The leaping gallop is characteristic of gazehounds (Greyhound, Whippet, Saluki, Borzoi, and Afghan) and Doberman Pinschers. The body loses all contact with the ground two times per stride. The first period of suspension is obtained by one thoracic limb; the second suspension is obtained two supports later by the diagonal pelvic limb. The sequence of supports in the leaping gallop is: right pes, left pes, left manus, and right manus.

BODY STRUCTURES--RUNNING

A dog's body may be specialized for many purposes such as digging, entering small underground tunnels, fighting, retrieving, or running down prey. The remainder of this chapter will be concerned only with certain factors related to the efficiency and effectiveness of the body structure for running.

Large dogs with body proportions similar to those of small dogs are not built as efficiently for locomotion as the smaller dogs; as the body length increases X times, body weight increases X^3 while muscular force increases only by X^2.

Efficiency in cursorial movement may be increased by (1) decreasing the vertical movement of the trunk, (2) decreasing the lateral movement of the body during forward motion, (3) reducing muscles that abduct, adduct, or rotate the limbs, (4) lengthening the distal limb segments relative to proximal segments, and (5) decreasing the vertical distance the distal ends of the limbs move from the ground.

The presence of only a rudimentary clavicle in an animal enables greater movement of the scapula relative to the thorax than in animals with well-developed clavicles. A deep, narrow chest further contributes to freedom of the scapula to pivot cranially and caudally. Such a movement of the scapula increases the effective stride and thus the animal's speed.

For efficient movement, a dog's pelvic and thoracic limbs should be in a straight line (when viewed from the cranial or caudal surface) from the humeral or coxal articulation to the ground. Since each joint distal to the humeral and coxal joints acts as a hinge joint, a deviation of bone laterally or medially would require more muscular effort for support and hence would be more fatiguing. Both thoracic and pelvic limbs should move cranially and caudally in a straight line during locomotion.

A thrusting force by a limb against the ground results in a movement of the body both forward and toward the opposite side (i.e., the right foot pushes the body cranially and left laterally). Fighting this LATERAL DISPLACEMENT with opposing muscles results in fatigue. Most running dogs bring their feet in toward the median plane (SINGLE TRACKING), which reduces lateral displacement (i.e., the distance between right and left manus and right and left pes is less on a running dog than on a standing dog). The limbs while forming a straight line (as observed cranially or caudally) incline medially. Many thick-chested, short-legged dogs (such as the Basset Hound) partially achieve this method of reducing lateral displacement by having a curved radius and ulna. By having widely separated feet, other dogs (such as the Bulldog) achieve stability at the expense of cursorial efficiency.

Vertical undulations of the vertebral column permit longer strides. Flexion of the vertebral column is accompanied by movement of the pelvic limbs cranially. Extension of the vertebral column is associated with movement of the thoracic limbs cranially; with each step of a rapidly galloping dog, the thorax and pelvis both rotate in the same direction as the limbs they support are moving.

Although the limbs of a running dog are straight when viewed cranially or caudally, the limbs during their supportive portion of the stride should not be straight when viewed laterally. For efficiency in running, the scapula should be set at a 45 degree angle to the long axis of the trunk; the scapula may normally pivot approximately 15 degrees during rapid locomotion. The humerus, which is optimally positioned at approximately a 90 degree angle to the scapula during the standing phase, may extend during locomotion to approximately a 150 degree angle with the long axis of the scapula. A vertical line drawn through the center of the scapula should intersect the metacarpal pad of a supporting limb. If the pad is cranial to the line the carpus would tend to sink, placing more strain on the carpal and digital flexors. If the pad is caudal to this vertical line, the dog will tend to travel on its toes, with continual danger of knuckling over or stumbling. The flexor angle of the cubital articulation would ideally approximate 130 degrees during the supportive phase of the stride. The flexor angle of the carpal articulation should be somewhat more than 180 degrees in order for this joint to take up the shock of ground contact (by sinking caudoventrally).

The pelvic limb of the dog functions to power the body forward. The pelvic limb is set to provide maximum thrust against the ground when the metatarsal pad is in a vertical line with the coxal articulation. The force that can be generated by the pelvic limb is determined by the ratio of the limb length with pad under coxal articulation and that of the fully extended limb. An angle of 150 degrees between the long axis of the lumbar vertebrae and that of the pelvis is nearly optimum. The flexor angle of the proximal femoral articulation should approximate 75-90 degrees. The longer the crus, relative to limb length, the more powerful the limb is likely to be. The pes should be at 90 degrees to the surface of the ground for optimum power (the dorsal surface of the German Shepherd pes is at a greater then 90 degree angle). A long metatarsus will provide greater power at the loss of endurance.

Respiratory System

FIG. 9.1. Schematic of the respiratory organs, dorsal view.

FIG. 9.2. Schematic of the nasal cavity, lateral view.

9 ROSTRAL PORTION

The respiratory system consists of organs that conduct gases (oxygen and carbon dioxide) between the blood and the external environment. The exchange of gases between the blood and the air around the organism is termed external respiration. At rest, an average dog breathes in, and out, a volume of approximately 175 ml of air, 10-30 times per minute; this external respiration is a diffusion process, i.e., air molecules move from an area of higher concentration in the ambient air to an area of lower concentration in the lung tissue and then from an area of higher concentration in the lung to an area of lower concentration in the ambient air.

By increasing the volume of the thoracic cavity--which results in a changing lung volume--the concentration of air molecules is decreased within the lungs, resulting in inspiration, or a movement of air from a region of high pressure (atmosphere) to a region of low pressure (lung). By decreasing the volume of the thoracic cavity--thereby decreasing the lung volume--the density of air molecules is increased, resulting in an outward diffusion of air molecules (expiration).

The respiratory organ system (Fig. 9.1) consists of the conducting airways--nasal cavity (1), nasopharynx (na"zo-far' inks) (2), laryngopharynx and larynx (lar'inks) (3), trachea (4), bronchi (5), and bronchioles (6)--and the gas exchange area, or alveoli (sing. alveolus; small hollow sac) (7).

The NASAL CAVITY (1, Fig. 9.2) is a paired space with constricted openings both rostrally and caudally. The paired vestibules form the rostral portion of the nasal cavity.

FIG. 9.3. Nasal cavity, with a portion of the nasal septum and walls of the right nasal fossa removed.

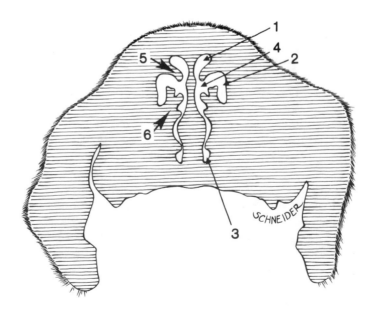

FIG. 9.4. Air passages, which constitute much of the nasal cavity.

Each NASAL VESTIBULE (antechamber) (2) is bounded and supported by cartilage; the surface of the nasal vestibule is a transitional zone between the pigmented skin of the NASAL PLANE (3) and the mucous membrane of the nasal cavity proper. Inspired air flows rapidly and at low pressure through the constricted orifice of the nasal vestibule; watery secretions from a number of nasal glands are discharged into the constricted orifice and are atomized into the air current. Small openings interconnect the caudodorsal portion of the nasal cavity with the frontal sinuses (4). Caudoventrally, the nasal cavity is continuous with the NASOPHARYNGEAL MEATUS (5).

The nasal cavity (Fig. 9.3) is divided by a median NASAL SEPTUM (1) into two fossae. Each NASAL FOSSA is subdivided by membrane-surfaced osseous projections into smaller air channels. Two of these osseous projections, named conchae, are present in the rostral portion of the nasal cavity. The DORSAL CONCHA, or nasoturbinate (2), is a ventral osseous projection from the nasal bone; the long dorsal concha is also a rostral projection of one of the ethmoid conchae. The greatly convoluted or scrolled VENTRAL CONCHA, or maxilloturbinate (3), projects dorsomedially from the maxillary bone into the nasal fossa. The rostral noncoiled enlargement of the ventral concha is the ALAR FOLD (4). An opening, the NASOLACRIMAL OSTIUM (5), is present in the ventromedial surface of the alar fold; the NASOLACRIMAL DUCT (6) drains orbital secretions from the LACRIMAL SAC (7) through the osseous lacrimal canal into the nasal vestibule. A second ostium of the nasolacrimal duct may also be present.

The rostral portion of each nasal fossa is subdivided by the conchae (Fig. 9.4) into dorsal (1), middle (2), ventral (3), and common (4) nasal meatuses. The DORSAL NASAL MEATUS (1) is the portion of the nasal fossa dorsomedial to the dorsal concha (5). The MIDDLE NASAL MEATUS (2) is the lateral airway situated between the dorsal concha and the ventral concha (6). The VENTRAL NASAL MEATUS (3) is the ventral air channel situated ventromedial to the ventral concha. The COMMON NASAL MEATUS (4) is the airway formed by the junction of dorsal, middle, and ventral meatuses.

A SAGITTAL SECTION

FIG 9.5. Conchae of the left nasal fossa: sagittal section (A) indicating levels of transverse sections B and C.

B TRANSVERSE SECTION

C TRANSVERSE SECTION

The middle, ventral and common nasal meatuses of the midportion of the nasal cavity are nearly occluded by the greatly branched ventral concha (1, Fig. 9.5); the membrane-covered branches (LAMELLAE, sing. lamella) of the ventral concha form many smaller airways, providing an increased surface area for more efficient filtering and warming of inhaled air. The ETHMOID CONCHAE (2) are a series of turbinates or osseous scrolls that project rostrally from the CRIBRIFORM LAMINA of the ethmoid bone; they also attach laterally or dorsally to other lamina of the ethmoid bone. Ethmoid conchae are described as ENDOTURBINATES (3) or ECTOTURBINATES (4) based upon how far they extend medially toward the nasal septum (i.e., whether they are observable from the median plane with the septum removed). An endoturbinate is usually larger, projects farther medially, and is more easily observed within the nasal cavity from the median plane than an ectoturbinate. Several of the larger endoturbinates project rostrally and are easily confused with the ventral concha. A few ectoturbinates project caudodorsally into the frontal sinus. Many air channels (ethmoid meatuses) occur between the ethmoid conchae; the apertures of three compartments of the frontal sinus open into the ethmoid meatuses. Much of the caudomedial epithelial surface of the ethmoid conchae contains olfactory receptor cells.

The MAXILLARY RECESS (5, Fig. 9.5) is a large cavity situated between the orbital lamina of the ethmoid bone (medially) and the maxillary, lacrimal, and palatine bones (laterally). The thick membrane that surfaces the maxillary recess is quite glandular. The maxillary recess opens rostromedially into the nasal cavity between the rostral margin of the ethmoidal orbital lamina and conchae and the caudodorsal margin of the ventral conchae; the opening is termed the HIATUS (hi-a'tus; cleft) OF THE MAXILLARY RECESS (arrow, Fig. 9.5; 1, Fig. 9.6).

Much of the frontal bone is separated into a superficial and a deep bony layer by three air spaces (see p. 123) termed the frontal sinuses. As is true of all paranasal sinuses, the air-filled cavity of the frontal sinus opens into the nasal cavity; and is termed the APERTURE OF THE FRONTAL SINUS.

(DIFFERENCES TO BE NOTED IN THE CAT: A single frontal sinus occurs in each frontal bone.)

FIG. 9.6. Left nasal fossa, with ventral concha and portions of the ethmoturbinates removed, sagittal section.

ENTIRE SEPTUM

FIG. 9.7. Nasal septum, right lateral view.

The portion of the nasal cavity that conducts as a single tube all the air inhaled through both nasal fossae (Fig. 9.6) extends caudally from the ventral nasal meatus (2) to the nasal part of the pharynx (3). The lumen of this portion situated dorsal to the caudal portion of the hard palate (4), is nearly the same size as the constricted lumen of the nasal vestibule. The CHOANA (ko'a-nah, pl. choanae; funnel) (5) is the single opening formed by osseous structures separating the nasal cavity (rostrally) from the nasal part of the pharynx (caudally). The choana, formed by the palatine, vomer, and presphenoid bones, is dorsal to the caudal extent of the hard palate.

The rostral portion of the nasal septum (Fig. 9.7) contains cartilage (1). The osseous PERPENDICULAR LAMINA (2) of the ethmoid bone forms the skeleton of the caudal portion of the nasal septum. The VOMERONASAL (vo″mer-o-na′sal) ORGAN (3) is a small, hollow, blind-ending structure that occurs bilaterally in the ventral portion of the nasal septum. This hollow tube, which is surfaced partially by olfactory epithelium, may be observed in a transverse section through the rostral portion of the nose. The vomeronasal organ opens rostrally into the INCISIVE DUCT (4); a vascular pumping mechanism may move fluid into and out of the vomeronasal organ. The incisive duct connects the ventral nasal meatus, via the palatine fissure, to the rostral portion of the oral cavity.

ROSTROVENTRAL PORTION

FIG. 9.8. Schematic of the nasopharynx, lateral view.

The SOFT PALATE (1, Fig. 9.8) is a caudal extension from the hard palate that separates the PHARYNX (far'inks; throat) into a dorsal airway and a ventral food passageway. The NASOPHARYNX (2) is that portion of the pharynx dorsal to the soft palate. It connects with the nasal cavity through the choana (3) and with the laryngeal portion of the pharynx through the INTRAPHARYNGEAL OSTIUM, which is a transverse opening formed by the free caudal margin of the soft palate (4), rostrally, and the PALATOPHARYNGEAL ARCHES (5), laterally. The soft palate, elevated against the dorsal wall of the nasopharynx during swallowing, prevents food from entering the nasal cavity. The PHARYNGEAL OSTIA (6) of right and left AUDITORY TUBES are in the dorsolateral wall of the nasopharynx; the auditory tubes extend to the middle ear cavities and function in the equalization of air pressures on the vibrant partition (TYMPANIC MEMBRANE) between middle and external ears.

PHARYNGEAL TONSILS (1, Fig. 9.9) are inconspicuous paired lymphatic tissues situated on the dorsal surface of the nasopharynx (2) between and adjacent to the auditory tube openings (3). Pharyngeal tonsils have efferent lymph vessels that drain into the MEDIAL RETROPHARYNGEAL (behind the pharynx) LYMPH NODES (see pp. 395-97). Tonsils do not have afferent lymph vessels since they are directly exposed to foreign substances present in the pharynx.

FIG. 9.9. Rostrodorsal portion of the nasopharynx, all other soft tissues removed.

FIG. 9.10. Pharynx, larynx, trachea, and esophagus, with a portion of the pharynx and esophagus removed, dorsocaudolateral view.

FIG. 9.11. Laryngopharynx, rostral view.

The LARYNGOPHARYNX (1, Fig. 9.10) is that portion of the pharynx dorsal to much of the larynx and between the NASOPHARYNX (2) and the cranial end of the ESOPHAGUS (3). The dorsal tip, or apex, of the EPIGLOTTIS (4) projects into the intrapharyngeal ostium (5) during quiet respiratory movements; during panting or labored breathing the soft palate is elevated, allowing air to pass in and out of the mouth, thus circumventing the greater air resistance of the nasal cavity. Brachycephalic dogs have soft palates that extend caudally past the epiglottis; air movement between nasopharynx and larynx is hampered by this relative extension of the soft palate.

The grooves in the ventral wall of the laryngopharynx (Fig. 9.11), one to each side of the epiglottis (1), are termed PIRIFORM RECESSES (2). These recesses are important in the conduction of food through the laryngopharynx such that food does not enter the larynx. A fold of tissue, the ARYEPIGLOTTIC FOLD (3), connects the lateral margin of the epiglottis with the CUNEIFORM (ku-ne′i-form; wedge shape) PROCESS (4) of the arytenoid cartilage and assists in preventing food from entering the larynx.

The cartilaginous skeleton of the dog larynx (Fig. 9.12) consists primarily of one paired cartilage: the arytenoid (ar″e-te′noid) cartilage (1), and three unpaired cartilages: the epiglottis (2), thyroid (shield shape) cartilage (3), and cricoid (kri′koid; ring shape) cartilage (4).

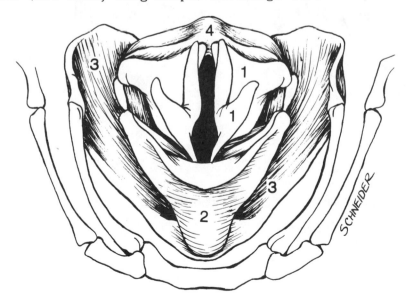

FIG. 9.12. Laryngeal cartilages and the hyoid apparatus, cranial view.

DORSAL VIEW

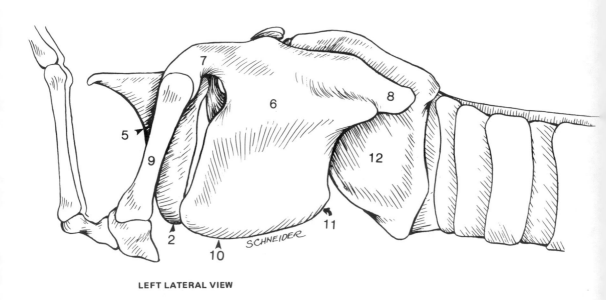

LEFT LATERAL VIEW

FIG. 9.13. Hyoid apparatus, laryngeal cartilages, and a cranial portion of the trachea.

The epiglottis (1, Fig. 9.13) is the farthest rostrally of the laryngeal cartilages; it is described as having an APEX (1), a BASE (2), right and left LATERAL MARGINS (3), and LARYNGEAL (4) and LINGUAL (ling'gwal; tongue) (5) SURFACES.

The THYROID CARTILAGE (6) is a U-shaped structure that forms the most lateral and ventral portion of the cartilaginous laryngeal skeleton. The right and left THYROID LAMINAE form the lateral walls of the U, with the open portion of the U directed dorsally. Rostral and caudal projections on the dorsal portion of the laminae are termed the ROSTRAL (7) and CAUDAL (8) CORNU (kor'nu, pl. cornua; horn). The rostral cornu articulates with the thyrohyoid bone (9). The cranial laryngeal nerve enters the larynx ventral to the rostral cornu. The LARYNGEAL PROMINENCE (10) is palpable on the ventral surface of the thyroid cartilage. The ventral portion of the thyroid cartilage is notched caudally; this median notch is named the CAUDAL THYROID NOTCH (11).

The CRICOID (ring form) CARTILAGE (12), the most caudal cartilage of the larynx, forms a complete ring around the airway. The cricoid cartilage is wide dorsally and narrow ventrally; the ventral portion is connected to the caudal thyroid notch by the CRICOTHYROID LIGAMENT (an important structure in the horse for surgical entry into the larynx). Much of the dorsal and lateral portions of the cricoid cartilage is positioned medial to the lamina of the thyroid cartilage (6). A small thyroid articular surface (13) is present on each lateral surface of the cricoid for articulation with the thyroid cartilage. Another small arytenoid articular surface (14) is present rostrally on each dorsolateral surface for articulation with the bilaterally paired arytenoid cartilage.

FIG. 9.14. Epiglottis, and left arytenoid and cricoid cartilages, left lateral view.

FIG. 9.15. Laryngeal and hyoid muscles, ventral view.

The ARYTENOID (laddle form) CARTILAGE (Fig. 9.14) is a paired cartilage situated medial to the lamina of the thyroid cartilage and between the epiglottic (rostrally) and the cricoid cartilage (caudally). Movement of the arytenoid cartilage relative to the other laryngeal cartilages results in teh production of noise of various amplitudes (loudness) and frequency (pitch).

Four cartilaginous processes of each arytenoid cartilage, which are of great importance in the functioning of the larynx, are the cuneiform, corniculate, vocal, and muscular processes. The CUNEIFORM (wedge form) PROCESS (1) is the most rostrodorsal projection of the arytenoid cartilage. The CORNICULATE PROCESS (2) is the conspicuous dorsal, hornlike process of the arytenoid. The VOCAL PROCESS (3) is a caudoventral projection of the arytenoid that provides an area of attachment for the vocal fold. The MUSCULAR PROCESS (4) is on the lateral surface of the most caudal portion of the arytenoid cartilage, near the surface that articulates with the cricoid cartilage.

(DIFFERENCES TO BE NOTED IN THE CAT: The arytenoid cartilage of the cat lacks corniculate and cuneiform processes.)

The intrinsic muscles of the larynx attach to the laryngeal cartilages; contraction of an intrinsic muscle produces movement of one cartilage relative to another, resulting in closure or opening of the space between the vocal folds. Seven intrinsic laryngeal muscles are present in the dog, six of which arise or insert on the muscular process (4) of the arytenoid cartilage and hence have arytenoideus as part of their name.

The CRICOTHYROIDEUS MUSCLE (1, Fig. 9.15), which does not attach to the arytenoid cartilage, may be observed on the caudoventral surface of the larynx, deep to the sternohyoideus muscle (2). It arises from the ventrolateral surface of the cricoid cartilage (3) and inserts on the caudomedial surface of the thyroid lamina (4). Contraction of this muscle, through innervation by the cranial laryngeal nerve, pivots the ventral portion of the thyroid and cricoid cartilages toward each other, indirectly producing a stretching of the vocal folds.

FIG. 9.16. Laryngopharynx, larynx, and cranial portion of the trachea, with the caudodorsal portion of the pharynx and esophagus removed, dorsal view.

FIG. 9.17. Right half of the larynx and cranial portion of the trachea, with the laryngeal mucosa removed, medial view.

Only two of the six muscles that attach to the arytenoid cartilages will be examined here; all six muscles are innervated by the caudal laryngeal nerve, a branch of the recurrent laryngeal. The CRICOARYTENOIDEUS DORSALIS MUSCLE (1, Fig. 9.16) is located on the dorsal surface of the larynx, ventral to some caudal pharyngeal muscles (2) and the cranial portion of the esophagus. Arising on the dorsal surface of the cricoid cartilage (3) and inserting on the muscular process of the lateral surface of the arytenoid cartilage, it is the only intrinsic laryngeal muscle responsible for enlarging (opening) the space between the vocal folds of each side. The dorsal cricoarytenoid muscle functions by drawing the arytenoid cartilage of each side dorsolaterally. Atrophy of this muscle, which results from damage to a recurrent laryngeal nerve (see pp. 502-5), results in an inability to abduct the vocal folds of the airway.

Another intrinsic muscle is the THYROARYTENOIDEUS MUSCLE, which extends between the median plane of the thyroid cartilage (1, Fig. 9.17), ventrally, and the muscular process of the arytenoid cartilage, dorsally. The VOCALIS MUSCLE (2) is a portion of the thyroarytenoideus that arises from the thyroid cartilage caudal and medial to the remainder of the thyroarytenoideus. The vocalis muscle is adjacent and caudolateral to the VOCAL LIGAMENT (3), which extends between the vocal process of the arytenoid (4), dorsally, and the thyroid cartilage, ventrally. The VOCAL FOLD is the membrane that covers the inner surface of the vocal ligament. Vibrations of the vocal fold (bilaterally), resulting from air rushing past these membranes, produce noise, which is then modulated by the remainder of the larynx, pharynx, nose, and mouth into barking, whimpering, and growling sounds of various tones.

The VESTIBULAR FOLD, or false vocal fold (1, Fig. 9.18), extends from the base of the cuneiform process (2), dorsally, to the cranioventral portion of the thyroid cartilage (3), ventrally. The ADITUS LARYNGIS (4), the opening into the larynx, is formed by the apical margin of the epiglottis, the aryepiglottic fold, and the membrane between the corniculate processes (5). The cavity of the larynx between the aditus laryngis (rostrodorsally) and the vestibular fold (caudally) is the LARYNGEAL VESTIBULE (6). The LARYNGEAL VENTRICLE (7) of each side is a lateral cavity, situated medial to the lamina of the thyroid cartilage, that opens into the larynx between the vestibular and vocal folds (8).

(DIFFERENCES TO BE NOTED IN THE CAT: The vestibular fold is thin and membranous. The feline larynx does not possess a laryngeal ventricle.)

FIG. 9.18. Right half of the larynx and cranial portion of the trachea.

The GLOTTIS is the vocal apparatus and consists of the vocal folds and the opening between the folds; the opening is named the RIMA GLOTTIDIS. The size of the rima glottidis varies with the respiratory cycle, widening during inspiration and narrowing during expiration. By adducting the vocal folds and closing off the rima glottidis during simultaneous contractions of the abdominal muscles, great pressures can be built up within the thoracic, abdominal, and pelvic cavities. These pressures are sufficient to cough up an irritant from the trachea into the mouth, sneeze an irritant out of the nose, force fecal material out the rectum, or aid in propelling a new puppy out into the world of the dog lover.

(The purring of a cat is a complex physiological mechanism present during both inspiratory and expiratory phases of respiration. Some 20-30 contractions per second by intrinsic laryngeal adductor muscles occur during purring. The rima glottidis is thus intermittently closed, periodically increasing then decreasing transglottal pressure. During inspiration in a purring animal, contractions by the thoracic diaphragm are interrupted 20-30 times. Laryngeal and diaphragmatic action potentials alternate. Air flow past the vocal folds produces the purring sound. Cats usually purr in the presence of humans although the sound may not be audible.)

FIG. 10.1. Transverse section through the neck.

FIG. 10.2. Schematic of relative positions of the
trachea and esophagus, dorsal view.

FIG. 10.3. Tracheal segment, left craniolateral view.

10 CAUDAL PORTION

The TRACHEA (1, Fig. 10.1) is situated dorsal to the sternohyoideus (2) and sternothyroideus (3) muscles and ventral to the longus colli muscles (4).

The trachea extends caudally from the cricoid cartilage (at the level of the axis) to the tracheal bifurcation into right and left principal bronchi (at the level of the 4th and 5th thoracic vertebrae). The level of the tracheal bifurcation varies somewhat with the phase of respiration. In the cranial cervical region the trachea (1, Fig. 10.2) is ventral to the esophagus (2); in the midcervical region it is situated to the right of the esophagus; and near the base of the heart it is again situated ventral to the esophagus.

The trachea (Fig. 10.3) consists of an outer wall of TRACHEAL CARTILAGE (1), ANNULAR LIGAMENTS (2), TRACHEALIS MUSCLE (3), and an inner mucous membrane. The U-shaped bands of tracheal cartilage are completed dorsally by the transversely oriented trachealis muscle (3), which is composed of smooth muscle fibers that connect the dorsal free portion of each cartilage band to that of the other side. Contraction of the trachealis muscle results in a constriction of the tracheal lumen (a parasympathetic effect). Annular ligaments encircle the trachea between consecutive tracheal cartilages, attaching adjacent cartilages to each other.

FIG. 10.4. Cranial thoracic aperture, cranial view.

FIG. 10.5. Caudal thoracic aperture, left lateral view.

FIG. 10.6. Thoracic diaphragm, cranial view.

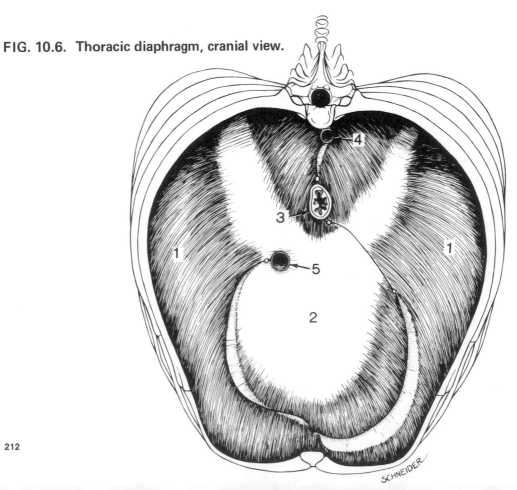

The THORACIC CAVITY is that potential space within the walls of the thorax, cranial to the diaphragm ("potential", because it is compactly filled by visceral structures). The internal layers of the thoracic walls are formed bilaterally by the ribs and intercostal muscles, dorsally by the thoracic vertebrae and intervertebral discs (plus the longus colli muscle in the cranial portion of the dorsal thoracic wall), and ventrally by the sternum and transversus thoracis muscles. The "inlet" and "outlet" of the thoracic cavity are termed the cranial and caudal thoracic apertures, respectively.

The CRANIAL THORACIC APERTURE (Fig. 10.4) is the oval "space" enclosed by the first pair of ribs and their costal cartilages (laterally), the 1st thoracic vertebra and longus colli muscles (dorsally), and the manubrium of the sternum (ventrally). Structures that course through the cranial thoracic aperture include the trachea (1), esophagus (2), right and left vagosympathetic trunks (3), right and left common carotid arteries (4), right and left recurrent laryngeal nerves, right and left phrenic nerves, right and left ventral rami of thoracic spinal nerves 1 and 2, and a number of blood vessels.

The CAUDAL THORACIC APERTURE (Fig. 10.5) is the area within the line formed by the diaphragmatic attachment to the 3rd and 4th lumbar vertebrae (1), costal arch (2), and sternum (3). The THORACIC DIAPHRAGM (Fig. 10.6) which divides the thoracic cavity from the abdominal cavity, is composed of a peripheral muscular portion (1) and a CENTRAL TENDON (2). A dorsal or lumbar part of the muscular portion attaches caudally to the lumbar vertebrae as the RIGHT and LEFT CRURA OF THE DIAPHRAGM. Three openings in the diaphragm through which structures pass between the thoracic and abdominal cavities are the ESOPHAGEAL HIATUS (3), the AORTIC HIATUS (4), and the VENA CAVAL FORAMEN (5). The cranial surface of the dome-shaped diaphragm projects cranially at the end of expiration approximately to the sixth intercostal space. The apex of the dome is within the ventral portion of the thoracic cavity. The diaphragm as the principal muscle of inspiration functions by lengthening the thoracic cavity; however, a paralyzed diaphragm does not critically debilitate an animal.

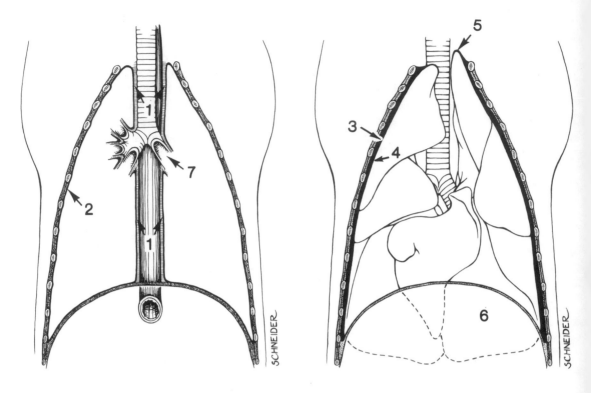

FIG. 10.7. Schematics of the pleural cavities, pleura, mediastinum, and lungs, ventral view.

FIG. 10.8. Tracheal bifurcation, principal and lobar bronchi.

The thoracic cavity is divided into right and left portions by a vertical connective tissue septum, the MEDIASTINUM (me″de-as-ti′num) (1, Fig. 10.7), which extends from the cranial thoracic aperture to the diaphragm at the caudal thoracic aperture. The internal surface of the wall of each portion of the thoracic cavity is lined by a thin, glistening moist membrane, the PARIETAL (wall) PLEURA (2), named according to its location as the DIAPHRAGMATIC, COSTAL, or MEDIASTINAL PLEURA. The pleura is attached to the deep layer of the deep fascia (endothoracic fascia) by subserous fascia (see p. 25). Lobes of the right and left lungs project from the mediastinum out into the right and left portions, respectively, of the thoracic cavity. Each pulmonary lobe is surfaced with a visceral (sing. viscus, pl. viscera) layer (3) of pleura (PULMONARY PLEURA), which is also tightly bound to pulmonary tissue by means of subserous fascia. The pulmonary and parietal pleura are held together by forces of capillary attraction and subatmospheric pressure. The normally nonexistent capillary "space" between pulmonary and parietal pleural layers is the PLEURAL CAVITY (4). When air is permitted to enter a pleural cavity (right or left), the bond is broken between the pleural linings of the thoracic wall and the pulmonary tissue; the lung and thoracic wall separate since each has a tension pulling it in opposite directions. Each lung (right and left) has an apex, a base, and a hilus. The PULMONARY APEX (5) is the cranial portion that extends toward the cranial thoracic aperture; the left lung extends farther cranially in the dog than the right. The PULMONARY BASE (6) is the concave caudal portion of the lung that makes contact with the diaphragmatic parietal pleura. The HILUS (7) is the area of the lung through which vessels, nerves, and lobar bronchi enter the lung.

A ridge of cartilage forms part of the medial wall of the two principal bronchi at their origin (Fig. 10.8). The ridge, or TRACHEAL CARINA (kah-ri′nah; keel) (1), representing the last tracheal cartilage, is often utilized during intubation of the bronchi. The right and left PRINCIPAL BRONCHI (sing. bronchus) (2) are short and have a structure similar to that of the trachea. Each divides into lobar bronchi, which enter the pulmonary tissue. The lobes of the lung are named in various species according to the presence of lobar bronchi, not according to the fissures present on the surface of the lungs. The right lung of the dog has a RIGHT CRANIAL LOBAR BRONCHUS (3), a RIGHT MIDDLE LOBAR BRONCHUS (4), a RIGHT CAUDAL LOBAR BRONCHUS (5), and an ACCESSORY LOBAR BRONCHUS (6). The left lung is supplied by a

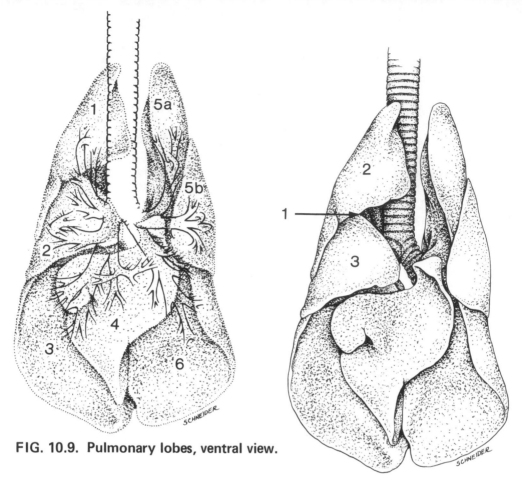

FIG. 10.9. Pulmonary lobes, ventral view.

FIG. 10.10. Pulmonary lobes, ventral view.

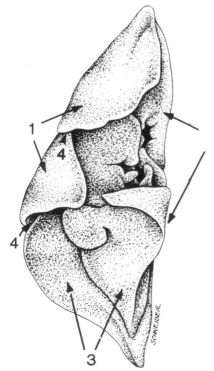

FIG. 10.11. Right lung, ventral view.

FIG. 10.12. Right lung, ventral view.

LEFT CRANIAL LOBAR BRONCHUS (7) and a LEFT CAUDAL LOBAR
BRONCHUS (8).   Each of the lobar bronchi subdivide into
segmental bronchi within the lobes of the lungs.

The lungs are divided by fissures into lobes, each of
which is named according to the lobar bronchus that supplies
it with air (Fig. 10.9). The right lung is larger than the
left. Four lobes are present on the right: RIGHT CRANIAL
(1), RIGHT MIDDLE (2), RIGHT CAUDAL (3), and ACCESSORY (4).
Two fissures are present on the costal surface of the right
lung, one between the cranial and middle lobes (CRANIAL
INTERLOBAR FISSURE) and one between the middle and caudal
lobes (CAUDAL INTERLOBAR FISSURE). One interlobar fissure,
the caudal interlobar fissure, is present in the costal
surface of the left lung dividing it into CRANIAL (5) and
CAUDAL (6) LOBES. The cranial lobe is subdivided by an
intralobar fissure into CRANIAL (5a) and CAUDAL (5b) PARTS.

The PULMONARY CARDIAC NOTCH (1, Fig. 10.10) in the
ventral border of the lungs is more pronounced on the right
side in the dog, where it is a wedge-shaped "space" situated
between the cranial (2) and middle (3) lobes of the lung,
deep to the fourth intercostal space. The heart is
vulnerable to cardiac puncture via the cardiac notch with
relatively little traumatizing of lung tissue. On the left
side, a small cardiac notch is situated between cranial and
caudal parts of the cranial lobe.

Surfaces of the lung are the COSTAL SURFACE (1), MEDIAL
SURFACE (2), DIAPHRAGMATIC SURFACE (3), and INTERLOBAR
SURFACES (4), each of which is self-explanatory (Fig. 10.11).
The diaphragmatic surface is the surface over the base of the
lung.

With the lungs fully expanded, the margins of lung
tissue formed by the ventral junction of costal and medial
surfaces, the VENTRAL MARGIN (1, Fig. 10.12), and the
peripheral portion of the diaphragmatic surface, the BASAL
MARGIN (2), form acute angles. The acutely angled ventral
and basal margins are positioned in recesses formed by the
parietal pleura.

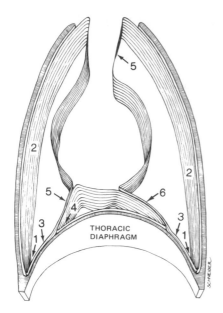

FIG. 10.13. Schematic of the pleural reflections, dorsal view.

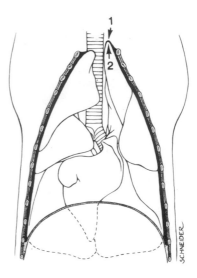

FIG. 10.14. Schematic of the thoracic cavity trachea, and lungs, ventral view.

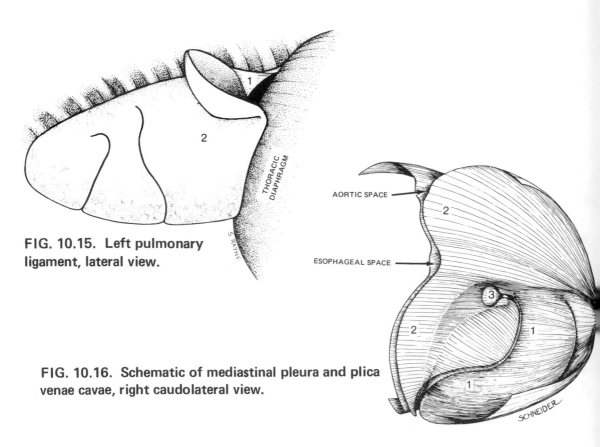

FIG. 10.15. Left pulmonary ligament, lateral view.

FIG. 10.16. Schematic of mediastinal pleura and plica venae cavae, right caudolateral view.

The COSTODIAPHRAGMATIC RECESS (1, Fig. 10.13) is formed by the caudal reflection of costal pleura (2) from the thoracic wall onto the diaphragm as diaphragmatic pleura (3). The costodiaphragmatic recess contains the basal margin of the lung. During inspiratory and expiratory movements the basal border of the lung slides caudally and cranially in contact with the parietal pleura of the costal and diaphragmatic surfaces. A surgical approach cranial to the line of reflection of the costodiaphragmatic recess would enter the pleural cavity; an incision caudal to the line of reflection would enter the peritoneal cavity of the abdomen. The MEDIASTINAL RECESS (4) is the portion of the right pleural cavity, between the caudal mediastinum (5) and the plica venae cavae (6), that contains the accessory lobe of the right lung.

The PLEURAL CUPULA (ku′pu-lah; small cup) (1, Fig. 10.14) is a cup-shaped extension of the pleural cavity of each side that extends cranially through the cranial thoracic aperture. The left pleural cupula extends farther cranially than the right. The apex (2) of each lung (cranial lobe) is situated in contact with the pleural cupula.

The PULMONARY LIGAMENT (1, Fig. 10.15) of each lung is a caudodorsal reflection of the visceral or pulmonary pleura from the caudal lobe (2) to the dorsal portion of the mediastinum. It is a caudally tapering continuation of the pleura that attaches the hilus of the lungs to the mediastinum.

The PLICA (pli′kah; fold) VENAE CAVAE (1, Fig. 10.16) is a reflection of mediastinal pleura to the right and dorsally from the mediastinum (2); the dorsal extent of the plica vena cava forms a sheath around the caudal vena cava (3). The accessory lobe of the right lung is positioned in the space between the plica and the mediastinum; since the caudal mediastinum is deflected to the left, the accesssory lobe appears to be on the left side.

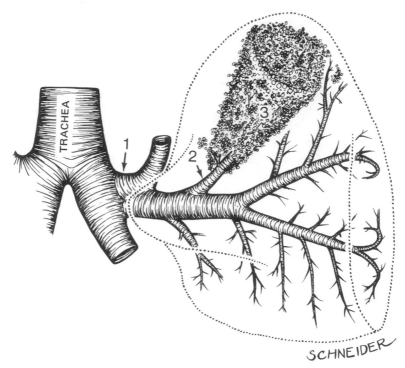

FIG. 10.17. Caudal portion of the left cranial
pulmonary lobe, ventral view.

FIG. 10.18. Schematic of the terminal airways,
alveoli, and their vasculature.

Each lobar bronchus (1, Fig. 10.17) divides into many SEGMENTAL BRONCHI (2) within the lung tissue. Each segmental bronchus and the tissue it supplies with air is a BRONCHOPULMONARY SEGMENT (3), a cone-shaped structure with its apex directed toward the lobar bronchus. Since the dog has relatively little pulmonary connective tissue, adjacent bronchopulmonary segments are not well separated and may evidence collateral ventilation. Within the bronchopulmonary segment, numerous consecutive branches occur, yielding smaller and smaller bronchi, each with less cartilaginous supportive content. Airways smaller than 1 mm in diameter are named BRONCHIOLES (sing. bronchiole). Unlike the larger bronchi, bronchioles do not contain cartilage in their walls; they are completely encircled by smooth muscle.

Pulmonary arteries (1, Fig. 10.18) carry blood toward the GASEOUS EXCHANGE AREA, or PULMONARY ALVEOLI (2), where it is oxygenated. Pulmonary veins (3) return the oxygenated blood to the left atrium for delivery to the body via the left ventricle. The conducting airways are supplied by blood primarily through the bronchial branches (4) of the bronchoesophageal artery (see p. 311). Some shunting of blood occurs between the two arterial systems.

The lung is a vascular filter for large blood-borne particles; particles ranging between 10 and 75 μm are delayed if not retained by the lung capillaries. Physiological emboli such as conglutinated blood cells, fat, bone marrow particles, placental tissue, and tumor cells are often trapped in the lung.

Digestive System

FIG. 11.1. Schematic of the oral cavity, transverse section.

HARD PALATE

TONGUE

SCHNEIDER

FIG. 11.2. Dental arches, inferior and superior.

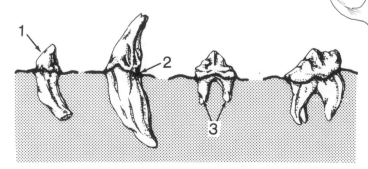

FIG. 11.3. Portions of teeth, lateral view.

11 ROSTRAL PORTION

The digestive system is composed of the digestive tract (mouth, pharynx, and alimentary canal) and associated glands (salivary glands, liver, and pancreas). The alimentary canal consists of the esophagus, stomach, and slender (small) and thick (large) intestines.

The mouth is composed of the oral cavity and surrounding walls: lips, teeth, hard palate, and rostral portion of the tongue.

The ORAL CAVITY (Fig. 11.1) consists of the ORAL VESTIBULE (1) and the ORAL CAVITY PROPER (2). The oral vestibule is the space external to the teeth and gums and internal to the lips and cheeks. The zygomatic and parotid salivary ducts open into the caudodorsal part of the vestibule. The walls of the oral cavity proper are the hard palate, dental arcades, tongue, and adjacent mucosa.

The teeth of the dog are present in two DENTAL ARCHES, SUPERIOR and INFERIOR (Fig. 11.2). Based upon structure, three types of teeth are present in the dog: INCISORS (1), CANINES (2), and CHEEK TEETH. Cheek teeth consist of PREMOLARS (3) and MOLARS (4), which are difficult to differentiate morphologically.

Each tooth (Fig. 11.3) consists of the DENTAL CROWN (1), or free distal portion; the DENTAL NECK (2), a slightly constricted portion at the gum line; and the DENTAL ROOT or ROOTS (3), the embedded portion. From 5 to 50 apical foramina are present in the apex of each dental root; these foramina open into the DENTAL ROOT CANAL, which in turn connects with the DENTAL CAVITY. The large dental cavity and

FIG. 11.4. Brachycephalic skull.

TABLE 11.1. Replacement of deciduous teeth in the dog

Pup teeth	Number	Age at replacement
Incisors	6 maxillary 6 mandibular	3-5 months
Canine	2 maxillary 2 mandibular	5-7 months
Premolar	1st maxillary 1st mandibular	Not replaced
	2nd-4th maxillary 2nd-4th mandibular	5-6 months

FIG. 11.5. Dental alveoli, inferior and superior.

wide root canal of the young tooth are partially and
gradually filled by DENTINE, thus narrowing the lumen. The
shape, position, and number of teeth vary in brachycephalic
dogs with shortened faces (Fig. 11.4).

   The dog, a DIPHYODONT (dif'i-o-dont; grow teeth twice)
animal, has two sets of teeth: deciduous and permanent. The
pup has no teeth during the first 3 weeks of life; in one
half of each dental arch, three incisor, one canine, and
three premolar teeth emerge through the gums between the ages
of 3 and 6 weeks. The deciduous set of teeth does not
contain molars. Thus the dental formula of the pup is 2(Di
3/3; Dc 1/1; Dp 3/3) = 28. The deciduous teeth are replaced
between the ages of 2 to 7 months by the permanent teeth:
three incisors, one canine, and three premolars for each half
of each dental arch (Table 11.1). Permanent teeth develop
along the LINGUAL SURFACE of the roots of deciduous teeth.
The blood supply of the deciduous tooth is reduced by
pressure of the adjacent growing permanent tooth; after a
time the deciduous tooth becomes loosened and is lost. The
BRACHYODONT (brak'e-o-dont"; short tooth), or low-crowned,
teeth are fully developed at the time of eruption through the
gums; only the roots continue to grow, thrusting the crowns
into their final position. Permanent teeth for which no
deciduous forerunners exist include the first premolar of
each arcade, two molars of each half of the superior arcade,
and three molars of each half of the inferior arcade. The
dental formula of the permanent dentition is 2(I 3/3; C 1/1;
P 4/4; M 2/3) = 42. The dog has its complete set of teeth by
8 months of age.

   The permanent incisors, canines, first (most rostral)
premolars of each arcade, and the most caudal inferior molar
(M 3) all have one root each (Fig. 11.5). The root of the
canine tooth is compressed laterally and is too large to be
easily extracted from the alveolus. The 2nd and 3rd
premolars of both arcades plus the 4th inferior premolar and
1st and 2nd inferior molar teeth have two roots each. The
superior 4th premolar is the SECTORIAL (CARNASSIAL) TOOTH,
which shears against the inferior 1st molar (the sectorial
tooth of the mandible). The superior 4th premolar and each
of the maxillary molars (M1 and M2) have three roots. The
relationship of the medial root of maxillary P4 should be
noted in reference to the maxillary recess: an abscess in
the two lateral roots may open through the maxilla and drain
onto the surface of the face; an abscess of the medial root
may drain into the maxillary recess.

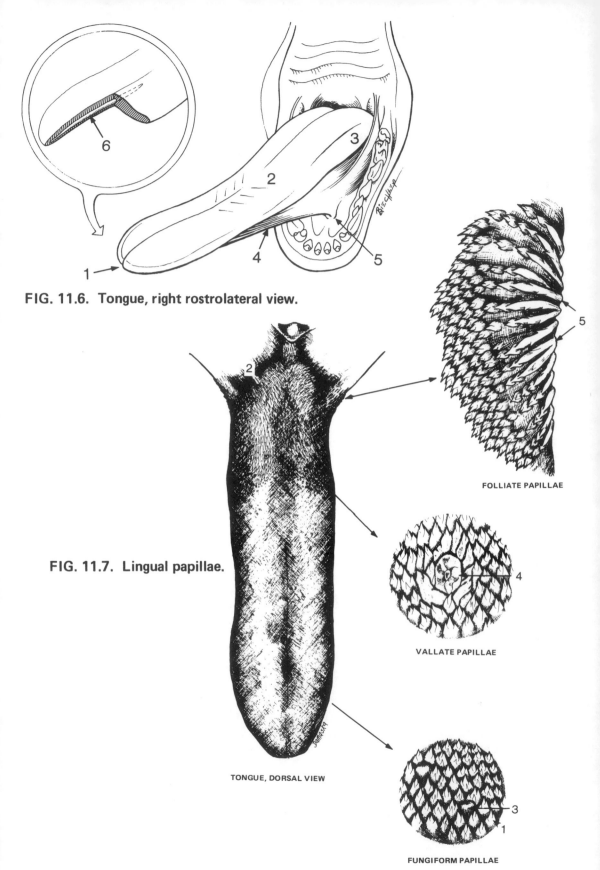

FIG. 11.6. Tongue, right rostrolateral view.

FIG. 11.7. Lingual papillae.

FOLLIATE PAPILLAE

VALLATE PAPILLAE

TONGUE, DORSAL VIEW

FUNGIFORM PAPILLAE

(FELINE DENTAL FORMULAE. Kitten: 2   Di 3/3; Dc 1/1;
Dp 3/2 = 26; adult: 2   I 3/3; C 1/1; P 3/2; M 1/1 = 30.
The premolars are numbered 2-4 in the maxilla and 3 and 4 in
the mandible. Only the superior fourth premolar has three
roots.)

The TONGUE forms much of the ventral surface of the oral
cavity proper and the oropharynx (Fig. 11.6). The tongue is
described as having an APEX (1), a BODY (2), and a ROOT (3).
The LINGUAL FRENULUM (4) is a median fold of mucosa
connecting the free portion of the tongue (ventrally) to the
floor of the oral cavity. The SUBLINGUAL CARUNCLE (5), one
on each side of the ventral portion of the lingual frenulum,
may be observed projecting rostrally; the mandibular and
monostomatic sublingual salivary ducts open into the oral
cavity through the sublingual caruncles. The LYSSA (lis ah)
(6) is a slender, wormlike structure oriented along the
median plane in the apical portion of the tongue.

LINGUAL PAPILLAE of five shapes are on the dorsal
surface of the canine tongue (Fig. 11.7). These structures
are filiform (thread shape), conical (cone shape), fungiform
(mushroom shape), vallate (cup shape), and foliate (leaf
shape). The FILIFORM PAPILLAE, (1) are on the rostrodorsal
two-thirds of the tongue; they do not have taste receptors.
The CONICAL PAPILLAE (2), shaped similarly to the smaller
filiform papillae, are over the caudal portion of the tongue;
they also do not contain taste receptors. The FUNGIFORM
PAPILLAE (3) are primarily on the rostral two-thirds of the
tongue; taste buds are present on the dorsal surface of the
papillae. VALLATE PAPILLAE (4) are four to six large, easily
observable papillae arranged in a V shape on the dorsal
surface of the tongue; the valate papillae demarcate the
junction of the rostral two-thirds and caudal one-third of
the tongue. Taste buds are also present in vallate papillae.
The FOLIATE PAPILLAE (5) are situated on the dorsolateral
margins of the tongue, rostral to the palatoglossal arch;
they also contain taste receptors. Tonsilar tissue is also
present within the dorsal mucosa of the root of the tongue;
however, this lymphatic tissue is not observable grossly.

(DIFFERENCES TO BE NOTED IN THE CAT: The filiform
papillae have elongate, caudally directed spines composed of
KERATIN. Foliate papillae lack taste buds.)

The extrinsic muscles of the tongue which have already
been studied (see p. 137), include the genioglossus,
hyoglossus, and styloglossus

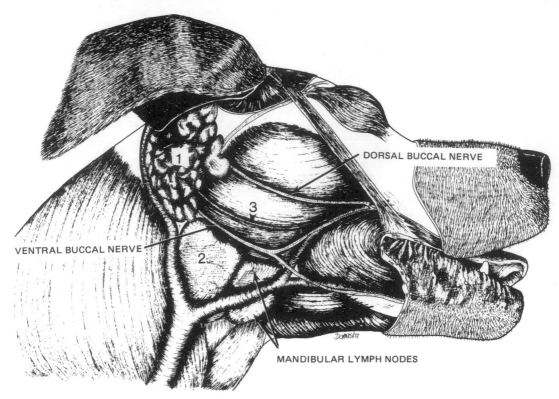

FIG. 11.8. Dog head, with skin and platysma muscle removed, lateral view.

DORSAL BUCCAL NERVE

VENTRAL BUCCAL NERVE

MANDIBULAR LYMPH NODES

FIG. 11.9. Schematic of the positions of salivary glands, right side of the skull.

The salivary glands include the parotid, mandibular, sublingual, zygomatic, and buccal glands. The PAROTID (1, Fig. 11.8) and MANDIBULAR (2) SALIVARY GLANDS are most easily observed. The PAROTID DUCT (3) crosses the surface of the masseter muscle and opens through the lip into the oral vestibule near the caudal surface of P4.

The ZYGOMATIC SALIVARY GLAND (1, Fig. 11.9), present in the orbit ventral to the eye and medial to the zygomatic arch, opens into the oral vestibule opposite the last molar tooth by means of four or five ducts; one major duct opening may be observed caudal to that of the parotid salivary duct. VENTRAL BUCCAL SALIVARY GLANDS (2), inconspicuous in most dogs, are present in the caudal and ventral portions of the cheek, adjacent to buccinator muscle fibers.

The mandibular salivary gland (1, Fig. 11.10) and the major portion of the sublingual salivary gland (2) are contained in a common connective tissue capsule; the ducts of both glands course rostrally between the mandible (laterally) and the tongue muscles (medially), to reach the sublingual caruncles (3). The major portion of the sublingual gland is part of the MONOSTOMATIC (one mouth) SUBLINGUAL SALIVARY GLAND (2). A series of salivary gland lobules (4) are positioned along the MAJOR SUBLINGUAL DUCT and open into the oral cavity proper either through the major duct (monostomatic) or via numerous minor sublingual ducts. These lobules, which have separate ducts opening into the oral cavity, are collectively named the POLYSTOMATIC SUBLINGUAL SALIVARY GLANDS.

(DIFFERENCES TO BE NOTED IN THE CAT: The parotid duct opens opposite the second upper cheek tooth into the oral vestibule. The cat has a MOLAR SALIVARY GLAND in the submucosal fascia of the inferior lip, near the oral commissure.)

FIG. 11.10. Schematic of the positions of the right mandibular and sublingual salivary glands, with dorsal portion of the right mandible removed, lateral view.

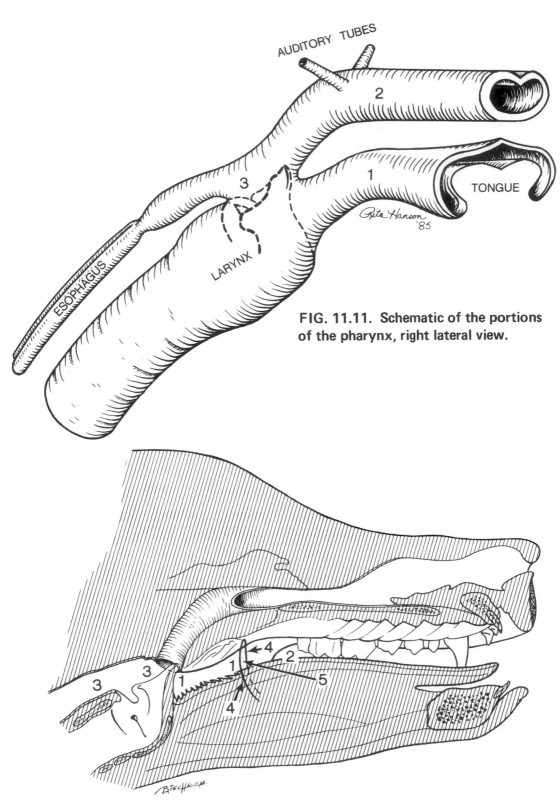

AUDITORY TUBES

TONGUE

ESOPHAGUS

LARYNX

Rita Hanson '85

FIG. 11.11. Schematic of the portions of the pharynx, right lateral view.

FIG. 11.12. Schematic of the pharynx, larynx, trachea, and esophagus as observed in a sagittal section, medial view.

The PHARYNX (Fig. 11.11) is subdivided into oropharynx (1), nasopharynx (2), and laryngopharynx (3) (see pp. 199, 201).

The OROPHARYNX (1, Fig. 11.12) is that portion of the pharynx between the oral cavity proper (2) and the LARYNGOPHARYNX (3). The PALATOGLOSSAL ARCHES (4), or membranous folds, extending between the base of the tongue and the rostral portion of the soft palate (more easily observed by pulling on the tongue), demarcates the caudal boundary of the oral cavity proper. The ISTHMUS (is′mus) FAUCIUM (5), or opening into the pharynx, is the transversely oriented space between the palatoglossal arches. The caudal portion of the oropharynx merges with the laryngopharynx at the level of the epiglottis and caudal border of the soft palate.

A TONSILAR FOSSA (1, Fig. 11.13) containing the PALATINE TONSIL (2) is present in the lateral wall of the oropharynx; the palatine tonsil drains by way of efferent vessels into the more caudally situated medial retropharyngeal lymph node (see p. 397).

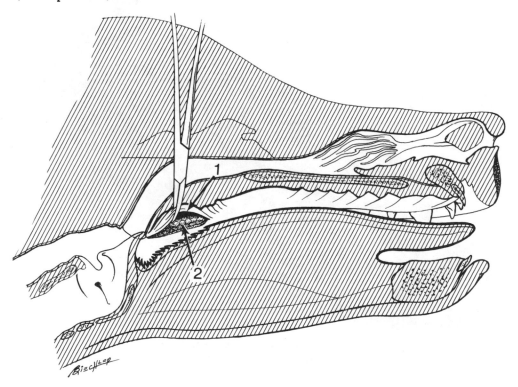

FIG. 11.13. Schematic of the pharynx, larynx, trachea, and esophagus as observed in a sagittal section, medial view.

FIG. 11.14. Left pharyngeal constrictor muscles, ventrolateral view.

STERNOTHYROIDEUS MUSCLE

ESOPHAGUS

THYROID GLAND

STERNOHYOIDEUS MUSCLE

FIG. 11.15. Pharyngoesophageal junction, with right dorsolateral esophageal and pharyngeal walls removed.

Various palatine muscles (which act upon the soft palate) and pharyngeal muscles (which act upon the pharynx) are present in the dog; of these, only three pharyngeal constrictors are described here (Fig. 11.14). The HYOPHARNGEUS (1), THYROPHARYNGEUS (2), and CRICOPHARYNGEUS (3) are paired muscles that arise from the thyrohyoid, thyroid lamina, and cricoid cartilage, respectively. The three muscles insert in series, from rostral to caudal, on the dorsal median raphe of the pharynx.

The caudal portion of the laryngopharynx (1, Fig. 11.15) is situated dorsal to the cricoid cartilage of the larynx. An annular fold of the mucous membrane, the PHARYNGOESOPHAGEAL LIMEN (li'men; boundary) (2), indicates the rostral extent of the esophagus.

Deglutition (swallowing) is a complex act of moving food from the oral cavity to the stomach. Once food enters the oropharynx an involuntary act of swallowing is initiated. The intrapharyngeal ostium is closed by elevation of the soft palate; the root of the tongue is raised against the soft palate; the larynx is drawn rostrodorsally, resulting in the epiglottis being passively hinged caudally; and the esophagus is dilated and drawn rostrally to receive the food. Semiliquid or liquid food passes around each side of the epiglottis and aryepiglottic membranes through the piriform recesses to reach the esophagus. Solid food may be thrown over the dorsal surface of the epiglottis; closure of the vocal folds (reduction of the rima glottidis) is an additional safeguard for the respiratory system.

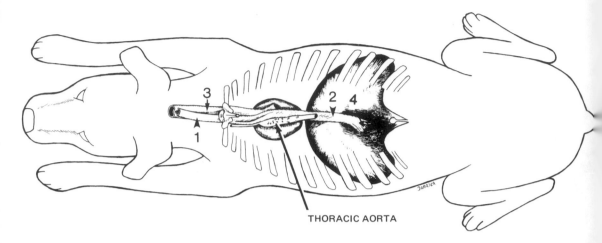

FIG. 12.1. Esophagus, dorsal view.

FIG. 12.2. Schematic of the peritoneum and mesentery.

12 CAUDAL PORTION

The esophagus (Fig. 12.1) is divided into cervical (1), thoracic (2), and abdominal portions. The cervical portion arises from the laryngopharynx at the pharyngoesophageal limen. The cricopharyngeus muscle forms a physiological sphincter (not well enough developed to be regarded as an anatomical sphincter). The cervical portion of the esophagus is at first (cranially) dorsal to the trachea (3) and then is situated to the left of the trachea (at the midcervical region). The esophagus is very close to the median plane in the midthoracic region, where it is situated within the mediastinum (between the right and left pleural cavities) and dorsal to the tracheal bifurcation. After passing through the thoracic diaphragm via the esophageal hiatus (4), a very short segment of esophagus is situated within the abdominal cavity.

The serous membrane that surfaces the wall of the abdominal cavity and the viscera (Fig. 12.2) is termed PARIETAL (1) and VISCERAL (2) PERITONEUM (per"i-to-ne'um, pl. peritonea; stretching around), respectively. The peritoneum provides a moist, slippery surface that facilitates digestive movements and prevents adhesions of viscera to the abdominal wall. Infections of the peritoneal cavity are minimized by the serous membrane (production of a fluid and cellular exudate in response to an infection) and lymphatic tissue (vessels, lymphatic foci, and nodes). Embryologically the parietal peritoneum is connected to visceral peritoneum ventrally by PRIMITIVE VENTRAL MESENTERY (3) and dorsally by PRIMITIVE DORSAL MESENTERY (4). Most of the ventral mesentery is absent in the mature animal; a portion is present between the stomach and liver, between the liver and the ventral median line of the abdominal cavity, and between

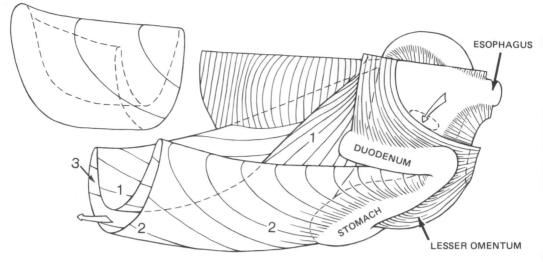

FIG. 12.3. Greater omentum and omental bursa, right lateral view.

FIG. 12.4. Liver, duodenum, pancreas, and epiploic foramen, right lateral view.

the urinary bladder and the ventral median line of the
abdominal wall. The dorsal mesentery is intact in the mature
animal and is named according to the structure it supports,
e.g., mesoduodenum, mesojejunum, mesoileum, mesocolon and
mesorectum.   The mesojejunum and mesoileum are collectively
known as the MESENTERY.   The PERITONEAL CAVITY is the "space"
between parietal and visceral peritonea.   This cavity
normally is only a potential space of microscopic thickness;
the amount of space shown in Figure 12.2 and the dissected
cadaver is very misleading.

The parietal peritoneum is attached superficially by
subserous fascia to the deepest layer of deep fascia, the
transversalis fascia (see p. 25).   Fat is stored in the
subserous fascia. The transversalis fascia is continuous
with the deep fascia of the thoracic cavity (endothoracic
fascia) through the three openings in the thoracic diaphragm
(esophageal hiatus, aortic hiatus, and vena caval foramen)
and through the "spaces" dorsolateral to the diaphragmatic
crura (lumbocostal arch).   Displacement of an abdominal
structure through the esophageal hiatus is termed a HIATAL
HERNIA.

The DORSAL MESOGASTRIUM, or portion of the mesentery
between the dorsal body wall and the stomach, is commonly
known as the GREATER OMENTUM (o-men'tum, pl. omenta; fat
skin) (Fig. 12.3). It arises from the dorsal body wall as a
double layer of serous membranes tightly adhered to each
other by connective tissue (i.e., the dorsal parietal
peritoneum reflects ventrally from the right and left sides
of the abdominal cavity to form the transparent double
serous-layered membrane). A DEEP PART (1) of the greater
omentum descends caudally to near the urinary bladder, then
reflects or loops cranioventrally as the SUPERFICIAL PART
(2); the "space" situated between the deep and superficial
parts of the folded sheetlike greater omentum is the OMENTAL
BURSA (3). Thus the greater omentum extends caudally as a
folded sheet between the intestines and the ventral abdominal
wall and between the intestines (craniodorsally) and the
urinary bladder (caudoventrally). The superficial portion of
the greater omentum attaches cranially to the greater
curvature of the stomach. The spleen and the left lobe of the
pancreas are within and supported by the greater omentum.
The spleen is in contact with the left abdominal wall. The
omental bursa is an extensive "space" that opens into the
greater peritoneal sac through the OMENTAL (EPIPLOIC) (ep"i-
plo'ik) FORAMEN (1, Fig. 12.4); the omental foramen is a
small, cleft like opening situated between the caudal vena

FIG. 12.5. Stomach, cranial view.

FIG. 12.6. Stomach in situ, caudal view.

FIG. 12.7. Stomach, with a portion of the parietal surface removed, cranial view.

cava (dorsally) and the complex of common bile duct, hepatic portal vein, and gastroduodenal artery (ventrally).

The STOMACH (Fig. 12.5), the largest dilatation of the alimentary canal, extends from the esophagus to the small intestine. The four parts of the stomach are the cardiac portion, fundus, body, pyloric portion, and pylorus. The CARDIAC (car'de-ak; relating to heart) PORTION (1), which arises from the esophagus, is the part that contains the pacemaker cells; these cells establish the inherent contractions of the stomach, the rhythm of which is modified by the autonomic and endocrine systems. The GASTRIC FUNDUS (2), a dome-shaped diverticulum adjacent and dorsal to the cardiac portion, is positioned dorsally on the left side of the abdominal region in serous contact with the diaphragm. The gastric fundus is apparent in radiographs since it is usually filled with air. The BODY (3) of the stomach is that portion between the fundus and pyloric portion. The PYLORIC PORTION (4) of the stomach is usually partly separated from the body by the ANGULAR INCISURE (5). The PYLORUS (pi-lo' rus; gate) (6) is the caudal portion of the stomach from which the small intestine originates.

The stomach has a GREATER CURVATURE (1, Fig. 12.6), which makes contact with the diaphragm dorsally, left-laterally, and ventrally. The LESSER CURVATURE (2) and the greater curvature of the stomach form nearly concentric arcs. The surface of the stomach directed dorsocranially toward the liver is the PARIETAL SURFACE. The VISCERAL SURFACE (3) is directed caudoventrally toward the intestines. When empty, the stomach is situated within the rib cage (cranial to the osseous caudal thoracic aperture); however, when full, the stomach distends and occupies the abdominal cavity as far caudally as the transverse level of the umbilicus.

Both the cardiac portion and pylorus of the stomach are structurally modified to regulate the passage of ingested matter. In the cardiac portion a circular layer of smooth muscle forms the CARDIAC SPHINCTER (Fig. 12.7), which anatomically is a weakly developed structure (physiologically it may effectively constrict the esophagealgastric junction). The opening from the esophagus through the cardiac sphincter is the CARDIAC OSTIUM (1). The pyloric portion is composed of the pyloric antrum and pyloric canal. The PYLORIC ANTRUM (2) is a slightly dilated region distal to the angular incisure of the stomach. The PYLORIC CANAL (3) is the caudal narrow part of the pyloric portion leading from the antrum to the pylorus. The pylorus contains a strong, well developed

FIG. 12.8. Stomach, duodenum, pancreas, and colon, dorsal view.

band of circular smooth muscle, the PYLORIC SPHINCTER; the PYLORIC OSTIUM (4) is the opening within the sphincter that connects the lumen of the pyloric canal with that of the cranial portion of the small intestine. Folds or wrinkles present over much of the internal surface of the stomach are named GASTRIC RUGAE (sing. ruga; fold) (5).

The DUODENUM (du″o-de′num or du-od′e-num) (Fig. 12.8), the first portion of the small intestine, is composed of a cranial, descending, and ascending portions. The CRANIAL PORTION (1) is the initial part of the duodenum situated between the pylorus and the cranial bend of the duodenum (this portion is often confused with the pylorus). The CRANIAL DUODENAL FLEXURE (2) is the bend in the duodenum that occurs near the level of the 9th and 10th ribs on the right side. The cranial portion of the duodenum and cranial duodenal flexure are relatively fixed in position by strong attachments to the liver. The DESCENDING PORTION (3) of the duodenum extends from the cranial duodenal flexure along the right side of the abdominal cavity to the level of the tuber coxae. The CAUDAL DUODENAL FLEXURE (4) is the bend of the duodenum between descending and ascending portions; this flexure is positioned near the right tuber coxae. The ASCENDING PORTION (5) of the duodenum extends from the caudal duodenal flexure across the median plane to an ill-defined DUODENOJEJUNAL FLEXURE.

The portion of the dorsal mesentery attached to the duodenum is termed the MESODUODENUM (6, Fig. 12.8). The portion of the mesoduodenum that attaches the descending duodenum to the dorsal body wall also contains and supports the RIGHT LOBE OF THE PANCREAS (7). The mesoduodenum of the ascending duodenum is attached to the mesocolon of the descending colon; this mesenteric attachment is called the DUODENOCOLIC FOLD (8).

FIG. 12.9. Caudal surface of the liver, parietal surface
of the stomach, and the lesser omentum.

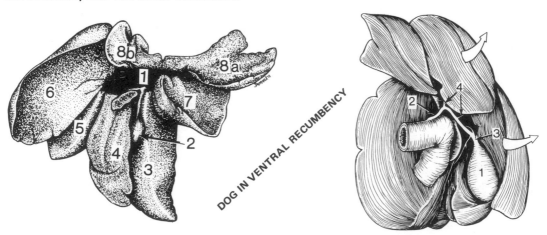

FIG. 12.10. Liver, caudal view.

FIG. 12.11. Liver, gall bladder, and biliary ducts,
right caudolateral view.

The LESSER OMENTUM (Fig. 12.9) connects the lesser curvature of the stomach and the cranial portion of the duodenum to the PORTA (entrance) OF THE LIVER (1). The portion of lesser omentum spanning the distance from stomach to liver is named the HEPATOGASTRIC LIGAMENT (2). The HEPATODUODENAL LIGAMENT (3) is the portion of lesser omentum between the liver and the cranial portion of the duodenum. The hepatoduodenal ligament is fused with the cranial portion of the mesoduodenum.

In young dogs the FALCIFORM HEPATIC LIGAMENT extends in the median plane from the liver to the ventral abdominal wall; in older dogs the falciform ligament may be observed as a fatty remnant on the deep surface of the abdominal wall in the umbilical region. The ROUND LIGAMENT OF THE LIVER, observed in some young dogs as an atrophied remnant of the umbilical vein along the caudodorsal edge of the falciform ligament, extends from the fatty tissue near the umbilicus toward the porta of the liver. A portion of the diaphragmatic surface of the liver is fused by connective tissue to the diaphragm. The CORONARY (crown) HEPATIC LIGAMENT is formed by a circular reflection of visceral peritoneum away from the liver mass onto the diaphragm as parietal peritoneum. Right and left lateral extensions (TRIANGULAR LIGAMENTS) of the coronary hepatic ligament are present as folds of mesentery.

From the porta of the liver (1, Fig. 12.10), ventrally and laterally, the liver is divided by deep fissures into lobes. Six lobes are present in the liver of the dog. The GALL BLADDER (2) is in a fossa between the RIGHT MEDIAL LOBE (3) and the QUADRATE LOBE (4). The LEFT MEDIAL LOBE (5) is in contact with the left surface of the quadrate lobe; the LEFT LATERAL LOBE (6) is the lobe situated farthest to the left. The RIGHT LATERAL LOBE (7) is positioned to the right of the right medial lobe. The sixth lobe is the CAUDATE LOBE (8), which is positioned dorsally on the right side. Two processes of the caudate lobe should be observed: the CAUDATE PROCESS (8a) is in contact with the right kidney, and the PAPILLARY PROCESS (8b) is in contact with the lesser curvature of the stomach.

The gall bladder (1, Fig. 12.11) is connected to the BILE DUCT (2) by the CYSTIC (bladder) DUCT (3). Ducts that conduct bile from the liver, where it is formed, are named HEPATIC DUCTS (4). The hepatic ducts combine to form a COMMON HEPATIC DUCT. The bile duct is formed by the combination of the common hepatic and cystic ducts. In the

FIG. 12.12. Stomach, duodenum, and pancreas, dorsal view.

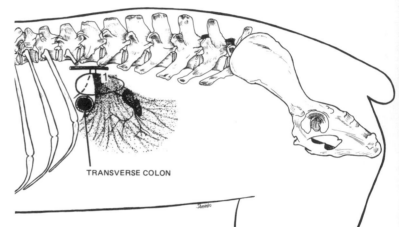

TRANSVERSE COLON

FIG. 12.13. Schematic of the root of the mesentery, left lateral view.

FIG. 12.14. Ileocolic and cecocolic junctions, ventral view.

dog some small ducts (HEPATOCYSTIC DUCTS) pass from the liver directly to the gall bladder. Much of the bile formed in the liver passes through the hepatic ducts and then up the cystic duct to the gall bladder for storage. When needed in the duodenum, bile is forced out of the gall bladder through the cystic duct and down the bile duct to the duodenum. The bile duct passes through the hepatoduodenal ligament to reach the cranial portion of the descending duodenum. After passing obliquely through the right dorsolateral wall of the duodenum, the bile duct discharges bile through the MAJOR DUODENAL PAPILLA, which is partially obscured by the mucosal surface.

The right lobe of the pancreas (1, Fig. 12.12) has already been observed in the mesoduodenum of the descending duodenum. The BODY OF THE PANCREAS (2) is the portion near the cranial duodenal flexure. The LEFT LOBE OF THE PANCREAS (3) is positioned in a deep portion of the greater omentum. The PANCREATIC DUCTS (4) interconnect within the pancreatic tissue. Pancreatic juice is usually carried into the cranial portion of the descending duodenum by means of two ducts: one duct opens into the duodenum through the major duodenal papilla with the bile duct, the other (a larger duct) opens into the duodenum through the mucosa 1-4 inches caudal to the major papilla.

The SLENDER (small) INTESTINE is composed of DUODENUM, JEJUNUM, and ILEUM. The jejunum and ileum, which are situated dorsal to the greater omentum in the caudoventral portion of the abdominal cavity, are difficult to differentiate. Both the jejunum and ileum are supported by mesentery, which allows them considerable movement. The mesenteries gather toward one area of attachment (dorsally) near the level of the 2nd lumbar vertebra (Fig. 12.13); this narrow area of attachment is the ROOT OF THE MESENTERY (1) through which the proximal portion of the cranial mesenteric artery passes.

The terminal portion of the ileum and the first part of the large intestine (ascending colon and cecum) are on the right dorsal side of the body (Fig. 12.14). The lumen of the ileum (1) is continuous with that of the ascending colon (2) through the ILEAL OSTIUM (3). The circular layer of smooth muscle around the ileal orifice forms the ILEAL SPHINCTER MUSCLE (4). The CECUM (5) is a blind-ending diverticulum off the first portion of the ascending colon. The lumen of the cecum is continuous with that of the colon through the CECOCOLIC OSTIUM (6); the CECAL SPHINCTER MUSCLE (7)

FIG. 12.15. Large intestine, dorsal view.

encircles the cecocolic orifice. LYMPH NODULES (8), which occur in the wall of much of the intestine, are quite noticeable in the gas-filled cecum of the dead animal.

(TO BE NOTED IN THE CAT: The cecum of the cat is a short, comma-shaped structure.)

The THICK (large) INTESTINE is composed of colon, cecum, rectum, and anal canal (Fig. 12.15). The short ASCENDING COLON (1) passes cranially in the right dorsal portion of the abdominal cavity to a transverse level near the root of the mesentery (2). A bend, the RIGHT COLIC FLEXURE (3), marks the junction of the ascending and transverse colons. The TRANSVERSE COLON (4) is transversely oriented across the dorsal portion of the abdominal cavity cranial to the root of the mesentery. On the left side, the LEFT COLIC FLEXURE (5) occurs dorsally between the transverse and descending portions of the colon. As the DESCENDING COLON (6) enters the pelvic canal it is named the RECTUM (7).

The ANAL CANAL (1, Fig. 12.16) is the short terminal part of the large intestine extending from the rectum (2) to the ANUS (3). It is surrounded by sphincter muscles: the EXTERNAL (4) and INTERNAL ANAL SPHINCTERS. The internal anal sphincter is composed of smooth muscle continuous with the smooth muscle of the rectum. The external anal sphincter is composed of striated (voluntary) muscle that encircles collectively the anal canal and the PARANAL SINUSES (5) of both sides (see p. 17).

COCCYGEUS MUSCLE →

RECTOCOCCYGEUS MUSCLE

LEVATOR ANI MUSCLE

FIG. 12.16. Caudal portion of the alimentary canal, left lateral view with part of the wall incised to reveal the mucosa.

FIG. 12.17. Pelvic girdle, deep muscles of the coxal articulation, and pelvic diaphragm, dorsal view.

RECTOCOCCYGEUS MUSCLE

FIG. 12.18. Pelvic girdle, tail muscles, and muscles in the ischiorectal fossa, caudolateral view.

The PELVIC DIAPHRAGM (Figs. 12.17, 12.18) is an important muscular and fascial structure in the caudal portion of the pelvic canal. Prolapse of pelvic viscera and perianal hernias are normally prevented, in part, by the presence of a strong pelvic diaphragm. The pelvic diaphragm also has an important role in terminating the act of defecation. The two striated muscles constituting the muscular portion of the pelvic diaphragm, the LEVATOR ANI (1) and COCCYGEUS (kok-sij'e-us) (2), may be located by cleaning fat out of the ISCHIORECTAL FOSSA (see p. 143). The levator ani is a broad, flat muscle that arises from the ventral floor and lateral wall of the pelvic cavity and inserts on the 4th to 7th caudal vertebrae. The coccygeus is a shorter, stronger muscle that arises from the ischiatic spine and inserts on the 2nd to 4th caudal vertebrae; thus the thicker coccygeus is lateral and slightly cranial to the dorsal portion of the levator ani muscle.

A third muscle associated with the caudal portion of the rectum/anus is the RECTOCOCCYGEUS MUSCLE (1, Fig. 12.19). As a caudal continuation of the outer smooth muscle of the rectum, it passes caudodorsally from the dorsal surface of the rectum to insert on the ventral surface of the caudal vertebrae.

FIG. 12.19. Rectum, anal canal, and paranal sinuses, dorsal view.

Urogenital System

FIG. 13.1. Schematic of the urinary system, dorsal view.

FIG. 13.2. Shape and position of the kidneys.

FIG. 13.3. Schematic of the kidney depicting the ureter, renal pelvis, renal diverticulae, and renal sinus.

13 FEMALE

The urinary system (Fig. 13.1) consists of the kidneys (1), ureters (2), urinary bladder (3), and urethra (4). The right kidney is ventrolateral to the 1st through 3rd lumbar vertebrae; the position of the left kidney, more variable than the right, is ventrolateral to the 2nd through 4th lumbar vertebrae. The URETERS are slender, muscular tubes that course caudally from the medial surface of the kidney to the dorsolateral surface of the urinary bladder. They are situated in the dorsal subserous fascia of the abdominal cavity, to each side of the major vessels (the ABDOMINAL AORTA and CAUDAL VENA CAVA).

(DIFFERENCE TO BE NOTED IN THE CAT: Right and left kidneys are approximately at the same level, L_2 through L_4.)

The KIDNEY is a bean-shaped structure with a convex lateral margin and a concave medial margin (Fig. 13.2). Since the parietal peritoneum covers its ventral but not its dorsal surface, the kidney is described as being retroperitoneal; one may remove a retroperitoneal kidney through a dorsolateral abdominal incision without incising the peritoneum (i.e., one does not need to enter the peritoneal cavity). The left kidney is less firmly attached to the dorsal body wall than is the right and is thus more mobile.

A depression, or RENAL HILUS (1, Fig. 13.3), is in the center of the concave medial margin through which vessels and nerves pass to and from the kidney. The hilus leads into a fat-filled cavity, the RENAL SINUS (2), which contains fat, blood vessels, and the expanded urine-receiving portion of the ureter (RENAL PELVIS). A fibrous RENAL CAPSULE (3) covers the surface of the kidney.

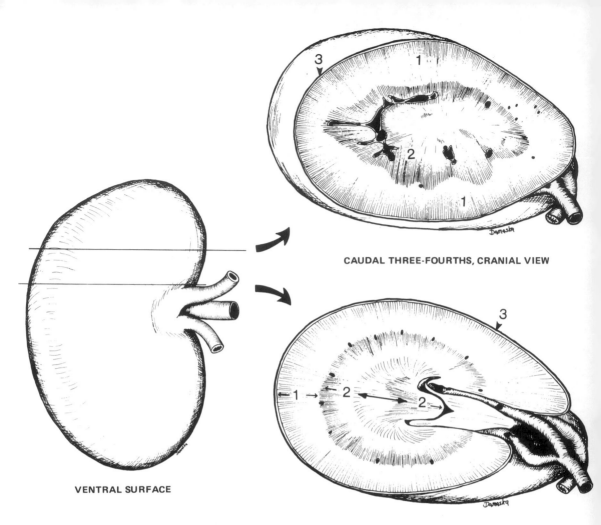

VENTRAL SURFACE

CAUDAL THREE-FOURTHS, CRANIAL VIEW

CAUDAL TWO-THIRDS, CRANIAL VIEW

FIG. 13.4. Right kidney.

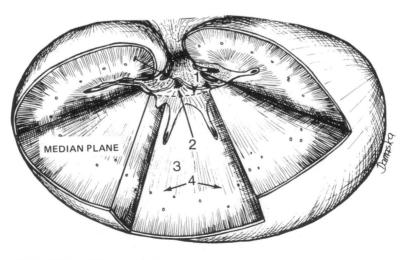

MEDIAN PLANE

FIG. 13.5. Kidney, with a portion of the renal cortex and medulla removed.

The kidney (Fig. 13.4) is composed of two major portions, the RENAL CORTEX (1) and the RENAL MEDULLA (2), both of which are grossly distinguishable. The renal cortex is a reddish brown, granular, superficial layer of the kidney situated between the renal capsule (3) and the renal medulla. It is within the renal cortex that blood under high pressure escapes as a filtrate from capillary tufts; the filtrate enters tiny tubules to be concentrated and carried toward the ureter as urine. The renal medulla is the light-colored, finely striated deeper portion of the kidney. The striations are due to the presence of many collecting ducts that convey urine toward the renal hilus.

If a kidney is sectioned through its median plane (Fig. 13.5), a rather simple renal medulla will be observed, which has a linear RENAL CREST (1) projecting into the renal pelvis (2). Urine drips out into the renal pelvis from duct orifices in the CRIBRIFORM (krib'ri-form; forms a sieve) AREA of the renal crest. Since the dog kidney is composed of a number of fused lobes, a sagittal section through the kidney yields an entirely different view of the medullary structure. The fusion of renal lobes is so complete that lobation is not grossly apparent either externally or in the cortex. The medulla (3) of each lobe (in a unilobate mammalian kidney or embryologically) is shaped like a pyramid, with its base (4) against the cortex and the apex, or RENAL PAPILLA, projecting into the renal pelvis. The renal papillae are fused in the dog, forming a median renal crest; however, to each side of the median plane the medulla of each lobe appears to be separate when observed in a sagittal section.

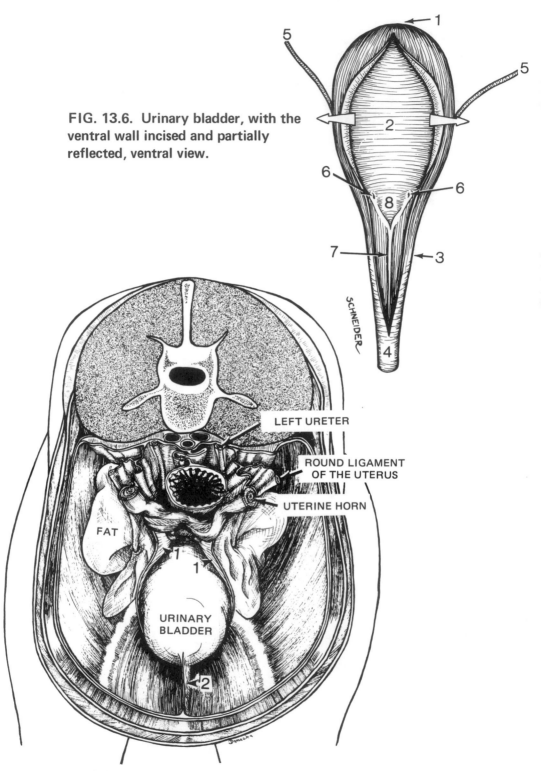

FIG. 13.6. Urinary bladder, with the ventral wall incised and partially reflected, ventral view.

SCHNEIDER

LEFT URETER

ROUND LIGAMENT OF THE UTERUS

UTERINE HORN

FAT

URINARY BLADDER

FIG. 13.7. Pelvic cavity of the bitch, cranial view.

The URINARY BLADDER (Fig. 13.6) is a highly distendable urine storage organ; it is situated within the pelvic cavity when empty and in the abdominal cavity when full. The regions of the urinary bladder are the APEX (1), BODY (2), and NECK (3). The body is the main portion of the urinary bladder; irregular bands, resulting from smooth muscle fibers deep to the surface, may be observed grossly in the walls. The neck of the urinary bladder is continuous with the URETHRA (4). The ureters (5) enter the dorsolateral surface of the urinary bladder near the neck. Because the ureters pass obliquely through the wall of the urinary bladder, the smooth muscle of the bladder acts upon them as a physiological sphincter. The URETERIC OSTIA (6) each open through a ridge on the dorsal internal surface of the urinary bladder; both of these ridges converge distally to form a dorsal ridge in the urethra, the URETHRAL CREST (7). The TRIGONE (tri'gon; triangular) OF THE BLADDER (8) is the area between the converging ridges of tissue.

The urinary bladder is supported by two LATERAL LIGAMENTS (1, Fig. 13.7) and one ventral MEDIAN LIGAMENT (2). The median ligament represents a caudal remnant of the ventral mesentery. The URACHUS (u'rah-kus), a vestige of the fetal allantoic stalk, is present in the median ligament; if it remains patent (open) in the newborn pup, urine may pass from the urinary bladder out through the umbilicus.

The urethra (1, Fig. 13.8) conducts urine from the urinary bladder (2) to the VAGINA (3). Smooth muscle of the urinary bladder extends into the urethra, forming a functional (not an anatomical) sphincter. Skeletal muscle, the URETHRALIS, is present in the urethral wall and forms a sphincter that is under voluntary control. The EXTERNAL URETHRAL ORIFICE (4) is the opening between the urethra and the vagina.

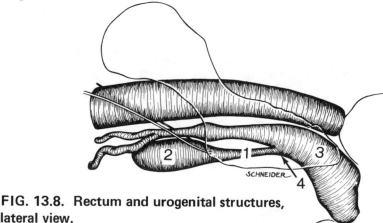

FIG. 13.8. Rectum and urogenital structures, lateral view.

FIG. 13.9. Vulva, caudal view.

FIG. 13.10. Urogenital tract of the bitch, dorsal view.

FIG. 13.11. Vulva, pudendal labia retracted.

FIG. 13.12. Pelvic viscera, with the left wall removed from the uterine cervix and vagina, left lateral view.

The external genital structure of the bitch is the VULVA (Fig. 13.9), which consists of the PUDENDAL (ashamed) LABIA (1) and the vulvar cleft, or RIMA PUDENDI (2). The rima pudendi is the opening common to both urinary and genital systems. The DORSAL (3) and VENTRAL (4) LABIAL COMMISSURES are the fusion lines of the labia, dorsal and ventral to the rima pudendi, respectively.

An incision (episiotomy) (e-piz"e-ot'o-me; cutting the vulva) through the dorsal commissure reveals the VESTIBULE OF THE VAGINA (Fig. 13.10), which extends from the rima pudendi to the URETHRAL TUBERCLE (1). A fossa in the ventral surface of the caudal portion of the vestibule is the FOSSA CLITORIDIS (2). The GLANS OF THE CLITORIS (3) projects caudodorsally into the fossa; the clitoris, consisting of CRURA, BODY and GLANS, is homologous to the penis of the male (see p. 279). The body and crura of the clitoris are within the wall of the vaginal vestibule. The urethral tubercle projects (slightly in nulliparous animals) into the vagina from the cranioventral surface of the vestibule; the external urethral orifice (4) opens into the vestibule through or under the urethral tubercle. The vagina (5) extends cranially for a considerable distance; longitudinal and transverse folds (RUGAE) in the vagina allow for its expansion. The caudal portion of the uterus may be felt as a hard, muscular UTERINE CERVIX (6). The UTERUS is composed of uterine cervix, UTERINE BODY (7), and RIGHT and LEFT UTERINE HORNS (8). An INTERCORNUAL LIGAMENT (9) connects the two cornua near their junction with the uterine body.

When catheterizing the urethra of a bitch, one needs to ensure that the catheter does not enter the blind-ending fossa clitoridis (1, Fig. 13.11).

A longitudinal slit in the lateral surface of the vagina reveals the FORNIX OF THE VAGINA (1, Fig. 13.12), a space in the vagina cranioventral to the intravaginal portion of the cervix. The small passage through the uterine cervix (2) is the UTERINE CERVICAL CANAL; the cranial and caudal openings into the cervical canal are named INTERNAL (3) and EXTERNAL (4) UTERINE OSTIA (sing. ostium; opening). The external uterine ostium is oriented caudoventrally. A muscular ridge extends caudally from the cervix along the dorsal wall of the vagina, protruding ventrally into the vaginal lumen.

FIG. 13.13. Muscles of the female perineal region and pelvic diaphragm, right caudolateral view.

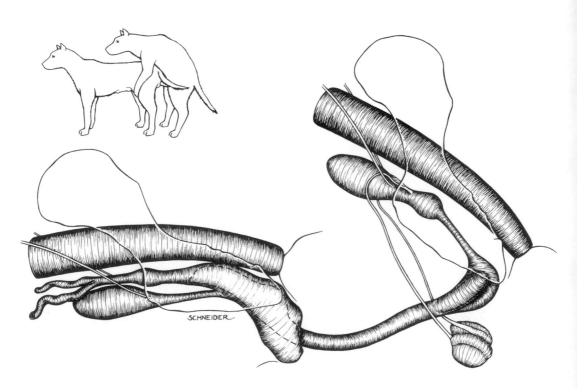

FIG. 13.14. Schematic of the initial phase of coitus, left lateral view.

Two muscles of considerable importance in the bitch (Fig. 13.13) are the CONSTRICTOR VESTIBULI (1) and CONSTRICTOR VULVAE (2). These striated muscles that encircle the vestibule and vulva comprise the BULBOSPONGIOSUS MUSCLE.

Constriction of the penile veins by the constrictors vulvae and vestibuli enhances erection in the dog. The enlarged distal portion of the penis (glans) in turn supports vascular engorgement of the female genital structures. The glans of the penis is intravaginal during coitus (Fig. 13.14). Ejaculation of sperm occurs within the first minute of coitus. Approximately 1 minute after intromission the male turns 180 degrees (Fig. 13.15) and remains "locked" from 5 to 45 minutes. During this time interval a voluminous sperm-free seminal fluid is ejaculated. The penis displaces the vagina dorsolaterally, with the rectum displaced to the opposite side. The uterine cervix is displaced as far cranially as the lumbosacral articulation.

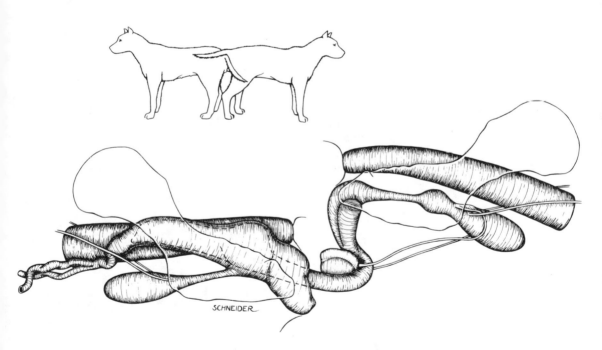

FIG. 13.15. "Locking" phase of coitus, lateral view.

FIG. 13.16. Right ovarian bursa and uterine tube.

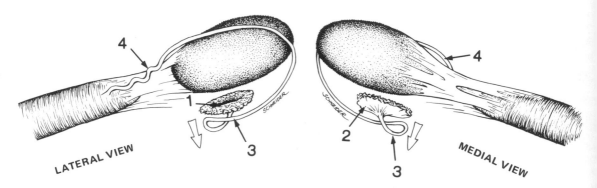

FIG. 13.17. Schematic of the right ovary, uterine tube, and initial segment of the uterine horn.

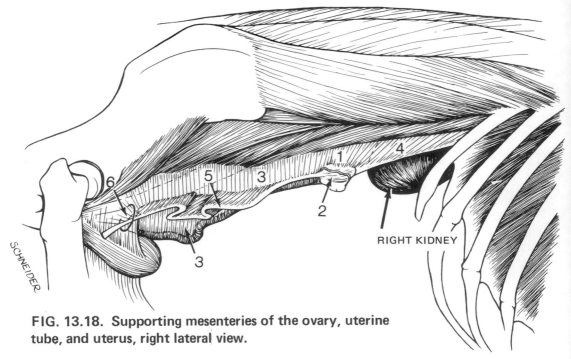

FIG. 13.18. Supporting mesenteries of the ovary, uterine tube, and uterus, right lateral view.

The cranial portion of the female reproductive system is difficult to visualize because of its small size and the serous membranous sac that surrounds the ovary (Fig. 13.16). The OVARIAN BURSA is a peritoneal space that contains the OVARY. A small slitlike opening (1) through the medial surface of the membranous sac connects the peritoneal cavity with the bursa. The UTERINE TUBE (2) of each side winds around within the wall of the membranous sac and merges caudally with the cranial extent of the uterine horn (3). The INFUNDIBULUM OF THE UTERINE TUBE is a funnel-shaped dilatation that opens into the ovarian bursa near the slit between bursa and peritoneal cavity. TUBAL FIMBRIAE (sing. frimbia; fringe) are extremely small fingerlike processes on the free edge of the infundibulum that partially protrude from the bursa into the peritoneal cavity.

The ABDOMINAL OSTIUM OF THE UTERINE TUBE (1, Fig. 13.17) is the opening of the ovarian end of the uterine tube into the infundibulum (2). Although grossly nondiscernible, a relatively wide initial segment is the AMPULLA (pl. ampullae; jug) OF THE UTERINE TUBE (3). The narrow portion between the ampulla and the uterine horn is the ISTHMUS OF THE UTERINE TUBE (4). Fertilization of the ovum occurs within the uterine tube.

The mesentery or peritoneal folds supporting the abdominal and pelvic portions of the female reproductive tract are fairly complex (Fig. 13.18). The MESOVARIUM (1) supports the ovary from the abdominal wall; the ovarian vessels pass from the dorsal abdominal vessels in the mesovarium to reach the hilus of the ovary. The MESOSALPINX (mes″o-sal′pinks) (2) is a fold of tissue arising from the lateral surface of the mesovarium; the uterine tube is contained within the mesosalpinx. The MESOMETRIUM (3) is a supporting mesentery, containing smooth muscle, that attaches the uterine horn and body to the abdominal wall. The BROAD LIGAMENT OF THE UTERUS, composed of the mesovarium, mesosalpinx, and mesometrium, allows considerable movement of the uterus. The ovaries, which are located near the 3rd and 4th lumbar vertebral levels, are also attached cranially to the transversalis fascia of the dorsolateral abdominal wall and thoracic diaphragm by the SUSPENSORY LIGAMENT OF THE OVARY (4). This ligament limits movement of the ovaries within the abdominal cavity. The suspensory ligament is continuous caudally with the mesovarium. The caudal extremity of the ovary is attached by the PROPER LIGAMENT OF THE OVARY to the cranial tip of the uterine horn. The ROUND LIGAMENT OF THE UTERUS (5) is a lateral fold from the

FIG. 13.19. Pelvic cavity, with the left os coxae removed, left lateral view.

RECTUM

FIG. 13.20. Caudal extension of the pelvic cavity, left view.

mesometrium; it passes through the INGUINAL CANAL (6), connecting the cranial tip of the uterine horn to the superficial fascia of the vulvar area.

The PELVIC CAVITY (Fig. 13.19) extends between the CRANIAL and CAUDAL PELVIC APERTURES. The peritoneal membranes and space are continuous from the abdominal cavity into the pelvic cavity. The cranial pelvic aperture is an osseous opening formed dorsally by the sacral promontory (1), ventrally by the cranial border of the pubic bones (2), and laterally by the arcuate lines (3). The caudal pelvic aperture is an opening formed dorsally by the 1st caudal vertebra (4), ventrally by the ischiatic arch (5), and laterally by the sacrotuberous ligaments (6) and superficial gluteal muscles.

Ventrally, the parietal peritoneum extends into the pelvic cavity for a very short distance before reflecting dorsally onto the neck of the urinary bladder (Figs. 13.20, 13.21). The peritoneal recesses formed by reflections of the parietal peritoneum onto the various pelvic viscera are termed excavations. Two ventral recesses, one on each side of the median ligament of the bladder, between the ventral wall of the pelvic cavity and the urinary bladder are the PUBOVESICULAR EXCAVATIONS (1). The VESICOGENITAL EXCAVATION (2) is the space formed by the reflection of visceral peritoneum from the dorsal surface of the urethra onto the ventral surface of the vagina. A dorsal reflection from the dorsal surface of the vagina onto the ventral surface of the rectum forms a space know as the RECTOGENITAL EXCAVATION (3). The portions of the rectogenital excavation situated dorsolateral to the rectum are termed the right and left PARARECTAL FOSSAE (4). In terms of craniocaudal orientation, the rectogenital excavation is more caudal than the vesicogenital excavation, which in turn is more caudal than the pubovesicular excavation.

FIG. 13.21. Schematic of the pelvic peritoneal recesses as observed in transverse section.

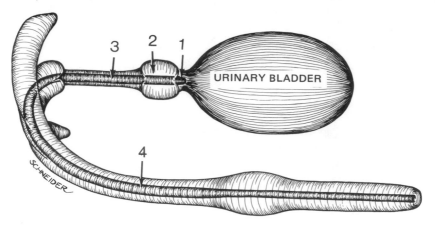

FIG. 14.1. Schematic of the urinary bladder, prostate gland, urethra, and erectile portion of the penis, right ventrolateral view.

FIG. 14.2. Schematic of the male genital organs, right caudolateral view.

FIG. 14.3. Prepuce, with part of the prepuce removed, left lateral view.

14 MALE

The urinary system of the male is quite similar to that of the female (see pp. 255-59); the urethra (Fig. 14.1) is modified both in its pelvic and spongy portions. The PELVIC PORTION is composed of preprostatic, prostatic, and postprostatic parts. The short PREPROSTATIC PART (1) of the urethra extends between the urinary bladder and the prostate gland; smooth muscle of the urinary bladder extends into the preprostatic urethra forming a functional internal sphincter. The PROSTATIC PART (2) of the urethra is described with the prostate (p. 277). The relatively long POSTPROSTATIC PART (3) is encircled by the urethralis muscle, a striated muscle. The SPONGY PORTION (4) of the urethra is described with the penis (pp. 279-81), with which it is associated.

The organs of the male reproductive system (Fig. 14.2) include the prepuce (1), scrotum (2), testis (3), epididymis (4), spermatic cord, ductus deferens (5), prostate gland (6), urethra (7), and penis (8).

The PREPUCE (pre'pyoos) (Fig. 14.3) is a sheath formed of modified integument. It consists of a hairy EXTERNAL LAYER (1) and an INTERNAL LAYER (2) that meet at the PREPUTIAL OSTIUM (3). The space between the internal layer and the glans penis is the PREPUTIAL CAVITY (4). A strong, fibrous SUSPENSORY LIGAMENT OF THE PENIS is present in the median plane between the abdominal wall (dorsally) and the penis (ventrally).

FIG. 14.4. Scrotum, with the left scrotal sac incised and the left testicle reflected.

FIG. 14.5. Scrotum, right testicle, and prepuce, with the right pelvic limb removed and the right vaginal tunic incised, right lateral view.

The SCROTUM (Fig. 14.4), a paired cutaneous pouch containing the TESTIS (pl. testes) (1), is composed of skin, DARTOS TUNIC (coat) (2), and fascia. The dartos tunic is a layer of smooth muscle closely adherent to the skin of the scrotum; it contracts in response to cold or mechanical stimulation. Much of the SCROTAL SEPTUM (pl. septa) (3), a median partition dividing the scrotum into two compartments, is also composed of the dartos tunic.

An incision through the scrotum reveals the PARIETAL LAYER OF THE VAGINAL TUNIC (1, Fig. 14.5). The VAGINAL TUNIC is continuous through the inguinal canal with the lining of the peritoneal cavity. The CREMASTER MUSCLE (2), a striated muscle arising from the caudal margin of the internal abdominal oblique, inserts on the parietal layer of the vaginal tunic. An incision through the parietal layer of the vaginal tunic reveals the VAGINAL "CAVITY" (3) and the VISCERAL LAYER OF THE VAGINAL TUNIC (4). The visceral layer of the vaginal tunic plus its contents (proximal to the testis) are termed the SPERMATIC CORD.

Blood vessels (1), lymph vessels, and nerve fibers from the abdominal cavity and the deferent (to carry away) ducts (2) from the pelvic cavity pass through the abdominal wall (Fig. 14.6) to reach the testes.

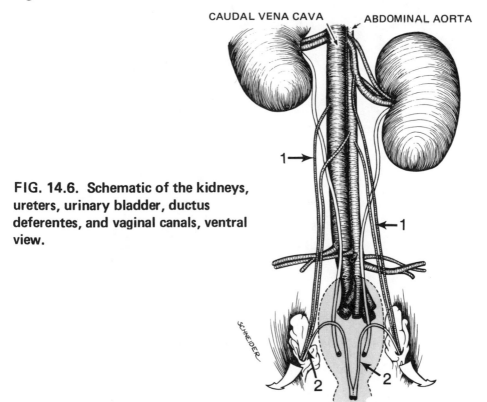

CAUDAL VENA CAVA   ABDOMINAL AORTA

FIG. 14.6. Schematic of the kidneys, ureters, urinary bladder, ductus deferentes, and vaginal canals, ventral view.

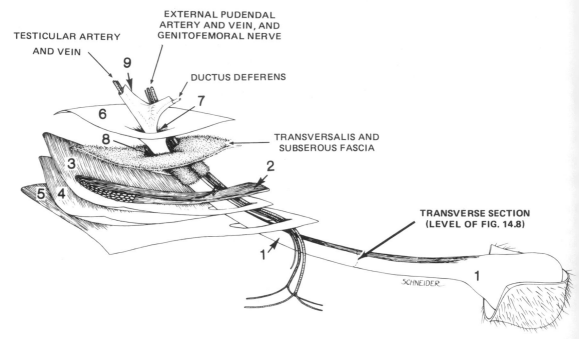

FIG. 14.7. Schematic of the right vaginal and inguinal canals and the structures that pass through the inguinal canal, medial view.

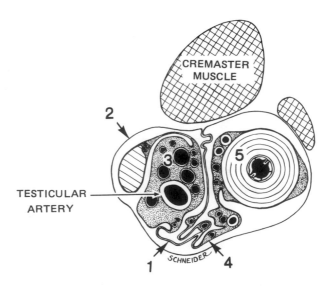

FIG. 14.8. Right cremaster, vaginal process, testicular vessels, and ductus deferens, transverse section.

The INGUINAL CANAL (Fig. 14.7) is a passage peripheral to the parietal layer of the vaginal tunic (1) and through or past the various layers of abdominal muscles: rectus abdominis (2), transversus abdominis (3), internal abdominal oblique (4), and external abdominal oblique (5). The reflection of parietal peritoneum (6) into the inguinal canal forms a serous membrane ring and canal, the VAGINAL RING (7) and VAGINAL CANAL. The reflection of fascia from the abdominal cavity into the inguinal canal, peripheral to the vaginal ring, is named the DEEP INGUINAL RING (8).

The MESORCHIUM (9, Fig. 14.7) suspends the testicular vessels from the dorsolateral wall in the abdominal cavity; in the vaginal tunic the mesorchium (1, Fig. 14.8) suspends the testicular vessels from the parietal vaginal tunic (2). The venous plexus formed by the TESTICULAR VEIN is called the PAMPINIFORM PLEXUS (3); this plexus has a role in heat exchange between the warm blood of the testicular artery and the cooler blood of the plexus. The MESODUCTUS DEFERENS (4) is a fold of tissue in the vaginal sac that supports the DUCTUS DEFERENS (5).

The lumen within that portion of the parietal vaginal tunic in the inguinal canal is the vaginal canal; the vaginal canal is patent and continues craniodorsally with the peritoneal cavity and caudally with the vaginal cavity. A SCROTAL HERNIA is a protrusion of an abdominal organ or tissue through the vaginal ring into the vaginal cavity, resulting in an elongated enlargement of the scrotal area. An INGUINAL HERNIA is a fold of mesentery or intestine that protrudes into the inguinal canal peripheral to the vaginal canal; an inguinal hernia forms a soft enlargement in the subcutaneous tissue to one side of the penis.

The TUNICA ALBUGINEA (al"bu-jin'e-ah), the outermost white, tough covering of the testis (of the ovary as well), and the visceral vaginal tunic are firmly bound to each other and are grossly indistinguishable as separate structures. A connective tissue mass within the testis, the MEDIASTINUM TESTIS, is connected to the peripheral tunica albuginea by connective tissue septa; these septa separate the testis into conical lobules. Each lobule of the testis is oriented with its apex toward the mediastinum testis and its base toward the tunica albuginea. SEMINIFEROUS TUBULES and interstitial cells are present within the lobules. Branches of the TESTICULAR ARTERY reach the lobules of the testis by passing through the mediastinum. The RETE (re'te, pl. retia; net) TESTIS is a network of interconnecting tubules within the

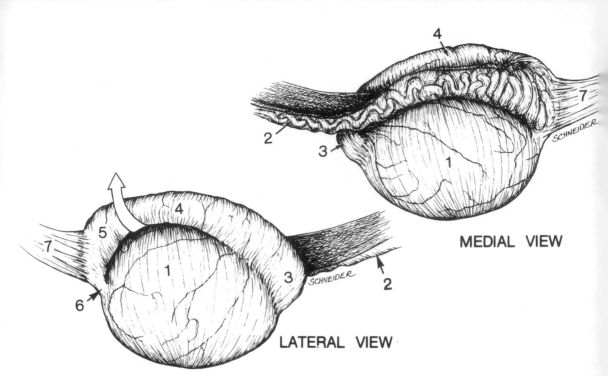

MEDIAL VIEW

LATERAL VIEW

FIG. 14.9. Right epididymis and testis.

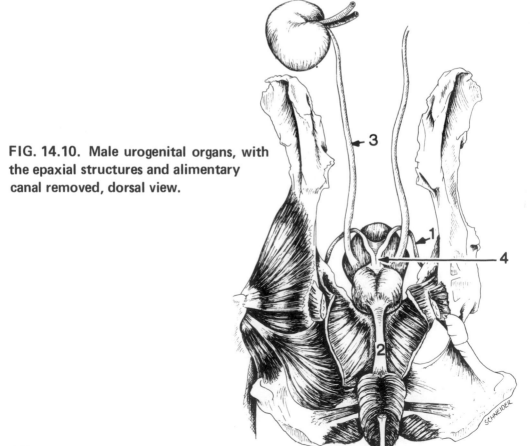

FIG. 14.10. Male urogenital organs, with the epaxial structures and alimentary canal removed, dorsal view.

mediastinum testis that collects the spermatozoa from the
seminiferous tubules and conducts them toward the epididymis.
The testes are abdominally located in the newborn pup; they
are near the deep inguinal ring at approximately 55-60 days
of fetal development and pass through the inguinal canal at
approximately 10-15 days of postnatal age.

The EPIDIDYMIS (pl. epididymides) (Fig. 14.9) is a
highly convoluted tube that collects spermatozoa from the
testis (1), stores them and then passes them on to the ductus
deferens (2). The HEAD OF THE EPIDIDYMIS (3) is the portion
of the epididymis at the cranial pole of the testis. The
spermatozoa pass from the testis to the head of the
epididymis. The BODY OF THE EPIDIDYMIS (4), the major
portion of the epididymis, is situated on the dorsal border
of the testis between the head and TAIL OF THE EPIDIDYMIS
(5), which is the portion situated on the caudal extremity of
the testis. The tail of the epididymis is continuous with
the ductus deferens. The caudal border of the testis is
attached to the epididymis by the PROPER LIGAMENT OF THE
TESTIS (6). The CAUDAL LIGAMENT OF THE EPIDIDYMIS (7), a
homolog of the round ligament of the uterus of the bitch, is
often very difficult to identify; it attaches the tail of the
epididymis to the parietal layer of the vaginal tunic (caudal
margin of the mesorchium).

The ductus deferens (1, Fig. 14.10) conveys spermatozoa
from the epididymis to the urethra (2). It arises from the
tail of the epididymis, passes cranially within the spermatic
cord, enters the abdominal cavity through the inguinal canal,
loops around the ventral surface of the ureter (3), and
enters the dorsal surface of the prostatic portion of the
urethra. Although grossly nondiscernible, the slightly
enlarged prostatic end of the ductus deferens (external to
the prostate) is the AMPULLA OF THE DUCTUS DEFERENS (4).

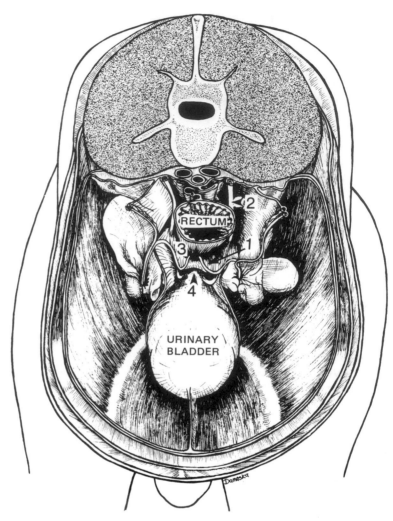

FIG. 14.11. Folds and recesses in the male pelvic cavity, cranial view.

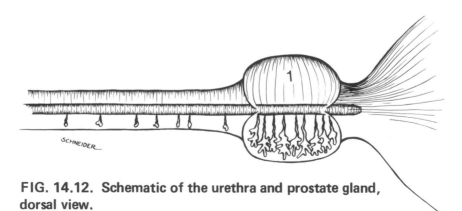

FIG. 14.12. Schematic of the urethra and prostate gland, dorsal view.

The paired ducti deferentes are suspended by a horizontal fold of peritoneum (1, Fig. 14.11) near their junction with the urethra. The caudal portions of the ureters (2) are also contained within this thin membranous fold. The rectogenital excavation (3) is dorsal and the vesicogenital excavation (4) ventral to this transverse fold (see p. 267).

The PROSTATE (pros'tate) GLAND (Fig. 14.12) is both around and scattered within the tissue of the pelvic urethra. The BODY OF THE PROSTATE GLAND (1) is divided by a median groove in the dog into right and left lobes surrounding the urethra. The prostate is an accessory genital organ that produces a milky alkaline fluid; this fluid neutralizes urethral acidity, aids in the activation of sperm, forms the bulk of the seminal fluid, and accounts for the characteristic odor of semen.

The internal dorsal surface of the pelvic portion of the urethra has a longitudinal ridge of mucosa. This ridge, the urethral crest (1, Fig. 14.13), terminates as the COLLICULUS (ko-lik'u-lus; small elevation) SEMINALIS (2), a mucosal elevation in the prostatic portion of the urethra. The urethral openings of the ductus deferens are in the colliculus seminalis. A number of small prostatic ductules open into the urethra on each side of the colliculus seminalis (if the prostate gland is squeezed, prostatic secretions may be observed entering the urethra).

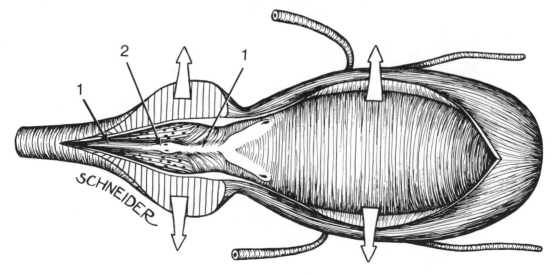

FIG. 14.13. Urinary bladder, ureters, ductus deferentes, prostate, and pelvic urethra, with a portion of the ventral wall of the urinary bladder and urethra removed, ventral view.

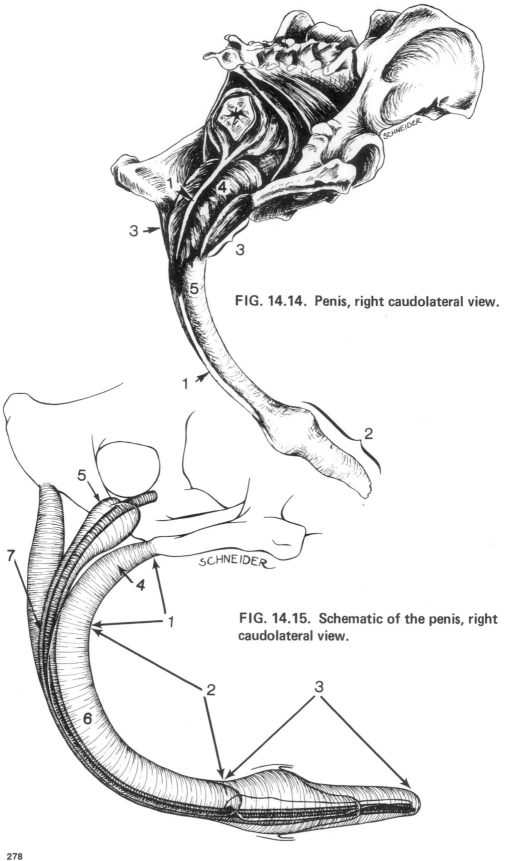

FIG. 14.14. Penis, right caudolateral view.

FIG. 14.15. Schematic of the penis, right caudolateral view.

The PENIS is composed of erectile, muscular, vascular, and nervous tissue. Paired (although seemingly single) RETRACTOR PENIS MUSCLES (1, Fig. 14.14) arise from the caudal vertebrae, pass around each side of the anal canal, and extend along the caudal and ventromedial surfaces of the penis to terminate near the glans penis (2). The retractor penis muscle is composed primarily of smooth muscle. The skeletal muscles of the penis include the ISCHIOCAVERNOSUS (is"ke-o-kav"er-no'sus) (3), BULBOSPONGIOSUS (4), and ischiourethralis. The ischiocavernosus muscle arises from the ischiatic tuberosity and terminates on the proximal ventral surface of the CORPUS CAVERNOSUM PENIS (5). The bulbospongiosus muscle is situated between the ischiocavernosus muscles of each side and deep to the retractor penis muscle; it partially encircles the urethra and the erectile CORPUS (pl. corpora; body) SPONGIOSUM PENIS in the proximal portion of the penis.

The penis (Fig. 14.15) is restrictively described by textbooks as consisting of erectile tissue that is subdivided into ROOT (1), BODY (2), and GLANS (3), with the root of the penis consisting of the CRURA OF THE PENIS (4) and the BULB OF THE PENIS (5). The crura of the penis attaches proximally to the ischiatic tuberosity and continues distally as the CORPORA CAVERNOSA PENIS (6). Each corpus cavernosum penis arches cranioventrally and converges with its member of the opposite side, forming the bulk of the body of the penis, ending at the proximal portion of the glans penis. The tough white connective tissue around the erectile tissue is the TUNICA ALBUGINEA of the corpus cavernosum. The bulb of the penis, a bilobed structure in the caudoventral portion of the pelvic cavity, is continuous distally in the penis as the slender erectile corpus spongiosum penis (7). The corpus spongiosum in the body of the penis is positioned ventromedial to the paired corpus cavernosum and contains the spongy portion of the urethra.

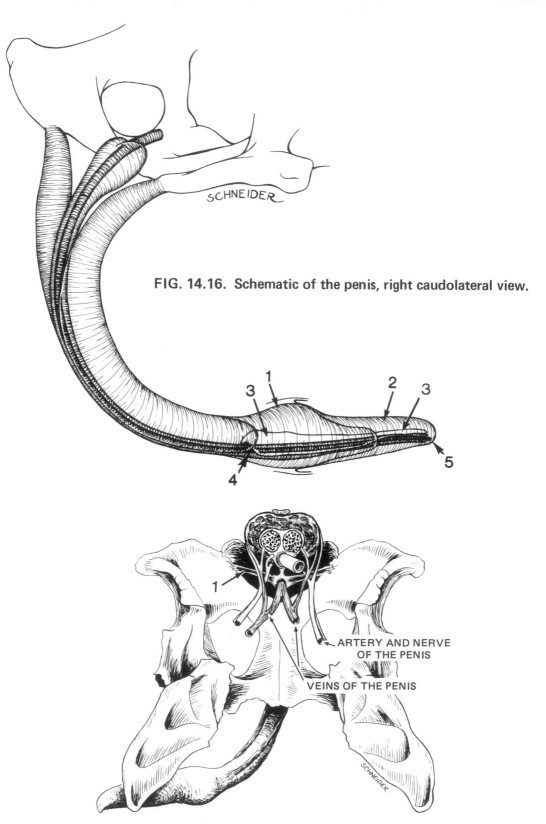

SCHNEIDER

FIG. 14.16. Schematic of the penis, right caudolateral view.

3   1   2   3

4   5

1

ARTERY AND NERVE
OF THE PENIS

VEINS OF THE PENIS

SCHNEIDER

FIG. 14.17. Ossa coxarum and root of the penis with associated
vessels, with muscles and cavernous tissue of the penis sectioned
transversely, dorsal view.

The glans penis (Fig. 14.16) is composed primarily of erectile tissue that is continuous with the corpus spongiosum penis. The large BULBUS GLANDIS (1) forms the proximal portion of the glans. It is this erectile tissue that is locked in the vagina of the bitch during coitus caused by vascular engorgement of the bulbus glandis and contraction of constrictor muscles of the vagina and vestibule; see p. 263. The external distal portion of the glans is formed by the PARS LONGA GLANDIS (2); vascular sinuses in the pars longa glandis are connected with both the bulbus glandis and the corpus spongiosum penis. Within the glans penis the corpus spongiosum penis (which surrounds the penile urethra) lies in a groove within the OS PENIS (3). The os penis, which provides support for the glans, is the distal continuation of the corpus cavernosum penis. The URETHRAL GROOVE (4), in the ventral surface of the os penis, prevents urethral expansion; urinary CALCULI (sing. calculus) often lodge in the urethra at the caudal (proximal) end of the os penis. The external urethral orifice (5) is in the distal ventral surface of the glans penis.

The paired ISCHIOURETHRALIS MUSCLES (1, Fig. 14.17) arise from the ischiatic tuberosities and insert on a fibrous ring, ventral to the bulb of the penis and dorsal to the ischiatic symphysis. Contraction of the ischiourethralis muscles results in a reduction of venous blood flow from the penis through the fibrous ring. This reduction in quantity of blood flowing from the penis is a major factor in the erection mechanism.

(DIFFERENCES TO BE NOTED IN THE CAT: The preprostatic part of the urethra is relatively long as compared to the dog. BULBOURETHRAL GLANDS are present adjacent to the bulb of the feline penis, deep to striated muscle. This muscle, a craniodorsal part of the bulbospongiosus, is continuous with the urethralis muscle. The flaccid penis is directed caudoventrally, a position that often leads to incorrect sexing by the cat owner. Small keratinized spines are present on the surface of the feline glans penis.)

Cardiovascular System

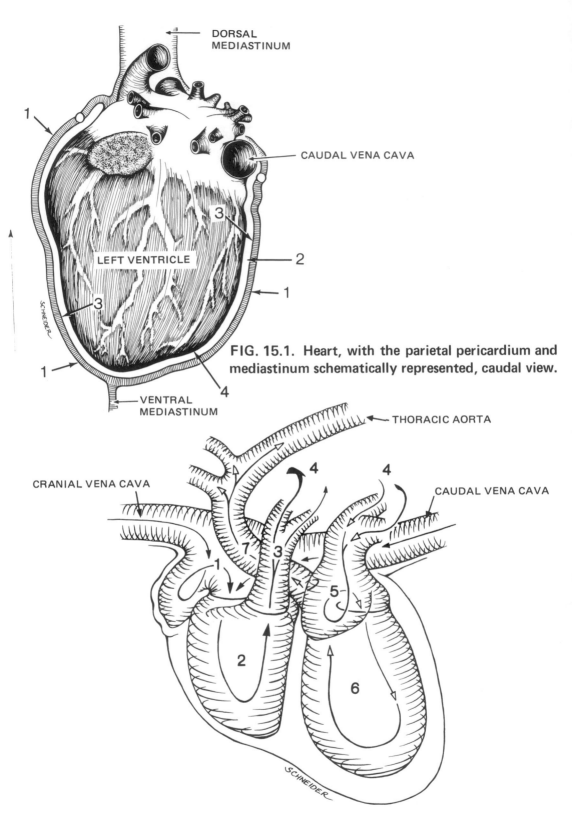

DORSAL
MEDIASTINUM

CAUDAL VENA CAVA

LEFT VENTRICLE

FIG. 15.1. Heart, with the parietal pericardium and mediastinum schematically represented, caudal view.

VENTRAL
MEDIASTINUM

THORACIC AORTA

CRANIAL VENA CAVA

CAUDAL VENA CAVA

FIG. 15.2. Schematic of the blood pathway through the heart.

15 HEART AND PERICARDIUM

The thoracic cavity contains the two pleural cavities and a third serous membrane-lined space, the PERICARDIAL CAVITY. The portion of the mediastinum superficial to the heart (Fig. 15.1) is lined by PERICARDIAL MEDIASTINAL PLEURA (1). The PERICARDIUM, composed of fibrous and serous layers and of the pericardial cavity (2), is situated within the mediastinum. The PARIETAL PERICARDIUM (3) forms the superficial wall of the pericardium and is composed of an external fibrous layer and an internal serous layer. An extension of the fibrous pericardium connects the pericardium to the diaphragm; this strong connective tissue band is the PHRENICOPERICARDIAC (phrenic: fren'ik; diaphragm) LIGAMENT. The deep wall of the pericardial cavity is formed by a visceral layer of serous pericardium, or EPICARDIUM (4), tightly bound to heart muscle. The pericardial cavity normally contains only a thin film of fluid positioned between parietal and visceral layers of serous pericardium.

The HEART is a four-chambered muscular structure positioned between venous and arterial systems (Fig. 15.2). Venous blood from the entire body (except for the lungs and some of the heart) enters the RIGHT ATRIUM (1) and then flows sequentially through the RIGHT VENTRICLE (2), PULMONARY TRUNK (3), pulmonary arteries/capillary bed/pulmonary veins (4), LEFT ATRIUM (5), LEFT VENTRICLE (6), and ASCENDING AORTA (7) and into all of the body (except for the alveoli).

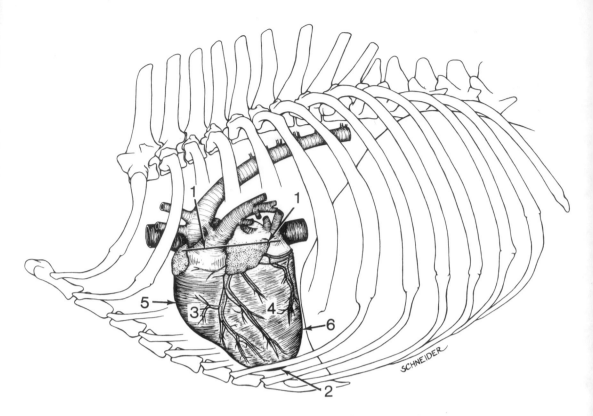

FIG. 15.3. Heart and major vessels in the thorax, left ventral view.

FIG. 15.4. Position of the heart in the thorax, relative to the thoracic limb.

The flattened BASE OF THE HEART (1, Fig. 15.3) is the wide craniodorsal portion of the heart through which major vessels enter and leave. The APEX OF THE HEART (2) is directed caudoventrally. The cranial portion of the base of the heart is situated at the approximate level of the 3rd rib; the apex is located near the 6th rib and slightly to the left of the median plane. The major portion of the heart is formed by the muscular right (3) and left (4) ventricles, each of which face both right and left thoracic walls since they are positioned more cranioventrally (right ventricle) and caudodorsally (left ventricle) than "right" and "left." The RIGHT VENTRICULAR MARGIN (5) forms the convex cranioventral surface of the heart, which is positioned nearly parallel to the curvature of the sternum. The LEFT VENTRICULAR MARGIN (6), which slopes nearly vertically from the base of the heart dorsally to the apex ventrally, forms the caudodorsal surface of the heart.

The tricipital margin of the brachium (see p. 59) overlies the transverse level of the 5th to 6th ribs (Fig. 15.4); therefore, all but the apex and caudal surface of the heart is medial or deep to the thoracic limb. When palpating the heart, maximum detection of the beat usually may be located at the left fifth intercostal space. The location for detection of sounds created by the four valves of the heart and the major vessels (shortly to be described) are as follows: left atrioventricular valve- left fifth intercostal space at the level of the costochondral junction; aortic valve- left fourth intercostal space, ventral to a dorsal plane through the humeral articulation; right atrioventricular valve- right third or fourth intercostal space, near the dorsal plane of the costochondral junction; and the pulmonary valve- left third intercostal space, ventrally near the sternum.

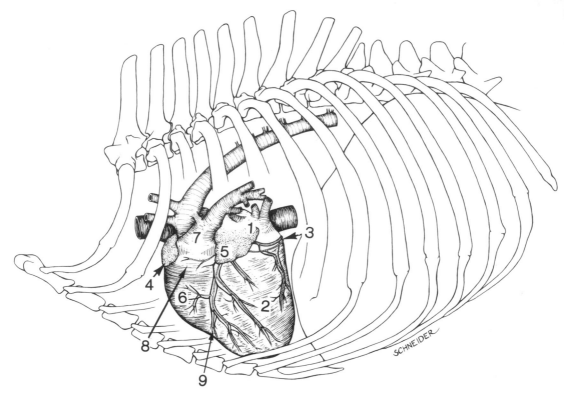

FIG. 15.5. Auricular surface of the heart.

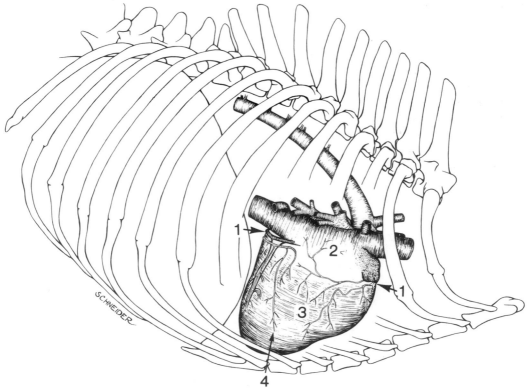

FIG. 15.6. Atrial surface of the heart.

The earlike appendages of both right and left atria are directed toward the left side of the thoracic cavity (Fig. 15.5). The appendages are termed AURICLES; thus the left side of the heart is described as the AURICULAR SURFACE. The left atrium (1) is separated from the left ventricle (2) on the auricular surface of the heart by the CORONARY GROOVE (3). The tips of right (4) and left (5) auricles are directed toward each other across the junction between right ventricle (6) and pulmonary trunk (7). This funnel-shaped junction is the CONUS ARTERIOSUS (8). The pulmonary trunk branches into RIGHT and LEFT PULMONARY ARTERIES, which supply the lobes of right and left lung, respectively. The fatty streak oriented from heart base to near the apex on the auricular surface is the PARACONAL INTERVENTRICULAR GROOVE (9), which contains a large branch of the left coronary artery and the great cardiac vein.

The ATRIAL SURFACE OF THE HEART (Fig. 15.6) is the surface related to the right ribs. The large coronary groove (1), a fat-filled area situated transversely with respect to the heart, marks the separation of the right atrium (a'tre-um, pl. atria; hall) (2), dorsocranially, from the ventricles (3), caudoventrally. The coronary groove, which contains the proximal portion of the coronary vessels, may be followed around the dorsocaudal aspect of the heart to the left side. Two or more fatty streaks, containing vessels, are on the ventricular portion of the atrial surface. One fatty streak on the right caudodorsal aspect of the heart superficial to the interventricular septum is the SUBSINUOSAL INTERVENTRICULAR GROOVE (4).

Thus a cardiac puncture from either right or left side may enter the somewhat flabby-walled right ventricle or the thick-walled, muscular left ventricle. A cardiac puncture also may enter the interventricular septum, with possible damage to coronary vessels that travel over the surface of the heart in grooves overlying the partition. A number of vascular branches also course over the surface of the ventricles at sites other than in the grooves overlying the septum.

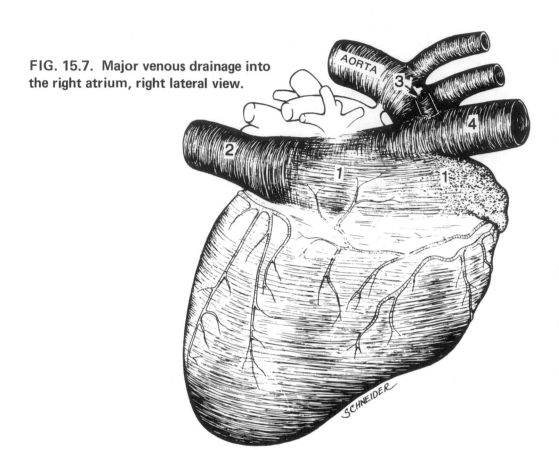

FIG. 15.7. Major venous drainage into the right atrium, right lateral view.

AORTA

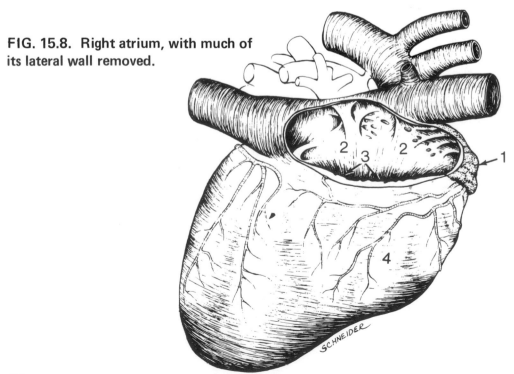

FIG. 15.8. Right atrium, with much of its lateral wall removed.

Four major veins drain blood into the right atrium (1, Fig. 15.7): three vessels from the body and one from the heart (for cardiac drainage see pp. 293, 301). The CAUDAL VENA CAVA (pl. venae cavae) (2) extends cranially from the dorsal portion of the abdominal cavity through the vena caval foramen of the thoracic diaphragm into the thoracic cavity; it discharges venous blood into the caudal portion of the right atrium. The RIGHT AZYGOUS VEIN (3), which collects venous blood from the vertebral canal and much of the thoracic and abdominal walls, crosses the right surface of the trachea cranioventrally and discharges venous blood into the right atrium or into the CRANIAL VENA CAVA (4). The cranial vena cava discharges venous blood, collected primarily from the head, neck, and thoracic limbs, into the cranial portion of the right atrium.

Due to subatmospheric pressures in the pleural and pericardial cavities, the atria, with intraluminal pressures equal to atmospheric pressure, are expanded, allowing venous blood to flow into them with little resistance. The right atrium by muscular contraction forces blood into the right ventricle; the blood is unable to back up into the major veins because blood pressure in the atrium is lower than that in the venae cavae.

The right atrium (Fig. 15.8) is composed of the small earlike RIGHT AURICLE (1) and the large SINUS VENARUM CAVARUM (2). An opening, the RIGHT ATRIOVENTRICULAR OSTIUM (3) discharges blood into the right ventricle (4).

FIG. 15.9. Medial wall of the right atrium and the ostia, which open into the atrium, right lateral view.

FIG. 15.10. Schematic of the conductive system of the heart, with much of the atrial surface removed, right lateral view.

The right atrium receives blood from three or four veins (Fig. 15.9). The OSTIA OF THE CRANIAL (1) and CAUDAL (2) VENAE CAVAE are at cranial and caudal ends of the right atrium. Blood coming into the atrium from the two venae cavae is directed ventrally by the INTERVENOUS TUBERCLE (3), which is situated on the medial wall of the atrium parallel with the long axis of the heart. The third point of venous discharge into the right atrium is the CORONARY SINUS (4), through which the great cardiac vein discharges blood collected from veins draining the surface of the heart. The coronary sinus is ventral to the ostium of the caudal vena cava. A small depression, the FOSSA OVALIS (5), is immediately caudal to the intervenous tubercle; this oval fossa is the remnant of the embryological opening (FORAMEN OVALE) between right and left atria. This foramen normally closes within a few weeks of postnatal life. Muscular bands on the internal surface of the right auricle are termed PECTINATE (comblike) MUSCLES (6); most of the pectinate muscles attach to the TERMINAL CREST (7), a ridge of muscle ventral to the ostium of the cranial vena cava. The ENDOCARDIUM is the thin glistening membrane that forms the inner or luminal surface of the four chambers of the heart.

The SINUATRIAL (SA) NODE (1, Fig. 15.10), or center from which each intrinsic beat of the heart originates, is in the terminal crest; the SA node cannot be observed grossly. The ATRIOVENTRICULAR (AV) NODE (2), also not grossly discernible, is in the medial wall of the right atrium (INTERATRIAL SEPTUM), cranial and ventral to the coronary sinus. From the AV node a conducting system of modified muscle fibers, the ATRIOVENTRICULAR FASCICULUS (3), courses distally through the interatrial septum, branches, and spreads distally near the luminal surface of the interventricular septum. Parasympathetic nerve fibers to the heart terminate primarily in the atria (many terminate on the SA and AV nodes), whereas sympathetic fibers terminate at many points distally in the ventricles.

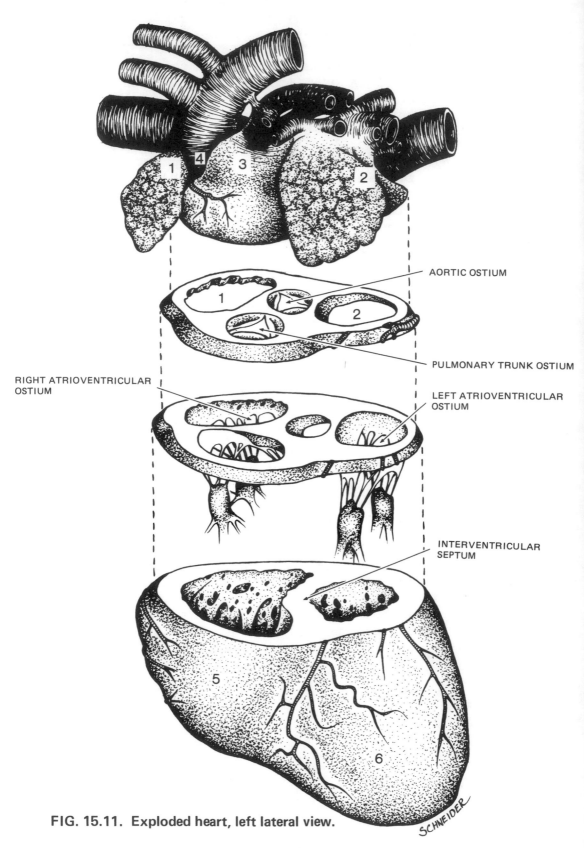

AORTIC OSTIUM

PULMONARY TRUNK OSTIUM

RIGHT ATRIOVENTRICULAR
OSTIUM

LEFT ATRIOVENTRICULAR
OSTIUM

INTERVENTRICULAR
SEPTUM

FIG. 15.11. Exploded heart, left lateral view.

Right (1, Fig. 15.11) and left (2) atria, the pulmonary trunk (3), and the ascending aorta (4) attach to a delicate "cardiac skeleton" that separates the preceding structures from right (5) and left (6) ventricles. This skeleton is composed in part of fibrous rings of collagenous tissue upon which four sets of valves attach.

The right atrioventricular ostium is bounded by the RIGHT ATRIOVENTRICULAR VALVE, which consists of two wide, thin flaps of tissue held open under tension by thin strands of tissue (Fig. 15.12). The flaps, or cusps, are named according to origin from the fibrous skeleton as parietal or septal. The PARIETAL CUSP (1) arises from the external atrial-ventricular wall; the SEPTAL CUSP (2) arises from the junction of interatrial and interventricular septa. Cone-shaped muscular projections from the INTERVENTRICULAR SEPTUM, called PAPILLARY MUSCLES (3), give origin to the fibromuscular CHORDAE TENDINEAE (4). Muscular ridges on the luminal surface of the ventricle are named TRABECULAE CARNEAE (kar´ne; fleshy) (5). A relatively thin fibrous cord spanning the lumen of the right ventricle from the septum to the parietal wall, termed the TRABECULA SEPTOMARGINALIS (6), serves both to provide support for the parietal wall and as a pathway of conducting fibers (part of the atrioventricular fasciculus) (pl. fasciculi; small bundle).

FIG. 15.12. Right atrioventricular valve and internal surface of the right ventricle, viewed from the right side.

FIG. 15.13. Conus arteriosus and pulmonary vessels, left dorsolateral view.

FIG. 15.14. Left atrioventricular valve, parietal wall of the left ventricle, and part of the aortic valve, viewed from the septal wall.

The funnel-shaped conus arteriosus (1, Fig. 15.13) portion of the right ventricle leads to the PULMONARY TRUNK OSTIUM, which is closed during part of the cardiac cycle by three SEMILUNAR (half moon) VALVULES (RIGHT, LEFT, and INTERMEDIATE) that form the PULMONARY TRUNK VALVE (2). The semilunar valvules are shaped like pockets, with the open portion of each pocket directed toward the distal end of the pulmonary trunk; backflow of blood opens the free margins of the three pockets against each other, closing off reentry of blood into the right ventricle. Nonoxygenated blood is carried from the pulmonary trunk through right (3) and left (4) pulmonary arteries to right and left lungs. Oxygenated blood returns from both right and left lungs through five or six PULMONARY VEINS (5) into the left atrium. In the left atrium the portion of the interatrial septum that overlies the fossa ovalis (see p. 293) may bear a small flap of tissue, the valvule of the foramen ovale. The left atrium pumps blood through the LEFT ATRIOVENTRICULAR OSTIUM into the left ventricle.

The left atrioventricular ostium (1, Fig. 15.14) is bounded by the PARIETAL (2) and SEPTAL (3) CUSPS OF THE LEFT ATRIOVENTRICULAR VALVE. Unlike the right ventricle, in the left ventricle the papillary muscles (4) arise from the outer or parietal wall. The AORTIC OSTIUM (5) is located near the center of the base of the heart. The AORTIC VALVE (6), which consists of three semilunar valvules (right, left, and septal), protects the aortic ostium from backflow of blood.

The dorsal portion of the interventricular septum, medial to the septal cusp of the right and left atrioventricular valves, is quite thin and membranous. Embryologically, this is the last portion of the interventricular septum to form; failure to close properly produces an interventricular foramen.

APEX OF THE HEART

FIG. 15.15. Heart and thoracic cage, caudal view.

FIG. 15.16. Branches of the ascending aorta and aortic arch, left lateral view.

The ascending aorta (1, Fig. 15.15) arises from the left ventricle (2) medial (deep) to the pulmonary trunk (3) on the left and medial (deep) to the right atrium (4) and cranial vena cava (5) on the right.

The aorta is descriptively divided into ascending aorta (1, Fig. 15.16), AORTIC ARCH (2), and DESCENDING (THORACIC and ABDOMINAL) AORTA (3). The slightly expanded origin (AORTIC BULB) of the ascending aorta and its cavity (AORTIC SINUS) gives rise to the first aortic branches, the RIGHT (4) and LEFT (5) CORONARY ARTERIES. The next branch of the aorta arises from the aortic arch and passes cranially and to the right across the ventral surface of the trachea. This large branch is the BRACHIOCEPHALIC TRUNK (6), which supplies blood to the head through both RIGHT and LEFT COMMON CAROTID ARTERIES and to the neck, right thoracic limb, and cranial part of the thorax via the RIGHT SUBCLAVIAN ARTERY. The next arterial branch off the aortic arch is the LEFT SUBCLAVIAN ARTERY (7).

The right coronary artery (1, Fig. 15.17) originates from the aortic sinus (2) distal to the right septal valvule and carries blood through the coronary groove of the atrial surface of the heart. Branches of the right coronary artery course distally over the surface of the right ventricle. The left coronary artery (3) carries blood from behind (caudolateral to) the left semilunar cusp to the coronary groove of the caudal auricular surface (partially covered by the left auricle).

FIG. 15.17. Aortic bulb, aortic sinus, and aortic valves, with the ascending aorta transected and removed, craniolateral view.

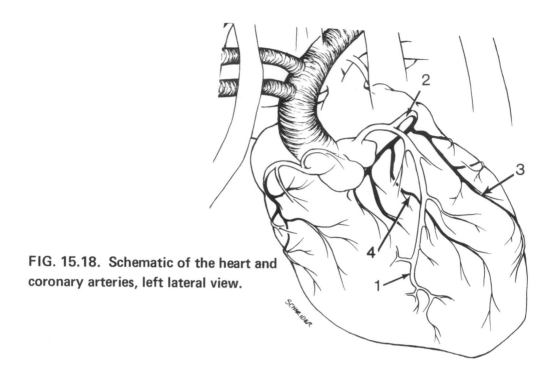

FIG. 15.18. Schematic of the heart and coronary arteries, left lateral view.

FIG. 15.19. Schematic of the heart and major veins that empty into the right atrium, right lateral view.

A PARACONAL INTERVENTRICULAR BRANCH (1, Fig. 15.18) of the left coronary artery carries blood through the paraconal interventricular groove. Another large branch, the CIRCUMFLEX BRANCH (2), continues toward the right side around the caudodorsal surface of the heart in the coronary groove. An INTERMEDIATE BRANCH (3) and a SUBSINUOSAL INTERVENTRICULAR BRANCH (4) course over the surface of the heart between the subsinuosal and paraconal interventricular grooves and in the subsinuosal interventricular groove, respectively.

The GREAT CARDIAC VEIN (1, Fig. 15.19) arises in the paraconal interventricular groove, courses around the caudodorsal surface of the heart in the coronary groove in association with the circumflex branch of the left coronary artery. It opens into the caudal portion of the right atrium ventral to the ostium of the caudal vena cava as the coronary sinus (2).

A fibrous band of tissue, the LIGAMENTUM ARTERIOSUM (1, Fig. 15.20) arises from the pulmonary trunk (2) near the bifurcation of the trunk into right and left pulmonary arteries, and passes to the aortic arch distal to the origin of the left subclavian artery (3). The ligamentum arteriosum is an embryonic vestige of the DUCTUS ARTERIOSUS, which acted to shunt blood from the pulmonary trunk to the aortic arch, thus bypassing the nonfunctional lungs of the fetus.

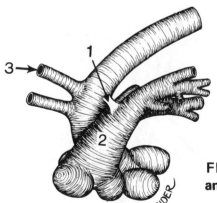

FIG. 15.20. Origin of pulmonary vessels and aorta, left lateral view.

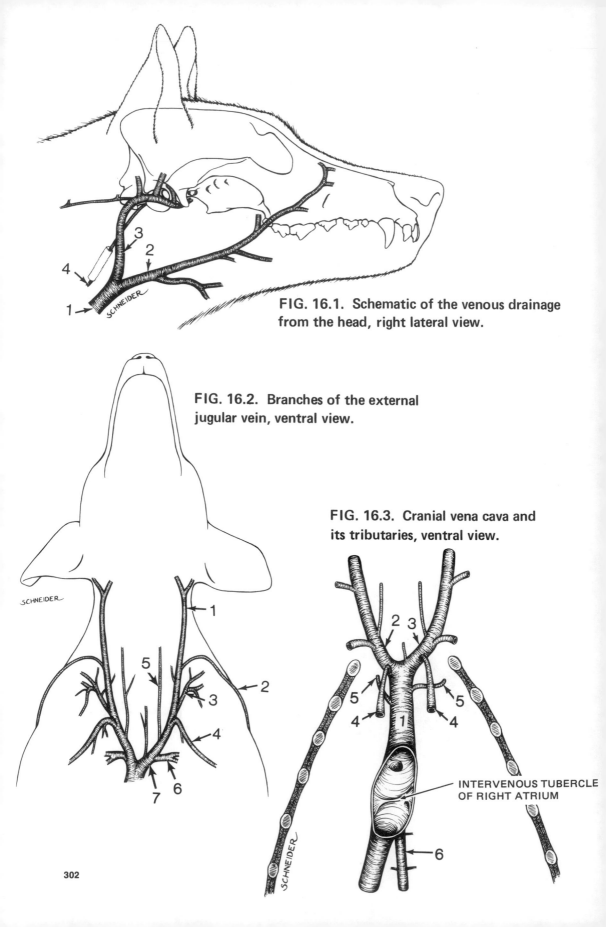

FIG. 16.1. Schematic of the venous drainage from the head, right lateral view.

FIG. 16.2. Branches of the external jugular vein, ventral view.

FIG. 16.3. Cranial vena cava and its tributaries, ventral view.

INTERVENOUS TUBERCLE OF RIGHT ATRIUM

16 TRUNK VESSELS

Most of the blood from the head (Fig. 16.1) drains caudally through the EXTERNAL JUGULAR VEIN (1). The LINGUOFACIAL VEIN (2), draining much of the surface of the head, and the MAXILLARY VEIN (3), draining much of the deeper portions of the head, join at the level of the 1st cervical vertebra to form the external jugular vein. The INTERNAL JUGULAR VEIN (4) drains some blood from the head through the carotid sheath.

In the caudal portion of the neck (Fig. 16.2), the external jugular vein (1) receives blood from the OMOBRACHIAL VEIN (2), a small superficial vein that drains blood from the thoracic limb (see p. 323). Near the level of the 1st rib, in the jugular fossa, the external jugular vein receives blood from the SUPERFICIAL CERVICAL (3), CEPHALIC (4), and internal jugular (5) veins. The confluences of external jugular and SUBCLAVIAN (6) VEINS of right and left sides forms the RIGHT and LEFT BRACHIOCEPHALIC VEINS (7).

THE CRANIAL VENA CAVA (1, Fig. 16.3), which is formed near the cranial thoracic aperture by the confluence of right (2) and left (3) brachiocephalic veins, receives venous blood draining through INTERNAL THORACIC (4), COSTOCERVICAL (5), and RIGHT AZYGOUS (az'i-gus; unpaired) (6) VEINS.

FIG. 16.4. Aortic arch and branches of the brachiocephalic trunk, left lateral view.

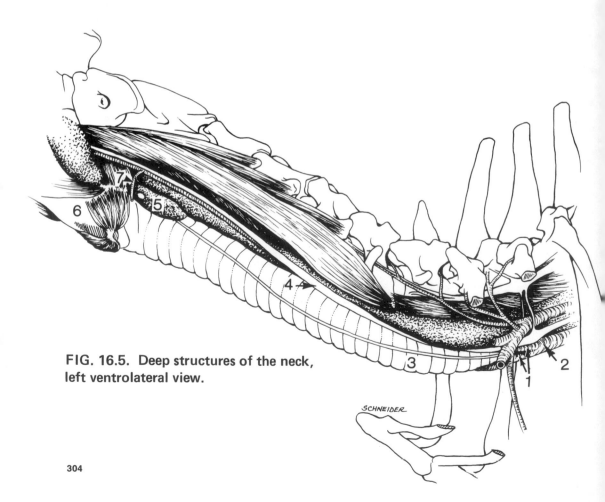

FIG. 16.5. Deep structures of the neck, left ventrolateral view.

The first four branches of the aorta (Fig. 16.4) have been described on page 299. They are the right (1) and left (2) coronary arteries off the ascending aorta and the brachiocephalic trunk (3) and left subclavian artery (4) off the aortic arch. The three main branches of the brachiocephalic trunk are the LEFT COMMON CAROTID (5), RIGHT COMMON CAROTID (6), and RIGHT SUBCLAVIAN (7) ARTERIES.

Both right and left (1, Fig. 16.5) common carotids arise from the brachiocephalic trunk (2) near the ventrolateral surface of the trachea (3). Each common carotid artery courses through the neck with the vagosympathetic trunk (4) and the internal jugular vein in the carotid sheath (see p. 25). Each common carotid artery supplies blood to the THYROID GLAND (5), the larynx (6), and the cervical portion of the trachea and esophagus by way of the CRANIAL THYROID ARTERY (7).

In the cervical region (Fig. 16.6) the RIGHT CAROTID SHEATH (1) is positioned between the longus capitis muscle (2) dorsolaterally and the trachea (3) ventromedially. The LEFT CAROTID SHEATH (4) is positioned between the esophagus (5) dorsomedially and the longus capitis muscle dorsolaterally.

FIG. 16.6. Positions of the carotid sheaths.

FIG. 16.7. Branches of the left subclavian artery, left lateral view.

FIG. 16.8. Bony thorax, illustrating the branches of the costocervical trunks, cranial view.

Both right and left subclavian arteries have similar branches although their origins are different; the right subclavian artery is a branch of the brachiocephalic trunk and the left subclavian originates from the aortic arch. The branches of each subclavian artery (Fig. 16.7) are vertebral artery (1), costocervical trunk (2), internal thoracic artery (3), and superficial cervical artery (4). All four arteries arise within the thoracic cavity near the level of the first intercostal space; the subclavian artery continues distally past the 1st rib as the axillary artery.

The VERTEBRAL ARTERY (1) passes dorsocranially into the neck between the longus colli and scalenus muscles. It passes through the transverse foramina of the cervical vertebrae in association with the sympathetic vertebral nerve. Branches of the vertebral artery pass through each intervertebral foramen and the lateral vertebral foramen, supplying blood to the meninges and blood vessels of the vertebral canal.

The COSTOCERVICAL TRUNKS (1, Fig. 16.8) course dorsally, lateral to the esophagus on the left side of the body, lateral to the trachea on the right side of the body, and lateral to the vertebral artery (2) near its origin on both sides. A cranial branch, the DORSAL SCAPULAR ARTERY (3), arises from the costocervical trunk, passes dorsally cranial to the 1st rib, and supplies blood to the serratus ventralis muscle. The other main branch of the costocervical trunk is a vessel that passes between the first two ribs and supplies blood to deep epaxial musculature via the DEEP CERVICAL ARTERY (4) and to the dorsal portion of the first several intercostal spaces via the THORACIC VERTEBRAL ARTERY (5, Fig. 16.7; 1, Fig. 16.9).

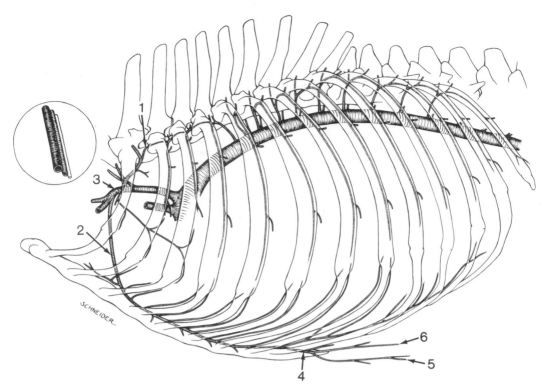

FIG. 16.9. Bony thorax and branches of the thoracic aorta, left lateral view.

FIG. 16.10. Bony thorax, illustrating the branches of the brachiocephalic trunk, subclavian, and axillary arteries, cranial view.

FIG. 16.11. Left axillary artery, lateral view

The INTERNAL THORACIC ARTERY (2, Fig. 16.9) courses caudoventrally from the subclavian artery (3), passing caudally between the transversus thoracis muscle and the costal cartilages. Branches of the internal thoracic artery supply the mediastinum, THYMUS, cranial portion of the phrenic nerve (PERICARDIACOPHRENIC ARTERY), ventral intercostal spaces (VENTRAL INTERCOSTAL BRANCHES), pectoral muscles, thoracic mammary glands, and ventral portion of the thoracic diaphragm. Near the eighth intercostal space, the internal thoracic artery passes through the diaphragm as the CRANIAL EPIGASTRIC (upon the belly) ARTERY (4), which divides at the level of the xiphoid process into two parallel, caudally coursing vessels, the CRANIAL SUPERFICIAL (5) and CRANIAL DEEP (6) EPIGASTRIC ARTERIES. The cranial deep epigastric is usually larger and may be observed on the deep surface of the rectus abdominis muscle. The cranial superficial epigastric is situated in the superficial fascia and may be quite large in the lactating bitch.

The SUPERFICIAL CERVICAL ARTERY (1, Fig. 16.10) arises from the subclavian artery (2) near the 1st rib and courses into the region of the cranial extrinsic limb muscles. Branches of the superficial cervical may be observed in the region of the superficial cervical lymph nodes (3) deep to the omotransversarius muscle, and in the area of the scapular notch (4), with the suprascapular nerve.

The AXILLARY ARTERY (1, Fig. 16.11) is the continuation of the subclavian artery (2) past the cranial surface of the 1st rib into the axilla (with the brachial plexus). A small EXTERNAL THORACIC ARTERY (3) is from the axillary artery and supplies the pectoral muscles. A LATERAL THORACIC ARTERY (4) courses caudally with the lateral thoracic nerve to supply axillary lymph nodes and latissimus dorsi, deep pectoral, and cutaneus trunci muscles. The arterial branches of the axillary and its continuation, the BRACHIAL ARTERY, are described with vessels of the thoracic limb (see pp. 325-29).

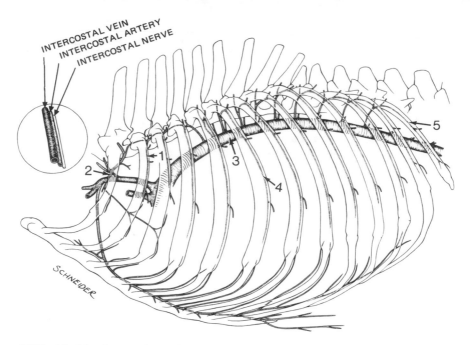

FIG. 16.12. Bony thorax and arteries supplying the thoracic wall, left lateral view.

FIG. 16.13. Branches of the intercostal arteries, caudal view.

FIG. 16.14. Bronchoesophageal arteries, left lateral view.

The first several intercostal spaces receive small DORSAL INTERCOSTAL ARTERIES (1, Fig. 16.12) from a branch of the costocervical trunk (2). The thoracic portion of the descending aorta (3) provides paired dorsal segmental branches to the caudal nine intercostal spaces and a branch to the portion of the body wall caudal to the 13th rib. The paired segmental arteries to the intercostal spaces are the dorsal intercostal arteries (4); the vessel caudal to the 13th rib is named, like the accompanying nerve, the DORSAL COSTOABDOMINAL ARTERY (5).

The dorsal intercostal arteries (1, Fig. 16.13) pass into the intercostal spaces and supply dorsal branches (2) to the vessels of the vertebral canal and to muscles and skin of the epaxial area; and lateral cutaneous branches (3), which appear superficially along the ventral border of the latissimus dorsi muscle (some of these lateral cutaneous branches supply the mammae). The dorsal intercostal arteries course along the caudal surface of each rib, superficial to the parietal pleura, and anastomose with the ventral intercostal branches (4) of the internal thoracic artery (5), forming a collateral circulation.

The BRONCHO-ESOPHAGEAL ARTERY (1, Fig. 16.14) is one or more vessels that may arise from the right 4th to 6th dorsal intercostal arteries or from the thoracic aorta. Although the broncho-esophageal artery usually arises from a right intercostal vessel, it crosses the left surface of the esophagus. This artery provides the main blood supply to the conducting airways of the lungs as well as esophageal branches to the thoracic portion of the esophagus.

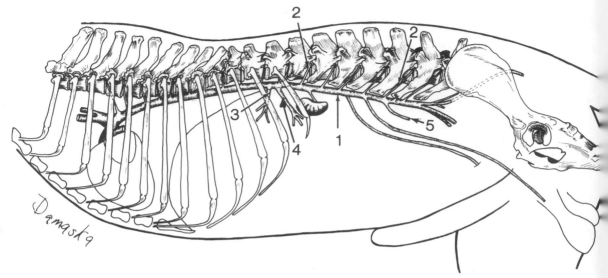

FIG. 16.15. Schematic of the body illustrating the parietal and visceral branches of the abdominal aorta, left lateral view.

FIG. 16.16. Paired parietal branches and the severed stumps of visceral branches of the abdominal aorta, ventral view.

The abdominal portion of the descending aorta, termed the ABDOMINAL AORTA (1, Fig. 16.15), supplies seven segmental, paired LUMBAR ARTERIES (2). Each lumbar artery supplies blood to a vertebra, to the vertebral canal and spinal cord, and to the muscles and skin of the epaxial area. Within the abdominal cavity, three unpaired arteries branch from the ventral surface of the aorta and supply viscera. The most cranial of the three arises at the level of the 1st lumbar vertebra near the aortic hiatus; this is the CELIAC (se'le-ak; belly) ARTERY (3), which supplies blood to the stomach, liver, and spleen (as well as other structures; see p. 369). The next caudal unpaired visceral branch is the CRANIAL MESENTERIC ARTERY (4), which also branches ventrally from the aorta at the level of the 1st lumbar vertebra; the celiac and cranial mesenteric arteries arise close together but diverge as the celiac artery passes cranioventrally and the cranial mesenteric artery passes caudoventrally. The cranial mesenteric artery supplies blood to the pancreas, duodenum, jejunum, ileum, cecum, and a portion of the colon. The third unpaired visceral artery, the CAUDAL MESENTERIC ARTERY (5), arises from the aorta at the level, approximately, of the 5th to 6th lumbar vertebrae. It supplies blood to the caudal portion of the colon and to the cranial portion of the rectum.

A large, paired parietal branch, the PHRENICOABDOMINAL ARTERY (1, Fig. 16.16), arises from the aorta caudal to the origin of the cranial mesenteric artery (2). Small branches supply the ADRENAL GLAND (3). It then divides, forming a CAUDAL PHRENIC ARTERY (4) and a CRANIAL ABDOMINAL ARTERY (5). Each caudal phrenic artery courses cranially, supplies blood to the thoracic diaphragm, and anastomoses with phrenic branches of the last several intercostal arteries (collateral circulation). The cranial abdominal artery supplies the abdominal wall of the middle abdominal region, anastomosing with the phrenic vessels cranially, with the epigastric vessels ventrally, and with the deep circumflex iliac artery caudally. Paired RENAL ARTERIES (6) arise from the aorta near the level of the 3rd lumbar vertebra; the origin of the right renal artery is cranial to that of the left. Two left renal arteries may be observed in some animals. Adrenal branches usually arise from each renal artery and pass cranially to the adrenal gland.

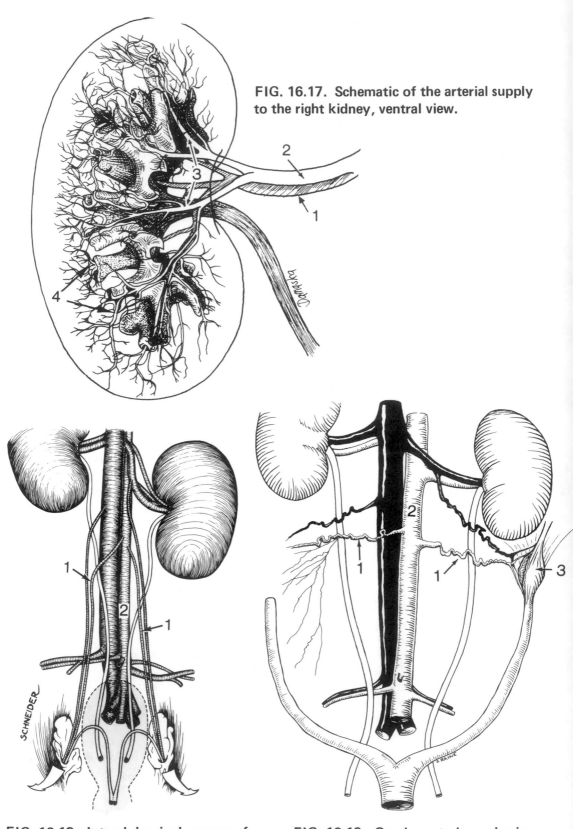

FIG. 16.17. Schematic of the arterial supply to the right kidney, ventral view.

FIG. 16.18. Intraabdominal course of the testicular arteries and veins, ventral view.

FIG. 16.19. Ovarian arteries and veins, ventral view.

The renal arteries usually divide into DORSAL (1, Fig. 16.17) and VENTRAL (2) BRANCHES prior to entering the kidney. The dorsal and ventral branches divide into INTERLOBAR ARTERIES (3), which course between renal pyramids to the corticomedullary junction. Each interlobar artery branches into a number of ARCUATE ARTERIES (4), which spread out over the renal medulla between cortical and medullary tissue. INTERLOBULAR ARTERIES arise from the arcuate vessels and pass at right angles toward the periphery of the cortex, which they supply with blood to be filtered.

In the dog paired TESTICULAR ARTERIES (1, Fig. 16.18) arise from the aorta (2) at about the 5th lumbar vertebra; the origin of the right testicular artery usually is cranial to that of the left. The testicular arteries pass through the inguinal canal and supply the testis with blood.

The paired OVARIAN ARTERIES (1, Fig. 16.19) of the bitch arise from the aorta (2) similarly to the testicular arteries of the male. The ovarian artery and its branches are usually very tortuous; these vessels supply blood to the ovary, wall of the ovarian bursa (3), and uterine tube. A small UTERINE BRANCH of the ovarian artery forms an anastomosis with the uterine artery, thus supplying some of the uterus with blood.

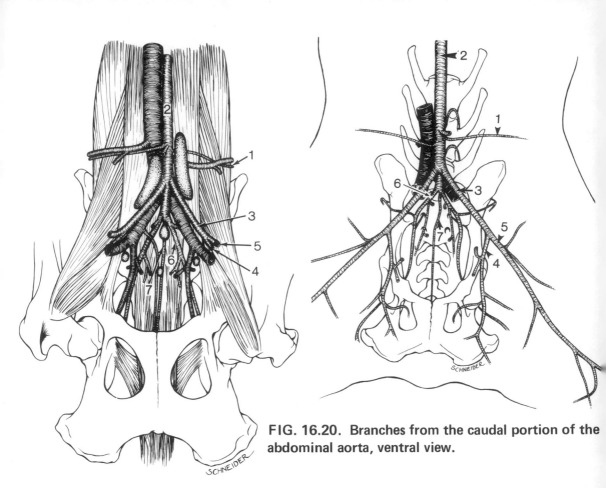

FIG. 16.20. Branches from the caudal portion of the abdominal aorta, ventral view.

FIG. 16.21. External iliac artery and its branches right pelvic limb and external iliac artery, medial view

The paired DEEP CIRCUMFLEX ILIAC ARTERY (1, Fig. 16.20) arises from the aorta (2) at the approximate level of the 6th lumbar vertebra. Its origin is usually slightly caudal to that of the unpaired caudal mesenteric artery. The deep circumflex iliac artery, which may be observed superficially with branches of the lateral cutaneus femoral nerve (see pp. 429, 479), is the main blood supply for the caudodorsal portion of the abdominal wall and much of the skin of the craniolateral femoral region. The paired EXTERNAL ILIAC ARTERY (3) is a large branch of the abdominal aorta that arises near the level of the 6th or 7th lumbar vertebra and exits from the abdominal cavity through the VASCULAR LACUNA. The vascular lacuna of each side is a gap between the inguinal arch and the ilium. Major branches include the DEEP FEMORAL (4) and FEMORAL (5) ARTERIES. The abdominal aorta terminates as the internal iliac and median sacral arteries. The INTERNAL ILIAC ARTERY (6) provides blood to pelvic viscera (and some abdominal structures), to gluteal and caudal thigh muscles, and to the tail. The MEDIAN SACRAL ARTERY (7) continues into the tail as the MEDIAN CAUDAL ARTERY.

The distal continuation of the external iliac (1, Fig. 16.21) through the vascular lacuna (2) is the femoral artery (3), which supplies blood to much of the pelvic limb. The deep femoral artery (4) branches caudally away from the external iliac within the abdominal cavity; the PUDENDOEPIGASTRIC TRUNK, a ventral branch of the deep femoral artery, in turn provides caudal deep epigastric and external pudendal arterial branches. (In cases where the caudal deep epigastric and external pudendal arteries arise separately, a pudendoepigastric trunk is not present.) The CAUDAL DEEP EPIGASTRIC ARTERY (5) courses cranially on the deep surface of the rectus abdominis muscle; it forms an anastomosis with the cranial deep epigastric artery (collateral circulation). The EXTERNAL PUDENDAL ARTERY (6) leaves the abdominal cavity through the caudal portion of the inguinal canal.

FIG. 16.22. Left external pudendal artery of the male, with the left pelvic limb transected and removed, lateral view.

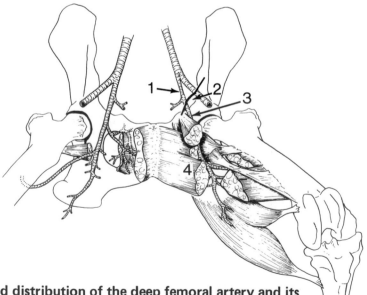

FIG. 16.23. Course and distribution of the deep femoral artery and its continuation and the medial circumflex femoral artery, ventral view.

Near the superficial inguinal lymph node (1, FIG. 16.22) the external pudendal artery (2) branches into CAUDAL SUPERFICIAL EPIGASTRIC (3) and VENTRAL LABIAL (bitch) or VENTRAL SCROTAL (4) (dog) ARTERIES. The caudal superficial epigastric artery courses cranially in the superficial fascia to supply blood to the caudal mammary glands (bitch) or preputial region (dog).

The continuation of the deep femoral artery (1, Fig. 16.23) through the vascular lacuna (2) is the MEDIAL CIRCUMFLEX FEMORAL ARTERY (3), which supplies blood to the adductor muscles (4) and to the nutrient foramen of the femoral bone.

The caudal vena cava (1, Fig. 16.24) collects venous blood from the caudal portion of the trunk through veins that parallel the pathway of arteries; the names of the veins are similar to those arteries with which they course. It should be noted that the LEFT OVARIAN (2) or LEFT TESTICULAR VEIN usually drains into the LEFT RENAL VEIN (3).

FIG. 16.24. Caudal vena cava and its abdominal tributaries, ventral view.

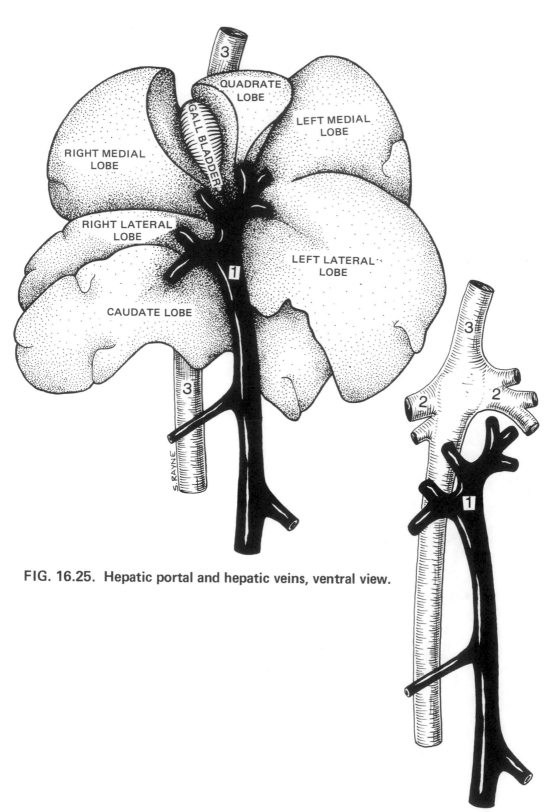

FIG. 16.25. Hepatic portal and hepatic veins, ventral view.

The venous blood of the hepatic portal system (Fig. 16.25) is quite separate from that of the caudal vena cava; blood collects into larger veins from capillaries in the pancreas, spleen, stomach, and small and large intestines and then passes through the HEPATIC PORTAL VEIN (1) into sinusoid capillaries of the liver. Blood is then collected from the sinusoids into terminal branches of a number of HEPATIC VEINS (2), which drain from the liver into the caudal vena cava (3) at a level near the vena caval foramen of the thoracic diaphragm. The branches of the hepatic portal vein are described with the visceral vasculature (see pp. 374–75).

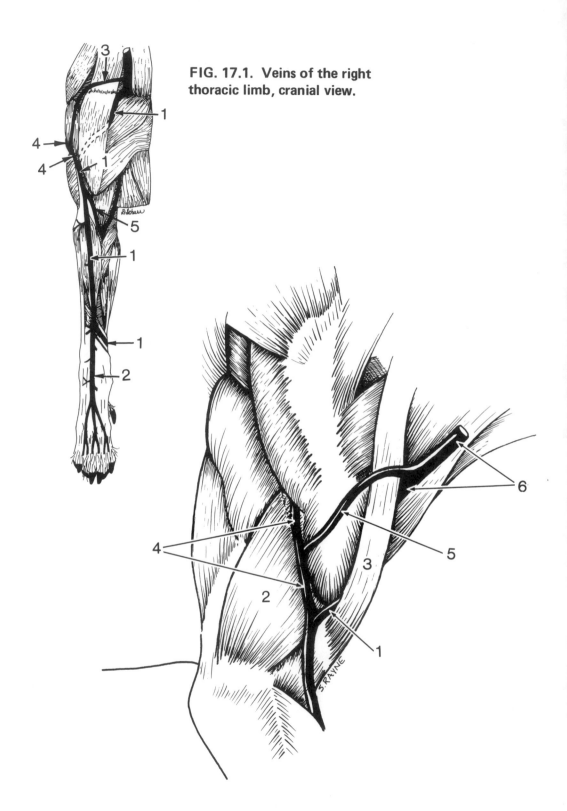

FIG. 17.1. Veins of the right thoracic limb, cranial view.

FIG. 17.2. Superficial veins of the right brachium, lateral view.

17 THORACIC LIMB

The venous system of the thoracic limb consists of two sets of vessels, one deep and one superficial. The deep set consists of veins that accompany arteries and are named accordingly. The superficial set (Fig. 17.1) consists of the cephalic (1), accessory cephalic (2), omobrachial (3), and axillobrachial (4) veins. The CEPHALIC VEIN (1) collects venous blood from the palmar surface of the manus, then passes dorsoproximally across the medial surface of the distal antebrachium to reach a position on the cranial surface of the antebrachium. The ACCESSORY CEPHALIC VEIN (2) arises in the dorsal metacarpal region and joins the cephalic vein on the distal cranial surface of the antebrachium. The cephalic and deeper brachial veins are interconnected at the level of the cubital articulation by the MEDIAN CUBITAL VEIN (5). Occlusion of the cephalic vein proximal to the median cubital vein (preliminary to venous injection) may not produce stasis of blood and vessel distension unless the median cubital vein is also occluded.

In the proximal brachial region the CEPHALIC VEIN (1, Fig. 17.2) passes from the superficial craniolateral surface of the triceps muscle (2) across the cranial border of the brachium, deep to the cleidobrachialis muscle (3), and joins the external jugular vein. The AXILLOBRACHIAL VEIN (4) is a large vessel that continues to course proximally from the cephalic vein on the lateral proximal surface of the brachium, then passes deep through the muscle mass caudal to the humeral articulation. The axillobrachial vein joins the axillary vein in the axilla. A branch of the axillobrachial vein that courses cranioproximally across the superficial surface of the cleidocervicalis is the OMOBRACHIAL VEIN (5), which discharges blood into the external jugular vein (6).

FIG. 17.3. Branches of the brachiocephalic trunk, subclavian, and axillary arteries, cranial view.

FIG. 17.4. Schematic of the tributaries of the left brachium as observed through the sternum and ribs, medial view.

The SUBCLAVIAN ARTERY (Fig. 17.3) is called the AXILLARY ARTERY when it exits from the thoracic cavity and enters the axillary space past the cranial surface of the 1st rib. The SUPERFICIAL CERVICAL ARTERY (1) arises from the subclavian artery near the 1st rib. Two proximal branches off the axillary artery are the external and lateral thoracic arteries. The EXTERNAL THORACIC ARTERY (2) courses with the cranial pectoral nerves and supplies blood to the superficial pectoral muscles. The LATERAL THORACIC ARTERY (3), which courses caudally with the lateral thoracic nerve, supplies blood to the axillary lymph nodes and the latissimus dorsi, deep pectoral, and cutaneus trunci muscles as well as the skin of the lateral thoracic region.

The axillary artery (1, Fig. 17.4) terminates as the SUBSCAPULAR (2) and BRACHIAL (3) ARTERIES. The brachial artery is located along the medial surface of the brachium, cranial to the brachial vein. The subscapular artery passes caudolaterally with the axillary nerve through the intermuscular septum between the teres major and subscapularis muscles; it provides a number of branches at the level of the humeral articulation, then courses caudodorsally along the caudal border of the scapula. Branches of the subscapular and superficial cervical arteries supply muscles, tendons, and joint capsule of the humeral articulation. The branches of the subscapular artery are the caudal circumflex humeral (4), thoracodorsal (5), circumflex scapular (6), and, in some dogs, the cranial circumflex humeral (7) arteries. The THORACODORSAL ARTERY (5) arises from the caudomedial surface of the subscapular and courses caudally with the thoracodorsal nerve to the latissimus dorsi muscle. Small branches off the subscapular artery arborize around both medial and lateral surfaces of the scapula, providing nutrient arteries to the scapula, and forming collateral circulation with branches of the superficial cervical artery. Arising from either the subscapular or the brachial artery, the small CRANIAL CIRCUMFLEX HUMERAL ARTERY (7) passes cranially on the proximal medial surface of the brachium, courses deep to the biceps brachii muscle, and forms a collateral circulation with the caudal circumflex humeral artery and a branch of the superficial cervical artery.

The CAUDAL CIRCUMFLEX HUMERAL (4) branch of the subscapular courses caudolaterally, supplying blood to the triceps brachii and deltoideus muscles; a descending branch, the COLLATERAL RADIAL ARTERY (8), accompanies the radial nerve to the level of the cubital articulation. The collateral radial artery provides the nutrient arterial branch to the humerus.

The brachial artery (1, Fig. 17.5) courses through the brachium on the medial surface of the medial head of the triceps brachii muscle between the musculocutaneus nerve (cranially) and the median and ulnar nerves (caudally). A DEEP BRACHIAL ARTERY (2) separates from the caudal surface of the brachial artery in the proximal portion of the brachium and supplies blood to the triceps brachii muscle. A small BICIPITAL ARTERY (3), which courses craniodistally from the

FIG. 17.5. Arteries of the left brachium, medial view.

brachial artery in the distal portion of the brachium, supplies the biceps brachii muscle. A branch of the brachial artery that courses caudodistally across the medial surface of the distal brachium, between the ulnar and the caudal cutaneous antebrachial nerves, is the COLLATERAL ULNAR ARTERY (4).

A small arterial branch arises from the cranial surface of the brachial artery (Fig. 17.6) near the level of the cubital articulation and courses craniodistally across the surface of the biceps brachii muscle to reach the cranial antebrachial region. This small artery is named the SUPERFICIAL BRACHIAL ARTERY (1) in the brachium and the CRANIAL SUPERFICIAL ANTEBRACHIAL ARTERY in the antebrachium. The cranial superficial antebrachial artery courses through the antebrachium as lateral (2) and medial (3) branches, one on each side of the cephalic vein, to supply blood to the dorsum of the paw. DORSAL COMMON and DORSAL PROPER DIGITAL ARTERIES receive blood via branches of the cranial superficial antebrachial artery (see p. 331).

FIG. 17.6. Superficial brachial artery and its branches: cranial view of the antebrachium and dorsal view of the manus.

FIG. 17.7. Arteries of the left antebrachium, medial view.

The TRANSVERSE CUBITAL ARTERY (1, Fig. 17.7) arises from the craniolateral surface of the brachial artery (2) near the deep surface of the distal end of the biceps brachii muscle.

The brachial artery courses deep to the pronator teres muscle to reach the antebrachium, where it terminates as it divides into two branches, the COMMON INTEROSSEOUS ARTERY (3) and the MEDIAN ARTERY (4). The common interosseous artery is a very short vessel that passes caudolaterally deep into the interosseous space between radius and ulna. The ULNAR ARTERY (5) is a branch of the common interosseous that courses caudodistally across the medial surface of the ulna. The ulnar artery and nerve course distally between the deep digital flexor and flexor carpi ulnaris muscles. A RECURRENT ULNAR ARTERY (6), which may arise from the brachial, common interosseous, or ulnar artery, courses caudoproximally and forms an anastomosis with the collateral ulnar artery (collateral circulation).

The common interosseous artery courses into the interosseous space where it divides into cranial and caudal interosseous arteries. The CRANIAL INTEROSSEOUS ARTERY passes laterally between the radius and ulna; the CAUDAL INTEROSSEOUS ARTERY (7) courses distally in the interosseous space, lateral to the pronator quadratus muscle. NUTRIENT ARTERIES to the radius and ulna arise from the common interosseous artery or one of its branches.

The median artery continues distally through the antebrachium in association with the median nerve. The DEEP ANTEBRACHIAL ARTERY (8) is a caudal branch to the flexor muscles. The RADIAL ARTERY (9) branches from the median artery craniodistally near the distal portion of the antebrachium.

(DIFFERENCES TO BE NOTED IN THE CAT: The brachial artery passes through the supracondylar foramen of the distal brachium. The common interosseous artery and omobrachial vein are usually not present.)

FIG. 17.8. Dorsal arteries of the right manus, dorsal view.

The cranial superficial antebrachial, median, radial, caudal interosseous, and ulnar arteries enter the carpus and contribute to the blood supply of the digits. Vessels of the metacarpus are located at four levels: dorsal superficial, dorsal deep, palmar superficial, and palmar deep. Superficial vessels of the metacarpus are named COMMON DIGITAL arteries and veins; deep vessels are named METACARPAL arteries and veins.

The dorsal arterial plan (Fig. 17.8) is as follows: the superficial DORSAL COMMON DIGITAL ARTERIES I-IV (1-4) supplied by medial (5) and lateral (6) branches of the cranial superficial antebrachial artery; and the deep DORSAL METACARPAL ARTERIES II, III, and IV (7-9) supplied by the radial artery (10) and a branch of the caudal interosseous artery (11). The designation of common digital or metacarpal arteries as I, II, III, or IV is made according to whether the artery is situated within the 1st, 2nd, 3rd, or 4th intermetacarpal space. Each metacarpal artery unites with the correspondingly numbered common digital artery in the distal portion of the metacarpus. Each of the four vessels thus formed interconnects with a palmar vessel and divides into two digital arteries. These dorsal digital arteries are named DORSAL AXIAL (12) or ABAXIAL (13) PROPER DIGITAL ARTERY II-IV according to digit number and whether it is on the side of the digit closest (axial) or farthest (abaxial) from the axis of the foot (see pp. 6-7).

FIG. 17.9. Palmar arteries of the right manus.

The palmar arterial plan (Fig. 17.9) is as follows: the superficial PALMAR COMMON DIGITAL ARTERIES I-IV (1-4) supplied by the median artery (5), with some collateral flow from the caudal interosseous artery; and the deep PALMAR METACARPAL ARTERIES II-IV (6-8), which receive blood from both the radial (9) and caudal interosseous (10) arteries. Palmar common digital and palmar metacarpal arteries of each intermetacarpal space join in the distal metacarpus. Each vessel thus formed has an arterial branch interconnecting with the corresponding dorsal vessel and divides into PALMAR AXIAL and ABAXIAL PROPER DIGITAL ARTERIES.

FIG. 18.1. Veins of the right pelvic limb, caudomedial view.

18 PELVIC LIMB

The superficial set of pelvic limb veins (Fig. 18.1) includes a medial and a lateral saphenous vein. The MEDIAL SAPHENOUS VEIN (1), which is formed distally by cranial (2) and caudal (3) branches, accompanies the saphenous artery and nerve in the crus; the medial saphenous vein joins the FEMORAL VEIN (4) in the distal medial femoral region. The LATERAL SAPHENOUS VEIN (5), which is formed distally by cranial and caudal branches, discharges into the DISTAL CAUDAL FEMORAL VEIN (6) of the popliteal region.

FIG. 18.2. Schematic of the arteries that supply the left pelvic limb, lateral view.

FIG. 18.3. Arteries of the left pelvic limb, medial view.

The pelvic limb receives blood via branches of both the EXTERNAL (1, Fig. 18.2) and INTERNAL (2) ILIAC ARTERIES. Of these two vessels, the external iliac provides most of the pelvic limb with blood. The DEEP FEMORAL ARTERY (3), which arises from the external iliac within the abdominal cavity (see p. 317), passes out into the medial femoral muscles through the caudal portion of the vascular lacuna (4); the continuation of the deep femoral artery peripheral to the vascular lacuna is named the MEDIAL CIRCUMFLEX FEMORAL ARTERY (5). The medial circumflex femoral artery passes through fascia between the vastus medialis and pectineus muscles to supply the muscles of the area, the nutrient foramen of the femoral bone, and the articular capsule of the coxal articulation. The external iliac artery also passes from the abdominal cavity through the vascular lacuna, after which it is named the FEMORAL ARTERY (6).

Proximally in the femoral triangle (Fig. 18.3; see also p. 99), the femoral artery (1) may be felt for the purpose of taking a pulse. The following branches to the pelvic limb arise from the femoral artery (listed from proximal to distal according to origin): superficial circumflex iliac (2), lateral circumflex femoral (3), proximal caudal femoral (4), descending genicular (5), saphenous (6), middle caudal femoral (7), and distal caudal femoral (8) arteries. The SUPERFICIAL CIRCUMFLEX ILIAC ARTERY (2) branches from the lateral surface of the femoral artery in the proximal portion of the femoral triangle either separately from or in common with the LATERAL CIRCUMFLEX FEMORAL ARTERY (3).

The PROXIMAL CAUDAL FEMORAL ARTERY (4) is one of three caudally coursing muscular branches (proximal, middle, and distal); as it crosses the distal superficial surface of the pectineus muscle to supply blood to the adductor magnus et brevis and gracilis muscles, it is vulnerable to injury during surgery in the femoral triangle.

The terminal branches of the superficial circumflex iliac artery anastomose with those of the deep circumflex iliac artery; the terminal branches of the lateral and medial circumflex femoral arteries likewise form a collateral circulation. Branches of the superficial circumflex iliac artery supply blood to the sartorius, tensor fasciae latae, and rectus femoris muscles. Branches of the lateral circumflex femoral supply blood to the quadriceps femoris muscle, the articular capsule of the coxal articulation, and muscles of the gluteal region.

FIG. 18.4. Arteries of the right pelvic limb, caudomedial view.

The small DESCENDING GENICULAR (1, Fig. 18.4) and SAPHENOUS (sah-fe′nus) (2) ARTERIES usually arise from the femoral artery (3) either as a common trunk or close together. The descending genicular artery supplies blood to the cranial and medial genicular regions.

The saphenous artery courses with the saphenous nerve distally across the superficial surface of the genu, near the fascial cleft separating the sartorius and gracilis muscles. The positional relationship of nerve and vessels is the same here as in many other parts of the body, i.e., nerve-artery-vein (NAV). The saphenous artery divides into cranial and caudal branches on the medial surface of the proximal portion of the crus. The CRANIAL BRANCH (4) courses craniodistally to the flexor surface of the tarsus and supplies blood to the dorsal superficial surface of the pes (DORSAL COMMON DIGITAL ARTERIES I-IV). The CAUDAL BRANCH (5) courses distally along the fascial cleft separating the medial surface of the gastrocnemius muscle from the medial head of the deep digital flexor muscle; at the level of the tarsus, the caudal saphenous branch divides into medial and lateral plantar arteries. The MEDIAL PLANTAR ARTERY supplies blood to the superficial set of plantar vessels (PLANTAR COMMON DIGITAL ARTERIES II-IV). The LATERAL PLANTAR ARTERY supplies some of the blood to the deep metatarsal vessels (PLANTAR METATARSAL ARTERIES II-IV).

FIG. 18.5. Arteries of the right pelvic limb, caudomedial view.

The MIDDLE CAUDAL FEMORAL ARTERY (1, Fig. 18.5) arises from the caudolateral surface of the femoral artery (2) in the distal portion of the femoral region; it courses caudally and supplies the adductor magnus et brevis and semimembranosus muscles with blood. The middle caudal femoral vessel is usually smaller than the proximal caudal femoral artery (3) with which it forms a collateral circulation.

The DISTAL CAUDAL FEMORAL ARTERY (4) arises from the femoral artery immediately proximal to where the continuation of the femoral artery (as the popliteal artery) passes distally between the lateral and medial heads of the gastrocnemius muscle. The large distal caudal femoral artery courses caudally and breaks up into a number of branches that supply the popliteal lymph node, muscles crossing the flexor surface of the genu, and the skin of the area. Terminal branches of the distal caudal femoral artery form collateral circulations with the middle caudal femoral, proximal caudal femoral, medial circumflex femoral, and caudal gluteal (see p. 347) arteries.

The POPLITEAL ARTERY (5) is the distal continuation of the femoral artery through the fascia separating lateral and medial heads of the gastrocnemius muscle. It perforates the deep digital flexor muscle and enters the interosseous space between the tibia and fibula, where it divides, forming the CRANIAL TIBIAL ARTERY (6) and the very small CAUDAL TIBIAL ARTERY (7). Small branches of the popliteal artery supply the articular capsule of the genual articulation, the cruciate and collateral ligaments, and muscles of the area. The caudal tibial artery supplies blood to the deep digital flexor muscle. The cranial tibial artery, the larger of the two terminal branches of the popliteal artery, passes craniodistally through the interosseous space deep to the proximal portion of the fibularis longus muscle. It courses through the crus, with the deep fibular nerve, deep to the fascial cleft separating cranial tibial and long digital extensor muscles. The cranial tibial artery supplies branches to the nutrient foramina of the tibia and fibula, flexor muscles of the tarsus, and extensor muscles of the digits.

FIG. 18.6. Dorsal arteries of the left pes, dorsal view.

FIG. 18.7. Plantar arteries of the left pes, plantar view.

The cranial tibial artery (1, Fig. 18.6) on the distal cranial surface of the crus passes deep to the crural extensor retinaculum (2); the continuation of the cranial tibial artery in the flexor angle of the tarsus is named the DORSAL PEDAL ARTERY (3). This short artery terminates as two branches, which supply blood to deep vessels of both dorsal and plantar surfaces of the pes. The ARCUATE ARTERY (4), passes laterally, giving off DORSAL METATARSAL ARTERIES III and IV (5, 6). The DORSAL METATARSAL ARTERY II (7) is a distal continuation of the dorsal pedal artery. The PROXIMAL PERFORATING BRANCH II (8), a branch of the dorsal metatarsal artery II, passes between metatarsal bones II and III to reach the deep plantar surface of the pes. It unites with deep branches of the caudal saphenous arterial branch. The proximal perforating branch II is of nearly the same diameter as the dorsal pedal artery.

Near the level of the distal metatarsal region, the dorsal metatarsal arteries and the dorsal common digital arteries (9) unite to supply blood to the digits via AXIAL and ABAXIAL DORSAL PROPER DIGITAL ARTERIES (10). The dorsal metatarsal arteries are supplied with blood via the dorsal pedal artery; the dorsal common digital arteries are supplied via the cranial branch of the saphenous artery.

The plantar vessels derive blood from the caudal branch of the saphenous artery (1, Fig. 18.7) and the proximal perforating branch II (2). The superficially positioned plantar common digital arteries II-IV (3) are branches of the medial plantar artery (4). The deeply positioned plantar metatarsal arteries II-IV (5) transport blood supplied primarily by the proximal perforating branch II but also by the lateral plantar artery (6) (see p. 339).

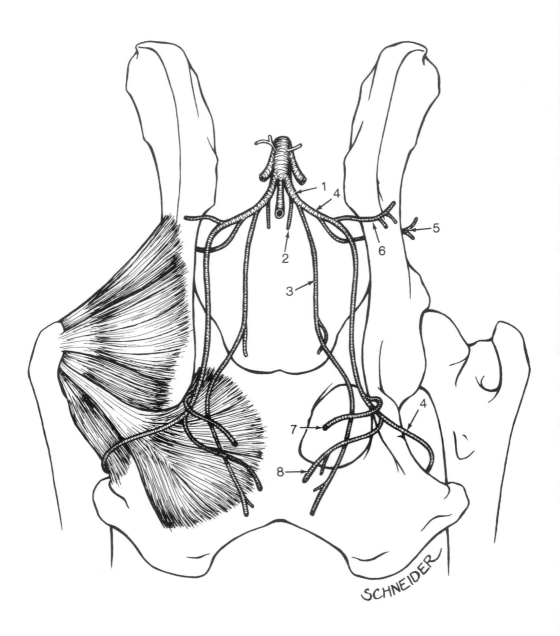

FIG. 18.8. Branches of the internal iliac and caudal gluteal arteries, dorsal view.

The internal iliac artery (1, Fig. 18.8) supplies blood to the pelvic viscera and to structures of the gluteal, ischiorectal, perineal, and caudal femoral regions. The visceral branches of the internal iliac, i.e., the UMBILICAL (2) and INTERNAL PUDENDAL (3) ARTERIES are described in the chapter on the pelvis and tail (see p. 347). The CAUDAL GLUTEAL ARTERY (4) arises as one of two terminal branches of the internal iliac artery, ventral to the sacroiliac articulation, and passes caudally out of the pelvic cavity in association with the ischiatic nerve. The other terminal branch of the internal iliac artery, the internal pudendal artery, is ventromedial to the caudal gluteal artery.

Branches of the caudal gluteal artery in the dog are the iliolumbar, cranial gluteal, lateral caudal, and dorsal perineal arteries. The ILIOLUMBAR ARTERY (5) branches laterally away from the caudal gluteal artery and crosses the ventral surface of the ilium to reach the gluteal muscles. It supplies blood to the psoas minor, iliopsoas, sartorius, tensor fasciae latae, and middle gluteus muscles.

The CRANIAL GLUTEAL ARTERY (6) branches laterally from the caudal gluteal artery and courses past the dorsal surface of the major ischiatic notch with the cranial gluteal nerve. It supplies blood to the middle gluteus muscle and forms a collateral flow with the iliolumbar artery.

The LATERAL CAUDAL ARTERY (7) arises dorsomedially from the caudal gluteal artery and courses caudally past the deep surface of the superficial gluteus muscle to enter and supply the tail. The DORSAL PERINEAL ARTERY (8) arises from the caudal gluteal artery within the ischiorectal fossa (near the origin of the lateral caudal artery) and passes caudally, where it supplies blood to the skin and fascia of the perineal region.

The caudal gluteal artery courses caudodistally through the lesser ischiatic notch, deep to the sacrotuberous ligament, to supply blood to the proximal portion of the caudal thigh muscles. Branches of the caudal gluteal artery may be observed with muscular branches of the ischiatic nerve.

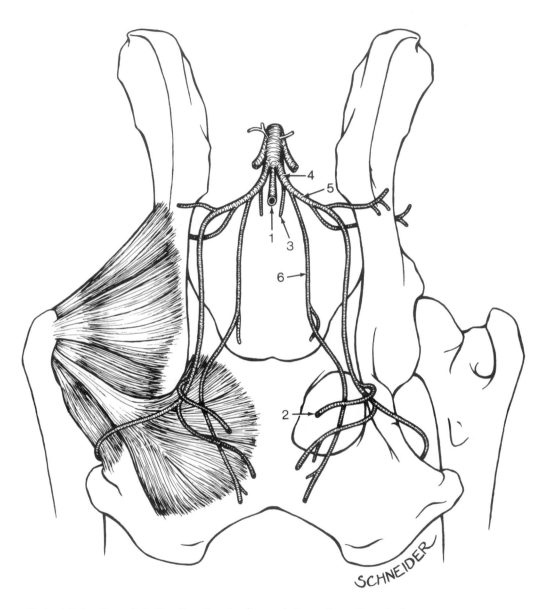

FIG. 19.1. Arterial distribution in the pelvic cavity, dorsal view.

19 PELVIS AND TAIL

Most of the vasculature of the pelvis is described on pages 317, 345 with vessels of the trunk and pelvic limb.

The MEDIAN SACRAL ARTERY (1, Fig. 19.1) supplies SACRAL BRANCHES that enter the ventral sacral foramina and continues caudally along the ventral surface of the tail as the MEDIAN CAUDAL ARTERY. The median caudal artery and the bilaterally paired LATERAL CAUDAL ARTERIES (2), branches of the caudal gluteal arteries, are the three major sources of blood to the tail.

A small UMBILICAL ARTERY (3) arises from the INTERNAL ILIAC ARTERY (4), near the division of the aorta, into paired internal iliac arteries and the median sacral artery. The umbilical artery courses ventrally along the lateral surface of the urinary bladder to supply some blood to the apex of the urinary bladder. The bilaterally paired umbilical arteries are remnants of vessels present during fetal life that carried blood to the placenta.

The two major branches of the internal iliac are the dorsolaterally situated CAUDAL GLUTEAL ARTERY (5) and the smaller, more ventromedially positioned INTERNAL PUDENDAL ARTERY (6). The branches of the caudal gluteal, described on page 345, are the iliolumbar, cranial gluteal, lateral caudal, and dorsal perineal arteries.

FIG. 19.2. Arterial supply to the pelvic viscera of the bitch, left lateral view.

FIG. 19.3. Arterial supply to the pelvic viscera of the dog, left lateral view.

The internal pudendal artery (1) is the major artery to the pelvic viscera and external genitalia (Figs. 19.2, 19.3). It courses caudally along the dorsolateral surface of the rectum (2). The first major branch, the VAGINAL (3, Fig. 19.2) or PROSTATIC (3, Fig. 19.3) ARTERY, courses caudoventrally to the pelvic viscera. Near the anus (in the ischiorectal fossa), the terminal portion of the internal pudendal artery divides into the VENTRAL PERINEAL ARTERY (4) and an ARTERY OF THE CLITORIS (5, Fig. 19.2) or ARTERY OF THE PENIS (5, Fig. 19.3).

In the bitch (Fig. 19.2) the vaginal artery (3) courses caudally to the vagina. The UTERINE ARTERY (6), a cranioventral branch of the vaginal artery that courses along in the mesometrium, supplies blood to the uterus. The cranial portion of the uterine artery anastomosis with a branch of the ovarian artery (see p. 315). The CAUDAL VESICULAR ARTERY (7) is a branch of the uterine artery that supplies blood to the urinary bladder; a URETHRAL BRANCH (8) supplies blood to the urethra; another small artery, the URETERIC BRANCH (9), passes cranially with the ureter. The MIDDLE RECTAL ARTERY (10) branches dorsally from the vaginal artery and supplies blood to the rectum.

(DIFFERENCE TO BE NOTED IN THE CAT: The uterine artery is close to the uterus in its mesometrial border.)

In the dog (Fig. 19.3) the prostatic artery (3) courses caudoventrally to the prostate gland. A ventral branch from the prostatic artery near its origin, the ARTERY OF THE DUCTUS DEFERENS (6), supplies blood to the ductus deferens. This artery supplies collateral flow with the testicular artery to the epididymis (collateral circulation). The CAUDAL VESICULAR ARTERY (7), a branch of the artery of the ductus deferens, is larger than the continuation of the parent artery. It supplies blood to the urinary bladder and forms a collateral circulation with the small cranial vesicular branch (11) of the umbilical artery. URETERIC (9) and URETHRAL BRANCHES of the caudal vesicular artery supply the ureter and urethra, respectively. The MIDDLE RECTAL ARTERY (10) is a caudodorsal branch of the prostatic artery that supplies blood to the rectum. The URETHRAL BRANCH (8) is a small vessel to the urethra that separates from the terminal portion of the prostatic artery.

FIG. 19.4. Arteries of the right ischiorectal fossa, caudolateral view.

FIG. 19.5. Arteries of the penis,
right caudolateral view.

FIG. 19.6. Arteries of the clitoris,
right caudolateral view.

The ventral perineal artery (1, Fig. 19.4) arises from the internal pudendal artery (2) near the anus and supplies blood to the rectum via the CAUDAL RECTAL ARTERY (3), and the skin of the perineum and scrotum (DORSAL SCROTAL BRANCH) or vulva (DORSAL LABIAL BRANCH). Paired VENTRAL SCROTAL or LABIAL VESSELS carrying blood supplied by the external pudendal artery (see p. 319) form a collateral circulation with the dorsal scrotal or labial vessels.

The blood supply to the penis (Fig. 19.5) is carried via the artery of the penis (1), a branch of the internal pudendal artery. The artery divides into three branches near the proximal portion of the penis. The ARTERY OF THE BULB OF THE PENIS (2) enters and supplies the corpus spongiosum penis and penile urethra. The DEEP ARTERY OF THE PENIS (3) supplies the corpus cavernosum penis. The DORSAL ARTERY OF THE PENIS (4) passes distally along the dorsal surface of the penis to supply the bulbus glandis, pars longa glandis, and prepuce. The DORSAL VEIN OF THE PENIS passes through a fibrous ring situated cranioventral to the bulb of the penis; a muscle, the ischiourethralis, arises from the ischiatic tuberosity of each side and inserts on this fibrous ring. Contraction of the paired ischiourethralis muscle results in occlusion of the dorsal vein of the penis and in engorgement of erectile tissue.

The artery of the clitoris (1, Fig. 19.6) supplies the clitoris with blood via three vessels.

FIG. 20.1. Veins of the head, right lateral view.

20 HEAD

EXTRACRANIAL VESSELS

A number of veins are situated superficially on the head of the dog (Fig. 20.1). Some of these vessels are observable on the live animal. The ANGULARIS OCULI VEIN (1) drains blood from the nose to the DORSAL EXTERNAL OPHTHALMIC VEIN of the deep orbital region (or vice versa, since it lacks valves). The DORSAL NASAL VEIN (2) of the dorsolateral surface of the nose joins with the angularis oculi vein to form the FACIAL VEIN (3), which drains caudoventrally over the surface of the face, deep to the levator nasolabialis muscle. A second nasal vein, the LATERAL NASAL VEIN (4), may be present and joins the facial vein caudoventral to the angularis oculi-dorsal nasal venous junction. The SUPERIOR LABIAL VEIN (5), which drains blood from the dorsal lip, joins the facial vein dorsal to the commissure (angle) of the lips. A deep vein that may not be easily observed is the DEEP FACIAL VEIN (6). It courses dorsomedially past the cranioventral portion of the zygomatic arch to connect the facial vein with the VENTRAL EXTERNAL OPHTHALMIC VEIN in the orbital or pterygopalatine fossa area. The INFERIOR LABIAL VEIN (7), superficial to and parallel with the mandible, drains into the facial vein at a point caudoventral to the oral commissure.

The LINGUAL VEIN (8), which drains blood from the tongue, passes caudally out of the intermandibular space through the caudal portion of the mylohyoideus muscle; the lingual veins of each side are interconnected by a venous arch superficial to the basihyoid bone. The lingual vein joins with the facial vein to form the LINGUOFACIAL VEIN (9) at a point ventral to the mandibular salivary glands and

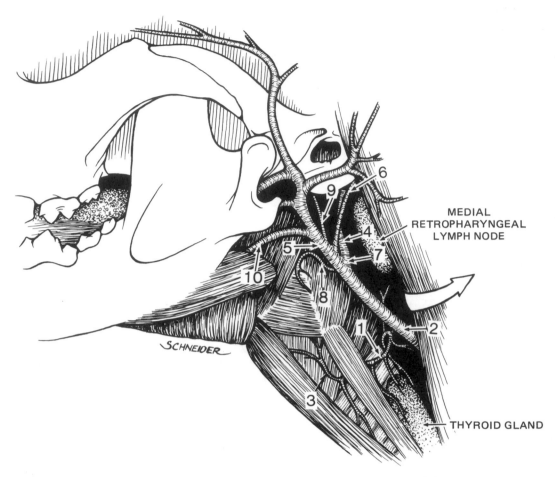

MEDIAL
RETROPHARYNGEAL
LYMPH NODE

THYROID GLAND

SCHNEIDER

FIG. 20.2. Branches of the common carotid and external carotid arteries, left lateral view.

caudal to the mandibular lymph nodes. At the transverse level of the caudal border of the larynx, the linguofacial vein joins with the caudoventrally coursing MAXILLARY VEIN (10) forming the EXTERNAL JUGULAR VEIN (11). The maxillary vein drains the cranium, orbit, and temporal and auricular regions.

The CRANIAL THYROID ARTERY (1, Fig. 20.2), a branch of the COMMON CAROTID ARTERY (2), originates dorsolateral to the second to third tracheal ring. A CAUDAL LARYNGEAL BRANCH (3) of the cranial thyroid artery courses with the caudal laryngeal nerve to the larynx. The medial retropharyngeal lymph node is dorsolateral to the carotid origin of the cranial thyroid artery. The common carotid artery courses rostrally past the deep surface of the mandibular salivary gland and branches, at a position dorsomedial to the rostral portion of the medial retropharyngeal lymph node, into the INTERNAL CAROTID (4) and EXTERNAL CAROTID (5) ARTERIES. The OCCIPITAL ARTERY (6) branches off the external carotid artery immediately distal to the origin of the internal carotid artery. The internal carotid artery may be distinguished from the occipital artery by the presence of a bulbous enlargement, the CAROTID SINUS (7), at the origin of the internal carotid, and the course of the internal carotid toward the tympanooccipital fissure (the occipital artery courses more caudodorsally, supplying branches to the deep cervical and occipital regions). Branches of the internal carotid artery form a portion of the cerebral arterial circle at the base of the brain; the cerebral arterial circle provides a major portion of the intracranial blood supply (see p. 365).

The CRANIAL LARYNGEAL ARTERY (8) branches ventrally from the external carotid artery, accompanying the cranial laryngeal nerve between hyopharyngeal and thyropharyngeal muscles, to supply blood to the larynx and pharynx. A small ASCENDING PHARYNGEAL ARTERY (9) branches rostrodorsally from the external carotid artery near the origin of the larger occipital artery; it provides a collateral blood supply to the cerebral arterial circle by anastomosing with the internal carotid artery near the foramen lacerum. The LINGUAL ARTERY (10) branches off the ventral surface of the external carotid artery and courses rostrally past the medial surface of the digastricus muscle. It supplies a branch to the palatine tonsil and enters the tongue through the genioglossus muscle in association with the hypoglossal nerve (cranial nerve XII).

FIG. 20.3. Branches of the left external carotid artery, left lateral view.

FIG. 20.4. Branches of the left caudal auricular artery, left lateral view.

The FACIAL ARTERY (1, Fig. 20.3) separates from the rostral surface of the external carotid artery (2) at a level caudal to the mandibular angle, deep to the digastricus muscle and superficial to the styloglossus muscle. A relatively large branch of the facial artery supplies the mandibular and sublingual salivary glands with blood. A branch of the facial artery, the SUBLINGUAL ARTERY, passes medial to the insertion of the digastricus muscle and courses rostrally along the medial surface of the body of the mandible in association with the mylohyoid nerve (a branch of cranial nerve V_3). The facial artery courses rostrolaterally through the fascial cleft between the digastricus and masseter muscles to supply blood to the cheek and to the superior and inferior lips.

The external carotid artery (2) courses dorsomedially toward the lateral surface of the tympanic bulla, gives origin dorsally to the CAUDAL AURICULAR (3) and SUPERFICIAL TEMPORAL (4) ARTERIES (caudal and rostral to the base of the ear, respectively), and continues rostrally as the maxillary artery (5). The superficial temporal artery branches from the external carotid at the rostroventral border of the annular cartilage of the ear, courses dorsally past the caudal surface of the zygomatic arch, and supplies blood to the parotid salivary gland; the masseter, temporalis, and rostral auricular muscles; and the palpebrae.

The caudal arricular artery (1, Fig. 20.4), a branch of the external carotid artery (2), courses caudally over the origin of the digastricus muscle, deep to the parotid salivary gland. In some dogs this artery's origin may be from the dorsal surface of the external carotid near the origin of the facial artery. The caudal auricular artery supplies the convex surface of the ear via LATERAL (3), INTERMEDIATE (4), and MEDIAL (5) AURICULAR BRANCHES.

FIG. 20.5. Arteries of the head.

The MAXILLARY ARTERY (1, Fig. 20.5) passes rostromedially by curving ventrally around the temporomandibular joint toward the caudal alar foramen. A branch of the maxillary, the INFERIOR ALVEOLAR ARTERY (2), passes into the mandibular foramen of the mandible and supplies blood to the roots of the mandibular teeth. By following the maxillary artery deeply toward the skull, several arterial branches may be observed. A large CAUDAL DEEP TEMPORAL ARTERY (3) arises and passes dorsally supplying the temporalis and masseter muscles. A small branch may arise from the maxillary artery and enter the temporal bone of the skull to supply the middle ear. A small MIDDLE MENINGEAL ARTERY (4) arises from the deep surface of the maxillary artery and enters the oval foramen; it supplies blood to much of the dura mater of the cranial meninges. The maxillary artery enters the caudal alar foramen, courses through the alar canal, and exits rostrally from the rostral alar foramen.

The maxillary artery emerges from the rostral alar foramen with the maxillary nerve. The first major branch (or two branches) of the portion rostral to the alar canal is the EXTERNAL OPHTHALMIC (of-thal'mic; eye) ARTERY (5). Branches of this artery anastomose with the internal carotid, middle meningeal, INTERNAL OPHTHALMIC, and INTERNAL ETHMOIDAL ARTERIES (some of these arteries are described with the intracranial vessels). The anastomotic branch with the internal ophthalmic artery is a major source of blood to the eye; two LONG POSTERIOR CILIARY ARTERIES reach the bulb of the eye, supplying seven or eight RETINAL ARTERIES to the retina, SHORT POSTERIOR CILIARY ARTERIES to the choroid, and EPISCLERAL ARTERIES to the sclera.

(DIFFERENCES TO BE NOTED IN THE CAT: A RETE MIRABILE, or plexus of arteries, arises from the maxillary artery in the deep orbital region adjacent to the round foramen and orbital fissure.)

FIG. 20.6. Branches of the maxillary artery in the right
pterygopalatine fossa, lateral view.

The maxillary artery (1, Fig. 20.6) courses rostrally between the medial surface of the zygomatic salivary gland and the superficial surface of the medial pterygoid muscle. A small ventral branch, the MINOR PALATINE ARTERY (2), courses ventrally over the palatine bone and supplies the soft palate. The DESCENDING PALATINE ARTERY (3) branches off the medial surface of the maxillary artery at a transverse level deep to the zygomatic salivary gland. The descending palatine artery divides rostrally into the sphenopalatine and major palatine arteries. The SPHENOPALATINE ARTERY (4) enters the sphenopalatine foramen, with the caudal nasal nerve, and supplies blood to much of the rostral portion of the nasal cavity. The MAJOR PALATINE ARTERY (5) enters the caudal palatine foramen, with the major palatine nerve, and supplies blood to the hard palate. A branch of the major palatine artery passes rostrally into the nasal cavity through the palatine fissure and forms an anastomosis with a branch of the sphenopalatine artery. The MALAR ARTERY (6) is a dorsal branch of the maxillary artery that arises near the maxillary foramen; it supplies blood to the lower and medial portions of the eyelids. The nasolacrimal duct and the conjunctiva also receive blood via the malar artery.

The continuation of the maxillary artery into the maxillary foramen is the INFRAORBITAL ARTERY (7). A number of small dental branches separate ventrally from the maxillary artery and enter small foramina of the maxillary bone; these dental branches, plus other branches arising from the infraorbital artery within the infraorbital canal, supply blood to teeth of the upper jaw. The infraorbital artery and nerve course through the infraorbital canal and exit rostrally through the infraorbital foramen. The branches of the infraorbital artery that course over the surface of the nose, deep to the levator nasolabialis, are the LATERAL NASAL ARTERIES; branches of the lateral nasal arteries anastomose with branches of the malar, facial, major palatine, and sphenopalatine arteries.

FIG. 20.7. Arterial supply to the brain and meninges, dorsal view.

INTRACRANIAL VESSELS

The blood supply to the brain of the dog is through a number of arterial channels (Fig. 20.7). The bilaterally paired VERTEBRAL ARTERIES (1) and INTERNAL CAROTID ARTERIES (2) provide the main source of blood to the brain. A vascular connection between the extracranial external ophthalmic artery (3) and the intracranial portion of the internal carotid artery provides an alternative blood pathway. There are other arterial connections between extracranial and intracranial vessels, which are not described here.

(DIFFERENCES TO BE NOTED IN THE CAT: The extracranial portion of the internal carotid artery is vestigeal in the adult cat. The occipital and ascending pharyngeal arteries, which supply blood to the cerebral arterial circle, are innervated by glossopharyngeal nerve fibers.)

The bilaterally paired vertebral arteries enter the vertebral canal, via the lateral vertebral foramina of the atlas, where they join with the VENTRAL SPINAL ARTERY (4), forming the BASILAR ARTERY (5). The single basilar artery passes rostrally along the ventral surface of the medulla oblongata to the junction with the bilaterally paired CAUDAL COMMUNICATING ARTERY (6). A number of paired arteries arise from the basilar artery and course laterally to supply structures of that portion of the brain caudal to the cerebrum.

The meninges of the brain are supplied with blood from ROSTRAL, MIDDLE, and CAUDAL MENINGEAL ARTERIES (which arise from branches of the ophthalmic, maxillary, and occipital arteries, respectively). The middle meningeal artery, which is most frequently injured in humans, supplies the meninges of most of the lateral surface of the cerebrum.

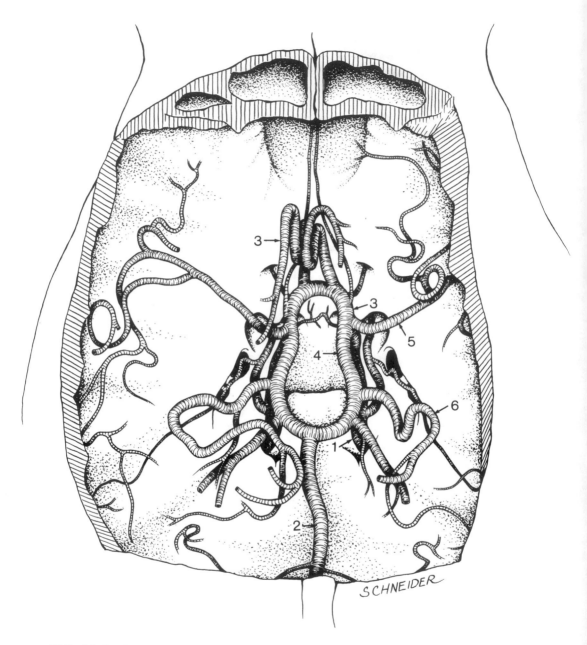

FIG. 20.8. Cerebral arterial circle, with the dorsum of the skull removed, dorsal view.

The cerebrum receives blood via the CEREBRAL ARTERIAL CIRCLE, an arterial circle around the hypophysis (pituitary) at the base of the brain (Fig. 20.8). It is formed primarily by two branches of the internal carotid artery (1) and the basilar artery (2). The rostral portion of the cerebral arterial circle is formed by the bilaterally paired ROSTRAL CEREBRAL ARTERIES (3), which curve around the cranial surface of the cerebrum within the longitudinal fissure. The rostral cerebral arteries supply blood to the medial portion of right and left cerebral hemispheres. The caudal portion of the cerebral arterial circle is formed by the right and left caudal communicating arteries (4), which anastomose with the single basilar artery situated in the median plane. The MIDDLE CEREBRAL ARTERY (5) arises from the lateral surface of the internal carotid artery at the internal carotid-cerebral arterial circle junction. It supplies much of the lateral surface of the cerebrum. The CAUDAL CEREBRAL ARTERY (6) arises from the lateral surface of the caudal communicating artery and courses caudolaterally to enter the groove between the cerebrum and cerebellum. The caudal cerebral artery of each side reaches the dorsal surface of the neural tissue, which connects right and left cerebral hemispheres, in the longitudinal fissure. Terminal branches of rostral and caudal cerebral arteries anastomose.

A number of large venous channels that do not contain valves are present in the cranium and vertebral column; a number of these venous sinuses are located in the outermost meningeal layer, the dura mater. The deep venous sinuses of the head receive blood from the brain, cranium, and scalp and carry it via other venous sinuses and/or veins to the MAXILLARY, INTERNAL JUGULAR, and VERTEBRAL VEINS and to the VENTRAL INTERNAL VERTEBRAL PLEXUS. Vertebral venous plexuses are paired vessels along the floor of the vertebral canal, superficial to the dura mater. Only a few of the venous sinuses are described here.

FIG. 20.9. Venous sinuses within the skull.

The venous blood of the dorsal surface of the cerebrum is collected into the DORSAL SAGITTAL SINUS (1, Fig. 20.9), which is in the long dural fold (the falx cerebri) in the longitudinal cerebral fissure. Blood from the dorsal sagittal sinus drains caudally into the bilaterally paired TRANSVERSE SINUSES (2) through the foramen of the dorsal sagittal sinus. The transverse sinus of each side carries the venous blood to the caudodorsal border of the petrous temporal bone, where it divides into a lateral TEMPORAL SINUS (3) and a medial SIGMOID SINUS (4).

Blood from the temporal sinus exits from the skull through the retroarticular foramen to reach the maxillary vein. The sigmoid sinus supplies blood to the ventral internal vertebral plexus through the condyloid canal and to the vertebral and internal jugular veins through the tympanooccipital fissure.

The CAVERNOUS SINUS (5), a venous pool in the floor of the rostral portion of the cranial cavity, encircles the hypophysis and may have a major role in brain temperature regulation. The venous plexuses of the orbits (external ophthalmic veins) are connected to the cavernous sinus, which in turn is connected to the sigmoid sinus. The terminal portion of the internal carotid artery, a portion of the middle meningeal artery, and the anastomotic branch of the external ophthalmic artery of each side pass through the cavernous sinus, where an efficient heat exchange is thought to take place between venous and arterial blood systems.

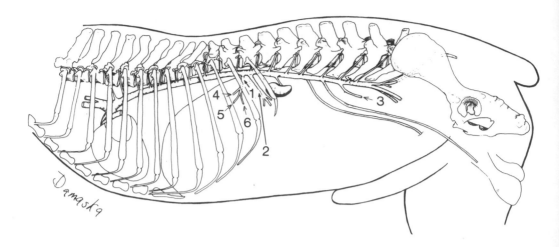

FIG. 21.1. Aortic branches to the abdominal viscera, left lateral view.

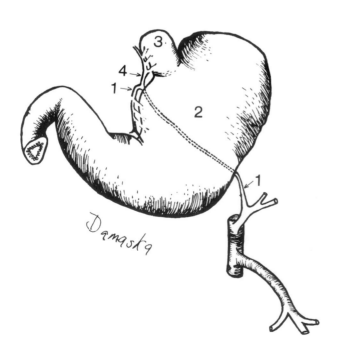

FIG. 21.2. Schematic of the left gastric artery, ventral view.

21 VISCERA

The thoracic viscera exclusive of the lungs (thymus, trachea and bronchi, esophagus, pericardium, mediastinal lymph nodes) receive blood through small arteries that are branches of the internal thoracic arteries, thoracic aorta, or dorsal intercostals (see pp. 309, 311).

Blood vessels to the abdominal viscera course from the abdominal aorta through the dorsal mesentery. Most of the abdominal viscera is supplied with blood by three large, unpaired arteries (Fig. 21.1): the CELIAC (1), CRANIAL MESENTERIC (2), and CAUDAL MESENTERIC (3) ARTERIES. Other blood vessels supply the adrenal glands, kidneys, ovaries or testes (see pp. 313-15), and that portion of the pelvic viscera extending cranially into the abdominal cavity (see p. 349). In the following discussion of the digestive tube the terms cranial and caudal may not imply position relative to the long axis of the body; they may instead imply position relative to the long axis of the digestive tube as though it were stretched out as a straight tube, with the esophagus cranially positioned and the rectum caudally positioned. Two of the three unpaired visceral arteries, the celiac and cranial mesenteric arteries, arise from the aorta and pass ventrally through the ROOT OF THE MESENTERY. The unpaired celiac artery branches to form three major vessels: left gastric (4), hepatic (5), and splenic (6) arteries (the left gastric and splenic arteries may share a short common trunk).

The LEFT GASTRIC ARTERY (1, Fig. 21.2) courses cranially to the stomach (2) where it supplies the cranial portion of the stomach and the esophagus (3). Distal to the point where the ESOPHAGEAL BRANCHES (4) are given off, the left gastric artery courses caudally along the lesser curvature of the

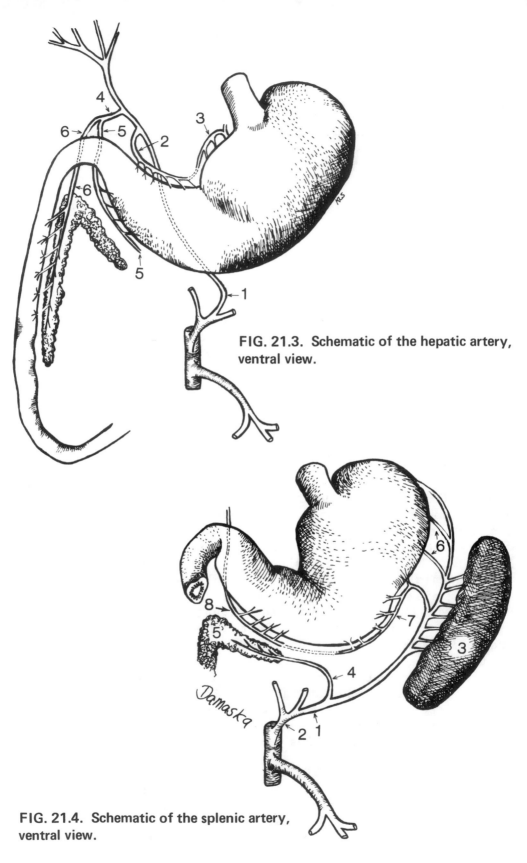

FIG. 21.3. Schematic of the hepatic artery, ventral view.

Damaska

FIG. 21.4. Schematic of the splenic artery, ventral view.

stomach, supplying blood to both surfaces (right or visceral and left or parietal). The lesser curvature of the stomach is embryologically the ventral surface.

The HEPATIC ARTERY (1, Fig. 21.3) courses craniolaterally, dorsal to the digestive tube, and supplies blood to the liver via several hepatic branches: right lateral, right middle, and left hepatic branches. The left hepatic branch divides to form left medial and left lateral branches; the cystic artery arises from the left medial branch of the left hepatic branch shortly before the latter enters the liver. In the portion of the ventral mesentery situated between the liver and the caudal portion of the stomach, the small RIGHT GASTRIC ARTERY (2) branches off the hepatic artery, or off a right hepatic branch, and supplies blood to the caudal portion of the lesser curvature of the stomach. The terminal branches of the right and left (3) gastric arteries anastomose along the lesser curvature of the stomach. The GASTRODUODENAL ARTERY (4) is a short branch of the hepatic artery that courses caudally toward the duodenum; after giving off a small RIGHT GASTROOMENTAL (gastroepiploic) ARTERY (5), the gastroduodenal artery is called the CRANIAL PANCREATICODUODENAL ARTERY (6). The right gastroomental artery supplies blood to the caudal portion of the stomach along the greater curvature (the dorsal margin, embryologically) of the stomach. The cranial pancreaticoduodenal artery supplies blood to the body and right lobe of the pancreas and to a cranial segment of the duodenum.

The SPLENIC ARTERY (1, Fig. 21.4) arises from the celiac artery (2) and supplies blood to the spleen (3). PANCREATIC BRANCHES (4) of the splenic artery enter the left lobe of the pancreas (5). Several SHORT GASTRIC ARTERIES (6) branch from the terminal portion of the splenic artery and supply the greater curvature of the stomach. A branch, the LEFT GASTROOMENTAL ARTERY (7), passes craniolaterally to the greater curvature of the stomach, then crosses caudally along the greater curvature to form an anastomosis with the right gastroomental artery (8).

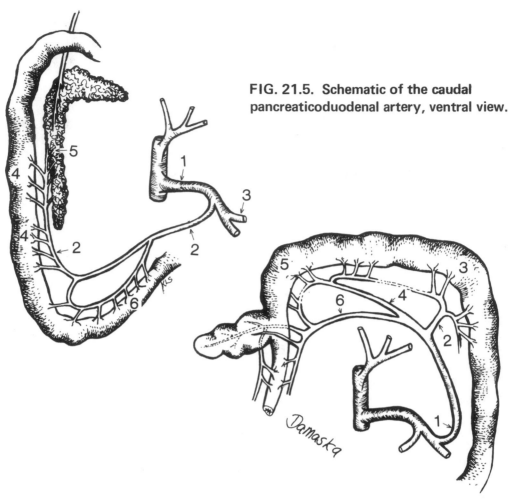

FIG. 21.5. Schematic of the caudal pancreaticoduodenal artery, ventral view.

FIG. 21.6. Schematic of the branches of the common colic trunk, ventral view.

FIG. 21.7. Schematic of the branches of the ileocolic artery, ventral view.

The unpaired cranial mesenteric artery (1, Fig. 21.5) passes ventrally to supply blood to most of the slender (small) intestine and to much of the thick (large) intestine. The first two branches of the cranial mesenteric are the CAUDAL PANCREATICODUODENAL ARTERY (2) and the COMMON COLIC TRUNK (3). The caudal pancreaticoduodenal artery supplies blood to the descending portion of the duodenum (4), which is on the right side of the abdominal cavity; the right lobe of the pancreas (5); and the ascending duodenum (6). The terminal branches of the caudal and cranial pancreaticoduodenal vessels anastomose.

The common colic trunk supplies vascular branches to the ileum, cecum, and much of the colon (Fig. 21.6). The major branches off the common colic trunk (1) are the middle colic, right colic, and ileocolic arteries. A great amount of variation occurs in the pattern and number of these vessels; however, by naming them according to distribution, no great difficulty should be encountered. The MIDDLE COLIC ARTERY (2) supplies the area of the left colic flexure (3), present craniodorsally in the left side of the abdominal cavity. The RIGHT COLIC ARTERY (4) supplies blood to the region of the right colic flexure (5), present craniodorsally in the right side of the abdominal cavity. Arching branches of the right and middle colic arteries supply the portion of colon between right and left colic flexures (the transverse colon); these arcuate branches anastomose. The ILEOCOLIC ARTERY (6) supplies blood to the terminal portion of the ileum, to the cecum, and to the most cranial portion (initial segment) of the colon.

The ileocolic artery (1, Fig. 21.7) divides into the colic branch, the cecal artery, and the mesenteric ileal branch. The COLIC BRANCH (2) supplies blood to the ascending colon, i.e., the cranial portion between the ileum (3) and the right colic flexure (4). The terminal branches of the colic branch and those of the right colic artery (5) anastomose. The CECAL ARTERY (6) crosses the right (dorsal) surface of the cecum (7) and provides most of the cecal blood supply; an ANTIMESENTERIC ILEAL BRANCH (8) courses along the distal (caudal) portion of the ileum on the opposite surface from the dorsal mesentery. The MESENTERIC ILEAL BRANCH (9) passes through the mesenteric attachment of the caudal portion of the ileum. A small CECAL BRANCH (10) arises from the mesenteric ileal branch and courses to the cecum.

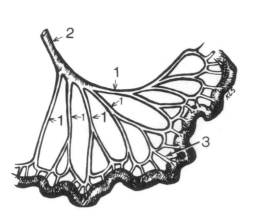

FIG. 21.8. Schematic depicting the distribution of several jejunal and ileal arteries.

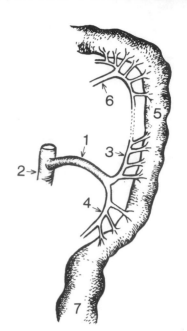

FIG. 21.9. Schematic of the caudal mesenteric artery, ventral view.

FIG. 21.10. Schematic of the tributaries of the hepatic portal vein, ventral view.

A series of JEJUNAL and ILEAL ARTERIES (1, Fig. 21.8) arise from the cranial mesenteric artery (2); these arteries supply the remainder of the slender intestine. Note that these arteries of the intestines branch in the mesentery as they approach the intestine; they join with adjacent branches of other arteries to form arcades. Straight branches from the arcuate vessels that pass to the intestine are termed VASA (sing. vas; vessel) RECTA (3).

The caudal mesenteric artery (1, Fig. 21.9) arises from the abdominal aorta (2) near the level of the 5th lumbar intervertebral disc. The two primary branches of the caudal mesenteric artery are the left colic (3) and cranial rectal (4) arteries. The LEFT COLIC ARTERY courses cranially in the mesenteric attachment (dorsal surface) of the descending colon (5); the terminal branches of the left colic artery anastomose with those of the middle colic artery (6). The CRANIAL RECTAL (pl. recti; straight) ARTERY passes along the mesenteric attachment of the rectum (7), supplying blood to the cranial portion of the rectum (see pp. 349, 351 for middle and caudal rectal arteries).

The HEPATIC PORTAL VEIN drains blood to the liver from much of the abdominal viscera. Upon entering the porta (entrance) of the liver, the hepatic portal vein divides into a smaller right and larger left branch. The sinusoidal capillaries of the liver receive blood from terminal branches of the hepatic portal vein.

The hepatic portal vein is formed by the GASTRODUODENAL VEIN (1, Fig. 21.10), which collects blood from the RIGHT GASTRIC, RIGHT GASTROOMENTAL, and CRANIAL PANCREATICODUODENAL VEINS; the SPLENIC VEIN (2), which collects blood from PANCREATIC, LEFT GASTRIC, SHORT GASTRIC, and LEFT GASTROOMENTAL VEINS; the CRANIAL MESENTERIC VEIN (3), which drains the CAUDAL PANCREATICODUODENAL, JENUNAL, ILEAL, and COMMON COLIC VEINS; and the CAUDAL MESENTERIC VEIN (4), which is formed by LEFT COLIC and CRANIAL RECTAL VEINS.

Lymphoreticular System

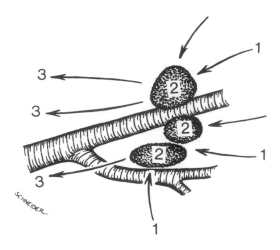

FIG. 22.1. Afferent lymph flow to and efferent lymph flow away from lymph nodes.

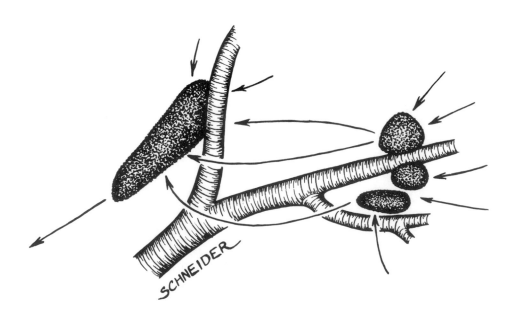

FIG. 22.2. Lymph nodes positioned in a series in a lymphatic pathway.

22 LYMPHATIC SYSTEM

Approximately 15% of the body weight is composed of interstitial fluid; this water, which is bound to the colloidal matrix between cells, is primarily derived from the blood vascular system. Approximately 40 ml/hr of this interstitial fluid is returned to the venous system in a 20 lb dog. The lymphatic system is a part of the circulatory system that functions to recirculate the interstitial fluid back into the bloodstream. Structures of the lymphatic system are generally present in all regions of the body except the central nervous system, bulb of the eye, bone marrow, and within skeletal muscle; however, lymphatic vessels are abundant in the fascial clefts between muscles.

The lymphatic system of the dog (Fig. 22.1) consists of LYMPH VESSELS, LYMPH NODES, and LYMPH NODULES. Lymph vessels are present as AFFERENT VESSELS (1), which drain extracellular tissue fluid toward lymph nodes (2), and EFFERENT VESSELS (3), which drain fluid from the lymph nodes and lymph nodules toward the venous system. When lymph nodes are interconnected in series, an efferent lymph vessel of one node is an afferent vessel for the next lymph node of the series (Fig. 22.2).

Lymph nodes and vessels are quite variable in both location and number; those groups of lymph nodes that occur constantly in the same region of all species and drain similar body regions via afferent lymph vessels are termed LYMPHOCENTERS. Lymph nodes filter out foreign substances from the lymph and produce lymphocytes and plasma cells (which function in the immune response of the body). The lymphatic vessels that drain interstitial fluid from the intestines function also to carry long-chain fats (stearic and palmitic acids) from the viscera to the bloodstream.

FIG. 22.3. Schematic of the lymphatic drainage into veins at the cranial thoracic aperture, ventral view.

FIG. 22.4. Schematic of the terminal portions of lymph capillaries.

FIG. 22.5. Schematic of the internal structure of a lymph node.

All efferent lymphatic vessels eventually drain into veins at the cranial thoracic aperture (Fig. 22.3). Efferent vessels in the region of the cranial thoracic aperture include RIGHT (1) and LEFT (2) TRACHEAL TRUNKS, the THORACIC DUCT (3), and the RIGHT LYMPHATIC DUCT (4). These lymph vessels drain into an external jugular vein (5), a subclavian vein (6) a brachiocephalic vein (7), or a combination of these structures. When describing the distribution of this highly variable system in subsequent paragraphs the term "cranial thoracic aperture" is used as a generality.

The smallest lymphatic vessels are termed LYMPHATIC CAPILLARIES and the largest are named LYMPHATIC TRUNKS, or PLEXI (plek′see, sing. plexus; braid or network) if they occur as branching networks. The terminal ends of lymph capillaries are closed, i.e., the capillary lumen is capped and not structurally open to the interstitial "space" (Fig. 22.4). Valves that prevent backflow of lymph are more numerous and effective in lymph vessels than they are in veins.

Lymph nodes (1, Fig. 22.5) are supplied by a number of afferent lymph vessels (2), which enter the node in the dog through the convex surface. One to several efferent lymph vessels (3) drain fluid from the concave surface or hilus of the lymph node. Blood vessels (4) also enter and leave the hilus of a lymph node; the walls of the smallest blood vessels (capillaries) within the lymph node are thickened, thus ensuring a greater degree of separation between blood and lymph.

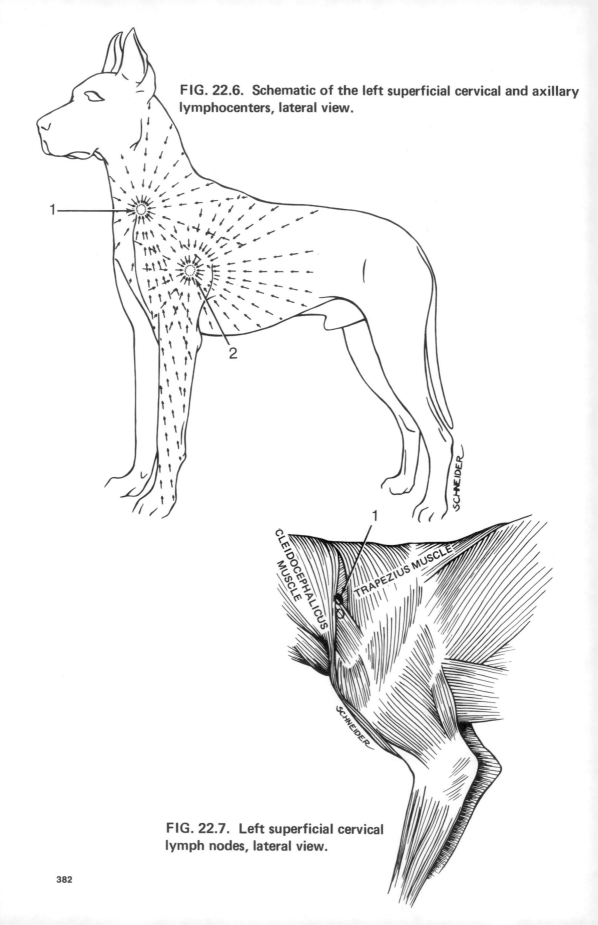

FIG. 22.6. Schematic of the left superficial cervical and axillary lymphocenters, lateral view.

CLEIDOCEPHALICUS MUSCLE

TRAPEZIUS MUSCLE

SCHNEIDER

SCHNEIDER

FIG. 22.7. Left superficial cervical lymph nodes, lateral view.

The thoracic limb and superficial structures of the cranial portion of the trunk are drained by lymph vessels (Fig. 22.6) carrying lymph to either the superficial cervical lymphocenter (1) or the axillary lymphocenter (2).

The SUPERFICIAL CERVICAL LYMPHOCENTER (Fig. 22.7) usually consists of two SUPERFICIAL CERVICAL LYMPH NODES (1), which are located deep to the omotransversarius muscle and cranial to the supraspinatus muscle. The superficial cervical lymph nodes drain the caudal surface of the head, lateral surface of the neck, ventral surface of the cranial thoracic region, and most of the thoracic limb. Efferent vessels drain deeply into the venous system at the cranial thoracic aperture.

The AXILLARY LYMPHOCENTER (Fig. 22.8) consists of PROPER (1) and ACCESSORY (2) AXILLARY LYMPH NODES situated in the axillary space superficial to the first to second and third intercostal spaces, respectively. Usually the accessory axillary and proper axillary lymph nodes are present as one node each (if the accessory axillary lymph node is present at all). The axillary lymphocenter drains fluid from the surface of the thorax and cranial portion of the abdomen and from much of the thoracic limb. The efferent vessels of the axillary lymphocenter course cranially around the 1st rib to enter the venous system in the region of the cranial thoracic aperture.

FIG. 22.8. Left axillary lymph nodes, lateral view with the left thoracic limb removed.

FIG. 22.9. Schematic of the left popliteal and inguinofemoral lymphocenters, lateral view.

FIG. 22.10. Right popliteal lymph node, caudomedial view.

SEMITENDINOSUS MUSCLE

The pelvic limb and superficial structures of the caudal portion of the trunk are drained by lymph vessels (Fig. 22.9) carrying lymph to either the popliteal (1) or inguinofemoral (2) lymphocenters.

The POPLITEAL LYMPHOCENTER (Fig. 22.10), which consists of one POPLITEAL LYMPH NODE (1), is situated deep to the biceps femoris muscle in the popliteal space. Afferent vessels of the popliteal lymph node drain the entire crus and pes as well as much of the lateral and caudal femoral regions. Efferent vessels from the popliteal lymphocenter pass either along with the ischiatic nerve or with the femoral blood vessels to drain into large lymph nodes (medial iliac lymph nodes) located near the origin of the external iliac vessels.

The INGUINOFEMORAL LYMPHOCENTER (Fig. 22.11) is usually composed of two SUPERFICIAL INGUINAL LYMPH NODES (1) situated in the superficial fascia, ventral to the cranial border of the pubic symphysis. In the bitch the superficial inguinal lymph nodes are termed MAMMARY LYMPH NODES since they receive afferent vessels from the caudal mammary glands; the superficial inguinal lymph nodes of the dog are called SCROTAL LYMPH NODES, even though they are located dorsal to the body of the penis and drain fluid from both the scrotum and prepuce. The superficial inguinal lymph nodes collect fluid via afferent lymph vessels from the caudoventral half of the trunk, from the ventral pelvic region (including the vulva or prepuce and scrotum), from the medial femoral and crural regions, and from the lateral femoral and gluteal regions. Lymph nodules are present in the surface layer of the prepuce. The efferent vessels of the superficial inguinal lymph nodes also convey their contents to the medial iliac lymph node.

FIG. 22.11. Left superficial inguinal lymph nodes, with the left pelvic limb transected and removed, lateral view.

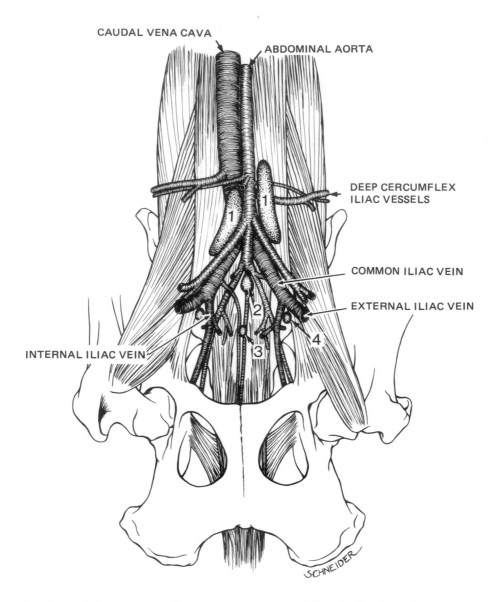

CAUDAL VENA CAVA

ABDOMINAL AORTA

DEEP CERCUMFLEX
ILIAC VESSELS

COMMON ILIAC VEIN

EXTERNAL ILIAC VEIN

INTERNAL ILIAC VEIN

SCHNEIDER

FIG. 22.12. Iliosacral lymphocenter, with the abdominal wall and viscera removed, ventral view.

The ILIOSACRAL LYMPHOCENTER (Fig. 22.12) in the dog is composed of three groups of lymph nodes within the abdominal and pelvic cavities (medial iliac, hypogastric, and sacral); these three groups of lymph nodes are situated adjacent to the external iliac, internal iliac, and median sacral arteries.

The MEDIAL ILIAC LYMPH NODES (1) are large nodes, one on each side of the abdominal aorta, between the origins of the deep circumflex iliac and external iliac arteries. Afferents carry lymph to the medial iliac lymph nodes from the inguinofemoral and popliteal lymphocenters, the hypogastric and sacral lymph nodes, and lymph nodes associated with the caudal mesenteric artery (caudal mesenteric lymphocenter).

HYPOGASTRIC LYMPH NODES (2) are situated along the medial surface of the internal iliac artery near the origin of the median sacral artery; the hypogastric lymph nodes are easily confused with SACRAL LYMPH NODES (3), which are positioned next to the median sacral artery. The sacral lymph nodes are considered to be a subgroup of the medial iliac lymph nodes. Afferent lymphatic vessels of the hypogastric nodes drain the structures supplied by vascular branches of the internal iliac artery--in particular, the rectum, anus, external genitalia, urinary bladder, urethra, uterus, prostate, and ductus deferens. The sacral lymph nodes are small nodes that filter lymph collected from the tail; they drain via efferent vessels into the medial iliac lymph nodes. Efferent vessels from the iliosacral lymphocenter drain cranially into small lymph nodes scattered along the abdominal aorta or into relatively large interconnecting vessels surrounding the aorta (LUMBAR TRUNK).

The ILIOFEMORAL LYMPHOCENTER in the dog usually consists of the ILIOFEMORAL LYMPH NODE (4, Fig. 22.12), which when present is positioned between the internal and external iliac veins as they converge to form the common iliac vein.

FIG. 22.13. Schematic of the celiac, cranial mesenteric, and caudal mesenteric lymphocenters, left lateral view.

The abdominal viscera is protected by three lymphocenters (celiac, cranial mesenteric, and caudal mesenteric) that filter fluid collected from the viscera (Fig. 22.13). Efferent vessels of the cranial mesenteric and celiac lymphocenters drain into the CISTERNA CHYLI (kie'lie; juice) (1), a dilated cranial continuation of the lumbar trunks dorsolateral to the abdominal aorta at a level between the 1st and 4th lumbar vertebrae. The caudal mesenteric lymphocenter drains via efferents into the lumbar trunk (2), the medial iliac lymph nodes, or into small scattered lumbar aortic lymph nodes.

The CELIAC LYMPHOCENTER consists of two HEPATIC LYMPH NODES (3), one on each side of the hepatic portal vein; SPLENIC LYMPH NODES (4), along the splenic vessels; GASTRIC LYMPH NODES (5), near the right gastric artery when present; and PANCREATICODUODENAL LYMPH NODES (6), in mesentery supporting the pancreas and duodenum.

The CRANIAL MESENTERIC LYMPHOCENTER consists of large JEJUNAL LYMPH NODES (7) and RIGHT (8) and MIDDLE (9) COLIC LYMPH NODES. The jejunal lymph nodes are present usually as two elongated nodes that receive afferent vessels from the jejunum and ileum. The right and middle colic lymph nodes are positioned along the correspondingly named vessels. Circular lymph nodules, approximately 3 mm in diameter, in the walls of the cecum and colon are quite visible in the gas-distended large intestine. The efferent vessels of these nodules drain into the colic lymph nodes.

The CAUDAL MESENTERIC LYMPHOCENTER is represented by several CAUDAL MESENTERIC LYMPH NODES (10) that receive afferent lymphatic flow from that portion of the intestine served by the left colic and cranial rectal vessels. Afferent vessels from lymph nodules in the wall of the descending colon and cranial portion of the rectum carry lymph to the caudal mesenteric lymphocenter.

The small lumbar aortic lymph and renal nodes (some 17 or more) form the LUMBAR LYMPHOCENTER. These lymph nodes filter lymph carried through afferent vessels from the parietal peritoneum, kidney, adrenal glands, ovaries and testes, and epaxial structures and the efferent flow from the medial iliac lymph nodes via the lumbar trunk. Efferents of the lumbar lymphocenter drain into either the lumbar trunk or into the cisterna chyli.

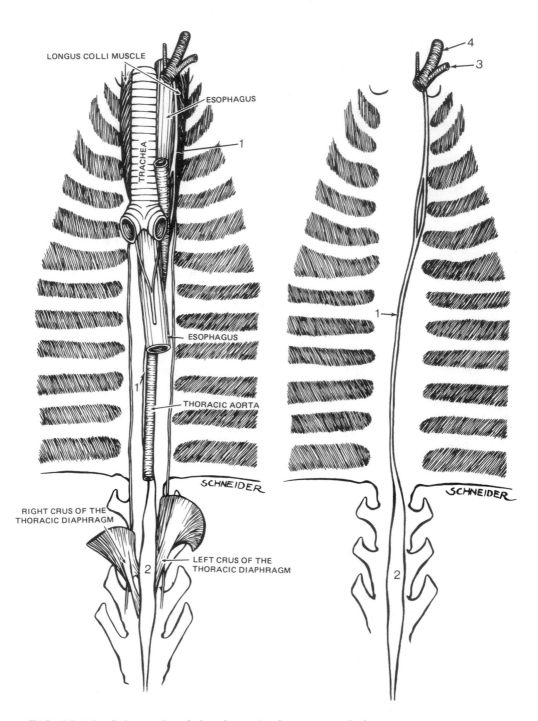

LONGUS COLLI MUSCLE

ESOPHAGUS

TRACHEA

1

4

3

ESOPHAGUS

1

THORACIC AORTA

1

SCHNEIDER

SCHNEIDER

RIGHT CRUS OF THE
THORACIC DIAPHRAGM

2

LEFT CRUS OF THE
THORACIC DIAPHRAGM

2

FIG. 22.14. Schematic of the thoracic duct, ventral view.

The THORACIC DUCT (1, Fig. 22.14) is the thoracic portion of the large lymphatic vessel that carries lymph along the dorsal wall of the abdominal cavity, i.e., it extends from the cisterna chyli (2) to the cranial thoracic aperture, where it joins a vein. The thoracic duct arises from the cisterna chyli between the right and left diaphragmatic crura and courses cranially along the right dorsal surface of the thoracic aorta (here it may be a plexus rather than a trunk). At approximately the level of the 6th thoracic vertebra it passes craniolaterally to the left across the dorsal surface of the aorta. As observed from the left, the thoracic duct cranial to the heart courses cranioventrally in the groove between the esophagus and left longus colli muscle to the area where the left subclavian (3) and external jugular (4) veins join. The thoracic duct terminates as a single or branched vessel, and it may discharge into any of the veins near the cranial thoracic aperture; however, it most likely will discharge its contents into the venous system near the junction of left subclavian and left external jugular veins.

Within the thoracic cavity are four lymphocenters (dorsal thoracic, ventral thoracic, mediastinal, and bronchial). The DORSAL THORACIC LYMPHOCENTER, if present in the dog, is represented by INTERCOSTAL LYMPH NODES in the 5th to 7th intercostal spaces, near the intervertebral disc. Afferent drainage is from the parietal pleura, epaxial structures, and thoracic wall; efferent flow is to the cranial mediastinal lymph nodes of the mediastinal lymphocenter.

FIG. 22.15. Sternal and cranial mediastinal lymph nodes, left lateral view.

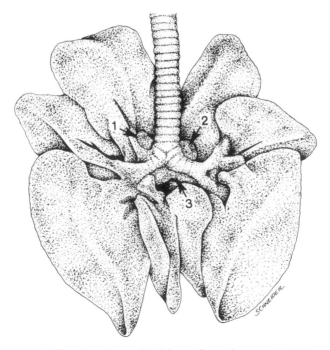

FIG. 22.16. Tracheobronchial lymph nodes, ventral view.

The VENTRAL THORACIC LYMPHOCENTER (Fig. 22.15) is represented by STERNAL LYMPH NODES (1), one on each side, that are positioned along the cranioventral surface of the internal thoracic artery (2). The sternal lymph nodes receive afferent flow from the parietal pleura, mediastinum, thymus, ventral thoracic wall, and thoracic diaphragm. Peritoneal fluid absorbed into afferent lymph vessels on the caudal surface of the thoracic diaphragm is conducted to the sternal nodes.

The MEDIASTINAL LYMPHOCENTER in the dog is represented by lymph nodes present only in that portion of the mediastinum cranial to the heart, termed CRANIAL MEDIASTINAL LYMPH NODES (3). These lymph nodes are scattered along the major vessels cranial to the heart (cranial vena cava, costocervical trunk, subclavian) and filter lymph received from the thymus, trachea, esophagus, and heart and the drainage area supplied by the costocervical trunk plus the efferent drainage of the dorsal thoracic and bronchial lymphocenters. Efferent vessels from the cranial mediastinal lymphocenter drain into the venous system at the cranial thoracic aperture.

The BRONCHIAL LYMPHOCENTER (Fig. 22.16) is composed of RIGHT TRACHEOBRONCHIAL LYMPH NODE (1), LEFT TRACHEOBRONCHIAL LYMPH NODE (2), MIDDLE TRACHEOBRONCHIAL LYMPH NODE (3), and PULMONARY LYMPH NODES. The small pulmonary lymph nodes are located near the terminal end of the primary bronchi, often within the angle of bifurcation of primary into secondary bronchi. The pulmonary lymph nodes receive afferent vessels from the smaller airways and lung tissue; efferent vessels carry fluid from the pulmonary lymph nodes to the tracheobronchial lymph nodes. The three tracheobronchial lymph nodes are situated at the tracheal bifurcation into primary bronchi: a node adjacent to the right azygous vein at the right craniolateral surface of the tracheal bifurcation, a node on the left craniolateral surface of the tracheal bifurcation, and a V-shaped node between the primary bronchi near their origin from the trachea. Efferent vessels from the bronchial lymphocenter drain into the cranial mediastinal lymph nodes.

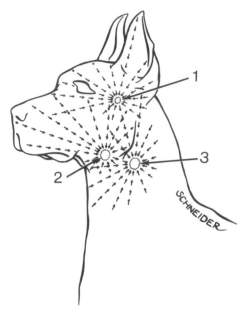

FIG. 22.17. Schemic of the left parotid, madibular, and
retropharyngeal lymphocenters, lateral view.

FIG. 22.18. Right parotid and mandibular lymph nodes, lateral view.

The lymph nodes of the head (Fig. 22.17) belong to one of three centers: parotid (1), mandibular (2), or retropharyngeal (3). The PAROTID LYMPHOCENTER (Fig. 22.18) in the dog usually consists of a single PAROTID LYMPH NODE (1) situated near and partly under the rostral border of the parotid salivary gland (2). The parotid lymph node filters lymph received from the surface structures of the nasal, frontal, orbital (including eyelids), and auricular regions; and from the temporomandibular joint, parotid salivary gland, and lacrimal gland. Efferents carry lymph to the retropharyngeal lymphocenter. Lymph nodules are present on the deep surface of the semilunar conjunctival fold (see p. 13).

(DIFFERENCES TO BE NOTED IN THE CAT: Two parotid nodes are the SUPERFICIAL and DEEP PAROTID NODES. The larger superficial parotid lymph node is on the caudal surface of the parotid salivary gland. The smaller deep parotid lymph node is deep to the rostral portion of the parotid salivary gland.)

The MANDIBULAR LYMPHOCENTER (Fig. 22.18) consists usually of two to three MANDIBULAR LYMPH NODES (3) situated on the surface of the head caudoventral to the masseter muscle and craniolateral to the basihyoid; these nodes are situated both within and dorsal to the angle formed by the bifurcation of the linguofacial vein (4) into lingual and facial veins. The mandibular lymph nodes receive lymph from the nasal, superior labial, inferior labial, mental, orbital (including palpebrae), zygomatic, temporal, masseteric, buccal, and intermandibular regions as well as from the tongue and temporomandibular joint. Efferent vessels pass from the mandibular lymph node to the retropharyngeal lymphocenter.

FIG. 22.19. Schematic of the right medial retropharyngeal, parotid, and mandibular lymph nodes, lateral view.

The RETROPHARYNGEAL LYMPHOCENTER (Fig. 22.19) of the dog is formed by the large MEDIAL RETROPHARYNGEAL LYMPH NODE (1) situated ventral to the transverse process of the atlas (2). Afferent lymph vessels carry lymph from the deep portions of the head and neck, deep portion of the external ear, salivary glands, larynx, cranial portions of the trachea and esophagus, and thyroid glands. Lymph nodules of the nasal and oral passages and PALATINE and PHARYNGEAL TONSILS of the pharynx drain into the retropharyngeal lymphocenter. The efferent vessels of the parotid and mandibular lymphocenters are also afferent vessels of the medial retropharyngeal lymph node. On each side, efferents of the medial retropharyngeal lymph node form a TRACHEAL TRUNK, which courses along the carotid sheath to the cranial thoracic aperture.

Three groups of lymph nodes situated along the trachea form the DEEP CERVICAL LYMPHOCENTER. When present, these small lymph nodes are observed as single nodes on each side of the trachea near the level of the thyroid gland (CRANIAL DEEP CERVICAL LYMPH NODES), middle third of the trachea (MIDDLE DEEP CERVICAL LYMPH NODES), and caudal third of the trachea (CAUDAL DEEP CERVICAL LYMPH NODES). Afferent vessels from the thyroid gland, larynx, trachea, and esophagus enter the deep cervical lymphocenter; efferent vessels from the deep cervical lymphocenter enter the tracheal trunks, thoracic duct, right lymphatic duct, or a major vein at the level of the 1st rib.

The RIGHT LYMPHATIC DUCT, when present, is a combination of the efferents of the superficial cervical lymph nodes and the right tracheal trunk.

Peripheral Nervous System

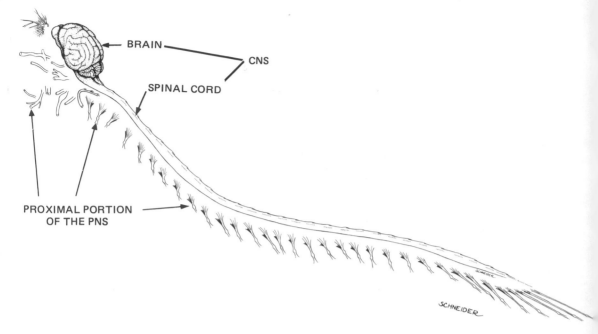

FIG. 23.1. Central and peripheral portions of the nervous system.

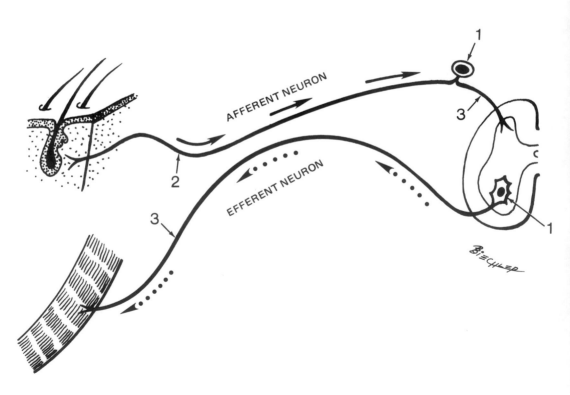

FIG. 23.2. Portions of neurons of the peripheral nervous system.

23 INTRODUCTION

Although the nervous system is one unit both functionally and structurally, it is arbitrarily divided into two major divisions (Fig. 23.1): the CENTRAL NERVOUS SYSTEM (CNS) and the PERIPHERAL NERVOUS SYSTEM (PNS). The CNS consists of the BRAIN and SPINAL CORD. The PNS consists of CRANIAL NERVES and SPINAL NERVES. The nervous system is composed of cells specialized for receiving stimuli and conducting waves of excitation (nerve impulses). These nerve cells (NEURONS) are present in living tissues throughout the body. Neurons are not the only cell type present in the nervous system. GLIAL (neuroglial) CELLS are various cell types (present throughout the nervous system) that support the functions of neurons but do not have specialized powers of irritability and conductivity.

Each neuron (Fig. 23.2) is composed of a NEURON BODY (1) and various processes. DENDRITES (2) are processes that transmit impulses to nerve cell bodies; AXONS (3) are processes that transmit impulses away from the nerve cell body. A transverse section of an axon or a dendrite is microscopic in size; however, many neuronal processes are quite long, e.g., those processes that span the distance between the distal portions of the manus or pes and the spinal cord.

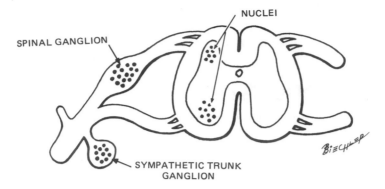

FIG. 23.3. Concentrations of neuron bodies in the CNS and PNS.

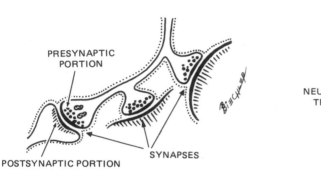

FIG. 23.4. Diagram of three synapses.

FIG. 23.5 Diagram of a myoneural junction.

FIG. 23.6. Diagram of the meninges and epineurium.

Localized concentrations of nerve cell bodies within the brain and spinal cord are termed NUCLEI (sing. nucleus) (Fig. 23.3). Those nerve cell bodies that are situated peripheral to the CNS are usually located in specific places with numerous other cell bodies of other neurons; these accumulations of nerve cell bodies in the PNS are called GANGLIA (sing. ganglion).

Three general types of cells stimulated by impulses carried by a neuron are other neurons, muscle cells (skeletal, cardiac, and smooth), and gland cells.

Neurons that excite or inhibit other neurons do so at cellular junctions named synapses. The most common type of mammalian SYNAPSE (Fig. 23.4) is an area where a very fine cleft separates two neurons and chemical transmitters produced by the one diffuse across to and irritate the other. Neurons that excite skeletal muscle cells do so at MOTOR ENDPLATES, or MYONEURAL JUNCTIONS (Fig. 23.5); during stimulation, chemical transmitters pass from the neuron to the muscle cell across a narrow cleft at the motor endplate.

Both divisions of the nervous system, central and peripheral, are encased in a protective tissue layer. The layer around the CNS is in the form of three membranes, collectively termed the MENINGES (Fig. 23.6). The outermost meningeal layer of the CNS, the DURA MATER (1), is continuous with the EPINEURIUM, or outermost covering of nerves belonging to the PNS. The other two layers are the delicate ARACHNOID MATER (2) and the PIA MATER (3).

The dog has 12 pairs of cranial nerves and approximately 36 pairs of spinal nerves (the caudal nerves are variable in number). It is through these neural pathways that information from the body parts reaches the CNS (afferent or sensory pathway) and by which impulses from the CNS reach their target or effector site (efferent or motor pathway).

AFFERENT NERVE FIBERS conduct impulses from receptors to the CNS; EFFERENT NERVE FIBERS conduct impulses away from the CNS to their terminations on muscle, gland, or other nerve cells.

FIG. 23.7. Diagram of a reflex arch.

AFFERENT NEURON

EFFERENT NEURON

EPINEURIUM

PERINEURIUM

NERVE FASCICLE

NONMYELINATED
NERVE FIBERS

NUCLEI OF
NEUROLEMMA CELLS

MYELINATED
NERVE FIBER

FIG. 23.8. Composition of a peripheral nerve.

Each sensory neuron of a peripheral nerve may have a hundred or more peripheral branches, some of which terminate in the skin and others that terminate on blood vessels, glands, muscles, and joints deep to the skin. Sensations received from the body by the CNS include exteroceptive, interoceptive, and proprioceptive sensations. Touch, pressure, temperature and noxious sensations from the skin are EXTEROCEPTIVE SENSATIONS. Perceptions of pain, burning, and pressure from visceral organs of the thorax and abdomen are INTEROCEPTIVE SENSATIONS. PROPRIOCEPTIVE SENSATIONS are those resulting from muscle tension and alterations in angulation of joints.

Generally, the fewer muscle fibers innervated by a single motor neuron the finer and more precise is the movement produced. The eyeball is an example of a structure that can be moved by very precise and coordinated muscular contractions.

Stimuli, either external to or within the body, elicit neurally controlled activity called a REFLEX. This involuntary response involves transmission of impulses over a REFLEX ARC usually consisting of a peripheral receptor or dendritic ending and its afferent neuron, one or more synapses in the CNS, and an efferent neuron (Fig. 23.7). Most actions of the dog involve reflexes, some of which include the: patellar tendon-stretch reflex, pupillary-light reflex, corneal-touch reflex, and carotid sinus reflex. Reflex activity frequently is modified by impulses originating from other centers in the CNS.

The epineurium is the superficial layer of connective tissue that forms a sheath or casing around a peripheral nerve (Fig. 23.8). A number of bundles (FASCICLES) of axons, each contained within its own connective tissue sheath or PERINEURIUM, are situated deep to the epineurium. Each axon is in turn ensheathed in a layer of cells, collectively named the NEUROLEMMA. Larger axons are insulated by a MYELIN LAYER, which is formed by spirals of the external cell membrane of the neurolemmal cells and is situated between the axon and the remainder of the neurolemma. Myelin is a white, glistening, fatty material that imparts to the nerve its white appearance. Neurons with little myelin are described as being NONMYELINATED. MYELINATED NERVE FIBERS transmit nerve impulses more rapidly than nonmyelinated fibers. Each axon and its neurilemma cells are supported by a thin connective tissue sheath called the ENDONEURIUM.

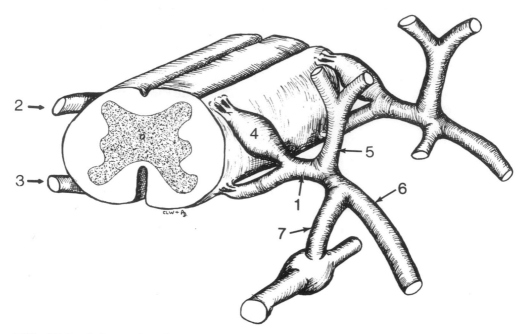

FIG. 23.9. Schematic of a segment of the spinal cord and the roots and proximal branches of a spinal nerve.

TABLE 23.1. Functional classification of neurons in spinal nerves.

	Direction of impulse	Functional class
Sensation		
Pain, temperature, touch	To CNS	General somatic afferent (GSA)
Fullness from distention of the alimentary canal Pain from lack of blood in the viscera	To CNS	General visceral afferent (GVA)
Changes in chemical content	To CNS	General visceral afferent (GVA)
Joint or muscle movement	To CNS	General proprioceptive (GP)
Action		
Fiber contraction in most skeletal muscles	From CNS	General somatic efferent (GSE)
Fiber contraction in skeletal muscle derived from mesoderm of the branchial arch	From CNS	Special visceral efferent (SVE)
Fiber contraction in smooth and cardiac muscle	From CNS	General visceral efferent (GVE)
Secretion by glands	From CNS	General visceral efferent (GVE)

Of the 36 pairs of spinal nerves in the dog, 8 are cervical (one more than the number of corresponding vertebrae), 13 are thoracic, 7 are lumbar, 3 are sacral, and 4-7 are caudal. The spinal nerves or their branches exit from the vertebral column bilaterally through intervertebral foramina; three exceptions to the preceding occur: the first cervical and first two sacral spinal nerves exit from the vertebral canal through foramina surrounded by bone.

Each spinal nerve (1, Fig. 23.9) is attached to the spinal cord by two roots, a DORSAL (2) and a VENTRAL (3) ROOT. Each root, in turn, is composed of a number of rootlets. Afferent impulses enter the spinal cord through the rootlets of the dorsal root of each spinal nerve. In each dorsal root an enlargement, the SPINAL GANGLION (4), is the result of an assemblage of nerve cell bodies of the sensory neurons contained in each spinal nerve. Efferent impulses leave the spinal cord through the rootlets of the ventral root of each spinal nerve. The nerve cell bodies of motor neurons are situated in the spinal cord. Distal to the junction of dorsal and ventral roots, the spinal nerve contains both sensory and motor nerve fibers.

A typical spinal nerve branches into two primary rami (dorsal and ventral) near the level of the intervertebral foramen; each of these primary rami conducts both afferent and efferent impulses. The DORSAL RAMUS (ra mus, pl. rami; branch) (5), typically as in the thoracic region, divides into a MEDIAL BRANCH, which innervates the spinal meninges and epaxial muscles, and a LATERAL BRANCH, which innervates primarily the skin. The VENTRAL RAMUS (6), supplies hypaxial structures. Most spinal nerves have a COMMUNICATING RAMUS (7) with the sympathetic portion of the autonomic nervous system; these junctions of spinal nerves with communicating branches occur near the intervertebral foramina.

Neurons are classified functionally (Table 23.1) according to the nature of the impulse (sensory or motor) and type of structure innervated (somatic or visceral).

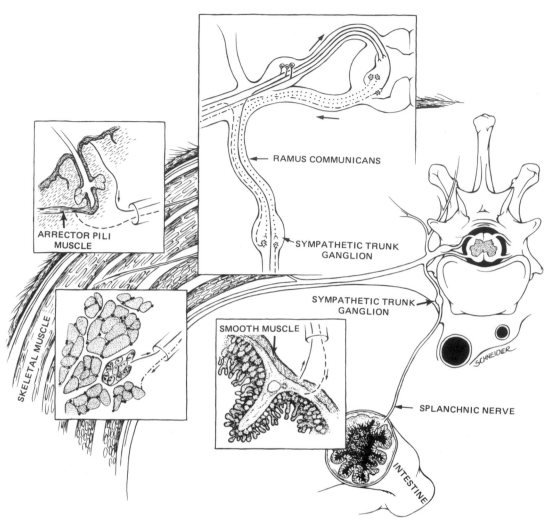

FIG. 23.10. Schematic of the pathway of sensory fibers from and motor fibers to the skin, skeletal muscles, and digestive tract.

Motor innervation of skeletal muscle (GSE) takes place through a one-neuron span from the CNS to the motor endplate (Fig. 23.10).   Sensory innervation from the skin, skeletal muscle, and joints (GSA) and from the viscera and visceral pleura and peritoneum (GVA) also occurs in a one neuron system spanning the distance from the receptor to the spinal cord.   Motor innervation of smooth muscle, cardiac muscle, and glands (GVE) occurs through a two-neuron span from the spinal cord to the effector site.   Another commonly used term for the GVE system is the AUTONOMIC NERVOUS SYSTEM (ANS); impulses of this important efferent system arise and exit from the CNS through four cranial nerves (III, VII, IX, and X), all the thoracic spinal nerves, the first five or six lumbar spinal nerves, and the sacral spinal nerves.

Efferent fibers to visceral structures arising from the brain through cranial nerves III, VII, IX, and X and from the sacral segment of the spinal cord form the PARASYMPATHETIC PORTION OF THE ANS, which is concerned with vegetative functions such as digestion and absorption.   Although the parasymphathetic nerve fibers arise from the craniosacral region of the body, some of them are distributed throughout the thoracic and abdominal cavities.

Efferent fibers to visceral structures that arise from the thoracolumbar portion of the spinal cord form the SYMPATHETIC PORTION OF THE ANS.   Although the sympathetic fibers arise from the thoracic and lumbar portions of the CNS, they are distributed with peripheral nerves and blood vessels to all parts of the body.   The sympathetic nervous system is concerned with the "flight or fight" state of the body.

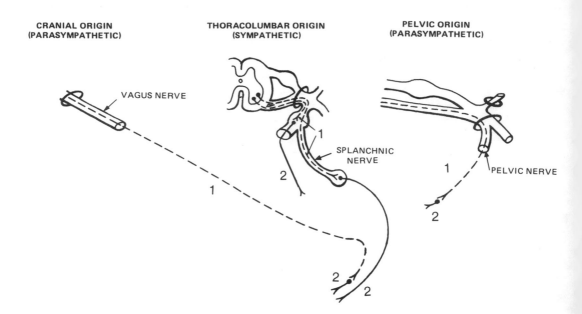

FIG. 23.11. Pathway of autonomic fibers.

Nerves observed within the thoracic, abdominal, and pelvic cavities are, with few exceptions, autonomic and contain GVE fibers; however, GVA fibers are also present in these nerves to the viscera. The GVE nerves in the major cavities of the body may be parasympathetic, sympathetic, or both; the individual fibers may be PREGANGLIONIC (1) or POSTGANGLIONIC (2, Fig. 23.11). Each of the divisions of efferent systems consists of two neurons connecting the CNS with the structure innervated. The nerve cell body of the proximal or preganglionic neuron is situated in either the thoracolumbar portion of the spinal cord (sympathetic), sacral portion of the spinal cord (parasympathetic), or brain (parasympathetic); the nerve cell body of the distal or postganglionic neuron is generally in a ganglion situated proximal to the structure innervated (sympathetic neuron) or in the structure innervated (parasympathetic neuron).

Anastomoses between blood vessels that course along in the connective tissue of peripheral nerves are so plentiful that a nerve may be freed from its attachments for a considerable distance (15 cm in some cases) during surgery without appreciable damage being done. Nerve fibers are organized in a "wavy" or undulating pattern in peripheral nerves. This undulating pattern permits the stretching of nerves without harm to individual nerve fibers; the perineurium is a tough layer of connective tissue that takes up most of the tension produced during stretching.

Nerves may be paralyzed in various degrees of severity by pressure. The more mild paralysis results from anoxia due to interference with blood flow. More severe paralysis may be due to destruction of axons and their connective tissue sheaths. Neural processes within peripheral nerves are capable of regeneration; this regenerative process is dependent to a large extent upon the integrity of the connective tissue sheaths surrounding the axons and nerve fascicles.

FIG. 24.1. Cervical intumescence, dorsal view.

FIG. 24.2. Left brachial plexus, lateral view.

24 THORACIC LIMB

The nerves that innervate the muscles, skin, and joints of the thoracic limb arise from or reach the spinal cord at the level of the 5th cervical through 1st thoracic vertebrae. Due to the many afferent and efferent neurons that pass between structures of the limb and spinal cord, this region is enlarged, nearly filling the vertebral canal. This localized enlargement of the spinal cord is termed the CERVICAL INTUMESCENCE (in"tu-mes'ens; swelling) (1, Fig. 24.1).

The ventral rami of a number of spinal nerves, usually C6, C7, C8, and T1, interconnect distal to the vertebral column, forming a tangle or network of nerve trunks. This tangle, called the BRACHIAL PLEXUS (1, Fig. 24.2), supplies nerves to the thoracic limb. A couple of nerves to the thoracic limb are direct continuations of the ventral rami and are not formed by the plexus, i.e., the intercostobrachial nerves are lateral branches of intercostal nerves (see p. 475). Distal to the brachial plexus, individual nerves supplying extrinsic and intrinsic structures of the thoracic limb may be identified; many of these nerves are formed by fibers from more than one level of the spinal cord. The spinal nerves that supply ventral rami to the brachial plexus exit from the vertebral canal between vertebrae as follows: C6--between the 5th and 6th cervical vertebrae; C7--between the 6th and 7th cervical vertebrae; C8--between the 7th cervical and the 1st thoracic vertebrae; and T1--between the 1st and 2nd thoracic vertebrae (Fig. 24.2).

FIG. 24.3. Brachiocephalic nerve,
cranial view.

SCALENUS

MUSCLE

A

B

FIG. 24.4. Branches of the left brachial plexus, lateral view.

The brachial plexus is situated within the axillary space at a level cranial to the 1st rib, ventral to the scalenus muscle, and dorsal to the pectoralis muscles. Those spinal nerves that innervate extrinsic structures of the thoracic limb include the brachiocephalic, cranial pectoral, long thoracic, thoracodorsal, lateral thoracic, and caudal pectoral nerves.

A muscular branch of the BRACHIOCEPHALIC NERVE (1, Fig. 24.3) enters the brachiocephalicus muscle near the clavicular intersection, cranial to the humeral articulation. A cutaneous branch of the brachiocephalic nerve innervates the skin of the cranial humeral region. The CRANIAL PECTORAL NERVES (2) are usually present as two nerves that pass ventrally to supply the superficial pectoral muscle.

The LONG THORACIC NERVE (1, Fig. 24.4) courses caudally on the superficial surface of the serratus ventralis muscle, which it innervates. The THORACODORSAL NERVE (2) courses caudally on the deep surface of the latissimus dorsi muscle, which it innervates. A superficial nerve, which may be confused with the more deeply and more dorsally situated thoracodorsal, is the LATERAL THORACIC NERVE (3). It courses caudally near the ventral margin of the latissimus dorsi and dorsolateral border of the deep pectoral muscles and innervates the cutaneous trunci muscle. Cutaneous branches, which pass from the lateral thoracic nerves to the skin, are fibers that reach the lateral thoracic from lateral cutaneous branches of intercostal nerves (INTERCOSTOBRACHIAL NERVES, see p. 475). Three or four nerve branches innervate the deep pectoral muscle; these CAUDAL PECTORAL NERVES (4) usually arise from the brachial plexus in common with the lateral thoracic nerve.

Other nerves to extrinsic muscles of the thoracic limb, some of which are described on page 473, include the accessory nerve (to the trapezius, omotransversarius, and cleidocephalicus muscles) and ventral branches of cervical and thoracic spinal nerves (to the cleidocephalicus, rhomboideus, and omotransversarius muscles).

FIG. 24.5. Branches of the right
brachial plexus, medial view.

FIG. 24.6. Nerves to the left
thoracic limb, medial view.

FIG. 24.7. Right shoulder dissected
to demonstrate the suprascapular
nerve, lateral view.

FIG. 24.8. Musculotaneous nerve
and deep structures of the left
thoracic limb, medial view.

Nerves to the intrinsic structures of the thoracic limb (Figs. 24.5, 24.6) are the suprascapular (1), subscapular (2), musculocutaneous (3), axillary (4), radial (5), median (6), and ulnar (7) nerves. Since these nerves may be involved in injuries of the thoracic limb or may evidence, through their loss of function, damage to the spinal cord, they are of considerable importance to the veterinarian. Nerves that distribute fibers to the antebrachial region and/or manus are the musculocutaneus, axillary, radial, median, and ulnar nerves.

The SUPRASCAPULAR NERVE (1, Fig. 24.6; 1, Fig. 24.7) courses around the cranial border of the scapula to supply the supraspinatus and infraspinatus muscles. Note that this nerve passes between the supraspinatus and subscapularis muscles to reach the scapular notch, through which it attains the lateral surface of the scapula. The suprascapular nerve is susceptible to damage from pressure applied to the craniodistal border of the scapula; a severely damaged suprascapular nerve will result in atrophy of the supraspinatus and infraspinatus muscles. The SUBSCAPULAR NERVES (2, Fig. 24.6) innervate the subscapularis muscle. Branches of these nerves will not be observed on the lateral or superficial surface of the scapula since they enter the deep surface of the subscapularis.

The MUSCULOCUTANEOUS NERVE (3, Fig. 24.6; 1, Fig. 24.8) courses down the medial surface of the brachium in contact with the biceps brachii muscle and in close assocation with the cranial border of the major artery of the arm (brachial artery). A small branch (2) of the musculocutaneous nerve separates off from the parent trunk, proximal and deep to the humeral articulation, and innervates the coracobrachialis muscle. On the proximal medial surface of the brachium a proximal muscular branch (3) of the musculocutaneus supplies the biceps brachii muscle. On the distal third of the medial surface of the brachium the musculocutaneous nerve splits into two branches; fibers of one branch (4) join with the median nerve (5) and are distributed distally with the various branches of the median nerve to carpal and digital flexor muscles. The other branch (6), a continuation of the musculocutaneous nerve, crosses the deep (lateral) surface of the distal portion of the biceps brachii, innervates the brachialis muscle at the level of the cubital articulation, and continues as a small cutaneous nerve. This MEDIAL CUTANEOUS ANTEBRACHIAL NERVE (7) supplies the skin on the craniomedial portion of the antebrachium.

FIG. 24.9. Nerves to the left thoracic limb, medial surface.

AXILLOBRACHIAL VEIN

CEPHALIC VEIN

CRANIOLATERAL VIEW

LATERAL VIEW

FIG. 24.10. Radial nerve and left thoracic limb.

The AXILLARY NERVE (1, Fig. 24.9) is a large nerve bundle that spans the axillary space to reach the caudomedial surface of the shoulder. It passes between the subscapular and teres major muscles at the level of the neck of the scapula, supplying muscular branches to the teres major, teres minor, deltoideus, and the caudal part of the subscapularis muscles. A fracture through the neck of the scapula may involve the axillary nerve. A portion of the axillary nerve, the CRANIAL LATERAL CUTANEOUS BRACHIAL NERVE, observed superficially between the deltoideus and lateral head of the triceps brachii muscles, provides innervation to the skin of the craniolateral surface of the brachium. Fibers of the cranial lateral cutaneous brachial nerve continue into the antebrachium as the CRANIAL CUTANEOUS ANTEBRACHIAL NERVE and provide innervation to the cranial surface of the antebrachium.

The RADIAL NERVE (2) is the largest and most important (in terms of locomotion) nerve of the brachial plexus. Within the axillary space, the radial nerve is parallel and adjacent to the common trunk (3) of the median and ulnar nerves. The radial nerve crosses the axilla to the caudal surface of the brachium where it enters the tricipital muscle mass, passing distally between the long and medial heads of the triceps brachii muscle.

Near the level at which the radial nerve enters the tricipital muscle, some muscular branches (1, Fig. 24.10) supply the long head, accessory head, and medial head of the triceps brachii muscle. The main continuation of the radial nerve courses distally between the triceps brachii and the brachialis muscles. The radial nerve and brachialis muscle are positioned in a spiralling pattern from the caudal border of the humerus (proximally) to the craniolateral border of the humerus (distally). The radial nerve provides muscular branches to the lateral head of the triceps brachii muscle and the anconeus muscle near the distal portion of the brachium.

Deep to the lateral head of the triceps brachii muscle, the radial nerve divides into superficial (2) and deep (3) branches. The SUPERFICIAL BRANCH OF THE RADIAL NERVE may be located in the fascia beneath the skin on the distal lateral surface of the brachialis muscle. It divides into MEDIAL (4) and LATERAL (5) BRANCHES. The smaller (medial) branch, which may be joined by fibers of the cranial cutaneous antebrachial nerve (of the axillary), is situated on the medial surface of the cephalic vein and craniolateral to the medial cutaneous antebrachial nerve (of the musculocutaneous).

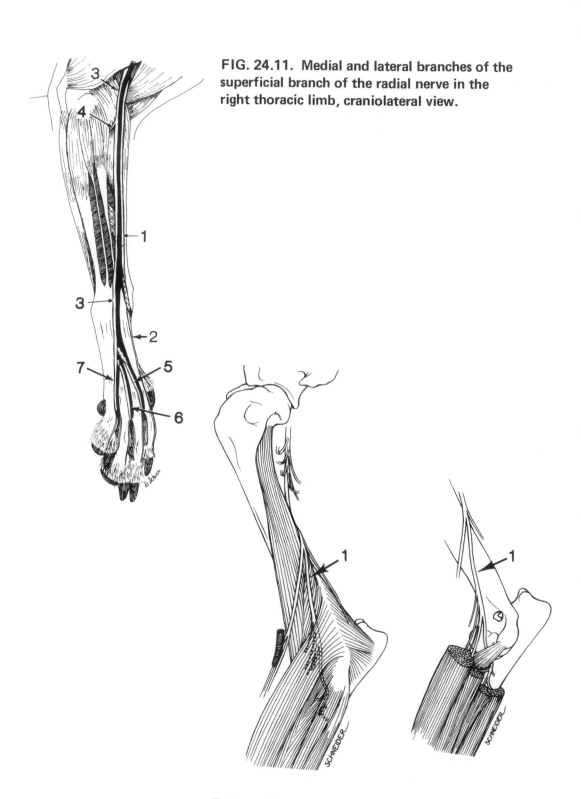

FIG. 24.11. Medial and lateral branches of the superficial branch of the radial nerve in the right thoracic limb, craniolateral view.

FIG. 24.12. Deep branch of the radial nerve and deep structures of the left thoracic limb, lateral view.

The medial branch of the superficial branch of the radial nerve (1, Fig. 24.11) in the metacarpal region is named the DORSAL COMMON DIGITAL NERVE I (2). (The designation of I, II, III, or IV is made according to whether the common digital nerve is situated superficial the 1st, 2nd, 3rd, or 4th intermetacarpal space.) The dorsal common digital nerve supplies the dorsal axial surface of digit I and the dorsal abaxial surface of digit II as the DORSAL PROPER DIGITAL NERVES. The lateral branch (3) of the superficial branch of the radial nerve courses along the lateral surface of the cephalic vein. Near the level of the cubital articulation the LATERAL CUTANEOUS ANTEBRACHIAL NERVE (4) arises from the lateral branch of the superficial radial to supply the skin of the craniolateral portion of the antebrachium. The lateral branch of the superficial branch of the radial nerve divides over the dorsal surface of the metacarpus into DORSAL COMMON DIGITAL NERVES II, III, and IV (5-7, respectively). Each of the dorsal common digital nerves divides, forming two dorsal proper digital nerves (e.g., dorsal common digital nerve II divides into two dorsal proper digital nerves: one supplying the dorsal axial surface of digit II and the other supplying the dorsal abaxial surface of digit III).

The DEEP BRANCH OF THE RADIAL NERVE (1, Fig. 24.12) enters the antebrachium deep to the extensor carpi radialis muscle and divides into a number of branches that supply the craniolateral (extensor) group of muscles of the antebrachium.

FIG. 24.13. Median and ulnar nerves of the left thoracic limb, medial view.

The MEDIAN NERVE (1, Fig. 24.13) is usually bound to the ulnar nerve (2) by connective tissue in the axilla and proximal brachial regions. The median nerve is positioned on the medial surface of the brachium, deep to the skin and superficial pectoral muscle, caudal to the brachial artery, and cranial to the ulnar nerve. At the transverse level of the cubital articulation, the median nerve, brachial artery, and ulnar nerve are quite superficially situated near the medial epicondyle (3) of the humerus; therefore, they are vulnerable to injury at this level.

On the distal medial surface of the brachium the COMMUNICATING BRANCH (4) OF THE MUSCULOCUTANEOUS NERVE joins the median nerve. The median nerve passes deep to the pronator teres muscle (5), where it provides nerve branches to a number of muscles of the caudomedial (flexor) muscle group. It continues distally along the antebrachium between the flexor carpi radialis (6) and deep digital flexor (7) muscles to reach the carpus.

(TO BE NOTED IN THE CAT: The median nerve passes through the supracondylar foramen.)

The ULNAR NERVE (2, Fig. 24.13) is situated along the caudal surface of the median nerve (1) in the brachium. The CAUDAL CUTANEOUS ANTEBRACHIAL NERVE (8) branches caudally away from the ulnar nerve in the distal half of the brachium; it courses superficial to the olecranon and the flexor carpi ulnaris muscle to reach a caudolateral position on the antebrachium. The main continuation of the ulnar nerve passes distally over the caudal surface of the medial humeral epicondyle to reach the flexor muscles of the antebrachium. Muscular branches of the ulnar nerve supply many of the caudomedial antebrachial muscles. In the proximal portion of the antebrachium the ulnar nerve is situated between the deep digital flexor (7) and flexor carpi ulnaris (9) muscles.

The median nerve (Fig. 24.14) branches in the metacarpal region to form the PALMAR ABAXIAL DIGITAL NERVE I and the PALMAR COMMON DIGITAL NERVES I, II, and III (1, 2, and 3, respectively), each of which divides into two PALMAR PROPER DIGITAL NERVES.

FIG. 24.14. Branches of the median nerve in the right manus, palmar view.

The ulnar nerve divides into two branches, a smaller DORSAL BRANCH (1, Fig. 24.15) and the larger PALMAR BRANCH (2). The dorsal branch of the ulnar nerve passes between the flexor carpi ulnaris and extensor carpi ulnaris muscles to reach the lateral surface of the distal antebrachium. The DORSAL ABAXIAL DIGITAL NERVE V (3) is the continuation of the dorsal branch. The palmar branch of the ulnar nerve passes through the carpal canal, where it divides into SUPERFICIAL and DEEP BRANCHES. The superficial branch of the ulnar nerve subdivides into the PALMAR COMMON DIGITAL NERVE IV (4) and the PALMAR ABAXIAL DIGITAL NERVE V (5). The deep branch of the ulnar subdivides into PALMAR METACARPAL NERVES I, II, III, and IV, each of which combines with a palmar common digital nerve before contributing to the formation of two palmar proper digital nerves.

FIG. 24.15. Branches of the ulnar nerve in the right manus, palmar view.

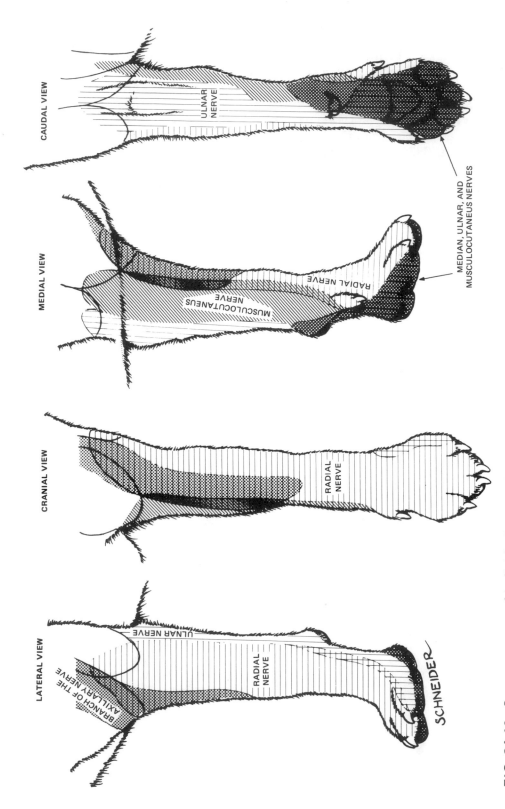

FIG. 24.16. Sensory nerves of individual nerves distributed to the skin of the left thoracic limb. (Modified from Kitchell et al. 1983. *Am. J. Vet. Res.* 41:61-76.)

The nerves that conduct innervation from the skin of the thoracic limb (Fig. 24.16) include the axillary, intercostobrachial, radial, musculocutaneous, ulnar, and median nerves. A summary of muscle and cutaneous innervation is given in Table 24.1.

TABLE 24.1. Innervation of the thoracic limb

Muscle	Nerve
Supraspinatus, infraspinatus	Suprascapular
Deltoideus, teres major, and teres minor	Axillary
Biceps brachii, brachialis	Musculocutaneous
Triceps brachii, anconeus	Radial
Craniolateral muscles of antebrachium (extensors of carpus and digits)	Radial
Caudomedial muscles of antebrachium (flexors of carpus and digits)	Ulnar, median, musculocutaneous

Region	Cutaneous branches*
Craniolateral brachium	Axillary
Caudal Brachium	Intercostobrachial
Caudolateral brachium	Radial
Cranial antebrachium	Axillary, radial
Lateral antebrachium	Radial
Caudal antebrachium	Ulnar
Medial antebrachium	Musculocutaneous
Palmar manus	Median
	Ulnar
Lateral manus	Ulnar
Dorsal manus	Radial

* The suprascapular, subscapular, lateral thoracic, thoracodorasal, and cranial and caudal pectoral nerves in the dog lack cutaneous afferent fibers.

Although a cutaneous nerve provides innervation to an area of skin, portions of the same area may also be supplied by several other nerves (zones of overlap). A more limited portion of this cutaneous area, innervated by a single cutaneous nerve, is termed the autonomous zone for that nerve.

FIG. 25.1. Caudal portion of the spinal cord, dorsal view.

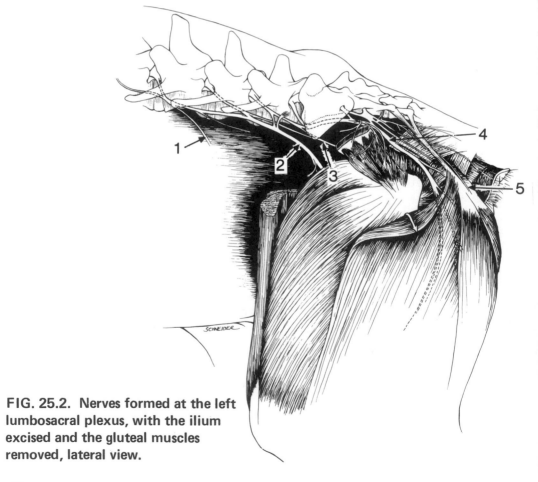

FIG. 25.2. Nerves formed at the left lumbosacral plexus, with the ilium excised and the gluteal muscles removed, lateral view.

25 PELVIC LIMB

The nerves supplying the pelvic limb are derived variably from the ventral branches of the last five lumbar and all three sacral spinal nerves. Because of the great number of neurons carrying information to and from the pelvic limb, there is also an enlargement in the spinal cord between the levels of the 4th lumbar and 2nd sacral spinal nerve-spinal cord junctions (3rd to 5th lumbar vertebral levels). Since the spinal cord extends caudally only as far as the 6th to 7th lumbar vertebrae in the dog, the second pair of sacral spinal nerves arises from the spinal cord at the level of the 5th lumbar vertebra (Fig. 25.1). This enlargement of the caudal portion of the spinal cord is termed the LUMBAR INTUMESCENCE (1). The ventral rami of lumbar and spinal nerves form a network of interconnecting fibers known as the LUMBOSACRAL PLEXUS.

The nerves, formed at the lumbosacral plexus that innervate structures of the pelvic limb (Fig. 25.2) include the lateral cutaneous femoral (1), femoral (2), obturator (3), lumbosacral trunk (4), and caudal cutaneous femoral (5) nerves. The LATERAL CUTANEOUS FEMORAL NERVE (1) passes through the psoas minor muscle and exits through the abdominal wall with the deep circumflex iliac vessel, reaching the superficial fascia near the ventral surface of the tuber coxae. Superficial branches of the lateral cutaneous femoral nerve supply the skin of the cranial gluteal, cranial femoral, and lateral genual regions.

(DIFFERENCES TO BE NOTED IN THE CAT: The spinal cord extends caudally, variably, to the level of the 6th lumbar to 3rd sacral vertebrae.)

SARTORIUS MUSCLE

VASTUS LATERALIS MUSCLE

FIG. 25.3. Left femoral nerve and pelvic limb, with the tensor fasciae latae removed, lateral view.

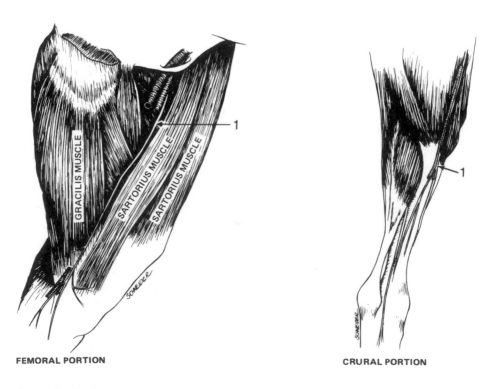

GRACILIS MUSCLE

SARTORIUS MUSCLE

SARTORIUS MUSCLE

FEMORAL PORTION

CRURAL PORTION

FIG. 25.4. Left saphenous nerve, medial view of the pelvic limb.

The fibers of the FEMORAL NERVE (1, Fig. 25.3) originate primarily from the 5th lumbar segment of the spinal cord. The femoral nerve is formed from the lumbosacral plexus within the iliopsoas muscle (2) and accompanies the iliopsoas muscle through the muscular lacuna to reach the pelvic limb. The major part of the femoral nerve is not observed superficially since it divides into a number of branches that enter the proximal portion of the quadriceps femoris muscle. The femoral nerve innervates the iliopsoas (the sartorius in some dogs) and extensor muscles of the stifle (cranial thigh muscles).

The SAPHENOUS NERVE (1, Fig. 25.4) is a branch of the femoral nerve, from which it separates within the iliopsoas muscle. In some dogs a proximal branch of the saphenous nerve supplies the sartorius muscle. The saphenous nerve is superficially positioned as it courses distally with the femoral vessels through the femoral triangle, across the superficial surface of the vastus medialis muscle, and on down the medial surface of the crus in close association with branches of saphenous blood vessels. Cutaneous branches of the saphenous nerve supply the skin of the medial femoral, medial crural, and dorsomedial tarsal regions. Digits I (when present) and II receive cutaneous innervation via the terminal branches of the saphenous nerve.

LEVATOR ANI MUSCLE

FIG. 25.5. Pelvic girdle and caudal portion of the lumbosacral plexus, caudodorsal view.

BICEPS FEMORIS MUSCLE

FIG. 25.6. Left lumbosacral plexus and pelvic limb, with the ilium excised and the gluteal muscles removed, lateral view.

SCHNEIDER

The OBTURATOR NERVE (1, Figs. 25.5, 25.6) is also formed from the lumbosacral plexus within the iliopsoas muscle. This nerve courses caudomedially to lie within the cranial pelvic aperture (pelvic inlet), deep to the ilium. It reaches the adductor muscles superficial to the os coxae by passing along the obturator groove and out through the obturator foramen. During parturition (particularly in large domestic animals or in certain breeds of dog such as the Boston terrier) the obturator nerves are susceptible to pressure as they are pressed by the fetus against the pelvic girdle. The obturator nerve innervates the external obturator, pectineus, gracilis, and adductor muscles.

The major nerve to the pelvic limb is the LUMBOSACRAL TRUNK (2, Figs. 25.5, 25.6), which arises primarily (via the lumbosacral plexus) from the ventral rami of the last two lumbar and first sacral spinal nerves (L6, L7, and S1). The lumbosacral trunk near its origin is situated in the dorsal portion of the pelvic cavity between the parietal peritoneum and the ventromedial surface of the ilium. In its caudolateral course to the major ischiatic notch the lumbosacral trunk branches, forming the CRANIAL GLUTEAL (3) and CAUDAL GLUTEAL (4) NERVES. The main extrapelvic continuation of the lumbosacral trunk, distal to the major ischiatic notch, is the ischiatic nerve (5). The cranial gluteal nerve arises from the lumbosacral trunk, crosses the dorsal surface of the ilium near the cranial margin of the major ischiatic notch with the cranial gluteal vessels, and innervates the middle gluteus, deep gluteus, and tensor fasciae latae muscles. The caudal gluteal nerve usually branches away from the lumbosacral trunk near the dorsal margin of the major ischiatic notch and supplies the superficial gluteal muscle. A muscular branch (6) from the lumbosacral trunk (or, more distally, from the ischiatic nerve) supplies the internal obturator, gemellus, and quadratus femoris muscles.

FIG. 25.7. Ischiatic nerve and its branches in the left pelvic limb, lateral view.

The ISCHIATIC NERVE (1, Fig. 25.7), a continuation of the lumbosacral trunk distal to the major ischiatic notch, consists of two large nerves bound together by connective tissue. These two nerves, the common fibular (peroneal) (2) and tibial (3) nerves, supply most of the intrinsic structures of the pelvic limb (those not supplied by the lateral cutaneous femoral, femoral, obturator, gluteal, and caudal cutaneous femoral nerves). The ischiatic nerve courses distally between the superficial and deep gluteal muscles, then between the biceps femoris (superficially) and gemellus, internal obturator, quadratus femoris, and adductor muscles (deeply). The ischiatic nerve is vulnerable in this location to careless injections made into the caudal thigh muscles. One or more large MUSCULAR BRANCHES (4) from the caudal surface of the proximal portion of the ischiatic nerve supply the biceps femoris, caudal crural abductor, semitendinosus, and semimembranosus muscles. A small proximal cutaneous branch of the tibial nerve passes distally with the caudal crural abductor muscle and provides sensory innervation to the skin in the popliteal region. A cutaneous branch of the common fibular nerve, either proximal or distal to the level at which the common fibular and tibial portions of the ischiatic nerve separate from each other, enters and passes through the biceps femoris muscle. This LATERAL CUTANEOUS SURAL (su'ral; calf of the leg) NERVE (5) passes through connective tissue between two portions of the biceps femoris muscle and supplies the skin of the lateral crural region. Another cutaneous nerve, the CAUDAL CUTANEOUS SURAL NERVE (6), arises from the tibial nerve a short distance distal to the origin of the lateral cutaneous sural from the common peroneal nerve. The caudal cutaneous sural nerve, located caudal to the tibial nerve, courses distally to the popliteal region, where the cutaneous nerve is associated with the caudal surface of the gastrocnemius muscle. The caudal cutaneous sural nerve divides into a number of small branches supplying the skin of the caudal tarsal region. One terminal branch passes craniomedially between the superficial and deep digital flexor tendons, joins the tibial nerve, and in some dogs provides innervation to the skin of the plantar metatarsal region.

The COMMON FIBULAR NERVE, located superficial to the lateral head of the gastrocnemius muscle and deep to the distal portion of the biceps femoris muscle, supplies the fibularis longus muscle with innervation and divides into two branches: the superficial (7) and deep (8) fibular nerves, both of which course distally through the crus parallel to each other, one more superficially and the other more deeply

FIG. 25.8. Branches of the superficial and deep peronal nerves in the left pes, dorsal view.

situated. The SUPERFICIAL FIBULAR NERVE (7), near its origin
from the common fibular nerve, is adjacent to the caudal
border of the fibularis longus muscle and superficial to the
lateral head of the deep digital flexor muscle; it courses
craniodistally deep to the fibularis longus tendon to lie
superficial to the long digital extensor tendon and proximal
extensor retinaculum.

A small branch (1, Fig. 25.8) separates from the
superficial fibular nerve (2), near the tarsocrural
articulation to course along the dorsolateral surface of the
tarsus and metatarsus. This small lateral branch is the
DORSAL ABAXIAL DIGITAL NERVE V. The superficial fibular
nerve branches over the dorsal surface of the tarsal bones
and proximal metatarsus to supply the superficial part of the
innervation to the digits. (The superficial nerves of the
metatarsal region are designated COMMON DIGITAL NERVES; the
deep nerves of the metatarsal region are designated
METATARSAL NERVES.) The dorsal nerves to the digits that
receive innervation via the superficial peroneal nerve are
the DORSAL COMMON DIGITAL NERVES II, III, and IV (3-5), which
are located in the second, third, and fourth intermetatarsal
spaces, respectively, and the DORSAL ABAXIAL DIGITAL NERVE II
(6). If a dew claw is present, the last named nerve would be
the DORSAL COMMON DIGITAL NERVE I. Each of the dorsal common
digital nerves divide into two DORSAL PROPER DIGITAL NERVES,
an AXIAL and an ABAXIAL NERVE.

The DEEP FIBULAR NERVE (7) also passes into the fascial
cleft separating the deep digital flexor muscle (caudally)
and the fibularis longus muscle (cranially). Branches of the
deep fibular nerve supply the fibularis longus, long digital
extensor, and cranial tibial muscles. The deep fibular nerve
courses distally with a major artery of the crus, the cranial
tibial artery (8), to the tarsocrural articulation where it
is situated deep and medial to the superficial fibular nerve.
The deep fibular nerve and cranial tibial artery pass
distally deep to the proximal extensor retinaculum. The deep
fibular nerve divides in the tarsal region to become DORSAL
METATARSAL NERVES II, III, and IV (9-11, respectively), each
of which combines with a dorsal common digital nerve (II,
III, or IV) to supply nerve fibers to the digits.

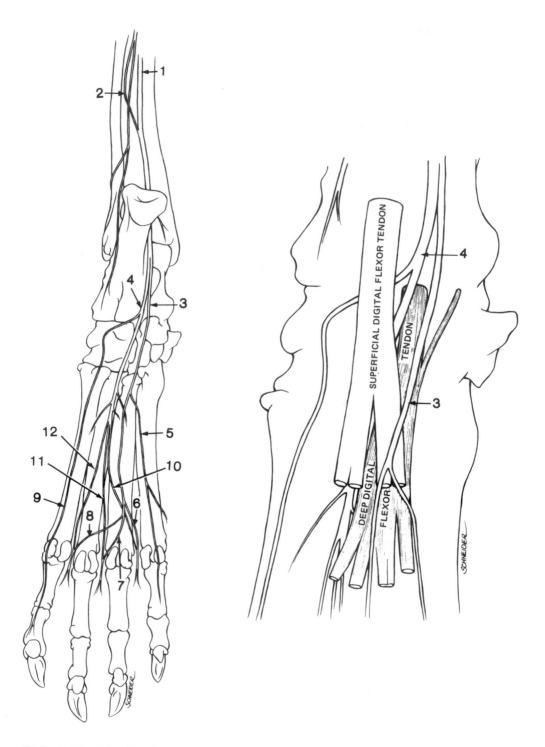

FIG. 25.9. Distribution of the tibial nerve in the left pes, plantar view.

The TIBIAL NERVE (Fig. 25.9) courses distally through the popliteal region and enters the crus between the lateral and medial heads of the gastrocnemius muscle. Muscular branches of the tibial nerve supply the gastrocnemius, superficial digital flexor, popliteus, and deep digital flexor muscles. In the crural region the tibial nerve (1) is situated between the superficial digital flexor and deep digital flexor muscles. Proximal to the tarsal articulation, a terminal branch (2) of the laterally situated caudal cutaneous sural nerve joins the tibial nerve. The tibial nerve separates into two nerves near the tarsocrural articulation: a smaller, more superficial medial plantar nerve (3) and a larger, deeper lateral plantar nerve (4), both of which pass distally across the medial surface of the calcaneus tarsal bone into the pes. The MEDIAL PLANTAR NERVE (3) courses through the tarsal region along the medial surface of the superficial digital flexor tendon. In the proximal metatarsal region the medial plantar nerve branches into the PLANTAR ABAXIAL DIGITAL NERVE II (5) and the parent trunk of the superficial plantar nerves of the distal metatarsus: PLANTAR COMMON DIGITAL NERVES II, III, and IV (6-8, respectively).

The LATERAL PLANTAR NERVE (4) passes distally into the fascia between the tendons of the superficial digital flexor and deep digital flexor muscles. It then branches to form the PLANTAR ABAXIAL DIGITAL NERVE V (9) and the deep plantar nerves of the metatarsus, PLANTAR METATARSAL NERVES II, III, and IV (10-12, respectively). The plantar metatarsal nerves combine with the plantar common digital nerves near the distal metatarsal region. The combined nerve trunks thus formed divide into PLANTAR AXIAL and ABAXIAL PROPER DIGITAL NERVES.

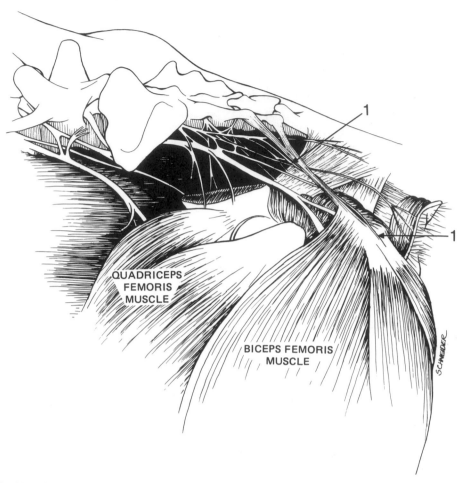

FIG. 25.10. Left lumbosacral plexus, with the ilium excised and the gluteal muscles removed, lateral view.

The CAUDAL CUTANEOUS FEMORAL NERVE (1, Fig. 25.10) courses caudolaterally, deep to the sacrotuberous ligament, in the ischiorectal fossa to appear superficially on the semitendinosus muscle at the ischiatic tuberosity. The terminal branches of the caudal cutaneus femoral nerve, the CAUDAL CLUNIAL (kloo′ne-al; buttocks) NERVES, supply fibers to the skin of the caudal and lateral femoral regions.

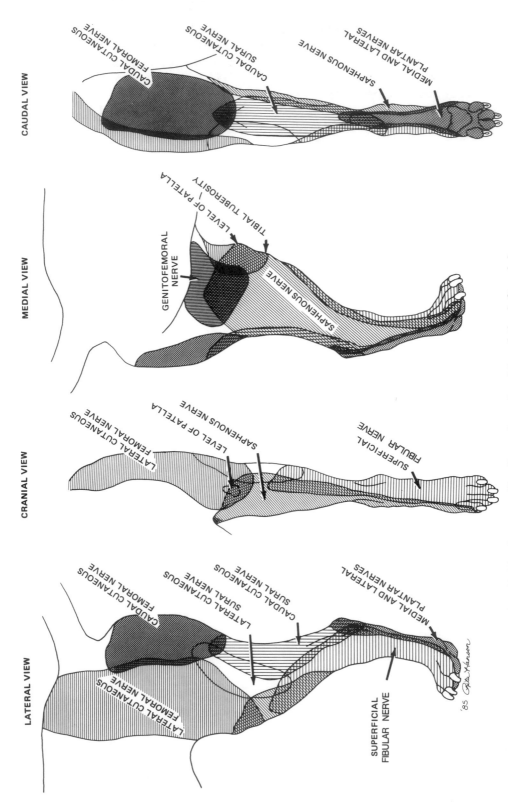

CAUDAL VIEW

CAUDAL CUTANEOUS
FEMORAL NERVE

CAUDAL CUTANEOUS
SURAL NERVE

SAPHENOUS NERVE

MEDIAL AND LATERAL
PLANTAR NERVES

MEDIAL VIEW

GENITOFEMORAL
NERVE

LEVEL OF PATELLA

TIBIAL TUBEROSITY

SAPHENOUS NERVE

CRANIAL VIEW

LATERAL CUTANEOUS
FEMORAL NERVE

LEVEL OF PATELLA

SAPHENOUS NERVE

SUPERFICIAL
FIBULAR NERVE

LATERAL VIEW

CAUDAL CUTANEOUS
FEMORAL NERVE

LATERAL CUTANEOUS
SURAL NERVE

CAUDAL CUTANEOUS
SURAL NERVE

MEDIAL AND LATERAL
PLANTAR NERVES

LATERAL CUTANEOUS
FEMORAL NERVE

SUPERFICIAL
FIBULAR NERVE

'85

FIG. 25.11. Sensory zones of individual nerves distributed to the skin of the left pelvic limb (based on correspondence with R. L. Kitchell, 1984).

   Nerves that conduct sensory innervation from the skin of
the pelvic limb (Fig. 25.11) include the lateral cutaneous
femoral; saphenous; and branches of the tibial, common
fibular, and caudal cutaneous femoral nerves. A summary of
muscle and cutaneous innervation is given in Table 25.1.

TABLE 25.1. Innervation of the pelvic limb

Muscle	Nerve
Middle gluteus, deep gluteus, tensor fasciae latae	Cranial gluteal
Superficial gluteus	Caudal gluteal
Quadriceps femoris, iliopsoas, sartorius	Femoral
Biceps femoris, caudal crural abductor, semitendinosus, semimembranosus	Muscular branches of the ischiatic
External obturator, pectineus, gracilis, adductor	Obturator
Internal obturator, gemellus, quadratus femoris	Muscular branch of the lumbosacral trunk
Craniolateral muscles of the crus (flexors of the tarsus, extensors of the digits)	Deep fibular
Caudal muscles of the crus (extensors of the tarus, flexors of the digits, popliteus)	Tibial

Region	Cutaneous branches
Cranial gluteal, craniolateral femoral	Lateral cutaneous femoral
Medial femoral and crural, dorsomedial tarsal	Saphenous
Caudal femoral	Caudal cutaneous femoral
Lateral crural	Lateral cutaneous sural
Caudal crural	Caudal cutaneous sural
Dorsal pes	Superficial and deep fibular
Plantar pes	Lateral and medial plantar

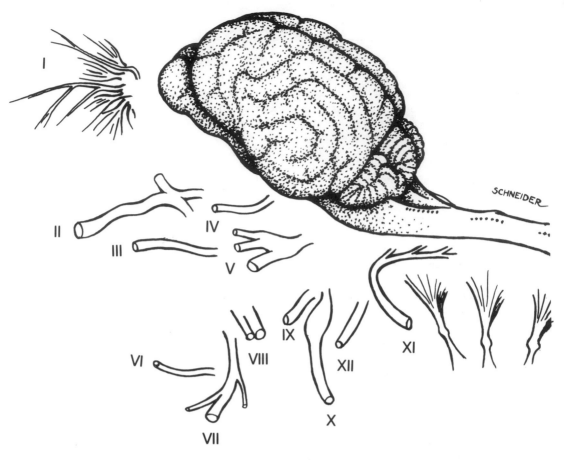

FIG. 26.1. Left cranial nerves I-XII, lateral view.

FIG. 26.2. Ventral internal surface of the skull with the stumps of cranial nerves I-XII exiting from the cranial cavity through foramina, dorsal view.

26 HEAD

The CRANIAL NERVES I through XII (Figs. 26.1; 26.2), numbered relative to their origin from the brain (rostral to caudal), are as follows: I = olfactory, II = optic, III = oculomotor, IV = trochlear, V = trigeminal, VI = abducens, VII = facial, VIII = vestibulocochlear, IX = glossopharyngeal, X = vagus, XI = accessory, and XII = hypoglossal.

A number of superficial nerve branches may be observed on the surface of the head deep to the skin, superficial fascia, and platysma muscle. Nearly all of these superficial nerves contain both efferent and afferent fibers; the majority of the superficial fibers to muscle are of the cranial nerve VII (facial), and most of the cutaneous fibers belong to branches of cranial nerve V (trigeminal).

FIG. 26.3. Schematic of the ventral surface of the cranial cavity illustrating the course of the facial and vestibulocochlear nerves in the petrous temporal bone.

FIG. 26.4. Schematic of the branches of the right facial nerve, lateral view.

FIG. 26.5. Branches of the right facial nerve, lateral view.

The FACIAL NERVE (1, Fig. 26.3) emerges from the cranial cavity by passing into the internal acoustic meatus (2) of the petrous temporal bone and exiting from the skull through the stylomastoid foramen (3). During its course through the temporal bone of the skull, small parasympathetic preganglionic fibers (4) branch away from the facial nerve. An auricular branch (5) of the vagus nerve joins with the facial nerve in the petrous temporal bone (see pp. 125, 461).

As the facial nerve emerges from the stylomastoid foramen, caudoventral to the ear, it branches deep to or within the parotid salivary gland into four or more large branches: the caudal auricular (1), ventral buccal (2), dorsal buccal (3), and auriculopalpebral (4) subdivisions (Fig. 26.4). The CAUDAL AURICULAR NERVES (1) arise from the facial nerve before or as the parent nerve emerges through the stylomastoid foramen, pass deep to the proximal lateral border of the auricular cartilage, and supply the caudal and dorsal auricular muscles.

The VENTRAL BUCCAL BRANCH OF THE FACIAL NERVE (1, Fig. 26.5) appears superficially between the rostroventral surface of the parotid salivary gland and the masseter muscle; it courses rostrally across the masseter muscle, superficial to the facial vein (2), and divides into two major components. One terminal portion of the ventral buccal branch (3) innervates the buccinator and orbicularis oris muscles of the lower jaw; the other terminal portion (4) passes rostrodorsally to combine with the DORSAL BUCCAL BRANCH OF THE FACIAL NERVE (5). The dorsal buccal branch courses rostrodorsally past the rostral margin of the parotid salivary gland and then superficially across the dorsal portion of the masseter muscle. Branches of the dorsal buccal branch innervate the buccinator and orbicularis oris muscles of the upper jaw. The AURICULOPALPEBRAL NERVE (6), deep to the parotid salivary gland, courses rostrodorsally, dividing into ROSTRAL AURICULAR (7) and ZYGOMATIC (8) branches. The zygomatic branch passes rostrodorsally over the zygomatic arch and temporalis muscle. Palpebral branches (9) of the zygomatic portion of the auriculopalpebral supply the orbicularis oculi muscle; the zygomatic branch also supplies the levator nasolabialis muscle with innervation. The rostral auricular branch passes dorsally near the rostral edge of the base of the ear, sending branches to the rostral auricular muscles. Near the stylomastoid foramen a branch nerve courses ventrally from the facial nerve to innervate the caudal portion of the digastricus muscle.

Cranial nerve V, the TRIGEMINAL NERVE (Fig. 26.6), divides into three large branches prior to exiting from the skull: the ophthalmic (1), maxillary (2), and mandibular (3) divisions.

FIG. 26.6. Ventral surface of cranial cavity, illustrating ophthalmic, maxillary, and mandibular divisions of right trigeminal nerve.

Subsequent to exiting from the cranial cavity via the oval foramen, the MANDIBULAR NERVE (Figs. 26.7, 26.8) branches into a dorsal and ventral trunk. The dorsal trunk of the mandibular nerve, containing fibers of the buccalis, masticatory, and pterygoid nerves, crosses the superficial surface of the lateral pterygoid muscle. The BUCCALIS NERVE (1) passes rostroventrally across the superficial surface of the lateral and medial pterygoid muscles to supply the mucosa and skin of the cheek. MASSETERIC and DEEP TEMPORAL branches of the MASTICATORY (2) NERVE innervate the temporalis and masseter muscles. The ventral trunk of the mandibular nerve passes between the lateral and medial pterygoid muscles, and divides into auriculotemporal, mylohyoid, inferior alveolar and lingual nerves. The AURICULOTEMPORAL NERVE (3) separates from the proximal portion of the mandibular nerve and curves ventrally around the retroarticular process before coursing dorsally to emerge on the surface of the head between the auricular cartilage and the masseter muscle. A branch of the auriculotemporal nerve is visible superficially between the zygomatic arch dorsally and the masseter muscle ventrally. Fibers from the auriculotemporal nerve, which join in parallel with branches of the facial nerve, supply cutaneous innervation to the auricular, temporal, zygomatic, and masseteric regions. The MYLOHYOID NERVE (4) courses ventrally (deep to the proximal portion of the mandible) to the digastricus muscle, part of which it supplies with fibers, and then along the medial surface of the mandible in association with the sublingual artery.   The INFERIOR ALVEOLAR NERVE (5) enters the mandibular canal through the mandibular foramen.   Small branches leave the inferior alveolar nerve within the mandibular canal to supply the roots of all the mandibular teeth.   Several MENTAL NERVES branch from the inferior alveolar nerve, exit from the rostral portion of the mandible through the mental foramina, and supply the lips and skin of the chin.   The LINGUAL NERVE (6) courses rostrally into the tongue.

FIG. 26.7. Schematic of the branches of the mandibular nerve, dorsal view.

FIG. 26.8. Branches of the right mandibular nerve with the caudal portion of the mandible removed, lateral view.

FIG. 26.9. Tongue and associated structures, with the left mandible removed, left lateral view.

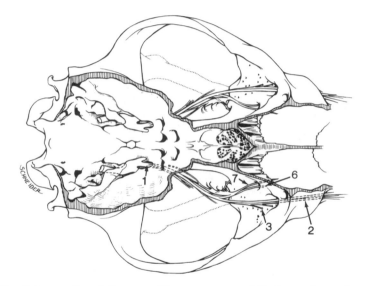

FIG. 26.10. Schematic of the maxillary nerve and its branches, dorsal view.

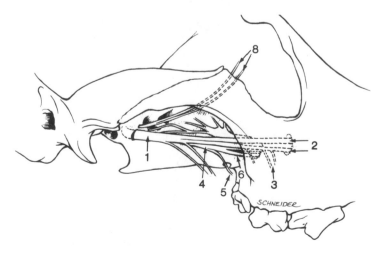

FIG. 26.11. Schematic of the maxillary nerve and its branches, lateral view.

The LINGUAL NERVE (1, Fig. 26.9), a branch of the mandibular nerve, passes rostroventrally medial to the mandible and lateral to the styloglossus muscle. It supplies fibers to the mucosa of a portion of the pharynx, the rostral two-thirds of the tongue, and the floor of the mouth.

The MAXILLARY NERVE (1, Figs. 26.10, 26.11) reaches the pterygopalatine fossa from the cranial cavity by passing into the alar canal through the round foramen and then rostrally out the rostral alar foramen. Within the pterygopalatine fossa the maxillary nerve is usually present as several nerves, two or three side by side and one deep. The superficial branches of the maxillary nerve are called INFRAORBITAL NERVES (2, Figs. 26.10, 26.11). Both the terminal maxillary and the infraorbital portions of this nerve supply sensory branches to the roots of the teeth. These sensory branches are the SUPERIOR ALVEOLAR NERVES (3, Figs. 26.10, 26.11). Branches of the infraorbital nerves exit from the infraorbital canal through the infraorbital foramen to innervate the skin of the upper lip and muzzle.

The deep branch of the maxillary nerve, the PTERYGOPALATINE NERVE (4, Fig. 26.11) courses rostrally and divides into the minor palatine, major palatine, and caudal nasal nerves. The MINOR PALATINE NERVE (5, Fig. 26.11) is a small branch that courses ventrally over the superficial surface of the medial pterygoid muscle to reach the soft palate, which it innervates. The MAJOR PALATINE NERVE (6, Figs. 26.10, 26.11) enters the caudal palatine foramen, travels through the palatine canal, and exits through the major and minor palatine foramina to innervate the soft structures of the hard palate. The CAUDAL NASAL NERVE (7, Fig. 26.10) enters the sphenopalatine foramen and supplies innervation to the soft structures of the nasal septum, ventral concha, and maxillary recess.

The ZYGOMATIC NERVE (8, Fig. 26.11) is a proximal branch of the maxillary nerve that often leaves the alar canal through a separate foramen (small alar foramen) dorsal to the rostral alar foramen. The zygomatic nerve passes into the apex of the cone-shaped muscular fascia, where it may be observed as two nerves (the ZYGOMATICOTEMPORAL and ZYGOMATICOFACIAL BRANCHES) on the lateral surface of the orbital muscles and fat. The zygomatic nerve supplies fibers to the lacrimal gland and to the lateral portion of the superior and inferior palpebrae.

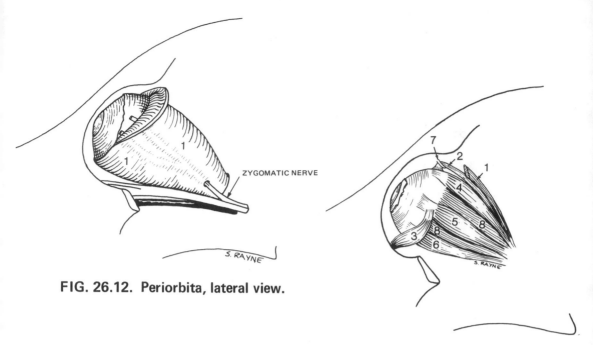

FIG. 26.12. Periorbita, lateral view.

ZYGOMATIC NERVE

S. RAYNE

FIG. 26.13. Extrinsic muscles of the eye, lateral view.

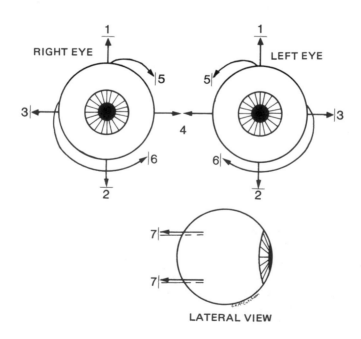

RIGHT EYE

LEFT EYE

LATERAL VIEW

FIG. 26.14. Schematic illustrating the points of insertion of extrinsic eye muscles on the bulb of the eye.

The extrinsic eye muscles; oculomotor, trochlear, abducens, optic, zygomatic, and ophthalmic nerves; and blood vessels of the eye are all enclosed by a cone-shaped muscular fascia, the PERIORBITA (1, Fig. 26.12).

The superficial set of muscles of the eye (Fig. 26.13), observed when the muscular fascia is removed, are the levator of the superior palpebra (1), the dorsal (2) and ventral (3) obliques, and four straight muscles. The LEVATOR PALPEBRAE SUPERIORIS arises from the skull near the optic canal and inserts as a flat tendon in the superior palpebra. The straight muscles are named according to their position relative to the optic nerve: DORSAL RECTUS (4), LATERAL RECTUS (5), VENTRAL RECTUS (6), and MEDIAL RECTUS. The four recti muscles arise from the skull near the optic canal and insert on the four surfaces of the eyeball (dorsal, lateral, ventral, and medial). The DORSAL OBLIQUE MUSCLE (2) arises from the skull near the optic canal, passes rostrally superficial and dorsomedial to the cone formed by the recti muscles, and inserts by a long tendon on the outer fibrous layer of the eyeball. Its tendon of insertion is anchored to the orbital surface of the frontal bone by a cartilaginous pulley or TROCHLEA (7); from the trochlea the tendon passes laterally to insert on the dorsal surface of the eyeball. The VENTRAL OBLIQUE MUSCLE (3) arises from the rostral portion of the orbital surface of the palatine bone and courses laterally around the ventral surface of the eyeball to insert on the lateral surface of the eyeball.

A cone of four muscle fascicles are positioned around the optic nerve deep to the four recti muscles. These fascicles are the RETRACTOR BULBI MUSCLES (8). They arise from the skull near the orbital fissure and insert on the eyeball posterior to the insertion of the recti muscles.

The extrinsic muscles, described briefly above, function as follows with respect to the anterior surface of the bulb of the eye (Fig. 26.14): 1) dorsal rectus - levates it, 2) ventral rectus - depresses it, 3) lateral rectus - pulls it laterally, 4) medial rectus - pulls it medially, 5) dorsal oblique - rotates or swivels the dorsal surface ventromedially , 6) ventral oblique - rotates or swivels the ventral surface dorsomedially, and 7) the retractor bulbi - pulls it posteriorly. When contracting simultaneously, the two oblique muscles pull the anterior portion of the eyeball medially.

FIG. 26.15. Nerves: trochlear, abducens, and branches of the ophthalmic, with several extrinsic muscles of the right eye removed, lateral view.

FIG. 26.16. Nerves: trochlear, abducens, and branches of the ophthalmic, dorsal view of the right eye.

FIG. 26.17. Right oculomotor nerve and its branches, with several extrinsic eye muscles removed, dorsal view.

The OPHTHALMIC NERVE (Figs. 26.15, 26.16) emerges from the orbital fissure and supplies afferent fibers to many structures of the orbital, nasal, and frontal regions via the FRONTAL (1), LACRIMAL (2), and NASOCILIARY (3) NERVES. The frontal nerve is sensory to the middle of the superior palpebra. Branches of the nasociliary are sensory to the medial commissure, cornea, bulbar conjunctiva, iris, and ciliary body; one branch, the INFRATROCHLEAR NERVE (4), is visible near the medial commissure, ventral to the trochlea.

In addition to the ophthalmic nerve, three other cranial nerves (oculomotor, trochlear, and abducens) provide innervation to periorbital structures. The oculomotor, trochlear, and abducens all emerge from the cranial cavity through the orbital fissure. These three cranial nerves (III, IV, and VI) innervate the seven extrinsic muscles of the eyeball and one of the superior palpebra.

Cranial nerve III, the OCULOMOTOR NERVE (1, Figs. 26.17, 26.18), enters the muscular fascia from the orbital fissure and courses along the ventrolateral surface of the optic nerve and ophthalmic blood vessels to innervate the levator palpebrae superioris; ventral oblique; and dorsal, medial, and ventral recti muscles.

FIG. 26.18. Right oculomotor nerve and its branches, with several extrinsic eye muscles removed, lateral view.

Cranial nerve IV, the TROCHLEAR NERVE (1, Fig. 26.19), upon entering the periorbita from the orbital fissure, innervates the dorsal oblique muscle. Cranial nerve VI, the ABDUCENS (ab-du'senz; to abduct) NERVE (2), after exiting from the cranial cavity through the orbital fissure, enters the periorbita and innervates the retractor bulbi and lateral rectus muscles. Retraction of the eyeball indirectly puts pressure on the base of the semilunar conjunctival fold, resulting in protrusion of the fold.

The numerous afferent OLFACTORY (cranial I) NERVES pass directly from the olfactory mucosa of the nasal cavity through foramina of the cribriform lamina of the ethmoid bone to the olfactory bulbs of the brain.

FIG. 26.19. Right trochlear and abducens nerves, with several extrinsic eye muscles removed, dorsal view.

Cranial nerve II, the OPTIC NERVE (1, Fig. 26.20), containing afferent fibers arising in the retina, passes through the optic canal to reach the brain. The optic nerve is deep to extrinsic muscles of the bulb of the eye.

FIG. 26.20. Bulb of the eye and extracranial portion of the optic nerve.

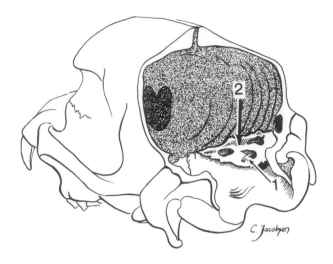

FIG. 26.21. Schematic of the position of the right vestibulocochlear nerve in the petrous temporal bone.

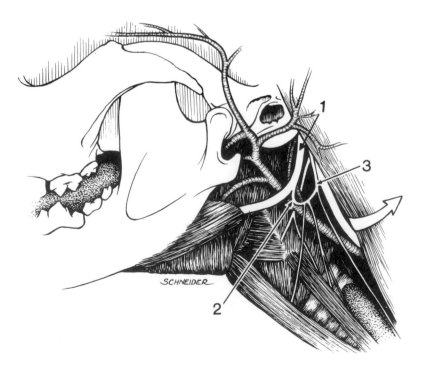

FIG. 26.22. Position of the left hypoglossal nerve relative to the carotid arteries, vagosympathetic trunk, and diagastricus muscle, lateral view.

Cranial nerve VIII, the VESTIBULOCOCHLEAR NERVE (1, Fig. 26.21), enters the internal acoustic meatus from the cranial cavity along with the facial nerve (see p. 447). The vestibular portion is concerned with balance and the cochlear portion with hearing. Neither the vestibular nor the cochlear portion of cranial nerve VIII may be seen on the superficial surface of the skull since both innervate structures of the inner ear, which is contained within the petrous temporal bone (2).

Cranial nerve XII, the HYPOGLOSSAL NERVE (1, Figs. 26.22, 26.23), exits from the skull through the hypoglossal canal. This nerve, medial to the accessory nerve and lateral to the vagus nerve at the canal, crosses the lateral surface of the external carotid artery and hyoglossal muscle to enter the tongue. The hypoglossal nerve supplies innervation to the extrinsic muscles of the tongue (genioglossus, hyoglossus, and styloglossus) as well as to the intrinsic tongue musculature. A small branch of the hypoglossal nerve (2, Fig. 26.22) forms a loop with a branch of the 1st cervical spinal nerve (3, Fig. 22.22). This loop is termed the ANSA (an'sah; handle) CERVICALIS (see p. 471).

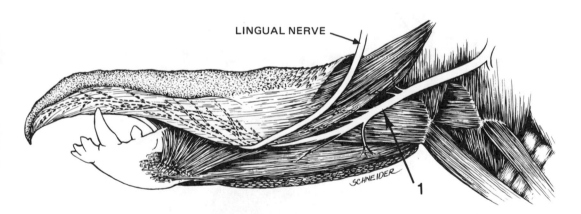

LINGUAL NERVE

SCHNEIDER

1

FIG. 26.23. Distribution of the left hypoglossal nerve in the tongue, with the left mandible removed, lateral view.

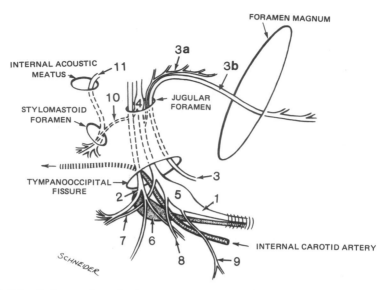

FIG. 26.24. Schematic of the positions of the facial, glossopharyngeal, vagus, and accessory nerves relative to each other and to the cranial cervical ganglion and internal carotid artery, lateral view.

FIG. 26.25. Schematic of the relationship of the facial and vagus nerves, caudal view.

Cranial nerve X, the vagus nerve, extends caudally into the neck, thorax, and abdomen; the vagus and its branches are closely associated with sympathetic fibers arising from the spinal cord in thoracolumbar segments. The VAGUS NERVE (1, Fig. 26.24) emerges from the tympanooccipital fissure in common with the glossopharyngeal (2) and accessory (3a, 3b) nerves. Nerve cell bodies of sensory fibers carried within the vagus are present in one of two ganglia; one ganglion is located proximal and the other distal to the tympanooccipital fissure. These two ganglia are called the PROXIMAL (4) and DISTAL (5) GANGLIA OF THE VAGUS. The distal ganglion of the vagus is closely united by connective tissue with an accumulation of sympathetic postganglionic nerve cell bodies, the CRANIAL CERVICAL GANLGION (6). Extracranial branches of the vagus to the head and neck regions include the COMMUNICATING RAMUS WITH THE GLOSSOPHARYNGEAL NERVE (7), PHARYNGEAL BRANCHES (8), and the CRANIAL LARYNGEAL NERVE (9). The cranial laryngeal nerve branches from the vagus at the level of the distal ganglion.

Within the skull an AURICULAR BRANCH OF THE VAGUS (10, Fig. 26.24; 1, Fig. 26.25) passes through a portion of the petrous temporal bone to join the facial nerve (11, Fig. 26.24; 2, Fig. 26.25). Sensory fibers of the auricular branch of the vagus reach the luminal surface of the external acoustic meatus with internal auricular branches of cranial nerve VII (3, Fig. 26.25). Irritation of the acoustic meatus by ear mites in young dogs may result in vomiting; the sensory inputs from the ear and the alimentary canal through the vagus apparently are not differentiated by the brain in the young dog.

Cranial nerve XI, the ACCESSORY NERVE, which has its origin both from the cervical portion of the spinal cord and the medulla oblongata, exits from the cranial cavity through the jugular foramen. Prior to emerging from the tympanooccipital fissure, the portion of the accessory nerve that originates from the medulla oblongata, the INTERNAL BRANCH (3a, Fig. 26.24), separates off and exits through the tympanooccipital fissure with the vagus nerve. The EXTERNAL BRANCH OF THE ACCESSORY NERVE (3b) passes into and through the sternomastoideus and cleidomastoideus muscles caudoventral to the mandibular salivary gland and dorsolateral to the medial retropharyngeal lymph node. The accessory nerve, which innervates the cleidomastoideus, sternomastoideus, sternohyoideus, omotransversarius, and trapezius muscles, is described with the trunk innervation (see p. 473).

The GLOSSOPHARYNGEAL NERVE (1, Fig. 26.26) enters the jugular foramen and exits from the skull through the tympanooccipital fissure. Two ganglia, PROXIMAL and DISTAL, of cranial nerve IX are present within the skull. The glossopharyngeal nerve divides to form several branches (pharyngeal, lingual, tonsillar, and carotid sinus). The PHARYNGEAL BRANCH (2) courses rostrally, medial to the stylohyoid, and with fibers from the vagus and sympathetic trunk forms the PHARYNGEAL PLEXUS. The pharyngeal plexus supplies the mucous membrane of the dorsal wall of the pharynx with fibers. The CAROTID SINUS BRANCH (3) courses caudoventrally to the bulbous origin of the internal carotid from the common carotid artery. The LINGUAL BRANCHES (4) supply the caudal one-third of the tongue with nerve fibers. The TONSILAR BRANCHES supply fibers to the lateral pharyngeal wall, including the palatine tonsil.

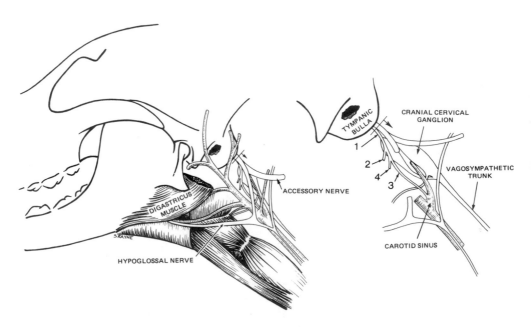

FIG. 26.26. Left cranial nerves IX-XII, cranial sympathetic ganglion, and internal carotid artery adjacent to the occipitotympanic fissure, lateral view.

Parasympathetic fibers originating from nerve cell bodies in nuclei of the CNS are carried from the brain by four cranial nerves: oculomotor, facial, glossopharyngeal, and the vagus. These parasympathetic fibers branch away from the four above-mentioned cranial nerves and join other nerves during their course to various glands and smooth muscle fibers.

Preganglionic parasympathetic fibers carried from the brain in the oculomotor nerve (1, Fig. 26.27) branch away from the oculomotor to reach the CILIARY GANGLION (2). The cell bodies of postganglionic parasympathetic neurons are present in the ciliary ganglion; parasympathetic axons (3) are distributed from the ciliary ganglion to the internal structures of the eyeball, where innervation results in constriction of the pupil and an alteration in the curvature of the eyeball, allowing the lens to become thicker.

FIG. 26.27. Schematic of the distribution of the parasympathetic fibers to the iris and ciliary body, lateral view.

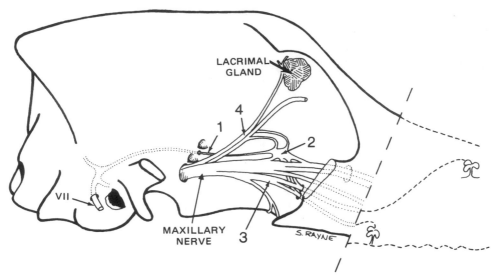

FIG. 26.28. Schematic of the distribution of parasympathetic fibers to the lacrimal, nasal, and palatine glands, lateral view.

FIG. 26.29. Schematic of the distribution of parasympathetic fibers to the mandibular and sublingual salivary glands, glands of the rostral portion of the tongue, and glands of the ventral oral mucosa, lateral view.

Parasympathetic fibers carried from the brain in the facial and glossopharyngeal nerves leave these nerves, exit from the skull, and join branches of the trigeminal nerve to reach the various salivary glands and glands of the nasal and oral mucosa.

Parasympathetic preganglionic fibers carried from the brain by the facial nerve exit from the skull through the minute pterygoid foramen as the NERVE OF THE PTERYGOID CANAL (1, Fig. 26.28). These preganglionic fibers synapse with postganglionic fibers in the PTERYGOPALATINE GANGLION (2), which is situated on the lateral surface of the medial pterygoid muscle, dorsal to the pterygopalatine nerve (3). Postganglionic parasympathetic fibers span the gap between the thin, flat pterygopalatine ganglion and the pterygopalatine nerve; postganglionic parasympathetic fibers may course in a retrograde direction to reach the lacrimal gland via the zygomatic nerve (4), or they may supply numerous nasal and palatine glands via branches of the pterygopalatine nerve.

The CHORDA (kor'dah; cord) TYMPANI (drum) (1, Fig. 26.29) is a small nerve that separates from the facial nerve (2), exits from the skull, and joins with the lingual nerve (3). The chorda tympani passes rostroventrally deep to the mylohyoid and inferior alveolar nerves to join the lingual nerve near the inferior alveolar-lingual bifurcation. The chorda tympani contains preganglionic parasympathetic fibers destined for the mandibular and sublingual salivary glands, preganglionic parasympathetic fibers to glands of the rostral two-thirds of the tongue and floor of the mouth, and afferent fibers from taste receptors in the rostral two-thirds of the tongue. Preganglionic parasympathetic fibers reach the mandibular and sublingual salivary glands by passing from the chorda tympani to the lingual nerve and then branching caudally, at the level of the styloglossus muscle, to enter ganglia near the glands.

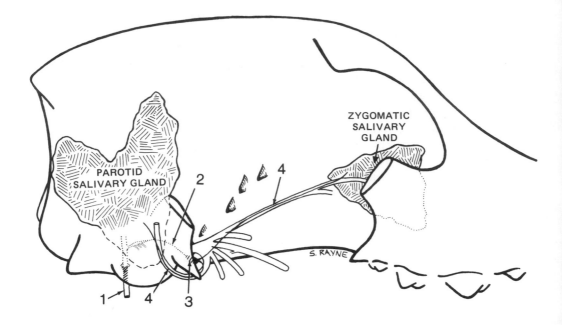

FIG. 26.30. Schematic of the distribution of parasympathetic fibers to the parotid and zygomatic salivary glands.

Preganglionic parasympathetic fibers (Fig. 26.30) also branch from the glossopharyngeal nerve (1) within the skull and pass out of the skull as the MINOR PETROSAL NERVE (2) to the OTIC GANGLION (3) near the oval foramen. Postganglionic parasympathetic fibers (4) join the auriculotemporal and buccalis nerves to reach the parotid and zygomatic salivary glands.

A number of the nerve fibers within the vagus are preganglionic parasympathetic fibers. Other fibers present within the vagus include GVA, SVE, SVA, and GSA.

(DIFFERENCES TO BE NOTED IN THE CAT: Striated muscle fibers of the lateral rectus and levator palpebrae superioris muscles insert on the third eyelid. Thus the third eyelid—semilunar conjunctival fold—may be drawn over the cornea of the cat independent of retraction of the eyeball.)

Some clinically useful reflexes are given in Table 26.1; a summary of the innervation of the head is listed in Table 26.2.

TABLE 26.1. Some clinically useful reflexes in the head

Structure stimulated	Stimulus	Sensory pathway	Motor pathway	Action
Cornea	Air	Ophthalmic of trigeminal	Auriculopalpebral of facial	Close palpebral fissure
Palpebrae				
Superior palpebra, medial commissure	Touch	Ophthalmic	Auriculopalpebral	Close palpebral fissure
Lateral commissure, inferior palpebra	Touch	Zygomatic of the maxillary division of the trigeminal	Auriculopalpebral	Close palpebral fissure
Retina	Movement toward the eye	Optic nerve	Auriculopalpebral	Close palpebral fissure
Retina	Light	Optic nerve	Oculomotor (parasympathetic fibers)	Constriction of pupil

TABLE 26.2. Summary of the innvervation of the head

Muscle	Cranial nerve	Primary branch	Secondary branch
Facial expression:			
Platysma, levator nasolabialis, orbicularis oris, orbicularis oculi, zygomaticus, buccinator, auricular	Facial		
Mastication:			
Close jaws — temporalis, masseter, medial and lateral pterygoideus	Trigeminal	Mandibular	
Open jaws — digastricus	Trigeminal Facial	Mandibular	Mylohyoid
Tongue:			
Genioglossus, hyoglossus, styloglossus, intrinsic	Hypoglossal		
Extrinsic eye:			
Dorsal rectus, medial rectus, ventral rectus, ventral oblique, levator palpebrae superioris	Oculomotor		
Dorsal oblique	Trochlear		
Lateral rectus, retractor bulbi	Abducens		
Extrinsic pharyngeal:			
Hyopharyngeus, thyropharyngeus, cricopharyngeus	Glossopharyngeal		
Extrinsic laryngeal:			
Cricothyroideus	Vagus	Cranial laryngeal	
Cricoarytenoideus dorsalis, cricoarytenoideus lateralis, thyroarytenoideus	Vagus	Recurrent laryngeal	Caudal laryngeal

Cutaneous or mucosal region	Secondary branch	Primary branch	Nerve
Dorsal and lateral nasal, superior labial	Infraorbital	Maxillary	Trigeminal
Inferior labial, mental	Inferior alveolar	Mandibular	Trigeminal
Cheek	Buccal	Mandibular	Trigeminal
Eyelids and cornea:			
Superior palpebra, medial commissure	Frontal Infratrochlear	Ophthalmic	Trigeminal
Inferior palpebra, lateral commissure	Zygomatic	Maxillary	Trigeminal
Ear:			
Tragic margin	Auriculotemporal	Mandibular, Major occipital	Trigeminal Second cervical
Concave surface		Internal auricular	Facial
Antitragic margin		Internal auricular Major auricular	Facial Second cervical
Convex surface		Major occipital Major auricular	Second cervical

TABLE 26.2. *(Continued)*

Cutaneous or mucosal region	Secondary branch	Primary branch	Nerve
Oral structures:			
Hard and soft palate, superior teeth and gums	Minor palatine Major palatine	Maxillary	Trigeminal
Ventral floor of the mouth, rostral two-thirds of the tongue (excluding taste), inferior teeth and gums, cheek	Lingual Inferior alveolar	Mandibular	Trigeminal
Taste receptors of rostral two-thirds of the tongue		Lingual — chorda tympani	Trigeminal — facial
Pharyngeal structures:			
Caudal one-third of the tongue		Lingual	Glossopharyngeal
Pharyngeal mucosa		Pharyngeal	Glossopharyngeal Vagus
Laryngeal mucosa		Cranial laryngeal	Vagus

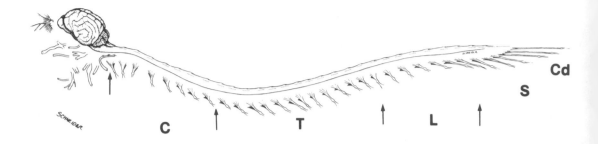

FIG. 27.1. Spinal nerves, lateral view.

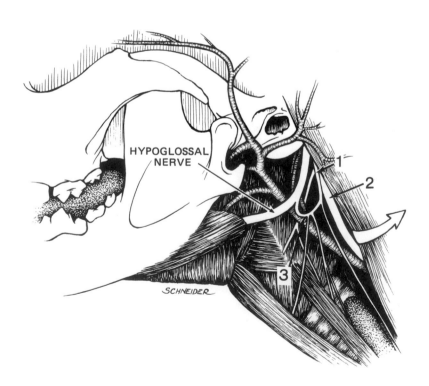

FIG. 27.2. Topographical relationship of the ansa cervicalis with the vagosympathetic trunk and carotid arteries, left lateral view.

27 TRUNK

The trunk is innervated by 8 pairs of CERVICAL, 13 pairs of THORACIC, 7 pairs of LUMBAR, and 3 pairs of SACRAL SPINAL NERVES (Fig. 27.1). Seven of the 8 pairs of cervical spinal nerves exit from the vertebral canal through intervertebral foramina (the 1st cervical spinal nerve emerges from the 1st cervical vertebra through the lateral vertebral foramen). Thus the cervical spinal nerves emerge from the vertebral column at intervals equal to the length of one vertebra.

The 1st (most cranial) cervical spinal nerve divides near the lateral vertebral foramen into a dorsal and ventral ramus. The dorsal and ventral rami of C1 usually do not reach the surface of the neck. The DORSAL RAMUS supplies epaxial neck musculature (including the capital obliques, dorsal recti muscles, the semispinalis capitis, and splenius). The VENTRAL RAMUS (1, Fig. 27.2) courses caudoventrally, initially deep to the medial retropharyngeal lymph node and distally next to the vagosympathetic trunk (2). The ventral ramus of C1 often forms a junction with a branch of the hypoglossal nerve, forming the ANSA CERVICALIS, or cervical loop (3). The ventral ramus of C1 innervates the sternothyroideus and sternohyoideus muscles.

FIG. 27.3. Surface of the head and neck depicting the position of the right accessory nerve and branches of the ventral ramus of the 2nd cervical spinal nerve.

FIG. 27.4. Left phrenic nerve, lateral view.

The part of the ACCESSORY (cranial XI) NERVE (1, Fig. 27.3) that arises from the cervical portion of the spinal cord is termed the EXTERNAL BRANCH (see p. 461). It courses caudally from the tympanooccipital fissure, through the sterno- and cleidomastoideus muscles, which it innervates, and on caudally deep to the cleidocervicalis and omotransversarius muscles. Branches of the ventral rami of a number of cervical spinal nerves (C2, C3, and C4) join the accessory nerve as the cranial nerve courses past them. The accessory nerve is the sole innervator of the trapezius muscle.

The roots of the 2nd cervical spinal nerve exit from the intervertebral foramen between the atlas and axis. The SPINAL GANGLION and the junction of dorsal and ventral roots are peripheral to the vertebral column. The dorsal ramus of C2 (the MAJOR OCCIPITAL NERVE) innervates the semispinalis capitis and splenius muscles, then supplies fibers to the skin of the caudal auricular and parietal regions. The ventral ramus of C2 courses caudoventrally between the sternooccipitalis and cleidomastoideus muscles. Superficially positioned adjacent to the transverse process of the atlas, the ventral ramus of C2 divides into a major auricular nerve and a transverse nerve of the neck. The MAJOR AURICULAR NERVE (2) courses craniodorsally to innervate the skin of the convex surface of the ear. The TRANSVERSE NERVE OF THE NECK (3) courses rostrally, superficial to the large veins of the head, supplying fibers to the platysma and the skin of the laryngeal and intermandibular regions.

Cervical spinal nerves 2-8 are characterized by relatively small dorsal rami, with medial subbranches supplying the skin of the dorsal cervical region and lateral subbranches supplying the epaxial muscles. Ventral rami of C3-C5 may be located deep to the omotransversarius muscle, through which they traverse. These ventral rami supply hypaxial muscles and the skin of the ventral and lateral cervical regions.

Caudal branches of the ventral rami of C5-C7 unite to form the PHRENIC NERVE (1, Fig. 27.4), which passes caudally deep to the 1st rib to innervate the thoracic diaphragm. The phrenic nerve of each side is situated within the lamina of connective tissue (mediastinum) separating right and left portions of the thoracic cavity, medial to the lungs and lateral to the base of the heart. On the surface of the diaphragm the phrenic nerve divides into ventral, lateral, and dorsal branches.

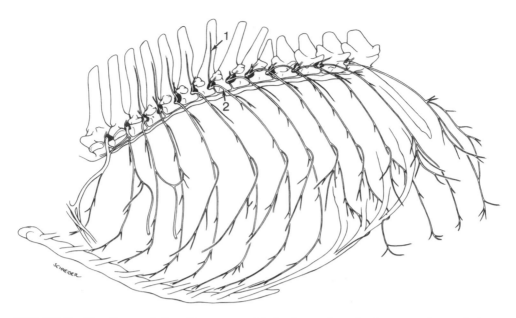

FIG. 27.5. Portions of the rib cage and left thoracic spinal nerves, lateral view.

FIG. 27.6. Branches of a thoracic spinal nerve, caudal view.

Each of the 13 THORACIC SPINAL NERVES (Fig. 27.5) exits from the vertebral canal through an intervertebral foramen immediately caudal to the corresponding vertebra (e.g., the 6th thoracic spinal nerve emerges from the vertebral canal through the foramen formed by the caudal vertebral notch of the 6th thoracic vertebra and the cranial vertebral notch of the 7th thoracic vertebra).   Each thoracic spinal nerve divides into a dorsal (1) and a ventral (2) ramus.

The DORSAL RAMUS (1, Fig. 27.6) of a thoracic spinal nerve bifurcates into medial and lateral branches.   The MEDIAL BRANCH (2) of the dorsal ramus supplies the epaxial muscles and the meninges of the spinal cord; the LATERAL BRANCH (3) courses dorsolaterally between the longissimus and iliocostalis muscles and divides into a MEDIAL CUTANEOUS (4) and a LATERAL CUTANEOUS (5) BRANCH.   Branches of the VENTRAL RAMI (6) of thoracic spinal nerves are MUSCULAR (7), LATERAL CUTANEOUS (8), and VENTRAL CUTANEOUS (9) BRANCHES.   The lateral cutaneous branches course laterally and may be observed superficially on the lateral surface of the external abdominal oblique muscle near the ventral border of the latissimus dorsi muscle.

The lateral cutaneous branches of T2 and T3 intercostal nerves are relatively large nerves that innervate the skin of the tricipital and olecranon regions; these nerves are named the INTERCOSTOBRACHIAL NERVES.   A number of the lateral cutaneous branches supply fibers to the thoracic mammary glands; these fibers are named the LATERAL MAMMARY BRANCHES. The ventral cutaneous branches of the ventral rami of the thoracic spinal nerves enter the skin in the sternal region. Nerve fibers that arise from the ventral cutaneous branches and innervate the thoracic mammary glands are termed the MEDIAL MAMMARY BRANCHES.   Each of the ventral portions of the last thoracic ventral rami are situated abdominally as the costal arch curves cranioventrally.

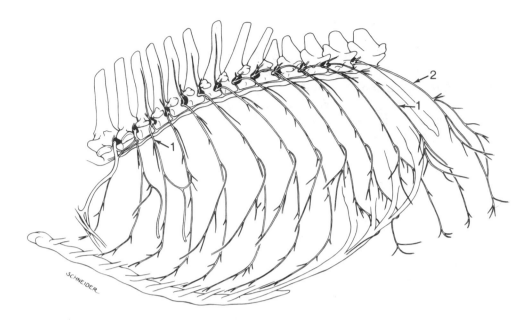

FIG. 27.7. Left intercostal nerves and the costoabdominal nerve, lateral view.

FIG. 27.8. Left costoabdominal and lumbar spinal nerves, lateral view.

Each of the ventral rami (1, Fig. 27.7) of the thoracic spinal nerves courses through the thoracic wall in contact with blood vessels next to the caudal border of the correspondingly numbered rib (the ventral ramus of the 1st thoracic spinal nerve is an exception since most of the nerve joins the brachial plexus). Since each ventral ramus of each thoracic spinal nerve is situated in an interval between two adjacent ribs, they are named INTERCOSTAL NERVES. The one exception to the intercostal location occurs caudally where the ventral ramus of the 13th spinal nerve is situated near the caudal surface of the last rib; the ventral ramus of T13 is named the COSTOABDOMINAL NERVE (2).

The seven LUMBAR SPINAL NERVES (Fig. 27.8) also divide into DORSAL (1) and VENTRAL (2) RAMI. The dorsal rami supply medial branches to the epaxial musculature and lateral branches to the skin of the dorsolateral lumbar and sacral regions. The lateral cutaneous branches of the caudal several lumbar spinal nerves are also known as the CRANIAL CLUNIAL NERVES. The ventral rami of the first several lumbar spinal nerves, oriented in series parallel with the ventral rami of the caudal thoracic spinal nerves, are named the cranial iliohypogastric (3), caudal iliohypogastric (4), ilioinguinal (5), lateral cutaneous femoral (6), and genitofemoral nerves. The ventral ramus of the 1st lumbar spinal nerve, named the CRANIAL ILIOHYPOGASTRIC NERVE (3), emerges deep to the abdominal wall from the quadratus lumborum. It innervates some of the parietal peritoneum and a segment of the quadratus lumborum, passes ventrolaterally through the dorsal aponeurosis of the transversus abdominis muscle, and divides into a lateral and a medial branch. The lateral branch passes through the internal abdominal oblique muscle to course ventrally between the two abdominal oblique muscles. This lateral branch innervates both oblique muscles, then passes through the external abdominal oblique as the LATERAL CUTANEOUS BRANCH, which innervates a vertical band of skin in the ventrolateral abdominal region. The medial branch courses ventrally on the superficial surface of the transversus abdominis muscles, which it innervates in part. A ventral portion of the medial branch innervates the rectus abdominis muscle in part and passes out to the skin as the VENTRAL CUTANEOUS BRANCH.

The ventral ramus of the 2nd lumbar spinal nerve, the CAUDAL ILIOHYPOGASTRIC NERVE (4), is similar in pattern and innervation to the cranial iliohypogastric nerve. It innervates the skin of the cranial femoral region. The ventral ramus of the 3rd lumbar spinal nerve is named the

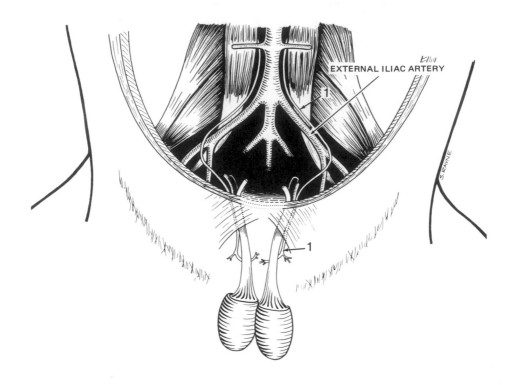

FIG. 27.9. Genitofemoral nerve and its distribution, ventral view.

ILIOINGUINAL NERVE (5); the ilioinguinal nerve, which also receives fibers from the 4th lumbar nerve, supplies cutaneous fibers via the lateral cutaneous branch to the skin of the craniolateral femoral region.   The LATERAL CUTANEOUS FEMORAL NERVE (6), formed primarily by the ventral ramus of the 4th lumbar nerve, courses laterally with the deep circumflex iliac vessels and supplies the lateral surface of the femoral and genual regions.

The GENITOFEMORAL NERVE (1, Fig. 27.9) contains fibers that arise from ventral rami of both the 3rd and 4th lumbar spinal nerves; the proximal portion of this nerve, deep to the abdominal wall, courses caudoventrally on the surface of the external iliac artery.   The genitofemoral nerve exits from the abdominal cavity through the inguinal canal to supply the cremaster muscle and the skin of the inguinal, medial femoral, and preputial regions in the dog, or the caudal abdominal mammary gland in the bitch.

The dorsal rami of the three SACRAL SPINAL NERVES exit from the vertebral canal through the dorsal sacral foramina. Each of these dorsal rami divides into a medial branch (supplying the dorsal muscles of the tail) and a lateral cutaneous branch.   The three lateral cutaneous branches of the dorsal sacral rami, named the MIDDLE CLUNIAL NERVES, innervate the skin of the superficial gluteal and proximal caudolateral femoral regions.

COCCYGEUS MUSCLE

LEVATOR ANI MUSCLE

SCHNEIDER

FIG. 27.10. Left pudendal nerve and its branches in the bitch, lateral view.

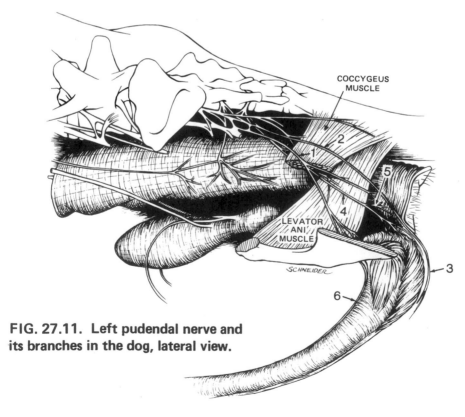

COCCYGEUS MUSCLE

LEVATOR ANI MUSCLE

SCHNEIDER

FIG. 27.11. Left pudendal nerve and its branches in the dog, lateral view.

The SACRAL PLEXUS is formed by ventral rami of the three sacral spinal nerves and by a contribution of fibers from the ventral rami of the 6th and 7th lumbar spinal nerves. The bilaterally paired PUDENDAL NERVE of the bitch (1, Fig. 27.10) arises from the sacral plexus and crosses the dorsolateral surface of the coccygeus muscle in association with the internal pudendal artery. The SUPERFICIAL PERINEAL NERVE (2), a branch of the pudendal nerve, courses laterally across the external anal sphincter and innervates the skin of the perineum and the dorsal vulvar region via DORSAL LABIAL NERVES. The DEEP PERINEAL NERVES (3) branch caudally off the pudendal nerve and innervate the urethralis, ischiourethralis, ischiocavernosus, constrictor vestibuli, and constrictor vulvae muscles. The CAUDAL RECTAL NERVE (4), usually a branch of a deep perineal nerve, innervates the external anal sphincters. The DORSAL NERVE OF THE CLITORIS is a branch of the pudendal nerve that innervates the body and glans of the clitoris.

The pudendal nerve of the dog (1, Fig. 27.11) courses caudally in association with the internal pudendal artery across the dorsolateral surface of the coccygeus. The superficial perineal nerve (2) and its terminal branch, the DORSAL SCROTAL NERVE (3), have a distribution similar to that in the bitch. The deep perineal nerves (4) innervate the retractor penis, urethralis, ischiourethralis, bulbospongiosus, and ischiocavernosus muscles. The caudal rectal nerve (5) innervates the external anal sphincter. The DORSAL NERVE OF THE PENIS (6) is the distal continuation of the pudendal nerve along the dorsum of the root and body and into the glans of the penis.

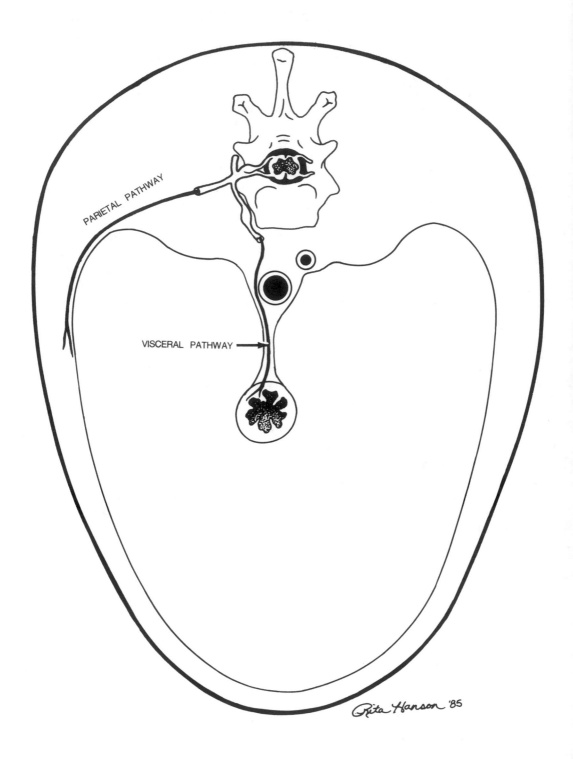

FIG. 28.1. Schematic of the pathways by which fibers reach the viscera and serous membranes from the spinal cord.

28 VISCERA

Nerves to the viscera contain both sensory and motor fibers. Sensory fibers from viscera are termed general visceral afferent (GVA); GVA fibers carry impulses from baro-, and chemoreceptors in blood vessels of the neck and thorax and from pain receptors in the thoracic, abdominal, and pelvic cavities. Impulses resulting from noxious stimuli may be carried from pleura and peritoneum through both visceral or parietal pathways (Fig. 28.1). The nerve cell bodies of afferent fibers belonging to both visceral and parietal pathways are situated in spinal ganglia of the various spinal nerves. The parietal pleura and peritoneum are associated with sensory endings that respond to tactile, thermal and chemical stimuli; impulses generated in the afferent fibers are carried through the same nerve trunks as are impulses from muscle and skin. In contrast to the parietal lining, touching or incising visceral structures is not perceived by the brain; pain in visceral structures is the result of a diffuse stimulation, as from distention of the gut or lack of blood (ischemia) in an area. The pain of a heart attack is largely due to ischemic cardiac tissue.

A sensation of pain in the viscera is often felt on the surface of the body (referred pain). Referred pain probably results when GVA fibers share a common termination in the CNS with general somatic afferent (GSA) fibers. The brain receives many more impulses over the GSA pathway and thus may not distinguish the GVA as a separate input. The surface area to which visceral pain is referred often has a common embryological origin with the visceral structure from which the pain impulse arises. Subsequent to the change in positions of many organs during development, visceral pain in the postnatal animal may be interpreted as coming from an area of the body some distance away from the irritated organ.

TABLE 28.1. A comparison of the two portions of the autonomic nervous system

Characteristic	Parasympathetic portion	Sympathetic portion
Number of neurons in series from CNS to effector organ	1 preganglionic 1 postganglionic	1 preganglionic 1 postganglionic
Location of preganglionic nerve cell bodies	Nuclei in the brain and sacral portion of the spinal cord	Nuclei in the thoracolumbar portion of the spinal cord
Location of postganglionic nerve cell bodies	In ciliary, pterygopalatine, otic, mandibular, and sublingual ganglia of head or near structures innervated in thoracic and abdominal cavities	In sympathetic trunk, cranial cervical, middle cervical, cervicothoracic, celiac, cranial mesenteric and caudal mesenteric ganglia
Function	For quiet, vegetative functions	For active, stressful situations

FIG. 28.2. Cervical and cranial thoracic portions of the left vagus, ventrolateral view.

The AUTONOMIC NERVOUS SYSTEM (ANS) is generally defined as the system of GVE fibers. The term GENERAL VISCERAL EFFERENT (GVE) describes motor innervation to visceral structures. VISCUS refers to an organ in one of the three large cavities of the body; however, in addition to viscera, the ANS supplies innervation to smooth muscle of blood vessels, smooth muscles of the eye, and many glands that are not restricted to the body cavities.

Anatomically and pharmacologically the ANS is divided into two units (Table 28.1): SYMPATHETIC and PARASYMPATHETIC. These two divisions are antagonistic in function, with the sympathetic portion of the ANS preparing the body for greater skeletomuscular activity and the parasympathetic portion preparing the body for quiet digestive-type activity. In general, each structure innervated by the sympathetic portion of the ANS is also innervated by the parasympathetic portion, and vice versa. Some exceptions to this dual innervation are sweat glands, arrector pili muscles, adrenal glands, testes, kidney, and smooth muscle of blood vessels, all of which receive little parasympathetic innervation. Continuous stimulation at a low level by both parasympathetic and sympathetic portions of the ANS produces a maintained state of partial contraction (tone) in visceral structures. Each portion can exert both positive and negative effects by either increasing or decreasing the number of impulses above or below the normal level.

The sympathetic nerve fibers extend from the thoracic and lumbar segments of the spinal cord to all regions of the body. The parasympathetic fibers extend from the brain and sacral segment of the spinal cord to visceral structures.

Each VAGUS (cranial X) NERVE (1, Fig. 28.2) extends caudally through the neck in association with fibers of the SYMPATHETIC TRUNK (2), which carry efferent impulses toward the head. The vagus and sympathetic trunk, bound together by connective tissue, are collectively named the VAGOSYMPATHETIC TRUNK (3). The sympathetic trunk is composed predominantly of preganglionic sympathetic fibers. The CRANIAL CERVICAL GANGLION (4) is an aggregation of nerve cell bodies, which are part of postganglionic sympathetic nerve fibers that are distributed with blood vessels and cranial nerves to nearly all parts of the head. Right and left vagus nerves separate from right and left sympathetic trunks near the level of the 1st ribs; a sympathetic ganglion, the MIDDLE CERVICAL GANGLION (5), may be observed near the level at which each vagus and sympathetic trunk separate.

FIG. 28.3. Thoracic portion of the right and left vagus nerves, ventral view.

The RIGHT VAGUS NERVE (1, Fig. 28.3) courses caudally ventral to the right subclavian artery and vein, the main vessels of the thoracic limb, giving off a number of branches as it passes caudally dorsal to the base of the heart. One relatively large branch, the RIGHT RECURRENT LARYNGEAL NERVE (2), curves craniodorsally around the right subclavian artery, then courses cranially toward the larynx in contact with the trachea and next to the right longus capitis muscle. The right recurrent laryngeal nerve innervates the esophagus and trachea. The RIGHT CAUDAL LARYNGEAL NERVE, a terminal branch of the right recurrent laryngeal, innervates all of the intrinsic laryngeal muscles on the right side except for the cricothyroideus. A number of nerve fibers branch from the vagus or recurrent laryngeal nerve near the base of the heart; some of these fibers are cardiac branches and some are bronchial branches. The LEFT VAGUS NERVE (3) separates from the sympathetic trunk near the left middle cervical ganglion and continues caudally past the base of the heart. The LEFT RECURRENT LARYNGEAL NERVE (4) curves dorsomedially around the aorta and then passes cranially toward the larynx between the trachea and esophagus. The branches of the left recurrent laryngeal nerve are the same as those of the right side.

Bronchial and cardiac branches arise from the vagus near the base of the heart. Both right and left vagi divide into dorsal (5) and ventral (6) branches dorsal to the caudal portion of the base of the heart. The right and left ventral vagal branches unite on the ventral surface of the esophagus to form the VENTRAL VAGAL TRUNK (7), which supplies fibers to the esophagus and then passes caudally through the esophageal hiatus of the diaphragm. Right and left dorsal vagal branches course along the right and left dorsolateral aspects of the esophagus, respectively, and fuse with each other near the thoracic diaphragm. The DORSAL VAGAL TRUNK supplies fibers to the esophagus and continues caudally through the esophageal hiatus with the esophagus and ventral vagal trunk.

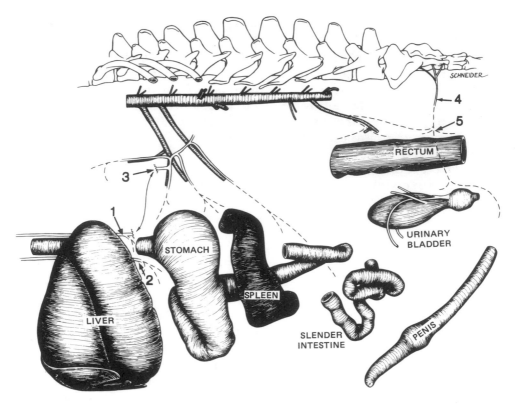

FIG. 28.4. Schematic of the distribution of parasympathetic fibers in the abdominal and pelvic cavities, lateral view.

FIG. 28.5. Some possible sympathetic pathways through which impulses may pass in going from the spinal cord to the effector site.

In the abdominal cavity, the dorsal (1, Fig. 28.4) and ventral (2) vagal trunks may be located along the lesser curvature of the stomach. The ventral vagal trunk supplies fibers to the liver, gallbladder, bile duct, pancreas, and parietal surface and pylorus of the stomach. The dorsal vagal trunk innervates the cardiac and visceral regions of the stomach as well as the pylorus. A CELIAC BRANCH (3) of the dorsal vagal trunk passes caudodorsally to a plexus around the origin of two major unpaired arteries that supply the viscera. Nerve fibers pass along these arteries and their branches to much of the abdominal viscera.

The PELVIC NERVE (4) carries parasympathetic fibers to the caudal abdominal and pelvic viscera; it also is a carrier of GVA fibers. The pelvic nerve arises as branches of the ventral rami of sacral spinal nerves. Right and left pelvic nerves each form a PELVIC PLEXUS (5) on the lateral surface of the caudal portion of the rectum within the pelvic cavity. Preganglionic parasympathetic fibers extend from the spinal cord through this plexus to reach the rectum, urinary bladder, uterus, descending colon, etc.

Preganglionic sympathetic neurons arise from the spinal cord and enter the sympathetic trunk ganglia between the 1st thoracic and 4th to 5th lumbar spinal cord segments. Although sympathetic fibers seldom arise from the spinal cord cranial to T1 or caudal to L5, they gain access to all areas of the body by leaving the sympathetic trunk to be distributed with cranial nerves, spinal nerves, and blood vessels.

Preganglionic neurons (1, Fig. 28.5) pass to SYMPATHETIC TRUNK GANGLIA (2) through COMMUNICATING RAMI (3); some of the preganglionic neurons synapse in the first ganglion entered, or in a sympathetic trunk ganglion located either more cranially or more caudally, while others synapse in a ganglion (4) located within the abdominal cavity. Postganglionic sympathetic neurons (5) pass through a communicating ramus to a spinal nerve and thus innervate glands of the skin or blood vessels of the body wall; pass to various parts of the body wall with blood vessels; or pass out to the viscera with blood vessels or nerves of the thoracic, abdominal, and pelvic cavities.

FIG. 28.6. Thoracic portion of the sympathetic nervous system, ventral view.

LEFT CRUS OF THE
THORACIC DIAPHRAGM

FIG. 28.7. Abdominal and pelvic portions of the sympathetic trunk, ventral view.

In the region of the thoracic inlet, medial to the 1st rib, each middle cervical ganglion, right and left (1, Fig. 28.6), is connected to a cranial cervical ganglion by the cervical portion of the sympathetic trunk (2) and to the CERVICOTHORACIC GANGLION (3) by means of the ANSA SUBCLAVIA (4). The ansa (or "loop") is a nerve that passes caudodorsally, around the ventral surface of the subclavian artery, from the middle cervical ganglion to the cervicothoracic ganglion. In general, preganglionic sympathetic fibers emerging from the spinal cord through thoracic spinal nerves cranial to T5 pass cranially in the sympathetic trunk, while those arising caudal to T5 pass caudally in the sympathetic trunk. Some of the preganglionic neurons pass cranially to synapse in the cranial cervical ganglion, while others synapse in either the middle cervical or the cervicothoracic ganglion. Postganglionic sympathetic fibers separate from the cervicothoracic ganglion, ansa subclavia, and middle cervical ganglion and pass to structures of the thoracic cavity or course along with blood vessels to the body wall. The VERTEBRAL NERVE (5) is a sympathetic postganglionic pathway or plexus that passes craniodorsally with the vertebral artery through the transverse foramina of cervical vertebrae; sympathetic fibers reach most of the cervical spinal nerves via the vertebral nerve.

The caudal continuations of right and left sympathetic trunks (Fig. 28.7), consisting of sympathetic trunk ganglia (1) and INTERGANGLIONIC RAMI (2), are situated along the dorsal surface of the thoracic, abdominal, and pelvic cavities. The sympathetic trunks are situated on each side of the vertebral column external or superficial to the parietal pleura (thoracic cavity) or parietal peritoneum (abdominal and pelvic cavities). At the approximate level of the 13th thoracic spinal nerve, a relatively large nerve arises from a sympathetic trunk ganglion and passes caudoventrally into the abdominal cavity past the lateral surface of the crus of the diaphragm. This MAJOR SPLANCHNIC NERVE (3) is adjacent and ventromedial to the lumbar continuation of the small sympathetic trunk, which also is situated lateral to the crus of the thoracic diaphragm.

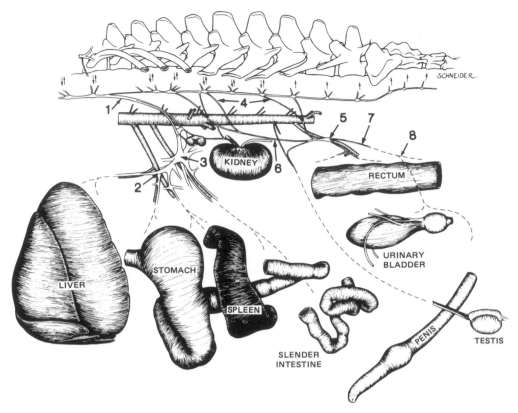

FIG. 28.8. Schematic of the distribution of sympathetic fibers in the abdominal and pelvic cavities, lateral view.

FIG. 28.9. Schematic of the relative positions of right and left sympathetic trunks and abdominal aorta, ventral view.

The major splanchnic nerve (1, Fig. 28.8) supplies fibers to the aorta, adrenal gland, and to the plexuses of fibers over the proximal portion of two of the major arteries to the abdominal viscera. These plexuses are named the CELIAC (2) and CRANIAL MESENTERIC (3) PLEXUSES according to the artery they are situated around. Sympathetic ganglia, CELIAC and CRANIAL MESENTERIC, are present in the plexus of sympathetic and parasympathetic fibers. Postganglionic sympathetic fibers course along with branches of these two arteries to the visceral structures they supply.

The sympathetic trunk is larger in the lumbar region than at the level of the caudal portion of the thorax. LUMBAR SPLANCHNIC NERVES (4) arise from a number of sympathetic trunk ganglia and course ventromedially to any of several ganglia or visceral structures. Lumbar splanchnics arising from ganglia at the 5th to 7th lumbar spinal nerve levels pass ventro-medially to the CAUDAL MESENTERIC PLEXUS and GANGLION (5). Fibers belonging to the INTERMESENTERIC PLEXUS (6) may be observed spanning the distance between the cranial and caudal mesenteric plexuses. Some postganglionic fibers are distributed with the femoral artery to the pelvic limb.

RIGHT and LEFT HYPOGASTRIC NERVES (7) are composed of predominantly postganglionic sympathetic neurons coursing from the caudal mesenteric ganglion (where their nerve cell bodies are located) to the pelvic plexus (8) on the lateral surface of the pelvic portion of the rectum. The sympathetic fibers course through the pelvic plexus to reach the various pelvic visceral structures; some postganglionic fibers pass out to the pelvic limb with the ischiatic and femoral nerves.

The right and left sympathetic trunks (1, Fig. 28.9) are more slender in the sacral region and tend to converge toward the median plane. Postganglionic sympathetic fibers pass from sympathetic trunk ganglia through communicating rami to sacral spinal nerves. The sympathetic trunks extend into the caudal region.

INDEX

THE TOWN HOUSE

By Norah Lofts

THE
TOWN
HOUSE

The Building of
the House

NORAH LOFTS

DOUBLEDAY & COMPANY, INC.

GARDEN CITY, NEW YORK

1959

Library of Congress Catalog Card Number 59–13680

Part One

MARTIN
REED'S
TALE

I

Few born serfs, like me, could tell you their birthdate, but I was born in that memorable year of 1381 when the peasants, armed only with the tools of their trade, supported by a few soldiers, back from the wars, and a few priests with hearts of compassion, rose up against their masters, against the laws and the customs that made a serf the property of his lord. They gave—according to the stories—a good account of themselves: the men of Kent reached London and forced the King himself to lend ear to their grievances. In the end, though, they were disbanded by trickery, sent away soothed by false promises, and the freedom they dreamed of did not come in their generation, nor the next. So, when I was born in the autumn of that year, 1381, I was born a serf as much the property of my Lord Bowdegrave as the horse he rode, and—at least until I reached working age—of less value; for his horse had an Arab strain, far more rare and precious than my Saxon peasant blood.

My mother died at, or soon after, my birth, and although some woman must have suckled me, or fed me with pap, I have no memory of it. For me life began in the forge, where my father worked and where I learned not to touch hot things because they burned, not to get in his way because his hand was heavy, and not to go too near the horses' heels. I was working the bellows—and doing it properly—when I was still so small that I had to stand on a great stone in order to hold them level with the fire.

For his work on my lord's horses and harness and field tools and armour on occasion, my father, being a villein, received no wage. He had his hut, a strip of land in each of the three open fields, and the right to eat his dinner at the lowest table in the hall. When he worked for other people he could make his charge in coin or in kind, and he was not unprosperous. Some years before the rising of 1381 there had been a great sickness in which many people had died; skilled smiths were not as common as they had been. On some manors my father could have hoped and tried, by industry and thrift, to have saved enough money to buy his freedom, but my Lord Bowdegrave was a lord after the ancient fashion and boasted that never, on any of his three manors, had he manumitted a serf for money. My father knew this and therefore, given the choice of a coin or payment in meat or drink, he would choose the latter, so in our hut we ate well and I grew taller and stronger than most of my kind.

Maybe my wits profited from the good food, too, for when the time came for me to learn the Catechism and Responses our parish priest praised me often, and in the end was taken with the notion of making a clerk of me. He was himself the son of a serf, base-born like me and set free by Holy Church, and he hoped to push me through the same door.

To my surprise my father was in favour of the plan. He was already showing signs of the dreaded smiths' palsy, that ungovernable shaking of the hands which results from the strain of lifting the heavy hammer and from the jar and thud of its fall. It was, as yet, slight, just a tremor which increased towards the end of the day, so that sometimes in the evening he would slop a little ale from his mug, but he knew what it heralded. He knew, too, that, on the manor of Rede, the old and the infirm had little to hope for. He would, of course, be entitled to a place by my fire, a share of the food of my table, but it would be a place and a share measured by the size of my family and the generosity or otherwise of the woman I married. He rightly reckoned that as the father of a celibate parish priest he would fare better, so, looking ahead, he allowed me time to take my lessons.

Learning came easy to me. I was, naturally, idle as all boys are, and earned myself many a buffet, but the priest said I had the makings of a scholar and would do him great credit in later years. As time went on I would relieve the tedium of the lessons by concocting questions which I hoped he would not be able to answer; the hope was justified more and more frequently. He had forgotten much of what he had learned. At last, in the summer before I was ten years old, he went to Norwich and bespoke for me a place in the monks' school there, where he had got his own learning. After that there was only one thing needed to set me on my way to clerkdom, and that was the permission of my Lord Bowdegrave to leave the manor and his service. The priest never doubted that permission would be given.

"My lord boasts that he has never sold a serf his freedom, but he will not hesitate to make a gift of you to Holy Church," he said.

My Lord Bowdegrave was seldom at his manor of Rede; he had two others, one in Lincoln, one in Kent. This last was his favourite, being within easier reach of London, but the others were visited each year immediately after harvest, at which time even the most trusty steward might go a little awry in his reckonings. Also, after harvest, when the great field was all a-stubble, was the best time of the year for hawking.

It was in the first week of October in the year 1391 that I first came face to face with the man who owned me. My face and hands had been scoured, my hair was newly shorn, and I was wearing a clean smock. I was very much frightened. The priest, who must have been—I now realise—a very simple and unworldly man, had warned me that my lord would surely wish to test my abilities. I must be prepared for questions; I must not answer hastily and without thought, nor must I answer slowly and thus appear stupid. Above all I must speak up so that I could be heard, and with the very greatest respect.

The steward had plainly prepared my lord for our appearance, for as we entered the great hall, he said, "Ah! The smith's son. I remember."

Fright boiled in my throat. I knew I could never answer a question, no matter how simple. Fright laid a heavy hand on my neck, so that my head was bowed, my eyes fixed on the rushes, fresh spread for my lord's visit.

Above me the voice asked one question.

"How many sons has the man?"

The steward said, "This one, my lord."

"Then he cannot be spared. Bad clerks are plentiful; good smiths are few." Thus briefly was my future, the priest's hopes, my father's old-age comfort disposed of. From my lord's verdict there was no appeal.

I was able then, for some reason, to raise my eyes and look into the face of the man whose lightest word was to us, his villeins, weightier than the King's law or the edicts of our Holy Father, the

Pope in Rome. It was a handsome, well-fleshed face, highly coloured; stern too, as befitted a man of consequence, but not ill-natured. From the height of his chair on the dais he looked down at me, and his light hazel eyes took my measure.

"You're a stout, likely-looking lad," he said, "far more fitted to handle a hammer than a quill." Having thus dismissed me, he lifted and crooked a finger and said, "A word in your ear, Sir Priest."

What the word was was not for me to know, but I noticed that from that day onward the priest favoured me no more but seemed rather to avoid me.

The priest may have suffered some disappointment. Now that I am older and know more, I can see that, having made the one great stride from serfdom to clerkdom, he had shot his bolt; he had ended as a priest in a small, poor parish. Had I become the scholar that he thought I had it in me to be, then he would have been more, for great scholars remember their teachers and many a man of small learning is immortal because he taught the rudiments to one who has become famous. But this, of course, I only guess at.

My father and I, on the other hand, suffered nothing so positive as disappointment. I had been dreading the discipline of the convent school and the break with everything I knew, the harder lessons, the competition with boys born free. And my father was consoled for the loss of a more secure old age by the thought that in the immediate future he would have my assistance at the forge. Also—and this I have seen proved many times in later years—it is seldom those who are oppressed who resent their oppression; they wear it as they wear their clothes. Serfs, when they rise against their serfdom, are always led by free-born men. There was nothing of resentment in us. My lord had spoken, and as he said, so it would be. I went back to the forge and the anvil; I began to take great pride in my strength, and later in my skill. Smith's work is a man's work, and it was quite as much to my taste as the question-and-answer work with the priest, who would drub my head if I erred.

So, year followed year; life went on in the old pattern. I grew, and I learned, toiling on the working days and making merry on holy days. I might well have lived and died at Rede, one of my Lord Bowdegrave's possessions, had I not fallen in love.

II

Love is not, it is rightly not, a thing for every day, for ordinary people. Love is for the minstrels and the singing men to make tales of. That way it is safe.

How often have I heard a singing man strum his lute and raise his voice:

> "A gracious fate to me, to me is sent;
> Methinks it is by Heaven lent.
> From women all my heart is bent
> To joy in Alyson."

There is a pleasant thought, set to a tunable air, and suitable for a singing man who means nothing by it. Pity the poor fool of a man who, in this our life, suffers such a fate; who goes mad and sets one woman above all others, above all else. I know whereof I speak, for such a poor fool was I.

Men of property choose women who will bring them good dowers; acres to link with their acres, coin to rattle with their own, or a good name to boast of, or some other advantage: poor men, when the itch comes upon them, take the wench who is handiest, or, if they are uncommonly prudent, have a care to pick one with sound limbs, sweet breath, and—so far as such things can be judged aforehand—an amiable temper. And they all do very well, since any woman can bear a child or boil a dumpling.

But I . . . I must needs fall in love!

There was, at first sight, no reason why my love for my sweet Kate should cause any upset. She belonged to our manor of Rede, and her father was, like mine, a villein. He was a shepherd and lived on the sheep run, over by the river in a remote and lonely place; and since Ancaster Church was nearer his hut than ours of Rede, he and his family went to Mass there; so I was twenty and Kate was seventeen before I noticed her, and then it was only by chance.

I was by this time a skilled smith and more active than my father, so when there was a job to be done at a distance I was the one to go; and on an April afternoon I was coming home from Ancaster, walking downhill towards the river where the steppingstones were, when I saw, on the Rede side of the stream, a child—as I thought—washing some linen in the stream. That was an ordinary sight enough on an April day when the body-clothes worn through the winter could be sloughed off and cleansed, and I took no notice until a woman came out of the shepherd's hut, walked towards the child, berating her as she walked, and then, snatching up a broken branch that lay nearby, began to lay on heavily.

That again was no extraordinary sight, and it was not for me to interfere between parent and child; only the priest, or perhaps the steward, had the right to do that. The little girl took the punishment without outcry and, for all I knew, deserved it. But after a moment, I, who all my life had seen women beating their children, was struck by the ferocity with which this woman went about the job. I splashed over the stones, and on the other side slowed my pace and at last stood still. The woman seemed to be in a killing rage, and the prevention of murder is every man's Christian duty. So I said:

"Have a care, good wife. Such heavy stripes might kill the little wench."

From what Kate told me later I have no doubt the woman would, sooner or later, have done that, but not out in the open under the eye of a witness. She gave me a savage look and laid on three more blows, as though to prove her right, but they were lighter ones, and then she threw down the branch and went stamping and grumbling away back into the hut.

My fate then made me go to comfort the child, and as soon as I was within arm's reach of her I saw that her smallness belied her years; inside the torn dress was the white curve and the pink bud of a girl's breast. I looked on it and was lost.

I am not a poet or a singing man to tell of love. When I think of what made her dearer to me than any other, I can only say that she was so small, so light and thin and small, like a little bird, a little rabbit. To the end of our days together I never grew used to the smallness of her, and my hands—sometimes against my will—always went gentle when they neared her. For the rest, her hair was the colour of new-run honey and her eyes as blue as a speedwell.

I held her close to me for comfort, and, dragging down the end of my sleeve, I dipped it in the water and wiped away the blood where the skin was broken. She cried then. That was ever her way;

to bear the blow, no matter how heavy, with fortitude, and then melt at a word or touch of kindness. When she was quiet again I asked for what reason her mother dealt so ill with her.

"She is not my mother. She is my father's new wife and she wishes me out of the house."

"To go would be better than to be treated thus roughly," I said.

"I cannot. The steward orders me to stay. I help my father with the sheep."

"Then he must stand between you and the woman."

"Ah, but she lays about him with her tongue," Kate said. "I should think shame to tell you what she says of us if ever he even looks at me kindly."

I held her in the crook of my arm and thought more rapidly than I had done for years, since I had done the last time the priest questioned me. Up to that moment the business of bedding and breeding had troubled me less than it does most men. One day, I had said to myself, I should marry and get a son to work in the forge when I, in my turn, began to shake and shudder, but it had never seemed an urgent or even a desirable business. There had never been a woman in our hut, and Father and I had managed very well; we were peaceful and better fed than most. But now I knew. . . .

"Be of good heart," I said, "and keep out of the woman's way as far as you can. I shall be back tomorrow, to see how you fare." I dared not say more lest I should raise a hope which it would be cruel to cast down. Rede, though in many ways a manor far behind the times, was well run, and the priest kept the Kin Book in order to make sure that no marriage was within the forbidden degree. There were the laws of the Church to be minded, and other, unwritten laws which ruled against the wedding of double cousins, that is, cousins related upon both sides. Experience had proved such unions to be bad alike for mind and body, harelips, fits, deafness, dumbness, and blindness had been the penalties of such near-incest in the past. So, on all properly managed estates, even the lowest hind had his "pedigree," and it must be consulted before leave to marry was given.

When I left Kate I went straight to the priest's house. I told him that I wished to marry Kate, daughter to the shepherd, and he said something which I always remembered.

"I have watched you, Walter, my son, and it has vexed me lest, all unwitting, I made a monk out of you when you were young, yet failed to bestow the benefit of clergy upon you. I was not to blame."

"I know that, Father. You had no cause to be vexed for me."

"You are twenty years old. Half your life is sped."

A cold thought for a man in love. I shuffled it off, looking at him; he had been in his middle years when he taught me.

"Ah," he said, "clerks live longer. That is the rule. Measure your years not by mine but by your father's. He lacks a year of his two score and he is an old man."

That was all too true. Oh, hurry, I said in my mind; open that Kin Book, give me leave to marry Kate, for twenty years is all too short a time. And yet, if we cannot marry, twenty years without her will last forever, they will last so long that I cannot live them out.

He used his finger on the page of parchment which, with other pages, all of slightly different size and tied by thongs onto a stave of wood, made up the book. Sweat broke out on my forehead and around my mouth. Weeks, months, years went by; and at last he lifted his head and said:

"You are no kin to her."

I thanked him as though he, and he alone, had arranged it.

It was too late, that evening, to disturb the steward; but early next morning, before he went out on his rounds, I went to him.

"Ha!" he said. "And about time too. By the Rood, I don't know what is happening to you young rascals. Too idle to breed! With labour so scarce, too." That reminded him of something else. "The wench must stay at her work," he said. "So she does that, nobody minds in which hut she sleeps. Except you, of course." He gave me a nudge and a leer. "You can tell shepherd that the bride fee will be two geese, rightly fattened. That being settled, I am sure you will have my lord's permission to marry. It is a pity that you must wait until his harvest visit."

That day I whistled as I worked, and as soon as I could down tools went, without waiting for my supper, over to the shepherd's hut and said to that weak-minded man, "I have, from priest and steward, permission to marry your daughter, Kate."

The woman looked pleased, but he grunted, and said something about talk coming cheap; he was a poor man with a wife and two children younger than Kate; where was the merchet coming from. He supposed I had never even thought of that; young men in their heat never remembered that every time a girl married the lord exacted his due.

"But I have remembered. Steward said two fat geese, and them I will provide."

"Three," he said, "can be fattened as easy as two. One for me, two for my lord, and the bargain is made."

"It is made," I said, and struck hands on it. "And now," I said, stepping back and including the woman in my stare, "any blow on Kate's body will be a blow on mine, and I will repay it fourfold." As I spoke I knotted my great fist and the muscle on my forearm leaped up and quivered. Shepherd bleated, like his own bellwether:

"The children have run overlong unmothered. Their new mother did no more than mend their manners."

His other children were boys, aged about seven and nine, and hardy looking. They bore no marks of ill-usage that I could see, whereas my poor Kate was all swollen and marked from yesterday's beating.

"Any correction that Kate needs from this day forward I will tend to," I said, smiling at her and feeling my heart go soft. "As for you boys, if the woman bears on you too hard, kick her back. You're two against one, or, if you, shepherd, had the courage of a louse, three. What did she bring as her marriage portion? A gelding iron?"

"Take your foot from my floor," the woman cried furiously.

"Gladly," I said, and, taking Kate by the arm, I drew her out and we went to a place where a bent hawthorn, just coming into flower, leaned over the stream. And there I held her close and we talked. I said:

"My pretty one, you shall be safe with me."

Safe with me. Yes, I said that. I looked down the years and saw her in our hut, eating fatly of food I had provided, growing smooth and sleek. She was so small and I was so strong; I would never even let her carry a bucket of water from the well. Her work as sheep-girl I could not order, but I would put fear into the shepherd, so that the hard tasks did not fall to her. She should be safe with me.

III

Now here is something which men born in free towns, or on the manors of more enlightened lords, may find hard to believe: or they will believe that it was true in times long past, not in my living memory. But I swear, by all that I hold holy, it was true at Rede.

It was a custom which our Norman masters brought with them. Having a little learning, I can give it its proper name, *jus primae noctis*, but we called it First Nights; and it meant simply that the lord of the manor had the right, if he so wished, to take any serf-born girl's maidenhead. Whether he exercised the right depended upon many things, the man's own lustfulness, age, or disposition, the way the girl looked, the fashion in the district. On many manors it was regarded as outmoded, like the Twelve Days of the Lord of Misrule at the Christmas season: but in this, as in other matters, my Lord Bowdegrave was old-fashioned, and here and there about Rede manor, and about his others I have no doubt, the long straight Norman nose, the cleft chin, the bright hazel eyes which were the visible sign of the Bowdegrave breed could be seen, incongruous in a peasant face, bearing witness that he had not only exercised his right, but done it potently. Of late years, however, age and an increasing heaviness—it took two stout men to heave him into his saddle by this time—had cooled his ardours, and for several seasons past he had contented himself with kissing the prospective bride if she were comely, or giving her a smack on the rump if she were otherwise.

Occasionally, during the weeks that followed my bespeaking of Kate, I thought upon this matter. It seemed to me impossible that any man, however old, however much he weighed, could look upon my Kate and not desire her. Yet, strange as it may sound to any not serfborn, I was not unduly disturbed. This matter of acceptance of circumstance cuts very deep. Think of those born humpbacked, deaf, blind. They accept their fate and bear it. I was born a serf. If my services were required even in the next village, Ancaster, to shoe a horse or mend a plough, I must ask the steward's permission before I could step across the boundary between Rede and Ancaster. Think how irksome that rule would be on any free man. To me it was nothing. In the same way it was . . . well, almost nothing, that the unlikely might happen and my Lord Bowdegrave should claim his First Nights right upon Kate. She would be mine for the rest of our lives. He could not be prevented. There lies the whole crux of the matter; what cannot be prevented must be borne, like unseasonal weather, mildew on wheat, murrain in cattle. Through May and June and the months that must drag until our lord's harvest visit, every time I thought upon the matter I told myself: There is nothing I can do; it is unlikely that he will claim his right, but if he does what is one night?

That was a year of most remarkable fine weather. With the new moon of June the heat set in, and by mid-July the corn was ready for reaping. Without hitch or hindrance, without so much as a summer shower to halt it, the harvest went on, and before the end of August, a full month early, the stubbles were cleared. My Lord Bowdegrave, informed of this, put forward his visit, and my time of waiting was cut from October to September.

I had ruled myself well. To a degree the season had been in my favour; hay-time and harvest are busy times for smiths, and this year, since they followed so hard on one another's heels, I was doubly busy. Also Kate's father, resenting, perhaps, my words about the gelding iron, had sent Kate farther and farther afield as pasture became scarce. So I saw her but rarely. However, late in August, the grass having grown again on the lowland by the river, the flock came home, and one night, under a lopsided moon, she and I lay together.

It was sin; but she was guiltless. God and all the saints are witness to that. I did it deliberately, courting all blame. I had heard that day, somewhere in the yard, that my lord was on his way to Rede, and I thought: He is old and clumsy, and he does not love her. She is very small. There may be hurt and it is better that I, who love her . . . That was part of my thought, but not all. There was the reined-in desire of the last five months, and there was the wish to forestall, to be first, despite all custom.

Afterwards I took her face between my hands with their calloused palms and blackened nails and I said, "Now you belong to me."

So then my Lord Bowdegrave came to Rede and there was much commotion, with the paying of the rents and the taking of tallies of all his stacks and beasts and flitches and honeycombs. Then, one fine morning, Kate and I were called into the hall, just as, long ago, my father and I had been called when it was to ask consent for me to go to the monks' school. Walking over the fresh rushes, hand in hand with Kate, I was grateful that that consent had been refused.

I had warned Kate not to make herself look pretty. I still, in my serf's heart, admitted the old lord's right, but by the mere action of forestalling him I had taken a step out of bondage. I had risen up,

under the moon, and said, "You belong to me"; later I saw the
falseness of that. If you lay claim to a piece of land, you should
be able to prove your right in the face of all men; if you cannot
do so, any man who trespasses there does you more wrong than
if he walked on common land. I was anxious, therefore, that she
should not appear in the hall with her hair newly washed and
streaming over her shoulders, wearing the wreath of flowers which
marked the bride-to-be. Kate had laughed and asked, "Shall I smear
wood ash on my face?"

Even had she done so it would not have hidden the fine shape-
liness of her bones, the thickness of her honey-coloured hair, or the
blue of her eyes. I saw the old man look at her; first with that
pitiable, old-man lustful look, wishing he were ten, twenty years
younger; then in another fashion. Even as the steward hastily
named us, Walter, the smith's son, Kate, the shepherd's daughter,
no relation according to the Kin Book, I saw the old man straighten
himself and shift a little in his seat.

"Both of this manor, which will neither gain nor lose labour
thereby," chanted the steward.

"Have done," said my lord. He dragged his eyes away from Kate,
and, shifting a little more, turned to me.

"You're my smith, eh?"

"Yes, my lord."

"Then this is an ill choice, surely. You need a wench capable of
working the bellows for you at a pinch, and breeding good strong
boys. This little maid is altogether too fine and delicate for your
purpose." His face had grown fat and purple since I last looked at
him; in it his eyes shone, his lips were wet, with lechery. He leaned
forward a little and reached out his great mottled hand to take Kate
by the wrist.

"I can find you better employment; in the still room of my house
at Abhurst. You'd like that, eh?"

Without giving her time to answer—for what did it matter
whether she said yes or no?—he said to the steward, "Have her
ready to ride, pillion to Jack or Will, when I go."

To describe a moment of boundless rage, folks often speak of
"seeing red." A true word. I saw red then. My Lord Bowdegrave,
the chair upon which he sat, the tapestry on the wall behind him,
the steward standing by, were all gulped up before my eyes in a
great red wave, into which I plunged my fist with all my weight

behind it. I felt, but did not see, the smash of my knuckles upon the great leering face. The next instant something hit me across the back of my skull, and the redness gave way to a burst of sparks and then to blackness.

The utter black pricked out with stars, and there I was, lying flat on my back with my face to the sky. There was not an inch of me that was not in pain. My hide had been broken in a score of places, and the whole of my body was set stiff in a case of dried blood. Somebody had given me a monstrous fine thrashing. I moved myself carefully and found that none of my main bones were broken; then I rolled over on my face and was sick and felt better for it. Bit by bit I came to myself. I was stark, stripped of my hose and shirt, and I lay on the dung-heap. Left for dead, I thought to myself. Remembering what I had done, and why, it struck me that maybe I should have been better dead, which thought, naturally, brought me fully back to life. I gathered myself together, piece by piece, and reeled into the forge which was handy, and where we always kept a bucket of clean water to slake our thirst. Feeling my way to it, I dipped the horn mug and drank again and again, taking in, with the cool blessed water, the full sense of the plight I was in. I must get away, and I could not go naked. I staggered away to our hut.

There was a strong smell of onions, and the fire upon which my father had cooked his supper was still a small pink glimmer on the hearthstone. He lay in his bed. I threw a handful of dry sticks on the embers, and as the flames leaped he moved, lifted his head, saw me, and crossed himself hurriedly, saying, "God betwixt me and harm."

"It's only me, Father."

"A ghost," he whispered.

"My living self." The flames gained power, and he could see me, horrid as any ghost, stripped and all bloody.

"I gave you up for dead," he said.

I was his son; we had lived together in fair amity for twenty years, and of late I had carried the weight of the work. I did not blame him for leaving me where I lay; I had done an unforgivable thing and he had his own safety to look to. But he had come home, cooked his onions, laid down to sleep. At the back of my mind something stirred, a whole thought in a breathing space. That was to be a serf. A serf had no right even to human feelings; it was only by throwing away all claim to human feelings that a serf could support his way of life. I had, this very morning, acted like a man, not a serf; and with what result!

"Small thanks to those who beat me that I am not dead. And if I am here by morning, dead I shall be." I forced my bruised, stiff limbs to move more briskly. I had dressed in my best to wait upon my lord, so now I must don my stinking working clothes. Then, because our hoard was hidden in the earth under his bed, I had to ask my father:

"Give me my share of the money we have saved."

He got up, grumbling.

"Less the price of the three geese your share is," he said.

"But I am leaving the geese with you. Father, I must go far away. Who knows what may befall me? A penny may mean life or death to me."

"And who is to blame for that?" Recovering from his fear of being visited by a dead man's ghost, he began to rate me. Mad, reckless, ingrate. That ever son of his should lift violent hand against his lord. Shame, shame, undying shame; and worse. Punishment for him for breeding and raising such a rogue.

"You showed your colours plain enough when you left me for dead on the dung-heap and came home and roasted your onions. You have nothing to fear. Who else, when I am gone, can shoe a horse within ten miles?"

"That is true," he said, comforted again.

Yet, when he had unearthed our little hoard, he divided the coins into two heaps, then took from mine the sum I had paid for the three geese and added it to his own. I protested at that.

"The sixpence for the geese should be laid aside first, then the sum should be divided. The way you have it now, you are twelve-pence to the good."

"You talk like the fool you are. You took out sixpence in April to buy the three geese. Now we divide into fair shares, and I take sixpence from your share and put to my own since I did not buy geese."

Nothing would make him see differently, and I dared not stay to beat it out with him. I took the twenty-one pence which was my share, put them, a half loaf, a piece of cheese, my knife, and a length of good cord into the little bag in which, when I worked away from home, I carried my noon piece, and then I was ready.

"You never saw me," I told him. "For all you know the crows picked out my eyes and the dogs ran off with my bones. If any speak to you of me, rail against me as you have just done."

I was on my way out, ducking at the low doorway, when he said in an uncertain voice, "God go with you, Walter." I remembered then that he was my father, growing old and tremulous, his working days almost numbered, and with no one now to depend upon. And he had taught me my trade without too much clouting. So I forgave him his supper, and the unfair division and made him a fair answer.

"God be with you," I said; and went out into the night.

I V

The river bank, near to the place where Kate had been washing that day, was dotted with clumps of gorse bushes. I chose one close to the path worn between the shepherd's hut and the stepping-stones where the family dipped their water, and there I hid myself. The gorse made an uncomfortable hiding place, but I was so sore all over that a few scratches mattered little. It was in my mind that I was most ill at ease. I had no certainty at all that Kate had been sent back home; it seemed far more likely that she had spent the night at the hall, in my lord's bed most like. But there was a faint, faint chance that she had come home, and I could not leave Rede forever without snatching at that chance.

Day dawned. A thin blue thread of smoke rose from the hole in the hut roof; the shepherd came out, eased himself by the wall, and went in again. Presently Kate herself came out, carrying a bucket. She must have cried all through the night; her face was swollen with tears. She looked stupid with misery and moved listlessly. When she was as near my bush as the path to the water would bring her I said, softly:

"Don't look round." I had debated with myself whether to say that first, or, "Don't be frightened." It seemed to me that a fright she would get over, whereas for me to be observed would be fatal. I quickly added, "Don't be frightened; and don't speak."

I cannot understand why all the mummers in the world—even

when it is the Blessed Virgin to be represented—should be men. Women are natural mummers. Apart from a slight start when she first heard my voice, Kate gave no sign at all. She walked down to the river, dipped the bucket, and came back, leaning sideways against the weight. Level with me, she set it down and stood rubbing her arm and shoulder, at the same time yawning heartily.

I jerked out a few words, telling her that I meant to slip away to the woods.

"I'm not asking you to come. Every man's hand will be against me. And you could live soft at Abhurst. But if you *want* to come, I shall wait in Tuck's Oak till dusk."

I was not being unselfish. At that moment, much as I loved her, I was not sure that I wanted her with me. I felt weak and sick and sore, and I was about to do something new and dangerous, something I had never heard of anyone else doing successfully. A man about to jump from a great height, or swim a wide stream in the dark, is better off without a woman clinging about his neck, however well beloved she may be. Yet in my heart, if not in my head, I must have wanted her to come, else why had I not made straight for the woods and got away under cover of darkness; why was I prepared to risk waiting all day?

Kate took up the bucket and moved away, and in a moment I heard the voice of her stepmother, intent now upon currying favour with one who shortly might have benefits to bestow.

"Give me that bucket," she said, her scolding voice overlaid with forced good humour. "You don't want blisters on your hands tomorrow."

They went indoors; the thread of smoke thickened. Soon, I judged, they would be breaking their fast. I began to move. I went on my belly like a snake, from gorse bush to gorse bush, keeping alongside the river until I was out of sight of the hut. Then I went to the water's edge and laid down my leather apron and the little round cap, which all careful smiths wear to save their hair from rubbing against the horses' hides and picking up the running itch. I walked into the water, careful to make clear footmarks in the mud. I waded downstream in the water until my legs were so benumbed that they failed me; then I climbed out and made for the woods. I hoped that I had broken the scent which the hounds and my lord's huntsman would soon be following. I hoped that my offcast apron and cap would look as though I had drowned myself.

Once safe in the great forest, I regretted having made tryst with Kate. "All for love," sing the singing men, and in their songs love risks all, conquers all, never doubts and never falters. But the Bible says, "All that a man has will he give for his life," and, for ordinary, frightened men like me, that is a true saying. I was in the forest by midday and could have made good progress during the hours of daylight, had I not promised to wait. I climbed Tuck's Oak and lay along a stout branch, sweating with fear at the thought of the hounds casting up and down the river bank. Would any see through my trick? Would the search be long enough and patient enough to pick up my trail again? I remembered the way my fist had smashed into my lord's face; he would feel the damage this morning; he would be after me for vengeance as well as for my value. The longest day's labour had never seemed so long as the few hours I waited; and they were few, for Kate came while it was still broad day. She brought a basket into which she had packed four goose eggs, some cold mutton, a loaf of bread, and some apples. She had thought to bring her winter's cloak.

At the sight of her, the realisation that she had chosen to be hunted with me, rather than to live at ease with our master, love leaped up in me again. I was glad that I had lain in the gorse and waited in the tree, and glad beyond all measure that she had come. I dropped from the bough, took the basket from her, and, holding her by the hand, set off in a southerly direction. She told me that the huntsman and two brace of hounds had found my hiding place in the gorse, followed it until it ended, and then, after casting about for an hour, returned. The man was carrying my cap and apron.

"And how did you get away so soon?"

"I said I must carry my father's dinner—for the last time. And for once she did not stand over me, weighing with her eye all that I put into the basket." She laughed. "Father said good-bye and he hoped that when I was in the still room at Abhurst I should remember that he was a poor man with several mouths to feed. I said I would. Then, when I left him, I came here."

"The hounds. If they are brought out on *your* trail?"

She laughed again. "The sheep always loved me. I had but to call and they would follow. They came after me almost to the wood's edge—Father was too busy with his dinner to mind them. When I was ready I turned and scattered them. It would be a rare hound that could scent me on ground sheep had been over twice."

"So it would. And you, my Kate, are rarer among women than that hound among hounds." I slackened pace long enough to kiss her heartily and then pressed on.

"Where are we going?" she asked.

"The only answer I can give you is away from Norwich. That is where they will seek us. So we must walk in the other direction until we reach a walled town."

That was another thing which every serf knew, it was part of his serf's heritage, the knowledge that if by some miracle he could ever escape from his manor and reach a walled town and there spend one year and one day, without being reclaimed or committing any offence against the town laws, then he would be a free man. Alongside this knowledge—which one might think any serf would try to use to his advantage almost as soon as he could walk—lay other knowledge all concerned with the risks and the difficulties and the ferocious punishments which awaited any who made an unsuccessful attempt. Once off his manor without leave, a serf was a marked man; for miles around a rider on a swift horse would raise the hue-and-cry, and while that was on any stranger would be challenged and asked to explain himself; when the runaway was overtaken he would be brought back, whipped, and branded. Such a fate few serfs were prepared to face in order to gain "freedom," which was just a word to them. The dues and the duties of villeinage might be heavy or light—it depended upon the lord of the manor, upon his steward or bailiff, upon old custom, but whether heavy or light they had worn calloused places upon the bodies and minds of the bondsmen, and, unless something out of the ordinary disagreeable happened, as it had happened in my case, no man in his senses would throw himself out into the unknown world. At least, so it was at Rede, which, as I have said before, was much behind the times in every way. I had never known a man to run away, and should never have done so myself had I not been driven. Having run, I intended, if possible, to make good my attempt.

I did not know then, though I know it now, that the great forest stretched, with but few large clearings, from the Wash to the Thames River, but I knew it was large and I hoped that Kate and I could stay in its shelter for a long time, and then perhaps emerge at Colchester, which was the only town besides Norwich which I knew by name. I knew it because of its oyster beds; every year, when my lord made his after-harvest visit, great creels of them were hurried up on horseback to lay upon his table. Where this town lay I did not know, except that it was southward, and my hope of reaching it was only a hope. For the woods, while offering shelter from the hue-and-cry along the roads, had dangers of their own. In the densest thickets there were wolves and the even more dangerous wild boars, and everywhere there were the game wardens. Merely by entering the forest, Kate and I were committing a felony and making ourselves liable to savage punishment, if caught.

All this we knew, yet, having found one another, we walked along in good spirits. On this first day of our journey the wood was mainly of beech trees, which do not encourage undergrowth. The great grey tree trunks rose straight and smooth as the pillars of a church, and under our feet was a carpet of leaves dropped in the autumns of bygone years. We travelled until a grey dusk was thick amongst the trees. Then I remembered stories of men who had been lost in fogs, or in forests, or in great open spaces like sheep runs and gone round and round, retreading the same path. Lest we do the same and find ourselves, in the morning, back at Rede, I called a halt. We threw ourselves down under a tree so old that its roots in places grew clear of the soil, making little low caves. We crouched in one, ate bread and mutton and apples, the first food we had ever taken together. I thought of that, blasphemously perhaps, thinking that it was a kind of communion; and as I did so Kate put up her hand and touched the twisted arch of root under which we sat.

"This is our very first house," she said.

Something began in my belly and swelled and swelled until it reached my head, I forgot all my fears, forgot our present plight and the future's uncertainties. I felt brave and powerful, tireless, undefeatable.

"You shall have better, sweetheart. I will build it myself, a snug, trig house, as sound as this tree." I reached out my longer arm and laid a finger on the tree trunk.

Kate laughed and said, "I'm glad you were touching wood!"

I laughed too. Rede seemed far away; here in the wood's quiet, with night gathering about us, we might have been alone in the world, another Adam, another Eve in a new Garden of Eden. We finished our meal and afterwards slept in each other's arms.

V

The next four or five days—that is so long as the food lasted—were
the happiest in my whole life. I can look back and see them, set
apart, glowing with something more than sunshine. Since then I
have never pitied idiots; for during that time Kate and I were
touched by idiocy, not set free from the dangers and cares of ordinary living, but somehow not properly concerned. It was as though
we had ceased to be Kate, daughter of the shepherd, Walter, son of
the smith, and become people in some minstrel's song, walking
through the greenwood, loving one another. "All for love."

The nature of the woods changed; the clear-floored beech trees
ended, and we came to the thick forest, with undergrowth of hazels,
brambles, and bracken, all closely woven. Sometimes we could turn
aside to seek easier passage, sometimes I had to go ahead, hacking
a way through with my knife. Still we moved on, careful to keep
the sun upon our left hand until it was high, walking into its eye
for an hour and then keeping it upon our right until it sank. We
were sparing of our poor provisions, eking them out with black-
berries and unripe hazelnuts, with sloes and crab apples that soured
our mouths, but even so we came to an end and were face to face
with the eternal problem of the poor, brought back to earth by the
question which is for all but the rich the first and the last question:
How shall we eat today? We learned, soon enough, that love is a
business for those with full bellies. No, maybe there I wrong Kate
and, through her, all women; I think they care more for love and
less for their bellies than men do. She stayed cheerful long after I
had begun to fret; she spoke gently and lovingly while my words
grew few and sharp from hunger.

We say, lightly enough, the words "starve to death." Put like that,
it sounds easy and brief enough, a man ceases to eat and he dies.
The truth is that he does not immediately die. Death by starvation
has many unpleasant stages. There is the belly pain, as though,
within you, some strange animal hungered and, lacking other
sustenance, gnawed at your vitals with sharp fangs. There is, following the pain, a constant desire to vomit, as though you would
turn your empty belly inside out, like a beggar proving his pocket

to be coinless. There is a shakiness in the bones, your hands fumble and grow clumsy, your knees give way. There is a ringing in your ears, as though bees hived there.

As our need to get out of the forest grew greater, we made less progress. We were weaker and we were forced to hunt. From the cord I made a rabbit snare, and we wasted hours sitting somewhere near, but out of sight, fretting over the loss of time and yet glad enough to have reason for inaction. I caught nothing.

Kate bore up bravely until we ate the hawthorn berries. They were plump and red and ripe and looked to us, in our hunger, as good as cherries. "Birds eat them," we told one another; and we ate them, in quantities. They did me no harm at all, but they turned Kate's bowels to water. Soon she was stumbling along, doubled over with pain and looking so wan that I was frightened. Up to that point we had been careful to make as little of ourselves as possible, but now I began calling as we went forward, cupping my hands to my mouth and uttering loud cries. Woodcutters, charcoal-burners, and game wardens lived in the forest, and now that we were starving the hope of falling in with some man with a heart of Christian charity loomed larger than our fear. Nothing answered me but my own voice, bouncing back from the trees. In all that time we saw nothing but one red deer, which flickered away like something seen in a dream.

We found no more hawthorn berries, but Kate's infirmity persisted; the time came when she could no longer walk at all, so I carried her; and I did not go straight forward, I took the easiest way. She never weighed much, but now she was variable. I'd pick her up and it was like lifting a kitten, so light she was; but as I went on she grew heavy and heavier. Sweat broke out all over my body, my heart hammered, my sight clouded. In the end I would set her down and fall prone, and she would creep away a little distance, behind the nearest tree or bush and then emerge, more deathly pale than ever. Through the ringing and buzzing in my ears a stern voice would say clearly, "Kate is going to die and you are to blame." Presently I would brace myself and try again. Again. Again. Making no progress, and the forest going on and on, and nobody in it but us.

From hunger sleep is no refuge; the starving do not sleep; they slip from one kind of misery to another; the gnawing pain goes on and so does the worry. I would lie down and think, imagine, dream, that a fine fat rabbit was kicking in my snare, then I would struggle up, shouting, to find that the piece of cord was still twisted about my wrist because I had lain where I had fallen and never set the snare at all.

It was a nightmare time.

Once I lifted Kate, turned dizzy, and only just set her down before I dropped her. She said, in a weak voice, gasping, "You can't . . . carry me . . . any more. Leave me. No need . . . for both . . . to die."

If I had had a known destination or any real hope of finding help, I might have been more tempted. But mere walking was not going to save me. Only a miracle could do that. I told her so.

"Only a miracle can save us now. And a miracle could happen here as well as at any other place." So I lay beside her for a little, gathering my strength, and then staggered a little distance and set my silly snare. That was the miracle I expected, a rabbit in my snare. As I set it I prayed, not in the manner I had been taught, but as though God were the steward and I were begging some small favour of him. "God, send a rabbit, please, God. A rabbit, God, please." The light was just beginning to fail; it was a time when rabbits were abroad.

When I got back to Kate she said, "I can smell . . . herrings roasting."

I almost wept then. I knew that delusion. It had been my companion for hours, days. As I walked I had smelt more food cooking than had ever been set on my lord's table; fat pork boiling with peas; roasting fowl; dried herring; new bread; seethed beef; dredged hare; onions.

"Poor Kate," I said. "My poor, poor Kate. Your hungry nose deceives you."

"But I can . . . can't you?"

I sniffed. I could smell it. A mouth-watering smell at any time. After the harvest of the earth came the harvest of the sea, and the dried herring would come in barrels to Rede. When the day's work was done Father and I would toast them, on long sticks, by the fire. We could have been doing it now, while Kate ate venison and syllabub at Abhurst.

Call me heartless knave if you will. But first go hungry for uncounted days; then make your own choice, love or a roasted herring. Lie weak with hunger on the ground and stare death by starvation in the face, and choose. If you say love, then I will call you saint and you may call me what you will. I am honest with myself. I wished myself back at Rede with a herring spluttering at the end of a stick, and Kate safe and full-fed in Abhurst.

I lay, wishing that, and the good smell continued. Presently I realised that never before in my delusions had the one kind of smell continued. Moreover, it grew more powerful. This, I thought, was because I was growing weaker, slipping farther and farther from reality. Perhaps, I thought, before we died we should taste food as well as smell it, God's final mercy. And from that I turned to thinking about dying, as Kate and I must do, unshriven, with all our sins upon us. Even the joys of our few happy days had been stolen. Unconfessed and unabsolved, they would weigh heavy in the scales. I was beginning, desperately, to try to recall the proper prayers for those on the point of departure when Kate nudged me.

"Go and . . . look. It can't . . . be . . . far away."

Even in that extremity my good strong body served me; lying prone, even in despair, had restored me. Standing up, without having to lift Kate, I found myself steadier than I could have hoped. Turning my head from side to side like a hound, and drooling water at the mouth, I set off in the direction from which the scent seemed strongest. A few paces brought me to a place where, in some time past, the forest trees had been felled. Where they had stood a coppice of bushes, elder and wild rose and hawthorn, had grown up. Close pressed and fighting with one another, they had woven themselves into a living wall. The strong scent of herrings roasting came from its farther side. I walked along the thicket, seeking an entrance, but there was none, and the scent grew fainter. I turned back and walked the other way. The fence continued, and the smell again faded. I was vastly puzzled. No house could be completely enclosed.

I staggered to the spot where the smell was strongest and threw myself at the bushes, thrusting my way into them bodily, hacking at them with my knife in a frenzy. The last line of them gave way before my onslaught, and I found myself standing at the top of a little bank, looking down upon a sight as astonishing as it was welcome. To left and right, as far as eye could see in either direction, ran a straight flat road, bordered on each side by thicket like that through which I had just forced my way. The road was thickly grassed, and at the point immediately below me stood a jenny ass with her foal. Nearby was a fire and over it, slung on a crossbar, the herrings. Standing guard over the whole was a little old woman with a donkey stick in her hand and an expression on her face that was at once terrified and defiant.

"Keep your distance!" she said. "I've nowt worth stealing, and if you come near I shall fetch you a clout."

I must have been a fearsome sight, bursting through the bushes, knife in hand, the bruises of my beating turning greenish yellow, the broken places now well scabbed, all in addition to my desperate, hungry look.

My wits were still with me, however. I did not move, but dropped the knife so that it fell down the bank almost at her feet.

"Good mother," I said, "I am no robber. We have gone astray in the forest and are like to die of hunger. Of your charity, let us eat." Then I remembered that I had money. "I am no beggar, either." I took out a penny and threw it after the knife.

" 'We,' " she repeated on a questioning note. "How many are you?"

"Myself and my wife. She is in worse case."

"All right then." She stooped and picked up my knife and the penny. "No tricks, though. I'm old, but I'm lively."

I turned and pushed my way back through the gap, widening it as best I could, and walked to where I had left Kate.

"Was . . . it true?"

For answer I bent and lifted her. Hope had given me strength, and I was able to carry her to the gap and pull her through it. The old woman was still on guard, but at the sight of Kate her manner changed.

"Poor creature," she said, and coming forward helped me to bring Kate down the little bank and place her by the fire. Then she quickly slid the herrings from the stick, cut great slabs from a round brown loaf, and said, "Lay to. And God send Grace on the food."

I ate as I had never eaten before, but Kate, after a bite or two, sickened again.

"Poor mawther. She has clemmed overlong. Her belly is shrunk. If only . . ." In her face, brown and wrinkled as a walnut, her faded eyes snapped and sparkled. "God be thanked," she said. "We have it!"

She routed about amongst her belongings and found a little wooden bowl.

"You must hold the donkey steady," she said to me. "She's not been milked this way afore."

If ever there should come a time when dancing bears are so common that they no longer draw a crowd, an old woman, a young man, and a jenny ass in milk should go the rounds. I was too anxious about Kate to be other than vexed by the performance and the time it took, but even then I could see its comical side, especially when the little foal, shrewd enough to see that it was being robbed, came butting in. However, at last we had a cupful of milk in the bowl. Kate drank it and it stayed down. The old woman slipped some more herrings on the stick.

"Maybe St. Christopher knew what he was about when he let my basket break," she said. I then looked at the two osier baskets which stood by the fire and saw that the bottom of one of them had given way.

"I'd have been a mile or two farther along the road if that hadn't happened," the old woman said. "Couldn't go scattering the good fish, so I thought I'd stop and mend it up while I could see; then I felt hungry and reckoned I'd eat first."

"And we smelt your supper and were saved," I said, looking at Kate, who was holding the bowl in both hands and sipping slowly, but steadily.

"Slip a bit of bread down with it, afore your belly shuts again," the old woman said, handing her a slice. Kate ate, obediently, and when that stayed with her too I knew the worst was over.

When I was full to bursting, I licked my fingers and offered to try my hand at mending the basket. I used a piece of the cord and some young hazel wands. Kate curled up under cover of her cloak and slept; the old woman and I sat by the fire. She had lost all fear of me by that time, and when I needed my knife for the work, handed it back with a grin.

"I was flummoxed to see you," she confessed. "Mostly I'm on the lookout for trouble, but on this bit of road I never seen another living soul, not in all the years I've travelled it. None else know of it, and I ain't likely to tell them."

It was a strange road, like none I ever saw before or since. Under the grass, which was shallow-rooted, were large flat slabs of stone, set edge to edge. I scraped away the grass to have a better look at it.

"It's a wonderful good road for a loaded donkey," said the old woman. "Pity there ain't more like it. I blundered on it by accident."

She told me how, years before, with another donkey, she had camped for the night on a common and waked to find that, despite his hobble, the donkey had strayed. She thought she could hear him moving behind some breast-high bracken, and, looking for him, had found the road.

"That was the end, all grown over and known to none. But it looked to me to run the same way as the other, so I reckoned I'd try it. And I'm glad I did. It's ten miles of easy going for the beast, and nice for a lone woman to have a spell with her mind at rest without fearing to be set upon. The ghosts I don't mind. They don't heed me, nor me them."

"Ghosts?"

"Aye. The like of no mortal men they are. Marching men, with short skirts, like a woman's but up to the knee, and shining helmets with brushes atop. There's great silver eagles on poles going ahead of them. I've seen them many's the time. The first time I was too scared to breathe, but I crossed myself and they went by without so much as a glance."

"You have a stout heart," I said.

"For some things. I'm feared of robbers. And of the time when I cannot get around to sell my herrings." She watched me work for a while. "By your hands," she said, "you're a smith. I've an idea that you broke your time and ran off to get married."

An apprentice who left his master before his time was up was in fault, but he was not the marked, hunted man that a serf was who had run from his manor, so I nodded.

"Ah well, there's good masters and bad. Was yours a beater?"

I nodded again, thinking to myself that in the morning I must warn Kate to tell the same tale.

"There's a smith in Baildon who *might* take you—if you was well spoke of by somebody he knew, like me."

"Would you so speak?"

"I might. You seem to me a decent sort of chap. And it'd cost me nowt."

"I should be grateful to you all my life," I said. "Is Baildon where you go to sell your herrings?"

"One of the places. It's a fine large town with the best market in these parts. And it's a long way from Norfolk," she added slyly.

"How do you know that I am from Norfolk?"

"By your tongue. Hereabouts we talk different. We sing our

words. Silly Suffolk, some call us, but in the old days it was Singing Suffolk. Still don't worry about that, we'll fash up a tale to explain. There, you've done a good job on that basket; good as new."

We were on the move early in the grey and rosy dawn, for the old woman was anxious to get on. She and I breakfasted on herrings, from which Kate still turned sickened away, but she ate heartily of the bread.

"The little mawther can ride the ass for a bit, you and I'll hump the baskets. We'll go faster that way."

Old and shrunken as she was, she set a fast pace, one which I, carrying one basket, could only just manage, and to which the donkey held unwillingly, urged on by a light blow now and again. The foal frisked along, light as a leaf, unaware that his unburdened days were numbered.

Three miles along the road we came to a wide-open space, which had also been cleared in some past time and was now all grass and self-sown bushes. Above the tangle some white columns rose, one complete, twice my height, and beautifully carved at the top. Others were broken.

"There's a good well here," the old woman said briskly. "This is where I aim to spend the night when I'm this way."

There was a well in Rede manor yard, but nothing like this one, all buried in bushes and weeds. This was a basin of that same white stone as made the pillars and shaped something like a church font, but one side was higher than the others and had a horse's head carved upon it, the water ran in a clear steady trickle out of the horse's mouth, into the basin. We all drank from it.

"Now we'll load the donkey and go in proper fashion," our guide said. That done, she took the animal's bridle and dragged it forward, through some bushes and a belt of trees, and in a few minutes we stood on a piece of common ground, beyond which was a sight that to me was new and most marvellous. When I say new, I mean to my *eyes*. Inside my head a picture something like it had formed when I had heard anything about Jerusalem. But my imagination had been small and mean compared with this reality. This town was walled, though in places the wall had been neglected and allowed to crumble; inside the walls were the crowded roofs of a multitude of houses, and rising above them were some great towers, taller than the highest tree I had ever seen. One in particular seemed to soar into the sky, with buttresses and pinnacles of extreme grace and beauty.

"That is Baildon Abbey," said the old woman, seeing me staring. "Don't stand goggling now. If Armstrong takes you, you'll have plenty of chance to look at it." She urged on the donkey and we left the common for the highroad, which was crowded with market-goers. There were men driving cattle and sheep and pigs, women carrying fowls and eggs and baskets of fruit and vegetables, other laden donkeys, people on horseback, even a litter or two.

"I didn't know," said Kate in an awed voice, "that there were so many people in the world."

"Any others with herrings; thass what I want to know," said the old woman. She looked sharply about her. "Not that I worry much," she went on contradictorily, "bringing fish this far is more of a trudge than most folks'd face. We go this way."

Directly ahead of us was one of the town's gateways; some people entered it, others swerved aside and followed a track worn close to the wall.

"A new order last year. Market dues used to be collected on the market place, but the poor fellows wore themselves out, walking round. So now us with stuff to sell walk round, to the north gate and pay as we go in. They chose that gate because it's nearest the Abbey—not so far to carry the bag!"

A monk—the first of his kind that I had ever seen—stood in the archway, accompanied by two ordinary men. As each marketgoer drew level with the monk he looked over the produce he carried and without a moment's hesitation decided whether the dues should be paid in cash or kind. He touched nothing: if cash were demanded, one of the laymen received it, if the due were to be paid in kind, the other took charge. It was all done swiftly and in order and in a singular silence. There was no haggling; the dues were paid in sullen silence and no one said much until out of earshot of the monk. At a safe distance grumbling began. I later learned that there was a kind of justice about the dues, ruled by the law of supply and demand. The monk might take, for example, a fowl from one woman and a pound of apples from another, unfair on the face of it; but inside the market that day fowls were plentiful and cheap, apples scarce and dear. From the basket that I had mended he demanded a score of herrings. Once out of earshot, our friend said sourly:

"There's robbers in all shapes, but them in cowls is the worst. They say that some of their takings come back again as alms and such, but I never took charity yet and never want to."

The market place was a great open square immediately in front of the Abbey's main gateway. Here on the cobbles some people took up a stand and began to cry their wares as a means of drawing attention; others moved to and fro amongst the townswomen who had come out to do their marketing. I saw several females of a kind new to me, well dressed, with rings on their fingers and elegant headgear, followed by maid- or menservants, carrying baskets. In my simple way I took them for great ladies, never having seen one, for if my Lord Bowdegrave had a wife he never brought her to Rede. It was a surprise to me to learn that all this grandeur appertained to the wives of burghers who had been successful in their various businesses, and an even greater surprise to know that these grave-faced, sedate women were in many cases breaking the law by dressing themselves so fine. In the towns ordinary folk had become so rich that they could afford to ape the nobility, and laws were passed saying at what rank one might wear velvet, satin, or the better kinds of fur. The laws were not heeded. In fact that was one of the first things I noticed about life in the town, the ordinary people were far less humble and conscious of their state than even the freemen on the country manors.

There was no other herring-seller in Baildon that morning so Old Betsy—as I heard her called—soon emptied her baskets. One man even made an offer for the donkey foal, to which she replied shortly that she'd think about selling it when the creature was weaned. Then she said to me:

"Come along, and I'll take you to Armstrong, and be on my way."

Leaving the Abbey behind us, we climbed a short steep street called Cooks Lane, in which almost every shop was a food shop, out of which came odours that set my mouth watering anew, and from there we turned left into a narrower lane that smelt of hot iron and scorched hoof-horn. The smithy was set back from the street and its wide thatch stuck out, supported by roughly trimmed tree trunks, so that the animals awaiting attention and the men with them were sheltered from rain or sun. The space was crowded, and the smith with three apprentices were working at full pelt. Old Betsy pushed her way in, leaving Kate to hold the donkey and beckoning to me to follow. When the smith, between jobs, straightened himself, he saw her and said:

"Thass no good, dame. You must wait your turn today. I'm too busy to draw breath."

"Then I'm doing you a favour. I've brought you my young kinsman, a good smith, in his sixth year. His master died, poor man, and his forge was took over by a man with four sons, so he wouldn't take over the 'prentices."

"You want I should take him, eh?" asked Armstrong, looking me over with a calculating eye.

"You'd be doing yourself a good turn."

"In his sixth year. I don't like other men's 'prentices, they ain't trained to my ways. Besides, though I got work, I'm short of room. These three lay all in one bed as it is."

"He'd find his own bed. He's married."

"What! In his sixth year! Scandalous."

"Thass different in Norfolk where he come from. They ain't so hardhearted; they make allowances for human nature."

"Let's see your work," Armstrong said, speaking to me for the first time. "Clap a shoe on this nag."

My hands were less steady, my movements less sure than usual, because so much depended upon how I showed, but I did the best job I could.

"Passable," Armstrong said, without enthusiasm, when I had done.

"Well, do you take him, or don't you?" Old Betsy asked shrilly. "We can't stand about all day, waiting on you."

"Tell you what I'll do," the smith said, narrowing his eyes. "I'll take him, but not as a six-year man. He go back to five; that'll give me a chance to undo the bad ways he've learned in Norfolk where everything is so different. He find his own bed, I give him his dinner and his dole at Christmas and Whitsun. Are you agreed?"

"Thass for him to say," Betsy said. She looked at me and managed to convey, without a word, that in her opinion I should be wise to accept the offer, since one in my position was not likely to get a better.

"I agree," I said, "and I thank you."

"Well you may," Armstrong said. "And all here will witness the agreement."

All the men within hearing nodded and said, "Aye. Aye."

"Start right in, then. How're you called?"

Mindful that I might even yet, even at this distance, be hunted, I renamed myself there and then.

"Martin, sir," I said.

I know now that amongst sailors there is a superstition that it is unlucky to change the name of a ship. Perhaps it does a man no good either.

VI

So I was established and had a footing, however humble, in the town, and could not be driven out as a vagrant, and Kate found work the next day in a bakehouse in Cooks Lane. The work was hard and heavy, the wages very small, but—and this meant much to us—she was allowed to bring away, at the end of her day's toil, a good quantity of unsalable stale bread.

We started off our life in Baildon in a lodging about which one of my fellow-apprentices told me, saying it was a cheap place. It was in a loft over a stable and contained six straw-stuffed pallets laid close together on the floor and a cooking stone under a hole in the roof. There was a trough of water in the yard below. The beds, at that time of the year, when people were on the move, were always occupied by travellers of the poorer sort, tinkers, drovers, tumblers, and bear-leaders, and by the humble pilgrims to St. Egbert's shrine in the Abbey. The loft had a stench of its own, a mingling of the stable smell from below, of years of careless cooking on the greasy hearth, of sweat and foul breath and human excrement; Kate and I found this irksome, for, though neither of us had been bred to be fastidious, we were used to fresh country air, and to stinks so accustomed as to be unnoticed. In this lodging place the stink changed from night to night and always, it seemed, for the worse. Still, it was a shelter, the cheapest one available, and, had I been earning only a little, we should have stayed there. As it was, what Kate earned just sufficed to feed us, and week by week I had to pay the rent out of my small store of money. I was ignorant of town life and had imagined that I might earn a coin or two by doing odd smith jobs for people, as Father and I had done in and around Rede: two things defeated that hope. For one thing Armstrong was a hard master, and we apprentices often worked far into the night; after the horses had all been shod and taken home we worked, by fire and candlelight on ploughshares and harrows, and chains, and spits and iron sconces. The other thing was that in towns all labour was organised into Guilds, which were communities of craftsmen, governed by strict laws, all of them aimed at upholding a monopoly. An apprentice to the smith's craft, for instance, was forbidden to work for hire outside the place where he was apprenticed. If he did so, he would be punished, and, worse yet, it would count against him when, his apprenticeship completed, he applied for journeyman status and admission to the Guild. The person who employed him would also be in trouble, since every Guildsman in the district would be against him, refuse perhaps to do the most urgent job for him for a period varying from a month to six, and, if the man himself were a Guildsman of another craft, his own members would regard him as a traitor. There were some forms of work which I would have been allowed to do. I might, for instance, have helped to drive cattle to market, or dig somebody's garden, but such jobs must be done in daylight, and I never had a daylight hour to spare. The smithy closed early on Saturdays, and then another rule came into force; every apprentice was bound to go and practise shooting at the Butts on Saturday afternoon; so I had only Sunday, when nobody wanted cattle driven or gardens dug.

I had not been in Baildon long before I saw that I had exchanged one servitude for another; in place of my Lord Bowdegrave I had a trinity of masters, Master Armstrong, the Guild, and money.

One wet October evening a man known as Tom the Juggler came to sleep in the loft. It was Saturday, one of the two market days, and he was grumbling that the weather had ruined his trade; people were not going to stand in the rain to watch his tricks.

"Another day like this," he said, "and I shall be sleeping in Squatters Row."

"Is that cheaper?" I asked, wondering whether all my inquiries had missed some useful piece of information. He laughed.

"It's free, you fool."

"Where is it?"

"Down by the Town Ditch. Grant you it stinks, but not worse than this. Only trouble is, the roof leaks."

"Maybe I could mend it. I'm handy," I said. He laughed again, as though at some wonderful jest.

Next day, when he took me along to the place he called Squatters Row, I understood his merriment.

It was at the rear of the Abbey, on the side farthest from the market place. It was a street, a good deal wider than any other in Baildon; one side of it was bounded by the Abbey's eastern wall, the other by the backs of houses, some of them slaughterhouses. The street sloped towards the centre and there ran the Town Ditch, the drainings of all the gutters and privies in the town, the blood from the slaughterhouses, the overflow from pigsties. It had, at some time long past, been decently covered in by an arched hood of stone, stretches of the cover still existed, but in the main it had given way. The stench was loathsome, but, as Tom the Juggler had said, not much worse than the loft when it was fully occupied.

"But I see no place to live hereabouts," I said.

"Use your eyes," he said; and pointed across the Ditch to the Abbey wall. It was heavily buttressed, and the buttresses stuck out to within a few feet of the Ditch, making, as it were, compartments with three walls. I looked along and saw that several of these compartments were occupied; most were open to the sky and to the Ditch, some were roofed over by pieces of sacking or sailcloth, supported at the front on poles.

A sick feeling of defeat squirmed in my belly, and when Tom the Juggler laughed I could have hit him.

"The north wind's the sharpest," he said. "You want to get the wall between you and it." I noticed then that he had brought along his pack. He crossed the Ditch at a place where the arch still held and chose his buttress, throwing the pack down.

"There're worse places. If you want to come back, say so, and I'll keep you the stall next door."

It was still raining, but the rain was coming on a wind from the west; I noticed that the tall wall of the Abbey sheltered the ground immediately below it to a distance of some feet. The buttress would keep off the north wind which brought the snow. I could do better than rig a flimsy bit of sailcloth on four posts; I could fix timbers to the wall and the buttress and lay a thatch over. I could make a fourth wall. With what little money I had left I could buy the materials for that work, and enough timber to make a table and two stools, straw and sacking for a mattress. All at once I could see the little hut completed, weatherproof, even snug. And ours alone.

After the lack of privacy in the loft, that in itself seemed a blessing.

"I shall stay. And I'm very thankful to you."

"Then your wife can cook my supper," said Tom the Juggler.

I hurried back to our lodging, where Kate was doing some washing, and told her I had found a place. I warned her that it was in a foul place and in the open, but that I had plans for it.

"Just so long as we can be alone at night," she said. So, when the washing was done, I led her to the spot and tried to make her see the little hut as I had seen it in my mind.

In our lodging we had been among the poor, now we had joined the destitute. Our permanent neighbours were a one-legged sailor who lived alone, a man who was deaf and dumb, his wife and four children who had not inherited his infirmity, an aged crone, who, when anyone would employ her, acted as midwife and layer out of the dead, and an evil-living young woman who twice a year was whipped through the streets for harlotry. As well as these, Squatters Row had a drifting population of people who had failed to find, or could not afford to pay for, a bed for the night. As the weather grew worse these grew fewer in number.

Before winter set in I had made a hut, just as I had planned; we had a table and two stools and a mattress stuffed with sweet fresh straw, much better than our louse-ridden bed in the loft, and, rough, humble, and cold as it was, it was, as Kate said, "our second house" and it became home to us. That we should be happy in such circumstances and that the meals we ate there—often no more than hunks of four-day-old bread thinly smeared with fat—should seem like feasts to us may sound strange, but is nonetheless true. We were young, we had our health, love was still lively and so was hope. If we were lucky, in a year and a day we should be free. In two years I should have served my time and be a journeyman, working for a daily wage. Then things would change. We had a great deal to look forward to. We had another advantage, too, and one which is, I think, sometimes overlooked when people think of living in great poverty; the smallest thing extra, or nicer than usual, was a wonderful treat. I remember Kate coming home with a skip in her step because, there being a shortage of stale bread, her mistress had told her to take a fresh loaf.

"Feel it," she said, thrusting it into my hand, "smell it." To the full-fed it would be a rare dainty indeed which could bring such pleasure.

The year and the day, so important to us, passed. On a September Sunday evening we could look at one another and say: We are free. On the Monday, Lord Bowdegrave could ride up to the forge where I worked, recognise me for his smith's son, and no more lay claim to me than he could to Master Armstrong. Only the serfborn can know or guess or even dimly imagine what that moment meant to us.

We were spending the evening as we, and many of our kind, spent all our free time in fair weather—gathering firewood on the fringe of the common ground. The forest there belonged, like most of the things around Baildon, to the Abbey of St. Egbert, and the Abbot granted the townspeople that privilege; any dead wood which could be found within thirty paces of the boundary might be collected and taken away. Kate and I were indefatigable woodgatherers; often through the past winter our less active or less provident neighbours had come to warm themselves, sometimes to cook, by our fire. On this evening we were making two faggots of what we had collected, a large one for my back, a smaller one for Kate's, when she said:

"Thanks to the Virgin, our child will be free-born."

God forgive me for the way my heart went plummeting down. A first child, indeed any child, should be a wished-for, a welcome thing. But I was earning no wage, nor should be for another year. It was Kate's meagre money and the bread she brought home that stood between us and hunger. And I had known all along that the work in the bakehouse was heavy, too heavy for her frail body; how long, with another burden within her, could she stay at work? And what would happen when that time was outrun?

There was that side to it; and there was another. It went hard with me to think that our child would be born, and live its first year, in a makeshift hovel by the brim of the Town Ditch. As month had followed month since our arrival in Baildon, I had hoped that God in His mercy was seeing fit to withhold parenthood from us until we had a home ready for a child.

Now all the cheer that the day had brought me failed and faded. Walking home, bowed under my faggot, I knew the first faltering of hope. I looked into the future and saw, not the neat little house in some more habitable part of the town, but Kate and I and our family condemned to live our lives out in that stinking place of outcasts.

Kate said, "Don't be angry." And that made me ashamed, remembering how, on a like occasion, the deaf-and-dumb man had beaten his wife until she was black-and-blue.

"I'm not angry," I said. "How could I be? It takes two to make a baby. But, Kate, I am worried."

"God and St. Katherine will take care of us—and the baby," she said. "They always have done. We've done very well so far."

"That is true. But I was looking ahead. You can't stay in the bakehouse when . . ."

"Then something else will turn up," she said, with the utmost faith. "You'll see."

Hating to drag her down into my own state of discouragement, I said no more. I only hitched my load a little more firmly onto my shoulders so that I could spare a hand to ease hers a little, thinking, as I did so, of the flour sacks, the loaves, the firing of the oven which she must manage, with none to help.

VII

Kate must have known about her state for some time before she told me in September, for the baby was born in February. The baker's wife had kept her on until Christmas and then told her not to come back, because it worried her, she said, to see Kate straining herself to do the work.

"Once your belly is out beyond the point of your nose when you stand upright, you should be careful," the woman said. "If you don't, the child'll come feet first."

Kate had argued that in the country women worked in the field sometimes until the very day the birth took place.

"Maybe, but I don't have to watch them," said the baker's wife.

All this Kate told me, making light of it and still saying that when one door shut God opened another. I could see, however, that she was a little dashed that another door had not opened already. And none did, just as I had feared. After Christmas was the worst time of the year to go looking for chance employment; even the markets grew small; there were few travellers and no pilgrims in the inns; housewives were saving their work for the spring. Everything was at a standstill.

Since September we had saved what we could, but it was pitiably little and we were once again on the very verge of starvation when that other door did open.

Ordinarily both Kate and I were out of our hut and away early in the morning, and did not return until late in the evening, so of the ordinary comings and goings of our neighbours we saw very little. Now, doomed to stay at home, Kate noticed that every morning the sailor with the wooden leg and one of the children of the deaf-and-dumb man left Squatters Row together just before midday and came back carrying food. She asked where they had been and was told, "To the Alms Gate."

"And the monks give you food? Would they give me some?"

"Brother Stephen would. Brother Justinius would not," Peg-Leg said. He knew all the rules. He explained the situation to Kate in his own simple words. The monks had plenty to give away. Baildon was a very rich Abbey and had in time past been heavily endowed by wealthy men who had sought favour in the sight of Heaven by remembering the poor in their wills. There had been a time when anyone, needy or not, deserving or not, could present himself at the Alms Gate and be fed; but after the great upheaval of the rebellion in the year when I was born, people in high places had become alarmed at this "indiscriminate charity," as they called it. They said it encouraged indolence and the habit of drifting from place to place. So a law was passed saying that alms were to be given only to those who were not able-bodied.

This was a law which admitted of varying interpretations. Some monks said that they had no time to waste on making a close physical inspection before handing out a bowl of peaseporridge or a hunk of bread, or who would split a hair of logic by arguing that a man in the throes of hunger could not rightly be said to be able-bodied. There were others who accepted the law as it read and made it an excuse for reducing the scope of their charity.

In Baildon, in the main, the law was accepted. Dummy, our deaf-and-dumb neighbour, for instance, could hope for nothing at the Alms Gate; he was able-bodied, that is, sound of wind and limb. Peg-Leg, on the other hand, was accepted as a responsibility, and so was Dummy's child, because she had been knocked down by a bullock running wild from the shambles and she had grown crooked.

A woman like Kate was a debatable case, and as, Peg-Leg said, it all depended upon which of the two almsgiving monks threw up the hatch in the Alms Gate which lay just beyond the Bell Tower. Brother Justinius argued that pregnancy was a natural state and that a woman heavy with child was in no sense disabled; Brother Stephen, on the other hand, counted heaviness of body and short-ness of breath as a disability.

"There you are," Kate said to me, after learning all this from Peg-Leg. "I told you we should be cared for."

She joined the miserable little crowd at the Alms Gate and came away, empty-handed or happy, according to which monk was on duty that day. Brother Stephen even carried matters so far as to now and then dole her out a double portion, saying, "You must eat for two."

I invented a tale that Master Armstrong had taken pity on me and offered me a breakfast piece in addition to my dinner. This meant that I went to work every day with an empty belly. In fact the dinners which our master provided were as scanty as he dared make them, and the weather being very cold and wet, I grew thin and low-spirited. Those who have never hungered think little of food, those who are hungry think of little else. I confess that there were many times between Christmas and the birth of my first son when I would have exchanged even my freedom to be back in the hut behind the smithy at Rede, with the fat pork cooking in the pot. I had to find another, a longer way home. Cooks Lane, the shorter way, was so full of mouth-watering smells; and then I would be home and Kate would have something left from her dole if it had been a good day with Brother Stephen at the hatch, and she would offer it to me and I could feel the wolf look come into my eyes.

However, the child was born, whole and sound. The old woman who was our neighbour—her name was Agnes—came and gave her assistance. And hardly was the baby born—it was a boy—before the old woman said:

"There, my dear, you've a fine lad and now you can claim your Trimble."

It was so early in the morning that I was still there, and I asked, "Her *what*?"

"Her Trimble," said Agnes. "God bless my soul. Where were you reared never to have heard of that saint among women, Dame Trimble?"

"Let me hear now," I said.

So, what time she bound the belly-band firmly about my son's raw naval, she told me about Dame Trimble as the story had been handed down a hundred years or more. A young girl, one of a large family reared in dire poverty, had gone to work for an old wool chandler, who married her and soon afterwards had died, leaving her well-to-do. She had no children of her own, but was all too well aware of the hardship which childbirth means to poor women. She was shrewd, too, and dealt wisely with the fortune she had been left, so that she died rich. She had founded a charity, now known familiarly as "The Trimble," by which any poor woman in Baildon —poor meaning any woman whose husband was not a full journeyman or its equivalent—could claim upon the birth of any child, meat, bread, and ale for forty days following, a woollen gown, a hood, and a pair of shoes.

"Dummy's wife is still wearing the one she got with her first," Old Agnes said. "She sold the others. There's a good market for such. And the food and drink are good too, very generous. Enough for the woman, and her man, and a bit over for the midwife if the family ain't too large, as in this case."

"Who hands it out?"

"The monks. At the Alms Gate. One of the parents has to take the child and show it. It's the father's job, though I've known mothers to crawl out on the second day, them with no men to rely on. Dame Trimble made no difference, she didn't even say *respectable* women."

So, on the next day, I had to forgo my dinner and run home and take the child to the Alms Gate. I felt silly and sheepish, expecting to be the butt for jeers, standing there with a baby in my arms; instead I found myself an object of envy. And well I might be. Brother Justinius was doling out the usual peaseporridge and bread, but at the sight of me he called out to someone behind him and bade me wait a little. Kate's Trimble, when it came, was food for a family, more food and better than I had seen at one time since I left Rede.

"The gown," Brother Justinius said, "according to the rules, must be of the woman's own choosing, and the shoes made to her measure. So they must wait. By what name is the child to be baptised?"

"Stephen," I said clearly. Kate had chosen the name, long ago, because Brother Stephen had been kind to her.

"These Norman names, how fashionable they grow," said Brother Justinius, with something sour in his voice.

I put on my most stupid, dull-witted look and said, "Norman is it? We thought it came from the Bible."

He gave me a sharp look. "It is to be hoped that you are not tainted with Lollardry, to be forever referring to Master Wycliffe's Bible."

"Master Wycliffe? I do not know him. Is he a Baildon man?"

"Oh, get along with you," Brother Justinius said crossly, and slammed down the hatch.

I hurried home to Kate with all the good food, and a little tale to make her laugh.

Dame Trimble's sweet charity carried us bravely through the next weeks; there was enough for Kate and me, and most often Old Agnes as well. Kate got back her strength and I gained some flesh. The baby throve surprisingly, and although he had been born a full year before my plans made me ready to welcome him, now that he was here I loved him very dearly.

April brought in the softer weather, with its one disadvantage to us who dwelt in Squatters Row; when the gutters of the upper town ran freely, the Town Ditch often brimmed over until its stinking waters lapped our doors. Still, summer was coming in, and by the first week in September I should have served my overlong apprenticeship and be earning. Hope stirred once more.

The town itself was growing; every market day brought more people. A shipowner from Bywater came inland and began to build a fine new house which employed a number of masons and carpenters. Master Webster, the chief wool merchant in the town, bought a new string of pack ponies. At the forge we were very busy. But when, at the end of six weeks, Kate began looking for work, she found it hard to come by. One reason was that she refused to leave Stephen in the charge of Dummy's wife, who had offered to look after him with her own, for twopence a week.

"I know her looking after," Kate said. "One of hers has been run down by a bullock, and one drowned in the Ditch. Stephen goes with me."

By that time I was beginning to be anxious again.

"If she had twopence a week for minding him, it would be to her own interest to keep him out of the Ditch. In any case it might be as well to leave him while you hunt for work, even if later, having proved your value, you took him with you."

Nothing, however, would persuade Kate from her course; she was sure the right job would turn up. And in mid-May she found work as a picker in Master Webster's woolsheds.

The fleeces were cut off the sheep in the spring and bundled up, just as they were, and brought into Baildon. Master Webster paid a price which took into account a certain amount of rubbish, burrs, caked dung, leaves, bits of stick and mud. The bigger merchants—many of them overseas in Flanders—paid so much a pound for clean wool, so the fleeces had to be picked over carefully. The picker knelt or squatted as she worked her way through the wool, and the unchanging position became tiring; the oil and odour of the fleeces saturated her clothes, her hair, her flesh even. Kate bore it cheerfully, saying that she was used to the smell of sheep, and that Master Webster had been kind about letting her take Stephen. When he could crawl, she pointed out, the woolshed would be a far safer place for him than the bakehouse would have been.

Alas, before Stephen could crawl, Kate was with child again. This time she was dismayed.

"There'll be only eleven months between them. If Stephen isn't walking, I shall have to carry them both to work."

"But I shall be earning," I told her.

She smiled as though it hurt her.

"I know. But there will be four to feed then."

She had carried Stephen cheerfully and willingly and never ailed much. This was different. She was sick and miserable. I was little comfort. To me there was something wrong, almost obscene about this begetting without being able to support. I was ashamed, and that made me peevish. It was at this time that something went out of our hut, something which had made it, despite its squalor, a happy home. Kate and I now seemed to take an unholy pleasure in making sharp remarks to one another. One day, when she was complaining, I said:

"I warned you, didn't I? You would have been better off at Abhurst."

She swung round on me like a swordsman.

"You mean you'd have been better off as an unmarried apprentice, with your feet under somebody else's table."

The weapon to wound was there, at my hand, and I seized it.

"If it comes to that, I *am* an unmarried apprentice," I said.

Kate shot me a glance of hatred and then began to cry.

"That's right. Throw that in my face!"

We had never been married. We had arrived in Baildon as man and wife and never dared risk drawing attention to ourselves by offering ourselves to be wed. There was that question, ordinarily so harmless, to us so dangerous, "Of what parish?" It would have been easy to lie, but Holy Church has a long arm. It might have occurred to the priest to make inquiries whether these unknown people were free to marry, and that would have been disastrous. Sailing under false colours, we had come into Baildon, voiced for by Old Betsy, and under those same false colours we must go on.

Now, sobbing bitterly, Kate poured out all her hidden shame and doubts. No wonder, she said, everything went wrong with us, living in mortal sin, as we were. And if she died in childbed, as well she might, she would go straight to Hell as a wanton. She went so far as to ask whether being born free could make up to Stephen and the child that was coming for their bastardy.

Her distress distressed me. I said I was sorry for having spoken as I had, and we kissed and made up. But every quarrel—of which this was but a sample—took something from us which no reconciliation could fully restore. I understood, during the next few months, what makes men go and drink themselves silly in the alehouse. I should have done so, many a night, had I had any money.

VIII

The day dawned that brought the end of my apprenticeship. Nothing had been said overnight, but I had not expected any sign, for during my two years at Armstrong's I had seen an apprentice become a journeyman. (Journeyman does not mean a man who journeys to his work; it means a man who works by the day, *jour* being the Norman for day.)

It was one of those enchanted days of late summer touched by the first breath of autumn, golden and blue and heavily dewed, as I set out for work, carrying Stephen, as I had done for some weeks, and walking round by Master Webster's woolsheds. Even Kate was more cheerful this morning.

I went, as soon as I reached the smithy, to the nail where my apron usually hung. It was not there. I pretended great surprise and anxiety. Then the others gathered round me, chanting:

> "He's grown too big for his *apron*
> He'll have to get another one."

The reply to this sally varied with the nature and wit of the new journeyman. I said, "How can I get another. I've earned nothing yet!" and that was well received, with more laughter.

I then went to take up my tools. They too were gone, and again I pretended concern. They gathered round me.

> "He worked so hard for a dinner a day
> He wore his hammer clean away!"

The next remark was prescribed. I must turn round and cry in mock dismay, "What shall I do?"

Then they all bellowed, "Become a journeyman!"

After that there was a moment or two of jollity, with good wishes and drinking, turn and turn about, from a jar of ale, which, according to rule, should be provided by the senior workman present. It was an understood thing that, on such a morning, the master should allow ten minutes for the little ritual. On this morning my apron and tools were returned to me, and I was, at last, I thought, a journeyman of the Smith Guild in Baildon town.

Presently Master Armstrong arrived, stood by my shoulder while I finished a job, and then said, "Step across the road with me. I've something to say to you."

The Smith's Arms stood directly across the road from the forge; we took a seat on the bench and Master Armstrong called for ale. This, I thought, was another stage in the process of being recognised as a journeyman. When the ale came I expected him to speak some words of salutation, but instead he took a deep draught and then wiped his mouth on the back of his hand.

"You ain't going to like this, Martin," he said. "But thass no good blaming me, nor nobody. Rules is rules and they hev to be kept. Last Guild meeting I brung up your name and said you'd done your time and was a handy skilled worker; but they ain't taking you."

The cobbled lane, the forge opposite with its smoky red fire, and the haunches of the waiting horses and donkeys began to rock and swing before my eyes, slowly at first and then faster, until all I could see was a blur. I realised that my eyes had filled with tears; I was about to cry, like a child. My throat ached and felt wooden. I lifted my mug and took a tiny sip and swallowing it eased me so that I was able to say:

"In God's name, why, master?"

"You worn't born here. And do you go back where you come from, you'll fare no better. There they'll hold agin you that you didn't do your full time there. See?"

At that moment it seemed like a cruel blow aimed at me personally by malignant fate. Later on I understood better and knew that I was but one of many men of all crafts who were, in the towns, superfluous to requirements. All through my lifetime, ever since the great rising of 1381, on all but the most old-fashioned manors the serfs had been buying themselves free and had thus been at liberty to apprentice their sons how they would. So every year more apprentices qualified to become craftsmen than old craftsmen died or retired, and those safely inside a Guild were casting around for excuses to keep the young men out. Often the excuse was flimsy, invented. In my case there was no need. I was a "foreigner"; my exclusion needed no cunning twist and would cause no searching of conscience on anyone's part.

"What's to become of me then?" I asked.

"Ah," Armstrong said. "Thass the question. But I got the answer. I'm sorry for you, Martin, and I'm making you this offer outa goodness of heart. You mind that. I brung this up at the Guild meeting, too, and they was all agreed. You can't be a full journeyman, nor claim the rate laid down for such. But you can go on as a *paid* apprentice, see? They looked up the rules, laid down in past years when there was a shortage of apprentices. They was paid then, anything between quarter and half the standard rate; and you being a handy sort of chap, I'd give you half."

I looked at him, and quickly away, lest he should see the loathing in my eyes. I'd had, from eating at his table and a hundred other little things, evidence of his meanness and cunning. Pretending to do me a favour, he had prolonged my apprenticeship for a year. Now, pretending to do me another, he was getting a skilled, finished workman at half rate.

But I had no choice. Half pay was better than no wage at all. I said humbly, "Thank you very much."

He jumped up quickly and said, "Let's to work then."

All that day, added to my own bitter disappointment, was the dread of the moment when I must tell Kate. She did not, however, weep or rail against Armstrong and the Guild; only the deepening of the lines in her face, the increased droop of her mouth, betrayed how shrewd the blow had been. I had dreaded her tears, and yet now, perversely enough, I wished she had cried. I might then have been moved to take her in my arms and comfort her. Once in a hard winter I saw a tree entirely encased in a coating of ice. Our poverty and our worries, and our defeated hopes, were putting a similar casing around our souls. Soon we should have lost even the memory of love, and be dull, plodding work animals, no more.

Kate had said miserably that there would be but eleven months' difference in the age of our children, in fact there was less than that, for Robin came into the world a little before time, a small, ailing baby, unlike Stephen. When I carried my second son to the Alms Gate I was the subject of coarse jests about being such a quick worker. "Do you get any faster," one man said, "you can knock off work and live on your Trimble."

This time Kate sold her woollen gown and the hood. Since her place in the woolshed had not been filled, she dragged herself back to work at the end of a week, frail as she was.

"That way we shall get something in hand," she said fiercely. "We can save my wage so long as the Trimble lasts. With two to feed—and God knows how many more on the way. . . ."

"There'll be no more, Kate." That was a promise which would cost me nothing to keep. I was not like my neighbour Dummy, who could go through the performance which ended with a baby while feeling nothing for the woman he bedded with. Yet, though our joy in one another had been lost, somewhere between Stephen's birth and Robin's, we were still a unit, we two against the world, as helpful to one another as we could be, a good wife, a good husband, good parents so far as our means allowed. Kate still washed and mended and cooked. I mended the roof and hunted for firewood, and every morning and evening I went to the woolshed so that I could carry the heavier child.

On one cold March evening, miserable with falling sleet, I found Kate awaiting me at the gate, with something of liveliness back in her face again. When I went to lift Stephen she stopped me, laying a hand on my arm.

"The ponies from Bywater have just come in," she said, "and without Old John. He dropped dead on the road. If you went to Master Webster now you might get the job."

It was a sensible suggestion; and Kate knew that ever since September I had longed for a chance to leave Armstrong; for I held in my mind the certainty that if he had stood up for me strongly enough, saying that he *needed* me as a journeyman, his word would have carried weight, even against the rules. Yet pride is a curious thing and will pop up in the unlikeliest places.

"But I'm a skilled smith," I said, without thinking. Those few words said it all. I'd strained and sweated, and waited and almost starved in order to be a smith, not a pack-whacker to a pony train.

"On half pay," Kate said.

I knew the need to defend myself. "Should I earn much more, if anything? Pack-whacking is an unskilled job; anybody can do it and that sort of job comes cheap."

"They get about. They pick up things. They do errands for people along the road and get gifts that way. I've seen Old John come in with food for a week." She tightened her arms about Robin and braced herself to move.

"If it's beneath you to care whether we eat or not . . ." she began sourly.

"I'll do it. Where shall I find him?"

"In his office. Through the yard, there, to the right, where the light is."

"You take the baby home," I said. "I'll bring Stephen." He could by this time walk a little, and holding his hand I went into the wool yard and knocked on the door.

The room inside served as office and living room, was well lighted and warm. Tally sticks stood in every corner. Master Webster stood by an open cupboard on whose shelves lay samples of wool.

"Well?" he said.

"I'm told that one of your pack-whackers is dead. I wondered if you would give me his job."

He pinched his upper lip between his finger and thumb, pulled it out and let it go again.

"You're a foreigner. I'd sooner hev a man that knew the roads."

"I could learn my way about, master," I said humbly.

"Wasting *my* time, meanwhile. You're the smith they wouldn't let into the Guild, ain't you?"

I nodded, gritting my teeth together, for I saw in this the beginning of a hard bargain. The man nobody wanted.

"Pack ponies are hard on their shoes," he said. "Now *suppose* I rigged up a forge, right here in the yard. Could you shoe the ponies as well as drive 'em?"

"Of course I could."

"It'd hev to be done on the quiet. Now and agin I'd hev to send a beast to Armstrong or Smithson, and if they queried why my trade dropped off, thass easy explained, ain't it? Pony's likely to cast a shoe anywhere."

"That is so," I said.

"Mark you," he said, "I'm doing you a favour. Making a job for you, you might say."

"I'm truly grateful."

"So you should be. Now, as to wages . . ."

I saw his fingers working as he reckoned. They tapped out a sum which was fourpence more than I was earning at Armstrong's. With a gallon loaf costing a penny, it was an increase worth considering; and I bore in mind Kate's words about a pack-whacker's chances to earn a little extra here and there. So I sold myself into another bondage for an extra fourpence a week.

IX

Within a week I was well aware of the advantages in my new job. For a trained craftsman, who had mastered his trade and passed his apprenticeship, to become a mere driver of pack ponies *was* a comedown, but it had its compensations. As Kate had said, we got into the country, and it was in the country that food was plentiful and cheap.

When I joined Master Webster's teamsters it was winter and we were not collecting the dirty fleeces from farms and sheep runs, we were carrying the picked-over wool down to Bywater.

Bywater was a small port, much smaller, we understood, than Dunwich or Yarmouth; but it had obtained, during the reign of the great King Edward III, one priceless privilege. It was allowed to export a certain amount of wool, in defiance of all the rules governing the staple. This was because at some critical moment during the King's wars with France, this small town's fishing fleet had chanced to be in harbour, and had been able to offer the King eighteen vessels for the transport of troops to France, shortly before the great Battle of Crécy. The privilege of being able to export wool freely was its reward.

The Bywater people often laughed and joked about the privilege, saying that, when King Edward granted them the favour, the limit he had set on their export had been far in excess of all the wool shorn in East Anglia, for Norfolk and Suffolk and Essex were not then reckoned to be sheep-rearing districts. The favour was, they said, "like giving a one-legged man permission to dance a jig." But things had changed since then; sheep runs had been established on many a ploughland, and in my time Bywater exported every bale of wool the license allowed.

Ships that set sail laden with wool returned with other commodities, and there were goods to be found in Bywater that could be obtained nowhere nearer than London. On the very first journey I made to Bywater we were stopped by an innkeeper at Nettleton. His little daughter was ill and he wanted an orange for her. She had once eaten an orange and all through her fever had craved another. I was lucky and found four, and when I delivered them into his hands on the return he almost wept with gratitude. He took me and my fellow-driver, a lively little hunchback called Crooky, into his house and gave us each a mug of his best October ale. Then he asked which would we rather have, sixpence apiece or our pick out of his storeroom. Crooky, who had no family and was a drinking man, chose the sixpence. I went to the storeroom and stared about at more stacked-up food than I had ever seen in my life.

"You mean I can have anything?"

"Anything you can carry. Could you have seen the little wench's face when I put the thing into her hands! Take what you like and call me still your debtor."

I chose a great ham, which, sliced into pieces by any of the keen knives in Cooks Lane and sold piecemeal, would have been worth four shillings.

"And I'd sooner give you that," said the innkeeper, when I had made my choice, "than the sixpence yon fellow took. The pig it came off fed on the scrapings of the plates, and drunk the wash-up water, and the smoking was done by the fire that we cook on. So it cost me nowt."

That was my first experience as a doer of errands. Others followed. Not all the people we obliged were so deeply grateful and wildly generous, but I always remembered a farmer's wife who had broken her needle. She lived a long way from the road we travelled and had twice walked the five miles and stood a whole morning in the biting wind to catch us on our way down to Bywater. She gave us the errand, and the money for two needles and asked us when we should be returning. We told her, and when we came clattering along, the unladen ponies trotting and thinking of their own stable, there she was, with two grey geese on long leads of plaited rushes.

She said, in a shamefaced way, "Would you take these in payment? The needles had to be paid for in coin, and I have no more, nor shall till the calves are sold. But they're good geese, right fat."

"A goose, for carrying a needle!" I said in astonishment. "Payment enough and over."

"But I can't walk to Bywater—the calves would starve; nor I can't sew with a goose, and my poor man's hose all agape. I'm much obliged to you both. Besides," she said, grinning, gap-toothed, "the geese cost nowt. Gander do his work for pleasure, goose lay the eggs. All summer they keep the grass down so I can walk dry-foot to tend the calves. Whass to a goose?"

I could have told her. To a goose there were some feathers to add to the collection in order, one day, to have a feather pillow. Then there was a fine hot savoury meal, and fat to spread on our bread on many a cold morning; and bones to boil, with an onion or two, into a heartening broth.

Oh, and there was more to it than that. There was me saying to Kate, "You were right. Snatching at Old John's job was the best thing I've done so far."

And there was Kate, with some of the worry eased out of her face, smiling at me with some of the old sweetness.

To the poor so little means so much.

When the sheep-shearing time began and we started making journeys to outlying farms and sheep runs to bring in the fleeces, there were more errands and more rewards. Now, with both of us in employment and a good deal of our food costing nothing, we began to lay aside a penny here and there, in the renewed hope of being able to hire a house somewhere far from Squatters Row.

There seemed no real reason why the secret of the work I was doing for Master Webster in addition to my pack-whacking should ever have been discovered. He was a very cunning man. He knew that the other drivers would soon notice if, bringing in a horse with a loose shoe, or an unshod hoof overnight, they found it wearing a bright new shoe in the morning. So he made a new rule, the teams were to be driven in rotation. In this way, in the course of a few days, I went out with each team, and, on our return to the stable, would take careful note of the state of the hoofs of the ponies with which I had made that journey. Crooky was well known to be unobservant and unheeding; he would leave a pony with a strained fetlock, or a sore back, and walk straight away to his drinking. I always walked away, just as lightheartedly, but, when there was a job to be done, I went back, late at night, was admitted by Master Webster, and went to work in the forge which he had set up in a little shed to which only I had the key. Every now and then, just to avert suspicion, a pony would be sent for shoeing to Armstrong or Smithson.

So, for six months Master Webster saved himself money and all was well.

One night, late in September, I had been working and was on my way when I turned a corner and ran into a man who was lolling there by the wall. He reeled and had so much difficulty in recovering himself that I judged him to be drunk and clutched at him, steadying him with my hands. His hands clutched at mine, and at the same time he fell against me, his face buried in the shoulder of my jerkin.

I said, "Hold up, man," or some such words, and he pulled himself straight, let go of my hands, and lurched off.

I thought no more about him until, four or five days later when I came in with a load of fleeces from Clevely and reached home, I found Master Armstrong sitting on one of our stools.

"I wanted to see you, Martin," he said. "Your wife said you might be back today, so I thought I'd wait a bit."

Kate turned from the hearth where she was cooking supper and over his shoulder made a face at me.

"Master Armstrong came yesterday and waited a long time," she said.

I had a wild hope that perhaps in the last six months he had missed me, had persuaded the Guild to admit me, or, next best thing, was now willing to re-engage me at a full journeyman's wage and be hanged to the Guild.

"What is it, master?" I asked.

"Thass this," he said. "You're doing Webster's smith work; and thass agin all the rules."

"Why should you say that?" I put on an astonished face.

"Now don't play no fool's game with me. We know. Smithson's first man, Nobby, ran into you the other night. Your hands was black; he'd washed his, but he gripped yours and blacked his, see? And you reeked of the forge."

"I did indeed, after he'd reeled against me, and so would any man. As for my hands—I'd just helped to unload twelve ponies, three hundred pounds of filthy fleeces apiece, marked with tar some of them."

Armstrong grinned. "You're a sharp one. Then how do you explain *this*? Ever since March, when you took up with Webster, that look like his ponies don't wear out their shoes. I noticed, Smithson noticed, but it worn't till we put our heads together we knew we'd *both* been done. I reckoned he was doing the jobs, he reckoned I was."

"Ponies don't mind where they cast a shoe," I said. "And you can't run a pack pony on three legs. We have to get work done at the nearest forge."

"That seem a rare rum thing that only this summer them ponies cast shoes so far afield so often. Me and Smithson, we still got our memories, mark you. 'Twasn't this way last summer, nor the one afore. Where's the difference? The difference is that Webster hev now got working for him the rascal I took and trained out of goodness of heart, and is now plying the trade I taught him to do honest men out of work."

That, in a way, I could deny. I wasn't doing it to spite honest men. I was doing it to keep myself alive. So I said, "That is not true, master."

"Thass true. And you know it. And now I'm giving you fair warning. There's ways of dealing with fellows who run agin the rules. Either you stop doing Webster's smith work, or we'll find a way to make you." He stood up and stamped out of our hut.

Kate pulled the pot to the side of the hearth and came and gripped my arm.

"Oh, Martin, what will they do?"

"Tackle Webster. He's a Guildsman too. He'll be savage at having to give up his fine penny-saving scheme and sack me. He never wanted to employ me anyway. He called me a foreigner."

"We never make any headway," Kate said drearily. "Every time we do a bit better and begin to hope, something happens."

Next morning, as soon as Master Webster appeared in the yard, I told him of Armstrong's visit and threat.

"Did you admit doing the work?"

"I denied it, but he is sure nonetheless."

"Then his case stands on the word of a drunken apprentice who ran into someone in the dark. And that against mine, mark you. We'll take no notice. The next pony to need a shoe shall go to Smithson, and that will keep him from siding too hearty with Armstrong. For the rest we'll go on as we were. It suits me well."

"It suits me. But Master Armstrong said there were ways of dealing with those who went against the rules."

"He said truly. But they must first prove that I'm breaking a rule. And of that I'm not so sure. I never seen any rule saying a man may not employ his private smith if he wants. I ain't flaunting the business, as you well know, there's nowt to be gained by falling out with your fellows. But first they must prove that you are doing smith work for me, and next they must prove thass agin the rules. And all that will take time. We'll go as we were."

By mid-October all that year's fleeces were in and our journeys to outlying places ceased. From then on, until winter weather closed the road, we carried the picked-over wool to Bywater, Lavenham, and Melford.

On our outward journeys, when the ponies were loaded, we never travelled after dusk. Wool was valuable and there was always the risk that the pony train might be set upon by rogues who could easily find, in any port, some ship's captain who was not too nice in his inquiries as to where the wool came from and whose it was. Our summer journeys were different, the raw dirty fleeces were not so immediately marketable, and to pick them over demanded some settled headquarters, which robbers lacked. In summer we often moved loads at night, but in the winter we only travelled after dark when the ponies were unladen and we were making for home.

Crooky and I were doing that, rattling along at a good pace, coming back from Bywater one November night. He rode the first pony, I the last, and we were urging the string along because there was fog about. We rode easily; having nothing of value to care for, our one concern was to get back home as soon as possible.

We reached a place where a narrow bridge spanned the river, some five miles out of Baildon. It was the same river which ran through Baildon and turned the Abbey Mill at Flaxham St. Giles. Once we were over the bridge, the river ran alongside the road on our left hand, and for us the bridge had become a landmark. Many a time Crooky and I, crossing it, had shouted to one another, "Nearly home."

This evening, Crooky, riding ahead of me, shouted back, "Nearly home!"

"God be thanked," I shouted back. I heard his pony's hoofs sound hollow over the bridge, and the next and the next. . . . I was almost on the bridge myself when something dropped in front of my face; it fell to my waist and there pulled tight and jerked me off the back of the pony, which kept up its trot. I shouted, "Crooky! Crooky!" but he didn't hear, or took no notice. And as I fell over the pony's tail and hit the road, blows began to shower down on me. The rope which had lassoed me held my arms fast, I was utterly defenceless. I remember thinking that this was how they dealt with those who went against the rules. Then somebody hit me on the leg, causing such sharp agony that I cried aloud. Another blow fell on my head, and the pain ceased.

When it began again I thought I was back at Rede. It was like waking from a dream, all about running away and trying to make a life in a place called Baildon, and having two children and a make-shift hut in Squatters Row. I was Walter, the smith's son, who had hit his lord in the face and must get away sharply if he wished to live. I tried to raise myself and a quiet voice said:

"You must lie still or you will undo my work."

I opened my eyes then and saw, not the dung-heap in Rede yard but a smooth whitewashed wall. Yet there was a connection with Rede—that same thirst which had sent me staggering to the bucket in our forge.

"I'm thirsty," I moaned.

"A good sign," said the quiet voice. And in a moment my head was lifted a little and the cool hard rim of a mug touched my lips.

Beyond it, hanging in space it seemed above me, was an old man's face, pink-fleshed, deeply wrinkled, with faded blue eyes, the whole enclosed in a monk's cowl.

"Brother . . . Brother . . ." I said in a fumbling way.

"Sebastian," he said. "I am the Infirmarian. You are safe and not much hurt except that your leg is broken."

He lowered my head and I lay still, thinking: My leg is broken. Broken bones will knit themselves together, but like a thread which has been tied they are shortened. I thought that. Then I remembered that what I had just lately thought to be a dream was real enough. I lived in Baildon, had a wife and two children, and had found it hard to make a living when I was whole and well. Henceforth I should be a cripple, a beggar.

"It had better been my neck," I said.

"And who are you to be giving orders to God?" asked Brother Sebastian, in a humourously rebuking voice. "You should lie there and be thankful. You could have lain in the road until you died, but for a mule's cast shoe. Brother Bartholomew was collecting the Nettleton rents and should have been home before Vespers, but he was delayed. So he found you. And here you are in experienced hands. I mended the leg of a lay brother who fell from a ladder two years since, and a bad job I made of it. But I know where I went wrong, and with you I have made good my error. Poor Edgar's set like a dog's back leg, but on yours I have tried a new trick. A broomstick, tied firmly in three places. Aha, that wayward leg may think to set all crooked, but governed by that broomstick it shall be."

"I am thankful," I said. Then I thought for a moment and asked, "Is it Thursday still?"

"No. The bell for Matins sounded half an hour ago. It is Friday."

"I have a wife. She expected me back for supper on Thursday. She will be worried."

"She knows. Brother Stephen recognised you and a message was sent. So calm yourself; lie still and be thankful and let your wounds heal."

Lie still, perforce, I must, but I was neither calm nor thankful. Brother Sebastian, along with his tender, careful ministrations to my body, tried to minister to my soul. He spoke often of faith in God, of the will of God, of the beauty and virtue of unquestioning acceptance. I listened with my ears, while my mind went its own way;

it was all very well for him, who had never had to grapple with the world, who if he hungered did it voluntarily and would be rewarded for his abstinence in Heaven. He could look down along the years—those few that remained to him—and see his life, peaceful, neatly ordered by the ringing of bells, pottering along until he died. I lay there, a young man yet, a man with a wife and two children, and saw myself limping and starving through the years.

Brother Sebastian and every other monk who came in contact with me showed me kindness. Brother Stephen sent frequent messages, and alms sometimes, to Kate, and every time she sent back word that all was well. My most urgent question—Is Master Webster holding my job open for me?—was either never asked, or never answered, or the answer suppressed.

"Time enough to fret about work when you are fitted to do it," Brother Sebastian would say.

Despite my fretting my flesh wounds healed and my broken bone knitted. The day came when Brother Sebastian removed the broomstick and, having allowed two more days for the limb to strengthen, helped me to stand up and test the virtue of his new experiment. Up to a point it was good. My leg was straight enough, but it had set quite stiff and about two inches shorter than the other. I walked, if anything, more clumsily and painfully than Peg-Leg.

The straightness was all Brother Sebastian cared about. Fingering my shin gloatingly, he said, "Thanks be to God who brought the broomstick to my mind. The stiffness will wear off with use, you will find. And I will myself make the shortness of that leg the subject of a Novena."

"Do you hope for a miracle?"

"Why not? I shall pray, and so must you, and you must have *faith*. Many much lamer than you have been restored at St. Egbert's shrine."

That, I knew, was true. The wealth and fame of Baildon Abbey was rooted in the miraculous reputation of the Saint. I knew his story by this time. In life he had been king of a tiny kingdom, part in Suffolk and part in Essex. This was in time long past, before one king ruled all England, in the dim ages, before the Normans came. Egbert's enemies had been the Danes, wild heathen men who had come to rob and burn and rape in that part of England that lay along the sea. In one of his battles Egbert had been captured; but he had been so doughty and valiant a foe that the Danes' leader had offered to make an ally of him, give him high rank in their order, provided he would abandon the Christian faith and worship the heathen gods. He had refused and been killed. The monks of Baildon—then a small, poor wooden convent—had sought for his body and buried it in their tiny church; and then the miracles had begun. Then had come the pilgrims in search of further miracles, and the gifts had poured in. The miracles could hardly be disputed. During my three years in Baildon there had been several; a young girl had been led to the shrine, jerking and twitching in the throes of St. Vitus's dance, and walked away in full control of her limbs; a man set fast in all his joints, just able to put one foot before the other, leaning on two sticks, had hobbled into the Abbey church and walked out, firm and upright, leaving his sticks laid across one another in the form of a cross at the spot where he had prayed and been healed. There were others, all well vouched for. But—and this is what stuck in my mind—both my afflicted neighbours, the deaf-and-dumb man and the man with one leg, had, in their time, asked a miracle and come empty away. And it seemed to me that Peg-Leg, at least, had asked the impossible. Had he really expected a brand-new leg to grow out of his stump, and how—all at once, or inch by inch? And had their failure been due to lack of faith in themselves?

I was not pondering these questions for the first time. I had often thought about them while I was working. I had come to the conclusion—which may be a blasphemous one—that St. Egbert's miracles acted, not on the affliction, but upon the person who was afflicted. The jumping, jerking victim of St. Vitus's dance, for instance, might have stood by the shrine and prayed and believed that St. Egbert was helping her to hold herself still, and in that belief held herself still and then known that if she could control herself for one minute she could do it forever. The same with the man who had stiffened. Maybe he had waked one morning a little stiff, and coddled himself and grown stiffer; maybe he liked to be pitied, maybe he welcomed and traded upon his affliction. Then a time came when he wished, for some reason, to be like other men, so he made his pilgrimage and, standing there, leaning on his sticks, thought that he could stand upright and unaided if he *tried*.

In such miracles I could believe. But in a miracle that would add two inches to my short leg, no.

However, all that day Brother Sebastian kept me on the move;

two other beds in the Infirmary were occupied, and he made me help to wait upon the invalids. After each clumsy walk he would say, "Rest now," and then, when I was rested, set me in motion again.

That evening he gave me an enormous supper.

"Eat heartily," he said. "Tomorrow I shall dismiss you and you will need all your strength." When I had eaten he said, "And now we will go and see what St. Egbert has to say."

I had noticed before that they always spoke of their Saint as though he were alive and aware.

For me it was a tiring and worrying walk. The Infirmary lay in a remote part of the Abbey, rightly, for often it housed sufferers from diseases which could be caught by others. We went along passages, up and down stairs, once across a piece of garden; and as I walked, my hand on Brother Sebastian's shoulder, I thought miserably that if this were the best I could do with aid, it did not matter whether Master Webster had held my place for me or not. I could never work as a pack-whacker again. And though I could perhaps at a pinch have stood on my toes on the short side, and plied my smith's trade, nobody would employ me now, even at half rate.

I was panting hard when we reached a great doorway with torches in sconces on either side, and with a small door set in the one half of the large ones.

"Get your breath," Brother Sebastian said. "And *pray!*"

We went up the steps and in at the small door. The vast church was but dimly lighted, just enough for us to see our way. The tall columns of the nave soared up into darkness, but at its end there was a light and a sparkle.

We walked towards it, side by side, Brother Sebastian silently in his soft cloth shoes, I going stamp and shuffle as I put down my good leg and then swung the stiff one round.

The light and the glitter came from two sources. There was the altar which lay beyond the reredos screen, and the shrine itself which was on this side, slightly to the left. There were candles innumerable, and their lights were taken up and thrown back at us, many times magnified by a thousand shining surfaces. The shrine, and this is true, was invisible under a thick pelt of gold and silver ornaments and jewels of every colour. Hundreds of people every year through hundreds of years had lain their offerings there. It was like looking at the sun at midday in the summer; my eyes blinked and squinted, unable to take in any one thing because the whole was so dazzling.

I was speechless with awe, but Brother Sebastian might have been in his own Infirmary.

"The Saint's real tributes lie there," he said, after giving me a moment to stare and wonder. He pointed to a space beyond the shrine, where sticks and crutches, leather neck braces, slings, and bandages lay all in a jumble.

"There, you have seen what he can do. Kneel down and ask him to act for you."

I tried. I tried to force out the prayer for the cure for the shortness of my leg, but it would not be. I found myself praying, with the utmost urgency: Let me find some work that I can do. Let me not be a burden on Kate. No other thought would come into my head, and I went on praying the same thing over and over, until at last Brother Sebastian touched me on the shoulder.

"We must not tire him," he said. And something impatient and evil moved in me. I wanted to cry: How can you tire someone who has been dead and at rest for hundreds of years? And I knew that there would be no miracle for me.

Brother Sebastian, after he had spoken to me, had moved away and was now on his knees on the step which led up from the nave to the choir stalls. I stood up and went, stamp, swing, shuffle, until I stood behind him.

The altar was a gold table, bearing a jewelled crucifix and two seven-branched golden candlesticks. It was backed by a screen, also of gold, divided into a number of oblongs, each one a picture, done in glowing colours and worked in some way I did not understand into the gold. There were three rows of them, twenty-six to a row. From where I stood it was impossible to see them clearly.

Brother Sebastian stood up. He knew he had failed, or I had failed, or St. Egbert had failed, and his manner took on a curious resemblance to that of a workman, say a smith, who has done a bad job and knows it and uneasily tries to divert attention by mentioning the weather or inquiring after the health of the customer or his family.

"You are looking at the screen. It is interesting. Come and regard it closely. It is one of our treasures." We went forward.

"Two hundred years old," he said. "You see, the pictures in the centre row represent scenes from the New Testament, those above and below, scenes from the Old. But each three have a common theme. How many do you recognise?"

I looked at the three pictures in the centre.

"In the middle," I said, "is the Crucifixion. Above it Abraham is prepared to sacrifice Isaac, but sees the ram caught in the thicket, and below is Jephthah keeping his vow by sacrificing his daughter. These three pictures have sacrifice as their common theme. Is that right?"

"Go on," he said.

I looked about. In many of the sections the light just shone back at me, off the surface of the gold and the inlaid colours, carrying no meaning. I was, after all, an ignorant fellow. Here and there a picture had meaning.

"On the left there. In the middle is Our Lord Jesus Christ feeding the five thousand. Above is the prophet Elijah and the widow woman of Zarephath with the unfailing barrel of meal and cruse of oil. Below, that same Elijah is being fed by the ravens."

"You are right. And what is the theme?"

"That God, if He wills, can provide."

"Right again. That is what I wished to point out to you, but you pointed it out to me. Bear it in mind. In a few minutes the bell will ring for Compline. Come, I will help you back to bed."

On the way back we neither of us spoke about the miracle which had not happened. Brother Sebastian talked about the altar screen, saying that, beautiful and valuable as it was, it was in the wrong place. It should be in some parish church where the priest could teach those who could not read the Bible truths by its means. Then he said suddenly:

"You have more learning than most. Where did you come by it?"

"I always heeded what our priest had to say."

"You should thank God for a good memory."

The good memory which so often reminded me how I had said to Kate, "You shall be safe with me." Something to be grateful for indeed.

That was my last night in the Abbey Infirmary, and it was a poor one. I slept in snatches, each full of strange and sometimes sinister dreams. Once I dreamed that my leg, like Peg-Leg's, was cut off at the knee and that St. Egbert answered my prayer for a miracle by causing me to grow a golden leg, very marvellous to look at, but too heavy for me to drag; I lay on Rede dunghill, unable to walk and lamenting the miracle. Then I dreamed that Kate and I and Stephen were *really* starving, sitting before our hut, bowed over with the pain in our bellies. A great bird came swooping down, carrying Robin's dead body in his bloody beak. Kate said, "It will be all right to eat this meat. It is a gift from God."

From these and similar wild dreams I woke sweating, to lie and face the old gnawing anxiety again until once more I fell into uneasy slumber. I was glad when the bell rang for Prime.

I rose and began to dress and found that my right shoe was missing. I hunted for it until the Infirmary servant brought the breakfast and then sat down to eat my porridge while it was still warm. I had almost finished when Brother Sebastian came hurrying in, carrying my shoe.

"The miracle!" he exclaimed. "The miracle, Martin. It happened. In my old head! Look." He held out my shoe onto which had been tacked, very neatly, another sole, two inches thick.

"Try it. Try it." He was as eager and impatient as a child. "The thought came to me at Matins, and I asked Brother Anthony, our shoemaker, if he could do the work. He stayed up and worked instead of going back to his bed. How is it now?"

I stood up and stood level.

"Most wonderfully easy." I began to thank him, but he cut me short.

"Thank St. Egbert, who put the thought into my head. Now, when the stiffness has worn off, you will hardly be the worse for your mishap."

Once more I tried to thank him. He stopped me again, tapping my hand with his finger.

"Wait. There was something else I had to tell you before you go. Now what could it be? Nothing to do with your leg or my work . . . that is why I have forgotten it. But I shall . . . Oh yes! Martin, you live in Squatters Row as they call it."

"Yes."

"Well, be warned by me. Begin to look for other accommodation. There is talk of clearing that wall and covering in the Ditch and making all tidy there. The Prior and the Cellarer were talking only yesterday. The Bishop of Dunwich came to visit and entered by the east gate and made some unfavourable comment. They're bound to take some action."

I'd had less than a moment to savour the joy of the shoe that mitigated my lameness.

"I don't suppose it will happen tomorrow or even next week," Brother Sebastian said kindly. "Our present Cellarer is too old to move quickly, but . . . well, I thought I would warn you."

I suppose I should have thanked him for that, too. As it was I took leave of him sullenly.

X

Kate's greeting of me was proof that our sharp words towards one another, the way we now lived, hardly touching one another, and all the worry and all the woe had not really set us apart. When I hobbled home she cried, partly at grief to see me so lame, but mainly with joy at seeing me again. She said how much she had missed me, how greatly she had longed to come and nurse me herself, and I in turn said that I had missed her very sorely, thought of her by day and dreamed of her by night. I could hardly tell her what form those thoughts, those dreams had taken.

Soon, however, I had to ask the question.

"And has Master Webster held my place for me?"

All the joy, the young-Kate look went out of her face, leaving the harassed, irritable one which was her everyday one nowadays.

"No. He put a new man on the very next Monday. I went to him, Martin, I spoke for you. I went on my knees, and I cried. He took no notice. Then I lost my temper and told him flatly he was ungrateful when you'd been hurt beating off robbers on his behalf."

"They weren't robbers," I said. "There was nothing to steal that night—except the ponies, and they made no attempt upon them. They let Crooky go by, and the ponies, until the last that I was riding. I think even Crooky knew."

"Knew what?"

"That I was to be set on. You were here, Kate, when Armstrong said they had ways of dealing with those who went against their rules."

"But they might have killed you."

"They probably meant to. In any case, lying out all night I should have died. It was only lucky chance that I was found."

"Then they're murderers. And they should be punished."

"Who by?"

"The law. The constable."

"I have no evidence against anyone. Whom could I accuse? It was dark and foggy. I never saw a face, or heard a voice."

"Then if it was Armstrong's men, it was because you were doing Webster's smith work and he should have stood by you."

"Maybe in a way he has; maybe he put on the new man just until I was better."

Kate shook her head.

"No, I made sure of that. And he seemed so against you, somehow. I think he would have sacked me, simply for being your wife, but Margit got married and left us shorthanded on the floor."

"Why should he be against me? I always served him well. I shall come along in the morning and see him."

"I don't think it will do a ha'porth of good," Kate said.

In the morning I dropped Kate and the children at the door of the woolshed and went to look for Master Webster. He was in the stables and the moment he saw me his face darkened.

"What d'you want?"

I forced myself to be meek.

"I've come back to work, master."

"Not here. I've no use for blabbermouth jugheads."

"Me?" I was never more astounded. I was of sheer necessity the soberest man who ever wore shoe leather, and I never talked to anyone. Even Kate hadn't known why I worked so late so often, until Armstrong had come and let it out.

"Yes. You. You got yourself tipsy in the Smith's Arms and bragged about what you were doing here after dark."

"I haven't been in the Smith's Arms since the day Armstrong broke it to me I couldn't join the Guild. Who's the liar who said he saw me there? I'll break his neck!"

"Shouting at me won't mend matters. This was all gone into at a full meeting of Guild aldermen."

"What was? You know yourself, I told you at the time, that I was spied on and reported to Armstrong and that he came and saw me and threatened me. You said take no notice and go on as we were."

"Nobody spied on you. You made that up when you realised,

sober, what you'd said in your cups. And it was a poor reward for my pandering to you."

"Pandering to me?"

He fixed his eyes on some point behind me, over my shoulder, and said in a wooden way which told that he was repeating something said before, "You wanted to keep your hand in—on the smith work—and I was silly enough to let you shoe a pony now and then. For practice, against the time you hoped to get back into the craft. Ain't that right? Out of charity I did it."

I saw his plump red face, the eyes avoiding mine, the lips moving, spilling out the lies; and then the red mist came down and blotted it out. I could feel, beforehand, the supreme pleasure of smashing my knuckles through the mist and onto that well-padded jaw. But this time I held my hand. Hit him and, shorthanded or not, he would give Kate her quittance, and what she earned was, at this moment, all there was between us and starvation.

Whirling about, at the back of my mind was the thought that free men can suffer humiliations deeper and more hurtful than any a serf can ever know. In order that Kate and Stephen and Robin should eat tomorrow—for myself I did not care, I never wanted to eat again—I must accept this lie. I could see exactly what had happened; the Guild aldermen had held a solemn conclave; Webster, a member of the Woolman's Guild, had offended the Smiths by using me, a non-member, to do smith work; and the Smith's Guild had committed, not a fault, but a breach in manners, by spying upon Webster. So there had been a meeting of all the aldermen, intent only upon smoothing the whole thing over. Webster had lied about employing me, and Armstrong had denied the spying. No matter what it took of lies and falsity to do it, the firm, unbroken face which the Guilds as a whole presented to the world outside must remain uncracked. Throw lies, throw a living man's body into the breach, and then seal it over with cakes and ale and renewed vows of brotherhood and fair dealing.

And I, for the sake of a loaf of bread, dared not speak.

Jesus Christ! I said to myself. If only a miracle could happen and I could deal with them all as they have dealt with me, with joy would I rub their faces in the dirt!

I knew I was like a child, beaten by his father, thinking, *When I grow up!* But there was this difference. The child will surely grow.

I went out on the hunt for work. The town was growing in size and business was flourishing, but work was hard to find. Out in the country more and more acres of arable land were being turned into sheep runs, and one man could tend the sheep where twenty had been needed to plough and sow and reap. Those put out of work came flooding into the towns, so that there were three men for every job. A good deal of the work going forward was building, and with my stiff leg and built-up shoe I did not look a likely digger, or climber of ladders. I was passed over again and again.

Soon, alongside Dummy and Peg-Leg, I was waiting at the town gates every morning, ready to fight for any despicable little job that might be going, to hold horses or walk hounds while their owners went into the Abbey to visit the shrine, to carry baggage, to lead the way to inns. Sometimes, standing there amongst the riffraff, I would think how far I had fallen, a smith, a craftsman who had served his time. By comparison my father's life, bound as he was, had had dignity and purpose. I'd run a long way and borne a great deal and got nowhere.

Now and again, having done a job and taken the meagre pay, I would go into the country and buy apples or plums or eggs on some day that was not market day, and come back and hawk them through the streets. The walking tired me and I grew lopsided, since the easiest way was to hitch the whole right-hand side of my body when I swung that leg forward. Dummy's brood, on the rare occasions when they were sufficiently full-fed to feel sportive, took to imitating me behind my back, as they did Peg-Leg.

I never passed on to Kate the word that our very hut was threatened, but some time during that summer the old midwife and layer-out, Agnes, came back from making a baker named Barnaby ready for his grave with news which seemed to excite her. She said that Barnaby had left all his money for the building of some almshouses and that as soon as they were standing everybody in Squatters Row was to move into them. It was strange to hear how that drunken old slattern, who lived under a piece of torn sailcloth, spoke of having a house again as though that was the one thing she wanted. But nothing came of it. The Barnaby houses were for eight widows whose husbands had been Guild members.

"And there goes my last hope," Agnes said, and went out and got herself most enviably drunk.

Dummy's wife said, "They are only one up and one down, they'd be no good to my lot. Laying heel to head, we go from here to there." She indicated the space between two buttresses.

So Squatters Row went on just as before, and that summer we had a new kind of visitor. The pilgrims brought their own parasites, bear-leaders, tumblers, dancers, and singers, but this was something different, a travelling friar, poorly dressed in a grey hood and gown of the coarsest stuff, and with his feet bare in the dust. At night he slept with the rest of us outcasts, between the buttresses, by day he went about preaching. He'd follow a performing bear or some other entertainer and wait until a crowd had gathered, and then he would call, in a very powerful voice, "Brothers! I bring you good news." His news was the Fatherhood of God, the brotherhood of man. The more frivolous, or the rough in the crowd, would jeer and pelt him, but he would stand his ground and sooner or later he would speak against the Abbey and the monks. He would say that it was wrong for professional religious to be great landlords; he decried all pomp and ceremony; he said that Christ only once in His life rode, and that on the back of a humble ass, how then could abbots and bishops, Christ's representatives on earth, go mounted and robed like temporal princes?

I do not doubt that he was honest and sincere. I suspect that his decrying of rank and power, his praise of humility and poverty were, in a manner, like the clapper, or the whistle by which other people gained the crowd's attention. For afterwards would come the real sermon, urging the virtues of charity and mercy, chastity and honesty, with many a text and story from the Bible to illustrate his point.

Moving around as I did, working or searching for work, I heard him often. Kate, shut away in the woolshed, had no such chance, so over supper I would tell her something of what he had said, or how he had been pelted.

One evening she fell thoughtful and after a time said, "He is a stranger and sounds good of heart. Could he *marry* us?"

"I don't know. If he has taken priest's orders, yes. But all monks are not priests, maybe all friars are not."

"You could ask him. Go now."

"Oh, not out there, with so many listening who think us married already."

"No. Get him out of earshot if you can. I know, bring him here, ask him to sup with us."

"But we've eaten," I said, looking at the bare platter.

"I should think my breakfast tomorrow, aye and every morning I have left to live, a small price for such a favour."

"So should I, of course. Of course," I said, and ran out into the night.

Squatters Row was fully occupied, and the friar had taken one of the least favourable places, midway between two buttresses, with no corner to huddle into. He was eating a slice of rye bread and when I proffered my invitation to supper he said:

"That is kind of you. I have enough here. Perhaps tomorrow . . . if you can afford it."

"Oh yes," I said. "Truth to tell my . . . my wife and I," I had to say that, for there were ears all about, "my wife and I wanted to ask you something . . . a favour. Would you come indoors with me? It is very near."

"Of course," he said, and heaved himself to his feet.

Inside the hut I closed the door, which hung awry from two hinges of leather which I had made, and wedged it close. In the faint light of the dying fire we all looked into one another's faces for a moment, none of us speaking. The friar broke silence, looking at the children in their bed by the inner wall.

"They are sick?" he asked gently.

"No, Father, asleep, I hope," Kate said. "My . . . this man and I have a confession to make and a favour to ask. We have lived as man and wife for four years now, but we were never married. . . ."

"And now you wish to be?"

"Yes," I said, "but not openly." I told him—not everything, but all he needed to know—of our circumstances; how we had intended to marry and been prevented through no fault of our own, and had come to the town as man and wife and then dared not betray our state.

"You have been living in sin; you know that?"

"We know. And we have suffered for it."

"And during this time you have performed your religious duties, always with this sin unconfessed and unabsolved?"

"Yes." He looked so grave that the consciousness of sin did come upon me. I must confess that in the rough and tumble of daily living the matter had troubled me very little; I had only thought of it occasionally as having been a mistake, the cause and reason for some of our misfortune.

"But you are free to marry? And during this time you have been faithful to one another?"

Kate said, "Always, Father." And I said, "Unswervingly." And that was true. I had never even looked with desire upon any woman save Kate and not for lack of temptation. During my pack-whacking days the chances had been plentiful.

"This can be mended then," the friar said. "Tomorrow you will both fast all day. At about this time in the evening I will come to you and you may make your confessions, and in that state of Grace you shall be wed. We will then break fast together."

We thanked him heartily and he went quietly away.

Next evening we fed the children and put them to bed early. Kate scrubbed the rough board which was our table top, and set out upon it the meat pie she had bought in Cooks Row, a fresh loaf, and a dish of red-cheeked apples. She was in high good spirits, calling this our wedding feast, and regretting that we had no wedding garments.

"Like the man in the Bible story," I said.

"But he was sent away. That can't happen to us."

We had left the door open and made up the fire with dry sticks which gave light but little heat; and in the light I looked at her with new, searching eyes, making compare with the girl who had entered the hall with me at Rede and roused an old man's lust. Hard work and poverty and misery had aged her by five times the four years that had gone by since then; her face was thin and lined, her hair rough and lustreless as hay. I thought how lightly the years would have touched her had she gone to Abhurst, and I remembered again those silly words, "My pretty one, you shall be safe with me."

"It's the Guilds that have ruined us," I burst out suddenly. "They threw me out to rot and when I refused to rot they broke my leg. Kate, I never meant it to be this way, I meant to take care of you and cherish you."

"And so you have," she said, and came over and put her arm about my neck and kissed me. "Few men are so careful about fetching water and carrying the heavy loads. Who else would have walked with me to work every day, to spare me? You say what *you* meant. I meant never to say a sharp word to you, and Heaven knows I've said many. But from tonight I start afresh."

I pulled her close. I felt tenderly towards her, though there was no desire in me.

"Few women," I said, "would have been so patient and worked so hard. Who else would have kept food on the table and washed and mended and made a home as you have?"

These were not romantic speeches, but they were sincere and more suited to our state than any flowery words could be. And I was angry that immediately afterwards my empty belly gave a loud rumble.

"I'm hungry too," Kate said. "All day I've been too much excited to notice, but now I am hungry and he is late."

Presently we were asking one another whether the friar could have forgotten us and reminding ourselves that he had spoken of breaking fast together; if he intended to fast with us, surely his own emptiness would make him think of us.

Kate began to fidget, going to the door to peer out and complaining that it was too dark to see.

"Go and see if you can find him," she said. I walked the length of the wall. I could not see the friar anywhere.

I went home again, and we waited.

It was after Curfew, so we dared not replenish the fire, and sitting in the dark the time stretched out endlessly, but at last it was eleven o'clock; we heard the bell tolling the hour.

"He isn't coming," Kate said.

"Something must have happened to him." I remembered how some of the rough people had jeered and pelted him. I remembered, too, that many of the things he had said about monasteries and the conduct of the monks were offensive enough to make the Abbot take action against him.

"Have you seen him at all today?" Kate asked.

"No, I've been off the streets all day today. I offered to guide some pilgrims to the Angel Inn, and while I was there I got a job sawing wood. I'm going there again tomorrow."

"He promised to come," Kate said, and the old complaining note was there in her voice again. "I really thought that at last we . . ."

I realised that marriage meant much more to her than it did to me; a woman who lives out of wedlock with a man is called a whore; there is no such damaging term for the man. I made a great effort to comfort her. First I said, fumbling about in the gloom for the knife and the meat pie:

"Let's have our supper. Everything looks worse when your belly is empty." And then, between the mouthfuls, I said what were perhaps the first fanciful words I had ever said.

"Kate," I began, "when Brother Sebastian took the broomstick off my leg and found that the bone had healed up short, he said he would pray for a miracle. We went together to St. Egbert's shrine and prayed there. Nothing happened to the bone in my leg, I didn't expect anything, so I wasn't disappointed; he was. But a few hours afterwards he thought about thickening the sole on my shoe, and when he told me about it he called that the miracle. You see . . . the thing you ask for comes, but not in the shape that you think. We thought that tonight the friar would come and marry us, but he didn't. Kate, really, if we could only understand it, we *were* married, that night by the river under the hawthorn tree . . . and tonight we were, in a fashion, married again when you said I'd been good about fetching water and I said you'd been good about mending and making a home. Try not to fret about the words that haven't been said over us. We are, in very truth, married."

"The friar himself said that we had lived in sin."

"Dummy and his wife were properly married, I've heard her boast of it to Loose Liz. Look how they live! Worse than animals. They make the beast with two backs, and as soon as a child comes of it he beats her black and blue. Their crooked child takes dole at the Alms Gate, and Dummy meets her on the way home and eats his fill without a thought for his wife's hunger. Kate, in all the time that I was a pack-whacker I never ate a mouthful of what I was given until I was back here and sharing with you. When the friar asked us had we been faithful to one another, we could both say yes, and truly. How could any ceremony make us more married than we are?"

She did not answer immediately; but after a moment she said, "All that is true; but there is another side to it. The friar said we were living in sin and that every time we went to Mass with that sin unconfessed and unabsolved we were sinning anew. And our being faithful to one another can't help them being bastards." Even in the dark I could see her arm fling out towards the bed where the children lay. "Nothing but ill-luck ever since we've been here, and now nothing but ill-luck to look forward to."

I pitied the misery that sounded in her voice, but it made me impatient, too. It may be true that misery loves company, but it finds its comfort in a different misery, not in a reflection of its own.

"I did my best and there's nothing more to do. Let's sleep and forget it," I said.

XI

That summer had been unusually wet and wet it continued over harvest, so that some of the poor thin crop was lost in the gathering, the sheaves standing mouldering in the fields. It was clear that bread would be scarce throughout the coming winter. Part of the blame for what happened next can be laid on the fear and ill-temper which this prospect roused in the hearts of all but the very rich. But something must also be blamed upon the friar, who had appeared in our midst, sown his seed of discord, and vanished; and a great deal of blame must be laid upon the Abbey, in particular the Cellarer, who dealt with many things affecting the good or ill-will between the monks and the townsfolk.

There were two rights which the Abbey held and which I had never, during my years in Baildon, seen exercised. One was the right to *all* the dung dropped within the town boundaries; that is not merely in the streets and market, but in stables and smithies and cowsheds and pigsties. This did not mean that all the dung went onto the Abbey lands, but it did mean that anyone who wanted to use his own manure on his own land or garden must buy it back, *in situ*, from the Abbey Cellarer. That this right had fallen into abeyance I knew from my years in the smithy. Master Armstrong had derived a small but steady income from the sale of dung dropped by horses waiting to be shod.

The other right was to demand that all corn within an area of ten miles should be ground at the Abbey Mill, which stood a little way out of town on the south side, at Flaxham St. Giles. That this right had not been exercised for many years was proved by the existence of another mill, on the north of the town, which was now being worked by the son of the man who had started it. Two easygoing Cellarers had followed one another in office.

Now, in this year of poor harvest, a new one was appointed, a young man, energetic and avaricious. One of his first acts was to have cried through the town the announcement that in future the Abbey Mill must be used for all corn grinding, and that the rights to the town's dung would be strictly enforced. Next day the Abbey servants, with a flat cart, went about the town, assessing every dung-heap and what was not paid for there and then was loaded onto the cart and taken away. The Cellarer himself, riding a grey mule, went out to the North Mill and curtly informed the young miller that he was welcome to grind any corn brought to him from any place more than ten miles distant from Baildon market place, but no other. That meant ruin to the miller, and two days later he drowned himself in his own millstream. The Church refused him burial and he went to a suicide's grave at the crossroads.

This story rang through the town, adding to the ill-feeling which the enforcement of the old rules had brought about.

Worse followed; for as soon as the monopoly of milling was assured, the charge for milling was raised. It had been one fourteenth, that is a pound of flour for every stone of corn ground, henceforth it would be two pounds—one seventh. This was bad for everybody, since it put up the price of bread.

Everywhere now people were speaking against the Abbey and the monks, and it was curious to hear, mixed with the straightforward grumbling voiced in their own simple words, the echo of the friar's accusations. Even those who had listened to him least had picked up from those who had given him their attention some phrases which sounded foreign on their tongues, "appearance of sanctity," "abuse of privilege," "temporal power," "private lechery." Many of them hardly knew what the words meant, but they did know that they were speaking against the Abbey and the monks, and whipping up the ill-feeling.

Nothing might have come of it, but in early November the Abbey officers arrested a man known as John Noggs, who kept a little ale-house just inside the west gate of the town. He had set up and been working a small hand mill, and his customers had been seen to arrive with sacks of corn and to depart carrying sacks of flour. The power to turn the stone was supplied by two simple-minded boys, and if it ground one hundredweight of corn in a full day's work that was its limit. Still the new Cellarer was a man rather to take account of the breaking of a rule than of the damage done by the breaking. He was also a man to judge the customers of the illicit mill equally guilty with the miller. Within the next few days several more arrests were made. One of those accused of cheating the Abbey of its rightful dues was a respectable, solid townsman who owned a cook shop, and one was a poor old woman who had gleaned diligently all through the harvest and taken her gleanings to be ground where the charge was lighter; the others I knew nothing of.

Immediately all the ill-feeling came, like a festering boil, to a head. The whole town was now united against the Abbey. Over most matters it was difficult to get the comfortably off to join with the poor, or the merely poor to join with the destitute, and there was a severance, always, between those within and those without the Guilds. Now the arrest of the pastry-cook, who was a Guildsman, was an affront to them all, the fate of the innkeeper-turned-miller was of concern to the middle sort, and the very poor were all agog in sympathising with the old woman. The sullen grumbling changed to a more active, though still vague feeling that "something should be done."

At this moment there popped up a very ancient fellow, half blind and more than half rambling in his wits, who could remember back to when he was a little boy, when on a somewhat similar occasion the townsfolk had all joined together and shown "them" that even "they" couldn't have everything their own way. The squabble then had concerned the taking of eels from the river—another Abbey right—and when the townspeople had done considerable damage to the Bell Tower and the main gate, the rules had been modified. The old grandfather, after years of obscurity, suddenly found himself the centre of attention. The little house of his granddaughter with whom he lived was always thronged with people anxious to hear his tale of what had happened seventy years ago. He conveniently forgot, or left out of his tale, anything which the townsfolk would not find agreeable, and the effect was to make them feel that they were a pack of powerful wolves who, for many years, had allowed themselves to be bullied by a few bleating old sheep and who had only to show their teeth to turn the tables. Very soon, before the arrested people could be brought before the Abbey Court, an attack on the Abbey was being planned.

I heard all about it. I was always moving about the town, here and there, in search of work. I was hungry and poor, one of the oppressed whose bread would be dear, whose feelings would veer towards the old gleaning woman. By the simple process of listening and saying nothing I learned a great deal. Sometime in November, at the dark of the moon, the Abbey was to be attacked. The monks

would then be in bed and sound asleep; they retired soon after
Compline, which was at seven in the winter, and slept until midnight when they were roused for Matins. It was not badly planned.
The postern gate in the great main gateway was to be forced by
means of a battering ram, and then a body of apprentices, armed
with the bows and arrows with which they practised on Saturday
afternoons, was to march in and demand the release of the pris-
oners. The aldermen of the Guilds, dressed in their livery, and un-
armed, but under guard of another group of apprentices and journeymen, were then to go and negotiate with the Abbot, or the
Prior, and get the charge for milling reduced again to one fourteenth and the claim on the dung waived. All this under threat of
real violence, letting the riffraff run wild through the Abbey, and
firing timbers and thatch. This, according to the old grandfather,
was how the townspeople had conducted their business seventy
years ago, and they had won what they asked for. Why shouldn't
it happen again?

Now it is true that an ordinary poor man like me can go through
a lifetime without once testing his loyalty to anything save his own
belly and his own family. In the main he cannot even be said to be
loyal to his own kind, since at any moment he is prepared to snatch
a job, or a crust, from another man exactly like himself; I had done
it many a time by the town gateway. But it is equally true that
some extraordinary circumstance may arise and the most simple
man must ask himself the question: Where do I stand in this matter? and the answer is there, clear and certain as soon as the question
is asked.

Such a testing point I had now reached, and there was no doubt
at all in my mind that I was with the monks. I had lived in the
town for over four years, and the only kindness that I had received
from anybody had come from within those Abbey walls. Brother
Justinius was mean; the increase in the milling charge made my
bread dear, but those facts looked small when placed beside the
alms Kate had received in both her pregnancies, the fair, just way
in which the Trimble charity had been administered, the careful
attention I had been given in the Infirmary, and the way Brother
Sebastian had devised and Brother Anthony had carried out the
scheme to make me less crippled.

I owed the Abbey a good deal. And I hated the Guilds, their
aldermen, their journeymen, and their rules.

At the same time I will not pretend I was ruled either by grati-tude or hatred. Expediency played its part. The old grandfather might remember only that the townspeople had gained their point about the eels; the fact remained that after seventy years the Abbey still governed the town; and even if the townsfolk had won back their right to go eel-fishing, the Abbey had retained every right that mattered. It seemed to me that I should do myself no harm by trying to get into favour with those who would surely get the better of the dispute in the long run. I might even contrive to put in a word for my little threatened house. If I warned the monks in time, they would be grateful and then I could say, "Please don't demolish my neat thatched hut with the rest of Squatters Row."

I was obliged to settle all these things in my mind rather quickly when it came to the point. After all the weeks of grumbling and plotting the decision to make the attack on the twelfth of Novem-ber was only settled on the evening of the eleventh. On the morn-ing of the twelfth I was helping a man to slaughter a pig; we had its throat cut and its guts out when the man's neighbour looked over the wall and passed the news. I stood for a moment with my filthy hands hanging idle and the scent of blood in my nostrils and ran through all the arguments again. The townsfolk who had never shown me any kindness at all, or the Abbey which had given me alms and mended my leg? The townsfolk who would never do me any good, or the Abbey which might grant me the right to go on living in my hut?

I made up my mind, and, striking my leg in a gesture of sudden comprehension, I exclaimed, "Holy Mother, my shoe! The monk Anthony is the only one who knows how to mend it. If trouble is brewing, I should get it done today."

The man I was helping gave a loud yelp of laughter and smote me on the back.

"Thass the way," he exclaimed. "Take the honey before you smoke out the hive. Get what you can out of the rogues. They'll hev more than shoes to mend tomorrow, I'll warrant."

I limped along to the Alms Gate and stood at the end of the little crowd who were drawing their dole. Brother Justinius was on duty, for which I was a little sorry; but when my turn came at last, I took off my shoe and, leaning against the hatch, said, "Brother Justinius, I have some information which is of importance to the Abbey."

I spoke softly, for there were some who, having snatched their dole, were eating it then and there.

The monk had his wits about him. Taking the shoe, he said in a loud, scolding voice, "What again! I declare you wear out more shoes than a tinker's ass! You'd think Brother Anthony had nothing else to do. Wait there."

He slammed down the hatch.

I curled my bare foot round the shin of my other leg and leaned against the wall. One by one those who were wolfing down their food finished it and wandered away; all but one, a stranger to me, his hand wrapped in a filthy, bloodied clout.

"Keep you waiting," he said, coming close to me. "Keep you waiting like you was a dog, for the bits they scrape off their plates." He cleared his throat and spat out his rancour.

"I must wait," I said. "Only the monk can mend my shoe."

"That may be. But if they was the kind brothers to everybody like they make out to be, wouldn't they say, 'Come in. Sit you down,' not, 'Wait there.' Same with the food. Why, once I heard a friar preach, telling about Our Lord Jesus Christ. . . ." He crossed himself piously. "*He* fed five thousand once, and He said, 'Sit down on the grass,' He said, 'and be comfortable.' And He didn't hev no hatches and waiting about till the hour struck. Fish He give them, too, and when their bellies wouldn't hold another bite He filled baskets for them to take away. Maybe you never heard that tale."

"I've heard all the tales," I said shortly, wishing he would take himself off.

"I'm a stranger here. I s'pose you don't know a place where I could lay, cheap, for the night."

"As it happens, I do." I directed him to the loft where Kate and I had lived during our first weeks in the town. I praised it, saying it was so good, so cheap that if he wanted to get a bed he should hurry. As I talked he began to unwind the rag from his hand. Under it flesh and bone were whole and sound.

"The monk will return in a minute. If you want to eat here tomorrow . . ." I said warningly.

He winked at me and hurried off. All poor men took it for granted that they were in league together, I thought. I was the one exception.

As soon as he had gone Brother Justinius opened, not the hatch but the whole door.

"Come in," he said.

The room was small and square with wide wooden shelves on the walls to left and right of the door. There were the remains of the loaves, and the big bowls of peaseporridge, cooked and allowed to set firm and then cut into sections. Someone in the crowd must have claimed Trimble too, for there was a joint of beef, glazed and brown without, pink and juicy within, which even at that nervous moment brought the water gushing into my mouth. I was meat-hungry. The thought struck me that had I stayed until that pig was dismembered, I should have been given a couple of trotters, or even maybe a hock.

"Now," Brother Justinius said briskly, "what is it that you have to tell?"

Tell him, I thought, and he would push me out, go to his immediate superior and say, "A man at the Alms Gate just told me . . ." How much would that profit me?

"It is for the ear of my Lord Abbot alone."

He looked at me. Kate went round my head and those of the boys every month with a pair of borrowed shears, and my time to be shorn was about due. Where I was not patched I was ragged, filthy from my last dirty job, and wearing but one shoe. A likely visitor for the Abbot!

"Who sent you?"

"Nobody. My own conscience compelled me."

He gave me a cold cynical look and said, "Oh, come along. What is it you have to say?"

"It is of importance. I can only speak of it to my Lord Abbot."

He said to me with great seriousness, "Do you know what you ask?"

And I said to him, with equal seriousness, "I know what I have to tell."

I could see him debating with himself whether or not to open the door and push me out. Finally he snapped out the one word, "Come."

He opened a door in the wall opposite the hatch and set off, at a great pace, along a stone passage, so cold with the stored-up chill of many sunless years that my teeth began to chatter. After what seemed to my bare limping foot a long walk, he stopped and threw open a door, saying in exactly the voice he had used before:

"Wait here."

The room was warm, with a good fire on the hearth and settles on either side. I went and warmed myself, slowly turning round like a roast on a spit, then I sat down. Something about the way I had been received, and this long waiting, started a doubt in my mind. Might it not have been wiser to stay with my own kind, outside these walls, thrown myself wholeheartedly into their plot, perhaps distinguished myself by boldness in the assault, so that they would say: This man must be admitted to the Guild forthwith; he is worthy to be a journeyman?

Well, it was too late now.

The door opened and another monk entered. I jumped up, forgetting my bare foot, lurched, and had to catch at the settle to save myself.

"I trust you are not drunk."

The voice was no more friendly than Brother Justinius', but it was different, cool, distant, very faintly amused. The face, narrow within the cowl's shadow, matched it, thin, sharply curved nose, arched brows above bright, intelligent eyes. There was nothing about his garb to mark him from any other monk, but I knew at once that I was in the presence of someone important.

"I am sober," I said. "I am lame without my shoe."

"And you have some tale to tell. What is it?"

"Are you my Lord Abbot?"

"No. But you must make do with me. I am the Prior."

It took all my courage to say again, "It is a matter of importance. It should be for my lord's ear alone."

"I *am* his ear. Come now, I am waiting."

I gave in and told him all that I knew. Except that his eyes narrowed a little as he listened, I might have been telling him that the weather was cold. When I had done, he asked one question.

"Why have you turned traitor to your fellows?" His tone was curious rather than accusing or malicious, yet it shamed me.

"I bear them a grudge for several wrongs they have done me. I was well treated in the Abbey Infirmary when my leg was broken. And I hope for a reward."

His glance brightened.

"I see. Well, rest assured that if your tale is true, you will be *well* rewarded."

"It *is* true. Why should I come and tell . . ."

"I have no time for that now. Wait here."

He went away, swiftly and silently. Soon the door opened again and Brother Justinius entered. Behind him were two men, servants, one of whom carried my shoe.

"Brother Anthony says that the upper hardly justifies a new sole, but it will last a little time. Put it on. Then these will show you the way."

He left us, and when my shoe was on one of the men said, "This way," and went ahead, the other fell in behind me. I suspected nothing. The two men might be on their way to town on some business, they might even have homes there and be about to return to them. I did notice that we were not going along the long cold passage that led to the Alms Gate, but there was nothing strange about that either. The Abbey had many entrances, and the Alms Gate, so far as I knew, was only used for its special purpose. Once we emerged into the daylight and crossed a paved courtyard, and I noticed that even out-of-doors the short winter light was waning. The next passage into which we plunged was almost dark. The man ahead of me stopped suddenly and threw open a door, and, instead of going through the opening himself, stepped aside and waited. The man behind me gave me a slight push and I went through the doorway, not into the twilit street as I expected, but into the pitch dark, full of a stench which even I, accustomed to the Town Ditch, found sickening. Before I could turn the door behind me slammed to with a horrid, final sound.

XII

Stupid bewilderment was, for a long time, the only thing I could feel. Why do this to me?

Afterwards came terror. I had heard—as who had not?—of the deep dungeons under great castles where men were thrown and forgotten, left to starve to death or be eaten by rats or go mad and beat their brains out against the walls. Those dungeons had a Norman name, "oubliettes," sinister indeed. Somehow I had never dreamed that an Abbey would have such a place. Even when Jack Nobbs and the others had been dragged off and imprisoned, I had imagined them in a less comfortable Infirmary. Now I knew. I was in even worse case than they were, for they were accused of an

offence, they would be brought to trial. I might very well just dis-
appear and never be heard of again. Nobody outside these walls
knew where I was.

Sweat of fear streamed over my body and dried cold as I thought
about Kate and the children. I had never supported them, but there
had never been a day when I had not somehow managed to contribute something to the household, even if it were only a bundle of
firewood; and I had kept the hut standing and moderately weatherproof. Apart from that most material consideration, there was
Kate's anxiety to worry over. Our first fond love had worn away, like
the nap from a woollen garment, but below, the fabric of unity was
still strong; if she had failed to come home one evening I should
have been distraught; I credited her with full as much concern
for me.

I should have said that it was impossible to find any spot in
Baildon out of the sound of the Abbey bells, but here the silence
was as complete as the darkness. The cold had driven me to burrow
into the heap of stinking straw, and I lay there for hours wishing
with all my heart I had kept clear of this business, imagining Kate
going home and waiting and wondering, waiting and worrying. For
a long time misery kept me from feeling hungry, but as the slow
hours dragged by the gnawing began in my vitals. I was schooled to
the feeling of not having had enough to eat, it was almost a constant state with me since my accident, but this was the painful
urgent need to eat *something*, anything, the need that will drive a
man to beg or steal. Presently, useless as I knew it to be, I was
beating with my hands on the door and shouting.

Nobody noticed, probably nobody heard me. I remained alone
with my fears and my hunger and the deadly cold which bit deeper
as my hunger increased. In the end I was driven back to the straw
again, and, comforted by the warmth, fell into a state which was
neither sleeping nor waking. Sometimes I was almost asleep, my
miseries of mind and body became a little blurred, and behind my
shut lids scenes from my past drifted by, small and very clear. Then
I would be jerked back to the straw and the hunger and the terror.

Once, thus jerked back, I had a new thought. I was going to die,
and I was afraid to die. Keeping alive had been such a struggle that
I had spared little thought for the state of my immortal soul; even
the friar's words about attending Mass while in a state of sin had
soon been, if not forgotten, pushed aside. Kate and I could not

suddenly absent ourselves, and we could not be married openly
without putting the brand of bastardy on the children, so we had
gone on as before and I had not worried about it until now. Now
not only that great sin but dozens of small ones must be remembered in torment. The lies I had told, one way and another! All
out of necessity, one might say, but each one a handing over of my
soul to the Devil, the Father of Lies. I had more than once stolen
things in the market—and never given the matter another thought.
It hadn't seemed sinful then, merely common sense, two eggs
slipped from a basketful while the owner turned her back meant
a meal for Stephen and Robin; I'd taken the nails that held my
hut together from Armstrong's stock—we made nails in slack hours
at the forge, and I had taken a few from a chest containing hundreds. Such petty pilfering I had not even confessed when I might
have done, they had weighed so lightly on my conscience. Now
they loomed enormous, and presently, thinking of death and the
Judgement, I reached the point where even my running from Rede
assumed the character of a sin. I was Lord Bowdegrave's property
and I had removed myself. . . .

Some remaining crumb of sanity became active then and I
thought: How ridiculous! How can a man steal himself? And I
laughed. The sound frightened me. I clapped my hand over my
mouth. Mad, mad! Locked up in the dark, starving to death, and
going mad. The next step was to beat my head against the wall and
add self-destruction to my other sins.

I was at the door again, beating on it and screaming, not this
time saying I was hungry, starving to death, this time begging for
a priest, beseeching them not to let me die with all my sins unconfessed and unabsolved.

As before nobody came.

Beating on the door and shouting had been too much for me in
my weak state; sweat poured off me again, my heart thudded so
hard that it struck sparks from my eyeballs. Without knowing that
I had fallen, I found myself on the floor. Then the cold struck
again and I crawled back into the straw, turned weakly warm, almost drifted into sleep again, and then was jerked back.

This time it was hope which tugged me. God was merciful. Jesus
Christ, in His earthly life, had been poor. Mary the Mother knew
how one felt about one's children and their hunger. I could pray
for pity and understanding and forgiveness.

So I knelt on the damp stone floor and prayed, passionately. I mentioned every sin I could remember, even my running away from Rede, which I could see now *was* a sin, in that it was evidence of my discontent with the condition to which it had pleased God to let me be born.

I prayed for hours. I prayed until the sweat ran down my face and dropped on to the floor and as it ran I began again.

"Sweet Jesus Christ, who in Gethsemane . . ." For He, too, knew the sweat of agony.

Then I swooned, or slept. From kneeling on the floor I was lying in the straw, which had, all at once, lost its stench. I was waiting for something, something of which I had been given warning, a pleasant and comforting thing.

What did I expect? Some voice in the silence, something luminous in the dark?

When it came it was merely a thought in my head. I *had* no soul. Serfs had no souls. They were treated like animals and they were animals. The pretence that we were immortal, with Hell to fear and Heaven to hope for, was simply a trick to make us well behaved.

How simple and how sensible, I thought. No master, no steward, however watchful, could keep an eye on us all the time, it is therefore greatly to their advantage to teach us, "Thou shalt not steal," and make us believe that thieves go to Hell.

Priests pretend too; it keeps the churches full and Peter's Pence rolling in. That must be true, because monks are religious men and if they believed that I had a soul they would never dare leave me to die here with my sins unshriven.

Strange as it sounds, the thought that I had no soul was the most comfortable notion that I had ever had. It removed the fear of Hell; it lifted all responsibility. I had lived as an animal and I should die like one. Like an old horse or a dog, past all use and a waste to feed any more. All this fuss about marriage, I thought. We coupled like dogs who don't expect to be chanted over; and as for those eggs . . . who calls it *sin* when a starving cat sneaks off with a fishhead?

Freed from the fear of Hell, I curled up in the straw and made ready to die.

Everything rocked a little, the darkness lifted, the walls melted away, and I was lying on the grass under the little crooked hawthorn tree, freshly green and white, just breaking into blossom. I could smell it, cool and scentless.

"You," I cried. And all at once I understood everything. Nothing to do with priests or sins or being forgiven, nothing to do with anything there are any words for. Just the beauty of the tree and my acceptance of it, promise and fulfilment all in one. And what there are no words for.

Now I could die.

All nonsense, of course.

The voices reached me first.

"Complete misunderstanding. 'Hold him safe,' I said. The order was perfectly clear."

"A gross mistake indeed; but that can wait. Brother Sebastian . . ."

"Hold the light a little closer."

Hot tallow dripped on my cheek; I opened my eyes and closed them again, the light struck so painfully.

"Why, this is the man Martin whose leg I mended. Give me the cup."

Something wet on my lips turned to fire in my mouth.

"Come, rouse yourself, man!"

". . . to reach such a state in little over twenty-four hours."

"Probably he was fasting when he was thrown in. Come, drink properly, wake up and drink. You waste more than you take."

The cool voice, which I recognised as the Prior's, said, "This noxious air, as much as the fast, is responsible for his state. Unless we move soon we shall all be insensible."

I made a great effort and mustered my voice.

"Why?" I cried. "Why did you leave me to die? I came to bring you warning."

"Drink," said Brother Sebastian, pressing the cup to my mouth again.

"Everything shall be explained presently," said the Prior. "Get him out of here, give him food. Then clean him and dress him anew. When he is ready, bring him to the Abbot's parlour."

Whatever it was they had given me to drink had gone to my head, so that my ears rang, and when at last they heaved me to my feet the floor seemed soft and yielding and a long way away. Brother Sebastian, carrying the candle, moved ahead, murmuring gentle encouragements. One of the men who ordinarily collected the market dues helped me along.

In a small warm room they sat me down and brought a basin and towel so that I could clean my hands before I ate. They served me barley broth, a roast capon, dried figs. Gradually my head cleared and my spirits rose. They seemed, after all, well disposed towards me. I had done them a service, been ill-used. . . . I began to think about reward, began framing in my mind the plea for my little hut. Surely now that would not seem much to ask.

"Now, Martin," said Brother Sebastian, "having restored the inner man, let us attend to the outer. That dungeon reek clings hard."

He led me to the laundry, where stone slabs, hollowed into basins, ran the length of one wall, and a great fire burned, with huge iron cauldrons swinging above. Hot water, tempered with cold, was poured into one of the basins. Brother Sebastian handed me a square of strong lye soap.

"I should get right in and wash all over, hair as well, if I were you. Our Abbot has a fastidious nose. Clothes will be brought you. I must get back to my duties. Fare you well."

The clothes, brought by a servant as I towelled myself, were such as I had never dreamed to wear, a rich man's clothes. Soft woollen shift, clinging close and warm from neck to knee and down the arms to the elbows, a fine linen shirt, hose and tunic of smooth grey cloth. The touch of them against my freshly scoured skin gave me a sense of well-being, of bodily ease that I had never known before. I had known its shadow once or twice, back at Rede when I was very young and a few of us boys had stripped and plunged into the river on a very warm sunny day, but we had come out and donned our creased, dirty clothes.

I remember thinking that the clothes themselves were a kind of reward, and that the shift was big enough for Kate to cut up and shape into warm garments for Stephen and Robin.

I was stooping to put on my old worn shoes when the door opened and there was a young monk, with a pink, girlish face and his sleeves rolled over his elbows. He had a pair of shoes in his hand.

"Made hurriedly and from memory. We trust they will fit."

They fitted much better than the old ones.

"Then . . . if you will come with me. . . ."

We went along passages, up and down steps, and at last came out into the open, where immediately I smelled the sour harsh scent of slow-burning wood, like that which fills a room where a log has rolled off the hearth. I stopped and sniffed and said:

"Did they get in then, after all?" If so, all my effort had been wasted and there would be no reward.

"Nobody got *in*," he said gently. "We were prepared and the main gate was reinforced. They tried to batter it down, and failed, so they set it afire. We welcomed its destruction, it was never worthy of its place. The new one is to be made from cedarwood from the groves of Lebanon." His voice took on a dreamy, ecstatic note. "Cedars are long-lived trees. It may even be that St. Egbert's new gate may be made from a tree which cast its shade over Our Lord."

"But you said you were prepared."

"Oh yes. Our Abbot has fifty knights to call upon; there was time to reach two of them, and their meinies. But our rule forbids us to strike the first blow. Once the gate was burned and the attackers were inside . . . then the archers and pikemen went into action."

"And drove them off?"

"Very easily, I believe."

Most cheerful news. "We were prepared," he said. "Time to reach two of them and their meinies." All thanks to me!

We were walking along a path, grey-paved, between two green lawns which ended in a laurel hedge through which the path went on. Behind the fence was a low stone building, made of dressed flint and owning a high, arched doorway, flanked by several windows in each side. The windows were glassed and just caught the last rays of the sinking sun.

At the doorway the monk halted.

"The Prior awaits you in the anteroom," he said.

I went in, blinking in the sudden light of a huge leaping fire and three or four candlestands. There was a long table in the centre of the room and at it a monk sat writing. The Prior stood at his elbow, reading every word he wrote. He gave me a brief glance of recognition, looked down again, and said:

"That will do well. Seal it."

The scribing monk took a bar of sealing wax, held it to a candle, dropped a great blob on the bottom of the parchment, and the Prior took up a gold seal and stamped it down. Then he rolled the parchment into a tube and said to me:

"There you are. Smelling sweeter, I trust. Follow me."

He opened a door at the back of the room and I followed him.

It was like walking into an oven, but the little figure seated in a chair close to the fire was all shrouded in fur, a great shawl of it lay across his shoulders, and another covered his legs. A woollen hood such as peasants wear in the fields in winter was pulled low over his ears and brow. His face was as brown and wrinkled as a walnut, and his lips a thin blue line. He looked a hundred years old. Only his eyes were lively.

The Prior went close to him and said in a high, penetrating voice, "My Lord Abbot, here is the man Martin, whom you wished to see."

Turning back to me, he said, "The Abbot is very deaf. Speak loudly or not at all."

In a high, thin monotone the Abbot said, "Ah yes, yes indeed. We owe you a great deal. I wished to thank you. Also I wished to hear why it was that you sided with us rather than with your fellows."

I said, in my loudest voice, "They refused me admission to the Guild."

He gave me an odd little smile and looked over my shoulder.

"What does he say?"

"He says that the townsfolk refused to admit him to the Guild."

"Ah, those Guilds. Most regrettable! Becoming so arbitrary. I'm not quite sure how far the Guilds were involved in last night's affair." He looked inquiringly at the Prior. "However. The Guild refused to admit you, so you turned against the Guild. And very fortunate for us that you did. Quite right of course in *any* circumstances." He nodded and smiled at me approvingly, and I thought that now was my chance.

"I had another reason, my lord," I said loudly.

Once again the Prior was obliged to repeat what I had said.

"Indeed. And what was that?"

I turned helplessly to the Prior, who said, with a sly smile, "Now you see the truth of what I said. I *am* my lord's ear. Very well, tell me and I will speak for you."

"They speak of clearing Squatters Row. I built a little hut there. I know I had no right to build, but I didn't know that at the time. It is the only home I have and it is not unsightly. I wondered . . . I mean I thought that if the information I brought you served your purpose, you might perhaps overlook . . . might allow my little hut to remain."

This stumbling speech the Prior compressed into two clear sentences. I watched the old man's face and saw with dismay that the request found no favour with him.

"The Cellarer tells me that the spot is a disgrace, a mere rubbish heap thrown up against our walls. It does not offend my eyes or nose, I never go abroad now. But we have visitors. What do *they* think when they see human beings living like pigs within arm's reach of the most splendid shrine in Christendom? The Cellarer tells me that nobody entering by the east gate can fail to see the place—and smell it."

It was, once again, a verdict against which there was no appeal. Forbidden to be a priest, I thought; forbidden to be married; forbidden to be a journeyman; and now, forbidden to remain in my hut.

"You have the parchment?" the old man asked the Prior.

"Signed and sealed, my lord."

"You see, we had thought of rewarding you by giving you what all poor men seem most to desire—a piece of land. Perhaps you know it—just outside the town on the south—the Old Vineyard they call it. The blight persists there, and I understand that we already have as much acreage under plough as we can handle. So it is yours, in perpetuity, in return for a red rose on the last day of June each year—a formality which shouldn't cause you any inconvenience. Give him his copyhold."

The Prior pushed the rolled-up parchment into my hand.

I tried to shout my thanks. Whether he heard or not, I could not know, but the Abbot nodded and smiled again. Then he said, "On the other hand it is poor gratitude which gives with one hand and takes away with the other. Also they tell me that the land is full of stumps, which must be cleared before it can yield any crop. What will you eat while you labour, and where will you live? I think," he said, looking past me at the Prior, "we should give him some money, too."

"As you wish."

"Give him fifty marks."

"My lord! Fifty marks is the scotage for the three Flaxhams in one year."

"Sir Alain and Sir Robert reached us, with their men, did they not? If that rabble had made an entry, it would have cost us fifty marks many times over. Fifty marks is no more than his due. Give it to him."

The Prior pulled aside a piece of tapestry hanging on the wall and opened the door behind it, went through, and closed the door carefully behind him.

I said, "My lord, I know not in what words to thank you."

The Abbot said, "It is useless to speak to me. For some reason, known only to God, I am deaf to all voices but *his*." He looked towards the door. "Very occasionally he thinks that gives him the right to dictate to me." He smiled and nodded his head.

I thought that if I could not speak I could act my gratitude, so I dropped to my knees, took the old man's thin cold hand, and kissed it. He withdrew it hastily and patted my shoulder.

"Don't let the aspect lead you to think that you can grow vines on that field. Six years ago the blight struck there and, though we rooted out every stump and ploughed it over and laid it fallow for a year and then planted strong new stock, still the blight remained. I went out to see for myself, I remember—one of my last rides. It was a sad sight—a very sad sight. Ah . . ."

The Prior returned, carefully closing the door again and drawing the tapestry over it. He carried a linen bag tied at the neck. He said to me, in the cool, amused voice which showed that he had recovered his composure, "My Lord Abbot must set high store on the people of Baildon. Our Lord Himself was betrayed for only thirty pieces. You have all this—and the Potter's Field as well!"

He could have said sharper things and caused me no twinge.

"Please," I said, "tell him how very grateful I am. All my life I have been so very poor . . . and lately lame as well. All that I have tried has been of no avail. Now I can begin again. I am so very thank . . ." I choked and tears came into my eyes.

The Abbot gave me one of his bright, shrewd glances.

"You would be wise—for your own sake—to conceal the source of your money."

I nodded to show that I understood, and the movement brought two tears spilling over.

"We are grateful to you," he said. "Go in peace."

The Prior came to the door with me.

"The east gate is nearest for you. Besides the great gate is closed."

The clerk, without being bidden, rose from the table and led the way. On this journey I saw several groups of pikemen and archers as well as a few men in armour, but they, like everything else, were just the background of a dream to me.

It was almost dusk. I intended to go to Webster's and fetch Kate and the children home, for the last time. I would put my arms about her and say, "Don't ask questions now, I will tell you everything when we are home, but, sweetheart, we are *rich!*" We would walk slowly down Cooks Row, that street which we so often avoided because of the sight and scent of food so far out of our reach, and we would buy everything we fancied. When we were home I would make a fire, not sparing the wood because in future we could have as much wood as we wanted. Over supper I would tell her the story and speak of what I planned. Dear Kate, she should never lift a finger outside her own house again.

Something sloughed off my soul, like the scab from an old sore, and all at once I was able to look beyond that happy supper table. Kate and I could go to bed together properly again. Another child would be welcome now. In every way we would start anew.

I reached Webster's gate just as one of the wool-pickers, a bent old woman with screwed-up, half-blind eyes, was coming out. She stopped by me and said, "Kate ain't bin to work today. Master's rare and vexed."

I turned and began to run, as quickly as I could in my new shoes, towards Squatters Row.

Interval

I

The man with the bear came into Baildon just before dusk. November days are short. They are cold, too, and the man, heavily muffled, thickset, and clumsy, might, in outline, almost have been another bear, forced to stay upright. As though to prove his claim to be human, he talked to himself as he walked. Very often children, keeping at a safe distance, would call after him, "Talk to yourself, talk to the Devil."

He was telling himself that leading a dancing bear was all right in the summer, but misery in winter. He said there ought to be a place where bears could be left at the end of September and collected at the beginning of April, well fed and kept in training. There was no such place. He reminded himself that even when a bear-leader had money for a lodging for himself and could find a place that had a stable where the bear could sleep, nine times out of ten they wouldn't have you in—horses didn't like the bear smell.

Every time he reminded himself of this, and felt the bitter wind, he looked at the bear with hatred and dragged viciously at the chain. Every time he did so, the bear looked at him with a curiously similar expression. In their imposed physical likeness to one another, in the flashes of hatred, and in their dependence each upon the other for the basic necessities of living, they were like an old married couple.

The man's name was Tom, and he was known on the roads as Pert Tom; the bear, neutered at the beginning of his training, was called Owd Muscovy.

As Tom had suspected, there was no lodging for man *and* bear; he took the rebuffs philosophically. It was some years since he had been in Baildon, but he remembered it well and knew of a fairly snug place in which to spend the night, a place where several people lived between the buttresses of the Abbey wall, and made their little fires and were willing—for a small consideration—to allow a stranger to warm himself and cook a bite of food. On his last visit there had been a woman, living behind a screen of tarred canvas, who—again for a consideration—had been willing to grant other favours. That, he remembered, must have been all of five years ago; probably she'd moved on, and in any case she would have aged. Still, in November a man couldn't be too particular.

When he reached the place it was very much as he remembered it, except that in one corner, between the wall and the buttress, someone had built a tidy little hut, with a thatch to its roof and a hole for a chimney, the hole carefully plastered round with clay to keep the straw from catching alight. Pert Tom looked at the place speculatively. If the owner of the place was good-hearted, he might find shelter for the night after all. At the moment the place was deserted and he wandered on, found some campers whom he remembered from his last visit—a very old woman and a deaf-and-dumb man and his wife, whose family had increased considerably—but the woman who had slept behind a piece of canvas and been willing to share her bed with him was not—to his disappointment—there.

"They laid onto her so hard last time she went to be whipped," the dumb man's wife explained, "that she mended her ways. She went off into the country to work in a dairy."

"What a cruel waste," Pert Tom said.

He began his preparations for the night, settling down in the corner opposite the little hut. He hobbled the bear by fixing the chain around one foreleg and one back, removed its iron muzzle, and gave it its supper. Always, wherever he was, he fed the bear first and when, as sometimes happened, there was only food for one it was the bear which supped and he who hungered. There was no sentiment concerned, he was capable of using the bear brutally, but to keep it in good fettle was simply common sense. When the beast had devoured its bread and honey, he slipped back its muzzle and went to sit by the dumb man's fire. But he kept his eye on the hut, and in the very last of the light saw a small woman, a girl almost, with two young children, enter it and close the door. He waited a little while, then, muttering that he was going to turn in, he went to the corner where the bear was asleep, lay down beside it, and waited again. He could see by the light that came through the ill-joined timbers of the hut that the young woman had got the fire going. At what he thought the right time he rose, went softly across the space, and knocked on the door. Kate opened it. Against the smoky red fire glow he saw the halo of her pale hair and missed the lines of worry and disappointment on her face. In his smoothest, most wheedling tone he said:

"I wondered if you could oblige me with a drop of hot water. I got a pinch o' ginger in my pack. With hot water and honey that make a rare warming drink. Ever tried it?"

"No," she said flatly. "I can let you have some water if you've got a crock."

He was trained to take in as much as possible at a glance. One sweep of his eyes informed him that, although, having a roof over her head, Kate might be said to be better off than he was himself, she was yet pitifully poor. The two children were eating bowls of water gruel, the very cheapest form of food, and they were eating it hungrily. But he noticed, too, that a mattress, made of sacking through which the straw was bursting, lay against the back wall, taking up indeed more than a half of the floor space. Better than lying on the bare ground in the open.

"I've got a bowl." In a moment he was back with it; he brought also his pinch of ginger and his pot of honey.

"I thought maybe the lil dears'd fancy a spoonful of the honey in their gruel," he said.

She was ashamed that even a stranger, begging at her door, should have seen how poor the children's supper was.

"You are kind; but they've finished now."

"Honey," Stephen said.

"Be quiet. Now, if you'll give me your bowl . . ." She took it, poured into it the small amount of hot water left over from the making of the gruel, and handed it back to him. Outlined against the hearth, her figure looked slim and shapely—too thin, but he wasn't fussy.

"I brung the ginger," Pert Tom said coaxingly. "If you never tasted it, you should. Go down right warm, like a fire in your belly."

"I believe you. I've no time to try. I have a lot to do and my husband will be home any minute."

She spoke the last words in a very clear, significant way.

"Well," he said in a deflated tone. "Thanks for the water."

He returned to his corner, drank his warming brew, choking a little, put his pack under his head and, cuddling close to Owd Muscovy for warmth, began to drift towards sleep as easily as an animal. Once, just before sleep took him, he was not unhappily aware of his woman-hunger, a mistake to drink the ginger, he thought, it was well known to heat the blood; if he'd known the woman was waiting for her husband and would refuse her share of the precious stuff, he'd have saved it for a more promising occasion. Then he was asleep.

The bear, stirring restlessly and grunting, roused him. He doubled his fist, thumped the heaving bulk beside him, and growled, "Lay down!"

The bear, ordinarily—and with good cause—extremely obedient, continued to stir and grumble, and presently Pert Tom was wide awake and aware that something was, if not wrong exactly, out of the ordinary. There was a distant noise which roused a confused memory of his soldiering days; and overhead the sky, without star or moon, was curiously light with a pinkish-yellow pulsing glow.

"You're right. Something's afoot," Tom said to the bear, and got to his feet, shivering in the brittle cold of the night. The confused noise sorted itself out into the sound of men shouting, some heavy thumping, and—was it possible?—the twang of bowstrings. Nearer, and quite distinct, came the sound of movement from the hut in the other corner. The pulsing light leaped again in the sky, and he could see the woman in the doorway.

There was something intimate about the two of them being wakeful at this hour of the night, and he forgave her for her earlier unfriendliness. He ambled over and said, "Whass going on?"

"They're fighting." He could hear that she had been crying. "And Martin must have gone and got mixed in it. He isn't home." She gave a sharp sob. "I never thought they'd do it," she said, a wild note creeping into her voice. "And I never thought he'd have so little sense. . . . If he's hurt . . . Oh, if only I knew!"

The sky lightened and darkened and the distant noise increased.

"'Sno use me going to look. I don't know your Martin."

"I know that. I want to go myself."

"Then why don't you?"

"The children. If I take them and he's hurt, then I've got both hands full and couldn't help. And if I leave them and they woke . . . with all this noise and nobody . . . The others have all gone to watch. They ran past minutes ago." She leaned forward and put a hand on his arm. "Would you watch them for me, just five minutes while I go and look or ask . . . ? Somebody must have seen him."

"I don't mind," he said, without enthusiasm.

"Oh, thank you! If the little one wakes, put his thumb in his mouth, but the big one, say Mother won't be a minute."

She was gone, running like a deer.

"So, after all, I'm *in*," Pert Tom said to himself, ducking his head and entering the low dark hut. He remembered, from his single searching glance, the position of the hearthstone and the fact that at one side of it lay a heap of dried twigs, and on the other some more solid pieces of wood. He took out his flint and tinder and soon had the fire alight. He squatted on his heels, warming his hands and the inner sides of his thighs. As the light strengthened he looked about him again. The two children lay against the wall, foot to foot, wrapped in a piece of woollen cloth. The unoccupied portion of the mattress, with another cloth crumpled across it, looked comfortable and inviting. He threw two pieces of wood onto the fire and went and lay down. He teased himself pleasantly with the idea of the woman lying here beside him, and dozed a little, losing all consciousness of time.

He roused when Kate came back.

She was no longer crying. The scene outside the Abbey gate had shocked her into calmness; she had been obliged to stare into the face of dead man after dead man in her search for Martin, fourteen in all, some horribly mutilated by arrows. She had not found him, nor anyone who had seen him lately, but a woman had told her that some of the men of the town had been inside the Abbey when the archers took them by surprise. She felt certain that Martin was there, dead; and mingled with her grief was a deep resentment that he should not only have joined the rabble in their stupid quarrel, but been in the forefront of the attack. When she thought of him lying dead she was ashamed of that feeling, but it was there just the same. Torn by two such conflicting emotions and denied the relief of tears, she had fallen into a stunned, somnambulistic state in which she was conscious of a single purpose—she must get home to the children. The sight of Pert Tom sprawled on the bed did not surprise her, although she had forgotten him, and when she had thought of the children had visualised them as being alone. She was past feeling anything so trivial as surprise; in a world where Martin was dead anything might happen.

Tom propped himself on one elbow and waited for her to speak. After a minute he said, "You didn't find him?"

Such a stupid question merited no answer. She sat down on one of the two stools and stared at the fire and presently said, "Why did he have to join them? They'd treated him as badly as they could. He was a good smith. . . ." As she spoke those words the tears almost came, for she saw Martin as he had been on that evening at Rede, striding back, full of youth and power, from his work at Ancaster and coming to her rescue. A hard bitterness dried the tears. "A *good* smith," she repeated, "but they wouldn't let him into their Guild. And then they broke his leg and lost him his job. He didn't have to side with *them*."

"How d'you know that he did?"

"If he didn't where *is* he? Never once since he lost his job has he been away for the night. And I know what he was doing today. Helping with a pig-killing, just over the Ditch. And I know what happened. . . ." She lifted her head so that the firelight shone in her eyes and on her lips. "He thought he'd get back in with them, show them what he was made of. The fool!" Grief and fury came together in the last word.

So far as Pert Tom was concerned, she might have been speaking in a foreign tongue. Lust was lively now and he saw every hope of gratification. He got to his feet and laid a heavy hand on Kate's clenched in her lap.

"Like ice," he said. "I'm gonna get my ginger and we'll put the pot on and hev a nice hot drink. Pull you together better'n anything."

She said nothing; when he returned she was sitting as he left her, staring into the fire. He was putting water into the pot and the pot in the heart of the flames when she said, as though continuing a conversation, "We never even said good-by." Then there was another long pause before she spoke again.

"It was all on account of me that he came here and was so wretched. He'd have been better off at Rede. He said so. No, I said that. I used to say a lot of things I didn't mean."

The water boiled and Tom made his brew, using the last of the ginger and stirring in the honey with a liberal hand.

"Here. You get that down. You'll feel better in no time."

"As though I could," she said, speaking directly to him for the first time. "Nothing could make me feel better except the sight of Martin coming in that door."

"Drink it and try."

She thought that in his dull un-understanding way he was trying to be kind, so she lifted the bowl and sipped and coughed.

"Go down so nice and warm, don't it?" He swilled his own with gusto.

Spices were so expensive that only the rich could afford to buy them for their flavour; to develop a market among the poorer people, the merchants had craftily spread the rumour of their aphrodisiac virtues. Pert Tom, because he was ready for Kate and warmed by his ginger, all too easily believed that the sip or two she had taken would render her complacent.

"Don't let it get cold," he urged her. She lifted the bowl and drank its contents in that same sleep-walking fashion. He waited another minute, then he said, "Don't fret. There's as good fish in the sea as ever came out."

"What do you mean?"

"This," he said; and took hold of her, his purpose quite plain.

She woke then and remembered that her first feeling towards him had been one of distrust. He was big and hot and heavy; he reeked of bear; it was like being mauled by a bear. He had his face at her breast—in dreadful parody of a nursing child—and she could feel the heat of his breath through her clothes. She pushed, but he only pulled her closer. She wanted to scream but knew it would be useless, there was no one to hear except the children. She went limp in his hold and let him pull her down on to the bed. Then she said:

"Wait," and made the first motion of unfastening her dress. Just as he'd expected, Pert Tom told himself. Then her hand moved, quick as a slithering snake, and she had snatched a piece of burning wood from the fire and was on her feet, standing over him, threatening him with it.

"Get out," she said.

He jumped up and stood hesitant, face to face with her in the tiny room. He had only to get hold of her arm and twist it. . . . But she jabbed at him with the flaming branch; the heat scorched his face and singed his beard. He backed to the door which opened outwards and was unlatched. With the opening of the door under the pressure of his body a draught of cold air came swooping in;

the flaming tip of the branch flared more fiercely and a piece of it dropped off and onto the edge of the straw-stuffed mattress which broke eagerly into flame.

Kate did scream then and tried to stamp on the new flame, but in a second her skirt was blazing. She threw the branch towards the hearth and stooped, smacking ineffectually at her skirt. Then she grabbed at the children, calling them by name, shaking Stephen awake and trying to lift Robin. They woke and shrank, screaming, nearer to the wall, away from the blazing edge of the mattress, the blazing of Kate's skirt.

"Help!" she screamed to Tom. "Help!"

It had all happened so quickly that he was still pressing his hands to his smouldering beard. But he had his wits about him. Save her, help her out, and what would be the result? Trouble. People were always ready to believe the worst of any stranger. She'd tell how the fire started and the least that would happen would be that he'd go to the lock-up; and nobody would care for Owd Muscovy. You could lose a good bear that way. Better let the bitch burn.

He put out his hand and pushed the door shut. It took another movement of air with it so that the flames leaped up with a hollow roar. Before he could have counted ten, before he dared withdraw his hand from the door, the inner side of the low thatch was alight.

He stepped back then to a safe distance. There was a moment when the woman and both the children were screaming together, then the thatch fell in on them, throwing out showers of sparks and little clots of burning straw. The screams stopped. There was a smell of burning flesh and then, after a minute, mingling with it, the stink of smouldering fur.

"Owd Muscovy!" cried Tom, and ran to the corner where the hobbled bear was plunging about, alight in a dozen places.

"Lay still. Lay! Down! Down! Down!" said Tom, beating at the thick greasy fur, tearing off bits of burning straw. He was not even conscious of the pain in his hands, he was so intent. The first lesson a bear-leader learned was that it did not pay to have too shabby or openly intimidated a bear; people liked to think that the bear was much stronger than any man and that but for the muzzle and the chain would tear its leader to pieces.

"Holy St. Ursula," Tom moaned. "You'll look like the moths hev been at you."

Even when his pelt was out of danger the bear, in whose early training fire had played a part, was nervous and shivering. Tom would have calmed him with an untimely offering of bread and honey, then remembered that he had taken the honey into the hut. All wasted and the ginger, too!

"And all over what?" he asked himself. "Slice off a cut cake that'd never've been missed. Silly bitch! What got into her?"

He looked back at the hut then. The poor flimsy timbers of its front and side wall had fallen inwards over the whole, and had almost burned themselves out.

"Need never hev happened," he said. "Could hev been as nice as nice."

In a mood of self-pity, and with no twinge of conscience, he again settled down beside the bear and slept so soundly that he did not hear the other residents of Squatters Row return from their sight-seeing.

With morning light shining on the ruin, the dumb man's wife and Old Agnes found the destruction of one small hut of far more interest and moment than the burning of the great Abbey gate which they had seen during the night. They asked the inevitable question, "How did it happen?" and Tom had his tale ready. He had waked to find the hut blazing and had done his best to save whoever was inside. He had his blistered hands, his scorched face, and raggedly singed beard to show. Nobody for a second doubted the truth of his story. Dummy's wife managed, without exactly saying it in so many words, to imply that such an accident could have been expected, if you couldn't have a proper house the only thing to do was to make your fire in the open, as she had done all these years. The accident, in fact, was the result of trying to set yourself up above your neighbours. Old Agnes, remembering that Kate and Martin had dealt more fairly with her over the Trimble than her clients ordinarily did, said that perhaps it was a mercy in disguise —if Martin were really dead; it was a hard world for widows and orphans.

Pert Tom was praised for his attempted rescue and sympathised with for having wandered into Baildon just at this time. Nobody would be in the mood to be amused by a bear's tricks today. The town was in mourning, some said nineteen men dead and many more injured. And all for nothing.

Tom believed that trade would be bad, and soon after breakfast was on his way towards the north gate of the town when he saw a new detachment of soldiers marching in. They moved with the dogged, flat motion of men who have marched through the night, so it was likely that they had come from a distance. The fighting seemed to be over, and they wouldn't be marched back without a rest. Soldiers were good customers, easily amused and very open-handed. He turned himself about and followed them back into the centre of the town.

The Market Square was scattered with the litter—some of it curiously irrelevant—that was left by street fighting. There were the spent arrows, the burned-out torches, the thrown-down clubs, and sticks which might be expected, but there were also bits of clothing, part of a wheel, a cooking pot, some grey wool on a spindle. Patches of blood showed where men had fallen dead or injured, but all the bodies save one had been removed. An old woman and a boy of about ten were struggling with the corpse of a heavy man, the old woman crying and hysterically admonishing the boy.

"Hold his legs higher. Higher. You're letting his bum drag on the ground."

Pert Tom remembered how, after the Battle of Radscot Bridge, he had come across a dead man with a ring on his finger. It was that ring which had enabled him to buy Owd Muscovy, a two-year-old, fully trained. He went carefully over this battleground and saw nothing worth salvaging except the spindle, which he put in his pack.

Inside the great stone archway the burned edges of the gate hung jaggedly. Two monks, their faces expressionless, as though every morning they measured up burned gateways, were using a yard-stick. Soldiers stood on guard all along the front of the Abbey, and inside Tom caught a glimpse of archers, pikemen, a man or two in armour. The soldiers he had followed had disappeared through the gateway, but soon others came out in groups of three or four and made off up Cooks Row towards the alehouses. He followed and was soon giving thanks to St. Ursula that he had decided to stay in the town. The bear's tricks were well received, especially his imita-tion of a pikeman's drill with a little cane for a pike, and by two o'clock in the afternoon Pert Tom had collected as much as was needed to live luxuriously by his standards for the next four days, which was as far as he ever looked ahead. He found an inn not yet discovered by the soldiers and therefore spared the sudden inflation of prices, and took a leisurely dinner of boiled beef and dumplings, apple pie and ale. Before he left he had his wooden bottle filled with ale, and on his way back down Cooks Row he did some pleasant shopping; a meat pie and five pickled onions for himself, a pot of honey, apples, bread for Owd Muscovy, half a pig's head for the wife of the deaf-and-dumb man whose fire he hoped to share again.

For the town this might be a day of mourning, but for Squatters Row, never in any real sense part of the town, it was a jubilant occasion. Old Agnes had laid out six that day and had four more to do tomorrow.

"Of course I could've done the lot today, but it don't do to hurry. If you make it look easy, they grudge your pay." She had bought bacon and ale for her supper, and was sharing Dummy's fire because she was too busy to make her own. Dummy had spent the day grave-digging and brought home a pig's trotter for each member of his family and ale for himself.

Just at dusk Peg-Leg arrived, begging to be told what had happened. He had been out of town for three days visiting a niece who lived in the country and had a tender conscience. Every now and then when he grew tired of the food doled out at the Alms Gate he would pay her a visit; she would feed him, mend his rags, call him "Uncle Jacob," and restore his self-esteem. Sometimes her patience and his good behaviour would last four, five days, a week; but sooner or later he would offend her and she would reprimand him, and he would return to Baildon, laden with the provisions which it eased her sense of responsibility to provide. On this evening, after an unusually brief visit, he was carrying a piece of pork, a dozen eggs, some flat oat-cakes sticky with honey, and a little sack of walnuts. He was easily drawn into the group and the tit-for-tat bargaining, promising a share of his pork when it was cooked in return for a piece of pig's head this evening, swopping some eggs for a mug of Old Agnes' ale and sharing out the walnuts amongst the children.

The air of festivity mounted until one child was bold enough to ask Pert Tom to put the bear through his tricks. Tom was not going to break an infallible rule for dwellers in Squatters Row.

"Owd Muscovy, he've earned his rest today. Tell you what I will do, though. I'll play you a tune on my whistle."

He played a merry tune, and the children began to hop and skip in time to it. Peg-Leg said, with a trace of wistfulness, "Nice to be young, and sound of wind and limb. I was a rare one at a hornpipe once on a time."

"Young!" cried Old Agnes scornfully. "I can shake a leg with the best. Aye, and after a full day's work, too."

Gathering up her skirts and exposing skinny legs like knotted twigs and huge flat feet, she began to caper, calling to Tom to play faster, to play louder. Dummy's wife sprang up to join her, and their antics made even the deaf-and-dumb man laugh; he rocked from side to side, making a hoarse wheezy sound, like a pair of bellows whose leather sides had cracked.

It was into this merry scene that Martin walked.

He saw first the black ruin of what had been his home. Breath and heartbeat stopped; then reason took control. A few yards away was the leaping fire, a crowd about it, laughing and dancing to music. They wouldn't be doing that if Kate and the children had been . . . No. The neighbours were celebrating a near-escape, Kate and the children were there . . . beyond the fire.

He walked towards it, and Old Agnes, spinning round, saw him, stopped dead, let her skirt fall, and stared. In a second they were all staring and silent; on the defensive, like cattle in a field when a strange dog enters. And he could now see beyond the fire. No Kate, no child of his.

"Holy Mother of God," Old Agnes said, "we thought you was dead, too."

"Dead." He repeated the word. "Too? D'you mean . . ." The rest of the question could not be spoken; his jaw jerked convulsively.

Old Agnes moved towards him and took him by the arm. She was suddenly sober and aware of how callous their behaviour must seem to him.

"Flared up in the night, your place did. But we thought you was dead too . . . she . . . Kate was running round, hunting for you and crying. And with all gone together there didn't seem much to grieve about."

He said, "Burned," but the shaking of his jaw mangled the word so that it emerged in a moan of anguish.

Agnes tightened her hold on his arm.

"Come and sit down, lad. Come to the fire and take a sup of ale. It'll ease you."

He pushed her off and took a few staggering steps back to the buttress which had been one wall of his home, and was now blackened by the flames which had destroyed it. He leaned his head against the cold stone and so stood.

He might have known. It was all part of his life's pattern; every small mitigation of misery had been immediately followed by some new misfortune. An hour ago he had been given the means to make his family safe and comfortable forever, so by some Devil's logic it was inevitable that now he should have no family.

He thought: She never had anything! And the tears came scalding into his throat and stayed there.

Back by the fire, where the silence continued, though the eating had been resumed, Old Agnes eyed Martin uneasily, and presently made her second imaginative leap in the day.

"Go and tell him you *tried*," she said to Pert Tom. "Tell him you did your best to save them. Show him your hands. It'll make him feel better to think somebody tried. Coming on us all playing the fool and making merry . . . Go on!"

Pert Tom rose and ambled over and stood beside Martin and said, "I did me best. Tried to save 'em. Burnt meself. Look."

Martin neither looked nor answered, but he put out his hand and laid it on Tom's shoulder. The bear-man could feel the ague-like shudder that ran through the other man's body, and, although he felt no guilt in the matter, something of Martin's deep misery was communicated to him.

"Once," he said, "a man that knew a lot about things towd me burning to death worn't as bad as it sound. Talking about holy martyrs, he was. He said the smoke sorta choked you and deadened your senses afore the fire took howd. Reckon thass true, too. They on'y screamed once."

Through the knot of pain in his throat, Martin said, "Pray God that's true." He used the expression from habit, out of earnestness. There *was* no God, or such things could never happen. How *had* it happened?

He forced out the question, adding, "She was always . . . so careful. I'd put in a good hearthstone, and clay round the smoke hole."

"I dunno. I woke up to find it all ablaze. Like I said, I tried, but that was too far gone, then. Burnt meself. Look." Once again he held out his hands. Some of the blisters had broken through hauling the bear's chain all day. All Martin could see was Kate, young and pretty, just as she was when she had come to join him under Tuck's Oak. But he managed to say:

"I'm deep in your debt for that much. Leave me alone now."

Tom went back to the fire.

"He hev took it to heart," he said to Old Agnes. "Pity. I know more'n one man'd think hisself well rid of his wife."

"They was different from most," said the old woman, thinking again of the Trimble.

The fire burned low, presently everyone save Agnes had left it. She took a good drink of her ale to give her heart and then filled the mug again and went to where Martin stood.

"Here," she said, "you drink this. I've had my losses, too, and I know what I'm saying. Ale'll ease you."

He made no move to take the mug, and she went on, "I been with death all my life, Martin, and folks in sorrow. Them that come out of it best take what comfort they can get and turn their minds to other things, even if thass only squabbling over the pickings. You can't bring Kate back, nor go to her till your time come. So you must bear up and comfort yourself."

"She never had anything; nothing but worry and misery and toil. And all my fault."

"Don't talk so daft," the old woman said sharply. "You couldn't help being poor. I never saw a man more ready to turn his hand to anything. I never saw a better husband neither. I've said that a dozen times, seeing you so careful about fetching the water and the firewood and all. Come on now, lad, don't add to your own load." She held the mug to him again. He took it, gulped down the contents, and handed it back.

"Now leave me," he said.

"You come and lay down," she insisted. "You can lay under my rug."

He said, "No," and flung himself down by the black ruin, the grave of all his love. The old woman sat down beside him, took his head in her skinny dirty claws, and eased it into her lap. Her kindness, or the ale—it was a long time since he had drunk anything but water—loosened something in him. Tears came, and with them words, such a flow of words as he was never to loose again. Everything he said was self-reproachful, all concerned with the ruin he had made of Kate's life, how he had promised that she should be safe with him and then robbed her of the only safety possible in

this unjust world. Old Agnes hardly listened. She stroked his head
and at intervals muttered a soothing word or two. "You couldn't
help that, lad." "Aye, I know, I've been through it myself, long
ago." "Ah, that's the way it is when you're poor." And once she
said, "Dying young's no real hardship. Plucked off the bough, clean
and sound. If you hang on, you rot. I've seen 'em, Martin, riddled
with rot, stinking like corpses, but still alive. Kate and your little
ones are safe from that, they're safe from everything now. We're
the ones anything could happen to. We're in worse case."

II

Pert Tom had been born into an age and a community as devoutly
mystical, as thoroughly religious, as any in the history of mankind.
As a baby he had been baptised, as a child put through his Catechism. As an apprentice the only holidays he had known, the only
landmarks in the year's toil, had been the festivals of the Church
and the Saints' days. As a soldier even his oaths had been religious,
since without belief there can be no blasphemy; and as a bear-
leader he had never spent a whole day without passing through a
town where a new church was building, or mingling with a group
of pilgrims on their way to or from some shrine, or hearing a friar
preach, some convent bell ringing.

Of it all he had absorbed and retained only one thing, as primitive and as personal as a savage's devotion to his household idol.
Pert Tom believed in St. Ursula. That same fellow-soldier who had
given him the information about the painlessness of death by burning had told him that St. Ursula was the patron saint of bears and
bear-leaders—an excusable piece of misinformation based upon the
likeness of the Saint's name to the generic *ursus*, meaning bear.
When a dead man's ring provided Tom with the price of Owd
Muscovy, he had thanked St. Ursula and adopted her as his personal deity. The Holy Trinity and the rest of the Saints seemed,
like most respectable people, to be against him and his fellow-
vagrants, but St. Ursula, whom he visualised as a stout, comfortable, vulgar, tolerant old woman, was firmly on his side. When a
cunning idea slid into his head, it came direct from her; any trick
he played had her nudging connivance; any luck that came his way

was her work. She did not, like the rest of them, set a poor man any impossible standard of virtue. She made no demands. She entirely understood that he had meant Kate no harm and that it had been necessary to lie about the burns on his hands and face. Proof of her understanding and partisanship was there, concrete, indisputable. Look how he had been rewarded!

By April of the next year Pert Tom had some vague conception of just how full and rich his reward was to be, and it occurred to him, for the first time, that he should make a gesture of recognition towards this Saint who had been so overwhelmingly generous to him. So when, with the spring, the fresh tide of pilgrims and tumblers and minstrels and vagrants came pouring into Baildon, he began to look out for an image-seller, and before long found one.

The image-seller was of grave, almost priestly mien. He carried a tray of meticulously fashioned, beautifully coloured little images and a box of holy relics. He wore a hat with cockleshells which indicated—in his case falsely—that he had made the pilgrimage to the Holy Land, and his box contained, amongst other things, a sliver of wood, purporting to be a piece of the true Cross, two thorns from Christ's crown of mockery, and a two-inch square of St. Veronica's handkerchief. Most of the figures on the tray were of the Virgin, the rest were of female Saints after whom girl children were named. What parent, having named a daughter Agnes, could resist buying for her an image of the Saint, with the lamb at her feet?

All the figures were made and fired and coloured at a pottery in Wattisfield, where clay had been dug and worked in Roman times, and they were all made by one old man, who, though he worked quickly enough to keep four salesmen on the road from April to September, as well as supplying two settled dealers, one in Norwich and one in Walsingham, never turned out anything shoddy or slapdash. True, the colours of the Saints' garments were a little gaudy, customers liked them that way, but the tiny faces were virginal and saintly, pearly-pale, and wearing one of two expressions, gently smiling or gently sorrowful.

On this bright April morning, Pert Tom, now a gentleman of leisure, with money in his pocket, halted and looked over the image-seller's stock. He would know his Saint when he saw her, buxom, red-faced, her interest identified by a bear, or perhaps a goad, spiked collar, or muzzle. There was no St. Ursula; the old man at Wattisfield knew his business; little girls in that district were named Catherine, Ethelreda, Winifred, Edith, Agnes, Elizabeth.

"You ain't got what I want," Tom said reproachfully.

"And who was you wanting?"

"St. Ursula."

"Here y'are." He proffered a St. Ethelreda with her daisy emblem.

"That ain't my St. Ursula. She'd hev a bear."

"A what?"

"A bear. Growler. Got a bit of flesh on her bones too."

"Oh. That one! Sold the last a day or two back. Great demand. Bring you good health, good luck. Tell you what, I'll bring one on my next round. I'll be back here for the Lammas Fair. You live here?"

He must ask that, for an unpopular outlandish Saint, with a *bear*, would be quite unsalable, and Pert Tom, though he had now been settled for five months and looked like being settled for the rest of his life, still had a vagrant look, something of the roadster about him.

"I live here. All right. I'll look out for you Lammas time."

There must be some special interest, something extra behind such choosiness, and it might be open to exploitation.

"Of course, if you *liked* and was prepared to pay for it, I could hev her made with a bit of genuine relic to it—strand of her own real hair or something. Only that'd cost you, naturally."

"How much?"

"Two shillings," said the image-seller tentatively, ready to abate the price should this odd customer flinch.

"I could manage that. But I want her *proper*, bear and all. Not one of them poor peaked-looking things."

"You should mind your tongue, remembering who these are. And if you want the hair, then you'll have to pay half down."

Tom paid, calling upon St. Ursula as he did so to witness how heartfelt was his gratitude that he should take such a risk.

Weeks after, on the morning of the Lammas Fair, he took delivery of his order with loud complaints.

The old man in Wattisfield, who was a dedicated artist, had disliked being given definite orders; he had protested that though he knew more about the Saints than any bishop alive he had never heard of a St. Ursula who had dealings with bears. There was only one St. Ursula, a virgin, who with eleven hundred other virgins had been martyred at a place called Cologne by some people called Huns. A virgin Saint, and virgin Saints were all slender, pearly-pale, yellow-haired, gently smiling or gently grave. He'd been making them for years and he *knew*. "Flesh on her bones," the very thought was a heresy.

"But, master, I told him two shillings and he paid one down. I promised him real hair."

Even the artist agreed that such a customer merited some consideration. But when it came to the point he could not bring himself to sacrifice his artistic integrity to the extent of making a Saint as buxom as a washerwoman. He made a solid-looking brown bear to crouch at the hem of the blue robe, and the inclusion of a flaxen curl cut from the head of his youngest granddaughter cost him no twinge of conscience at all. If people were such fools as to believe that their silver could buy hair from the head of a woman dead and buried for hundreds of years, they deserved to be cheated. What could not be cheated, or ever would be, was his own standard of workmanship.

"Poor starved-looking thing! But for the bear I shouldn't've known her," said Tom, handing over his money grudgingly.

Still, there it was, he had bought the best that money could buy, and St. Ursula, who had understood so much, would understand that the false representation was not his fault.

He carried the little image home and set it on a shelf in the room that was his, the first room that he had ever been able to call his own.

"Set you there," he said, "and enjoy all you was so kind as to give me."

He thought of how, in the next dark winter, when the snow fell and the mud lay thick in the roads, the flames would leap on the hearthstone and the howling wind would drop back, baffled by the thick walls and the stout shutters, by the heavy door and deep thatch of the house that was already known as the Old Vine.

No member of any Guild had laid a finger on the house. Martin had planned it and done much of the work, the rest had been done by unemployables like Peg-Leg and Dummy. The monks' Old Vineyard lay outside the town walls where the Guild rules did not hold.

It was a small house, two tiny rooms and a kitchen, but there was as much sound timber in it as in many three times the size.

The walls were made of oaken posts, planted at eighteen-inch intervals. Smaller beams were set aslant, joining the bottom of the one post to the top of the next, and the triangles thus formed were divided again, horizontally. The spaces were filled in with laths and the whole plastered over, once on the inside and twice on the outside. A brick chimney in the centre carried the smoke from both rooms and from the kitchen hearth.

"We'll have our own fire," Martin had said, already aware that although he had bonded himself for life to the bear-leader his enforced constant company would be intolerable. All that he had, all that he intended to have in the future, he was prepared to share with Tom, who had tried to save Kate, and with Old Agnes who had tried to ease his hour of misery, but his fire and his bed he must have to himself.

The little house stood at the lowest edge of the vineyard, close to the road, and adjoining it, sharing a wall with Martin's own room, was the new smithy, into which during the next summer season much of Armstrong's and Smithson's trade was to be diverted. Once the house and smithy were up, Martin's gang of cripples and misfits, who would work for any pittance and the certainty of one good meal a day, set to work upon a stable block, built of clod and wattle.

Pert Tom could see the reason for the house and for the forge where Martin was going to earn a living for them both, but the stables puzzled him.

"What d'you want them for?"

"I shall offer stabling, like smith work, at a price those in town can't match. To begin with, that is. Later I shall have horses of my own."

"And what d'you aim to do with them?"

"You'll see."

It was not a satisfactory answer, but one with which Tom must be content. To press a question was useless, although on that November morning when Martin had talked in stony-faced calm with Tom, one of his reasons for offering to take him into partnership was that he needed his company.

"There's not a man in this town that I can ever bring myself to talk to, except in the way of business, and that the least I can; and living that fashion a man could be struck with the dumb madness."

The other reason he had given was that he needed Tom's partnership as a screen for his own sudden possession of money.

"I've got it and I didn't steal it. More than that I can't tell you. Nobody could know what you've earned or saved over the years. It'd look natural enough for you to settle down, build a house and a smithy for me to work in, so that your old age would be taken care of. You could have come into Baildon with some such scheme in mind."

His real, his secret reason, the wish to share with Tom all that he should have shared with Kate, he never mentioned to anyone. Nor did he ever put into words his grudge against the town. When, at the beginning of the second summer season, a deputation of the Smith's Guild waited upon him and offered him full membership, even some seniority, admission at once as a master man, if he would cease undercutting prices, he gave no sign of the bitter, ironic amusement the proposal roused.

"I cannot see how that would work to my advantage," he said.

And this time, though the damage he was doing them was far more serious than that he had done by shoeing Master Webster's pack ponies, they hesitated about taking revenge by violence. For this there were two reasons, he had his gang of riffraff, the poor without a craft, the disabled, reinforced by tougher elements, an old soldier or two, one of Peg-Leg's shipmates, a half-crazy priest who had been unfrocked. They owed an almost feudal allegiance to Martin, who allowed them to build another, more solid Squatters Row at the back of his stables, who paid them when there was work to be done and fed them between times. And there was also a strong feeling throughout the town that Pert Tom and Martin, in becoming—as it seemed—tenants of a piece of Abbey land, had moved into the shadow of the protection of that august authority. It was an authority with which, at the moment, the townspeople had no wish to try another throw. After their failure in the previous November the Abbey seemed to delight in grinding their faces; even the rule concerning the eel-fishing had now been revived and was strictly enforced. The town as a whole had been laid under an obligation to pay a large part of the cost of the new gate and was groaning under the imposition. Not until many years had passed, and a King set an example, would the people of Baildon defy their Abbot again.

The suspicion that the Abbey looked with favour upon Pert Tom and Martin, who had taken a piece of unprofitable land off its hands, was confirmed by the story of an amazingly out-of-character behaviour upon the part of the new Cellarer. It concerned a horse, a young, strong horse, newly broken, and brought to Martin's forge to be shod for the first time. Its owner, an oldish peasant, was sitting on a bench waiting, when he clapped his hand to his chest, gave a loud groan, and collapsed. He was dead when he was picked up. It was evening when his eldest son came to remove the body, and before he left he said to Martin, slyly:

"Now they'll come round to pick the heriot, and they allust take the best beast. The horse is the best my father had. Would you let it bide—just till the dues are paid."

Martin looked the young man in the face.

"Ask me to stable your horse and I agree. I make part of my living by stabling horses."

He had no intention of involving himself, though he would have agreed that the heriot was a peculiarly heartless exaction, for it meant that when a villein's family lost its breadwinner it also lost —to its manorial lord—the most valuable of its possessions.

"Then will you stable my horse until I fetch it and pay what I owe. They'll take the cow for heriot—and she's dry in two teats."

Nine or ten days later the Cellarer rode up on his mule and beckoned Martin from the forge.

"We understand," he said, "that you have in your stable a horse which is, by heriot right, Abbey property."

So the peasant was an Abbey tenant and had underestimated the thoroughness of the system.

"There are several horses in the stable," Martin said.

"This one is young, freshly broken. Its owner died here, suddenly."

"I know the one. I'll fetch it."

"No." The Cellarer held up a plump hand. "In this case, because there was some dispute about the heriot—they offered a cow, fit only for beef—the Abbot himself took an interest. He said that if the horse was with you, it should remain. He has asked from time to time about the Old Vineyard and was interested to hear that you had laid the rest of the field down to barley. He thought the animal would be useful to you."

Every word of this singular conversation was audible to the men waiting on the bench outside the forge and was duly reported in the town. What, men asked themselves, was so virtuous about growing barley? And why had such a valuable present been made to Martin, with no mention of Pert Tom who was understood to be the tenant of the land? When all the questions had been asked, and all the speculations made, and the gossip finished, one thing remained in the memory—the Abbot took an interest in the Old Vineyard. Martin in his upward spiral towards success met, therefore, much less opposition than he might have done.

Part Two

OLD AGNES' TALE

I

I never knew my age by yearly reckoning, but a woman's life has milestones of its own, and by their measure I was an old woman, and had been for years, when Martin took me to live with him in the house at Old Vine and made me free with all that he had.

Before that, for more years than I can number, I'd lived in Squatters Row, amongst—save for a very few—the scum of the earth. For that I had only myself to blame, in the main. I'd had one knock as a young woman and never pulled myself up again. My family were decent country people, and my mother taught me her midwife's trade. When I married I got a good steady man, one of Sir Stephen Fennel's game wardens out at Ockley, where we had a tidy snug house on the edge of Layer Wood. We'd been married two years, and I'd just started a baby, when he died of a fever and the house was wanted for the man that took over his job.

What with the grief and the baby coming and all, I didn't act sensible; I went running round like a hen with its head off trying to find—not a job, as I should have done—but some little place to put my bits and pieces. That took some doing, and before I'd managed it, along came the bailiff and two men and put my furniture out. I never forgot that day; it was October and pouring wet, and there was my goose-feather bed that my mother had made, the chest my granny had left me, the chair my own father had sat down to die in, and all my other things, set out in the rain and the wind. I was like somebody crazy and stood there crying and howling.

After a bit one of the men came back and said he'd give a shilling for the lot. I took his shilling, got a ride in a wagon to Baildon, and went straight to an alehouse and got drunk. Whether it was that or the jolting in the wagon, I lost the baby the next day; and

after that there didn't seem anything to bother for, except to earn
enough to keep me in ale. I never tried for a steady job, or to try
to get myself a house again. Whenever I even thought about houses
I thought of the one I'd had, and how I'd kept it clean and aired
the bed in the sun and polished the chest and the chairs with bees-
wax. And yet I was a home-keeping body. All those years I never
heard of a pig-killing without my fingers itching to do the salting
and make the brawn and the sausages; I never smelt bread baking
without wishing I'd had a hand in it. I hated the way I lived and the
riffraff all round me; but all I ever did was get drunk and forget it.
When Martin took his knock, which was so much like mine, the
first thing I did was to offer him some ale and a chance to forget.

One knock didn't down him though, and the day came when he
looked for me and said Pert Tom the bear-man and he were setting
up in business together and had a house nearly built, and they
wanted me to go and look after it for them.

I said, "I don't know. I reckon it's too late by many a year. I've
lost all my housekeeping skills. And you've lived alongside me long
enough to know my weakness for ale."

"I don't ask for skill. All we want is food on the table and a
stitch put in now and again. And you're welcome to all the ale you
can drink, and to anything else you want."

"You want somebody younger."

"I want you," he said. So I said I'd try.

I hardly knew myself. I found there wasn't a thing I'd forgotten.
After all those years, living hand to mouth, I could still do things
just as I'd seen my mother do them, and been taught by her to do
them. Even her wonderful lardy cake I could make as though I'd
been doing it all my days. I made a little garden and grew herbs
and peas and beans and bushes of lavender and rosemary. As for
the ale, now that I was happy I could take a pot and be content
with that, just like anybody else.

It was like being born again, and it was all due to Martin who'd
taken me out of the gutter. I'd always liked him; he'd been very
generous over the Trimble; and now, what with the liking, and feeling sorry for him and admiring the way he worked and schemed,
I came to love him. He seemed like my own, the son I never had.

I had three happy, busy years. Then one morning I noticed that
my ankles were swelling. That was how Death first put his finger on

my mother. Later would come the blue lips, the shortness of breath. Then I'd be useless. And what would happen to Martin?

There were, I knew, dozens of women who would come and keep house for him and Tom; but there is a difference between keeping house and looking after. I kept house for Tom, I looked after Martin.

If Pert Tom came home soaking wet—as rarely happened, for he could pick his time for going abroad—I'd say to him, "Look at the mess you've brought in!" and let him sit down wet or dry as he chose. If Martin came in wet and would have gone to his room to get busy with his tally sticks or some such, I would say, "Oh no, you don't. You put off your wet things and on with these dry ones, and drink this hot broth before you so much as sit down."

Once—the winter he started his wool-buying, and should have gone to Kersey and had a heavy cold—I took away every stitch of clothing he had, so he had to stay in bed.

I looked ahead and I could even see the new woman making more fuss of Pert Tom than of Martin. For one thing Pert Tom was supposed to be the one with the money, and he was cheerful and joking, while Martin was glum, on the sour side, all wrapped up in whatever it was he was doing, no matter what it was. Martin worked as some men drink or gamble.

To me and to Tom he was civil enough, so long as we didn't take liberties; even Tom held him in some awe. To speak to him on such a private business was taking a liberty, perhaps, still I did it.

I asked him, "Did you ever give a thought to marrying again?"

He gave me one of those black looks of his. They'd come over him since Kate's death. Before that I'd seen him look miserable, or hungry, dog-tired, or angry, but this was something different; there was a sort of power to that look, so that it was as bad as having another man curse you.

"It'd put some purpose to all this work and getting gear together," I went on. "You'll end a rich man, with no one to take after you."

"I'll leave a fund to pay nosy old women to mind their own business."

"I know I'm old, and maybe I'm nosy, but I would like to see you settled. The past is over and done with. A new wife in your bed and a new boy in a cradle and . . ."

He gave me another, even blacker look, one that cut clean through me, turned on his heel, and went out. I never mustered the courage to speak of it again.

Still, there are more ways of catching a cony than running after it shouting. I put my wits to work.

I didn't know any respectable young women, and none ever came to the house. There had been a time, when Martin first looked like being successful, when the townsfolk would have been friendly —they even invited him to join a Guild, after all; but he would have none of that. He never went into anybody's house, and no one visited us. So where to start my matchmaking?

There was Peg-Leg. He was the black sheep of a very respectable family and had a niece, out at Clevely, married to a yeoman farmer that owned his fifty acres; she must have been a very decent sort of woman too, for, riffraff as Peg-Leg had become, she never cut him off. I talked to him frankly, telling him what I was looking out for.

He laughed at first.

"Do the man want a wife he'd find one hisself. He get about, don't he, he must see dozens. He've lived alone three year now, and I reckon he must like it."

"He's never given the matter a thought, being too busy, first with the forge and the stabling and now with all this wool. There's a difference between going out to find yourself a wife and seeing a neat pretty girl doing the jobs about the house, waiting on you and listening when you talk. If we could find the right girl, it'd come over him bit by bit, without any thinking."

"Well, maybe. I'll hev a talk to Winnie about it, next time I go over."

But I hadn't got endless time; I couldn't wait.

"I tell you what I'll do, Peg-Leg; I'll give you the money to buy yourself a ride, and to take your niece a present."

"Where'd you get it from?"

"The housekeeping. I handle all." I was proud of that.

"All right then. Only don't set your heart on it too much. You know the saying about the horse and water."

A day or two later he set off for Clevely and he must have been on his very best behaviour, for he stayed ten days, and when he came back he was as pleased as if he'd thought of the whole idea himself.

His niece's husband had a sister named Jennie, eighteen years old, and, said Peg-Leg, as pretty as a hedge rose as well as being skilled in the house. Peg-Leg had explained the situation, and the girl and her family were willing. So I said to Martin that the work was getting a bit much for me and that Peg-Leg had a niece who would come and help me.

"Where'd she sleep?"

"With me. There's room." My bed was in a kind of alcove in the kitchen, the chimney stuck out and there was just room for a bed between it and the wall.

"Not much room. If that was shored up stronger," he said, pointing up to a kind of wide shelf that ran across one end of the kitchen, and was used to store cheese and bacon and onions—all of which we used a lot of, feeding so many men their dinners.

"All right. Maybe that would be best. Thank you," I said.

So presently Jennie came; and she was as pretty as a hedge rose, and almost as quiet. Asked a flat question, she'd say yes or no as the case might be; and passed the salt she'd say, "Thank you." For a sensible young man with the itch in his blood that would have been enough; but being so quiet and shy made her seem younger than she was, while Martin was years older than his age. Across the gap he only gave her the kind of attention he'd have given a child.

There was a fair while she was with us and I made an effort and went into town and bought her a headdress, the prettiest I ever saw, made of stuff so thin it was like cobwebs on a frosty morning, all draped over two pointed horns. It'd make her look older, I thought, and it couldn't help but be noticed. It would have made any girl prink and toss her head and flutter her eyelashes and *be* noticed; but Jennie wore it as though it were a woollen hood to keep out the cold.

After six weeks I knew it was hopeless and sent her home. Then Peg-Leg said there *was* another girl he knew, a cousin of Jennie's, not so pretty, rather older, but lively. He'd seen her at his niece's too, and she was enough to make a cat laugh at times.

Her name was Kate. I said we must change that, and she was agreeable, she liked being called Kitty. Her skin was sallow and her hair the colour of mud, but she was cheerful and amusing, and every bit as good in the house as Jennie. Even Martin smiled at her sometimes, with the smile which came rarely nowadays and always looked as though it hurt him somewhere deep inside. However, after a bit he began to make excuses not to sit down at table with us; he'd say he was busy and would have a piece in his hand. I got tired of having Peg-Leg sidle up to the door and ask how things were going, when nothing was going at all; and also I didn't trust Pert Tom; all the little airs and graces, the jokes and the glances that were wasted on Martin, found a ready mark with the bear-man, so in the end I thought it'd save trouble if Kitty went home too.

Tom, who was sharp enough in his way, had seen what I was up to.

"You daft owd besom," he said. "Don't you know when you're well off? If Martin got married, his wife'd look round your greasy pans and show you the door."

"That wouldn't matter to me," I said, thinking of my legs and the way the swelling was creeping up. "I want to leave him *with* somebody before I die."

"I'm here, ain't I?"

"Fine help you are. You'd watch him work himself to death and never do a hand's turn."

"You can't say that. Didn't I take Owd Muscovy and my whistle, and go round gathering the crowd and yelling my lungs out about the cheap smith work and stabling to be found at the Owd Vine?"

"So you did. Three summers back. Just to get him more work than three men should've tackled!"

There was no love lost between Pert Tom and me. For one thing, after that first night I never believed that he burnt himself trying to save Martin's wife and children. I noticed next morning that the bear was burnt too; and it certainly hadn't tried to save anybody. Tom said it to boast and be admired, and it had paid him well. It seems that he'd saved a bit of money, not a lot, but enough to start a business with, and he wanted somebody to start up with that was capable of earning him a comfortable living for the rest of his life. Martin was just the man. It amused me, though, to see that, despite it being Pert Tom's money, Martin all along had stayed top dog, mainly on account of those black looks of his. Even while Martin was working from dawn to dusk in the forge and Tom was just idling about, Tom was never master. And later, when Martin went into the wool trade and had smiths working for him in the forge, and began to call himself with two names, Martin Reed, and was being called Master, the bear-man stayed plain Pert Tom.

Well, all I could do, having tried my hand at matchmaking and being acquainted with no other respectable young women, was to pray; and since by that time I couldn't get to church, the best I could do was to steal into Pert Tom's room now and again and painfully go down on my knees before the Virgin that he had there, calling her St. Ursula. I knew better; her cloak was true Mary blue, and she had the face of the Holy Mother. The bear was just there to show that even a savage beast could be tame in Her presence. At least, that is how I thought and believed while I was doing my praying that somehow or other Martin should find him a good steady wife that he could be fond of. Later on, when I saw what we got, I changed my mind, and I reckon Tom was right, that *was* St. Ursula and I'd annoyed her by calling her out of her name.

We got to June again and Martin was riding about, buying up fleeces. He'd been away two days and nights and was coming home for supper. I'd got a fowl on the spit, peas in the pot, fresh-baked bread, and a dish of little strawberries I'd bought from a hawker. Pert Tom was fidgeting about, wanting to begin, saying Martin had changed his mind and wouldn't be back that night; and I said I wouldn't cut the fowl and let the good juice run, just for him. It was well on into dusk and I'd lighted the candles when we heard the horse come in at the back and trot to the stable. Then we heard Martin, walking slowly.

"He's met with a mishap, or he's ill," I said; and I shuffled over to the door and opened it just as he got there. He'd got his arm round what I thought was a child and was helping her along. They were both smeared with mud and dripping with water.

"Oh, what is it? What happened?" I asked, the foolish way you do when surprised.

"Let's get in," he said. I pushed a stool close to the fire and he set her down. Her long black hair reached to the edge of the stool and water dripped from it to the hearthstone.

"I'll see to her," I said. "You go and put on some dry things. Tom, brighten the fire and mull some ale." It wasn't a cold night, fortunately, but the girl's teeth were chattering and Martin was all goose pimples.

I threw a blanket from my bed over the girl and stripped her, no hard task, she had on only a bodice and a skirt, such stuff and colours as no decent woman would wear. The bodice was made of red silk, frayed and worn web-thin in places; the skirt was all striped with different colours and had holes in it you could put your hand through. My work as midwife and layer-out made me knowledgeable about bodies, but I never, in all my time, saw a woman quite like this one. She was so thin, but not wasted thin, sinewy rather, square in the shoulder and narrow in the flank, more like a boy, and yet very dainty. And her legs, in proportion to her body, were the longest I ever saw.

I had a queer fancy, when I'd got her stripped and was rubbing her down, that this was the kind of body angels had perhaps, under the long robes, a body not tied down to any one sex.

At the same time I had a great dislike for touching her. I couldn't think why—for except for the river mud she was clean, cleaner than most folks I've had to handle. But she had the effect on me that mice have on some people, or cats, or harmless frogs. In the first instant, faced with a drenched woman, I'd snatched the blanket from my bed, but once it had been over her, touching her here and there, I knew I couldn't sleep with it again until it had been washed and hung in the air several times. I put my second shift on her— I was so well provided for these days I had three, just like a bride, and my best dress I gave her, too, knowing that I should never like them again. Shoes I couldn't lend her, mine were too big, and there was no need. I doubt if she'd ever worn shoes in her life; her feet were as hard as horn and so high-arched she could have stood on a good-sized pullet's egg without crushing it.

Martin came back into the kitchen, dressed dry and with his hair standing on end where he had rubbed it.

"All right now?"

"I am—thanks to you—very well."

Her voice wasn't like a woman's, either; it was deep, like a low note on a fiddle and she certainly wasn't from our part of the country.

Pert Tom poured out the hot, spicy-smelling ale, and the girl took her cup without saying "Thank you," and sat hugging it to her chest and staring into the fire. Martin took his and sat at his own place at the table.

"Well, what happened?" Tom asked. "Why was you both so wet?"

They seemed each to wait to let the other answer, and both spoke together when they did speak.

"I fell . . ." the girl began, just as Martin said, "I fished . . ." He stopped and allowed her to finish.

She lifted one long thin hand and laid it to her flat wet hair.

"I am doing my hair, making the water my looking glass, and I fall in."

"And you fished her out?" Tom said to Martin.

"That's so. Is supper ready?"

"And waiting," I said. "Pull that stool in."

"You are inviting me?"

"You're welcome to your supper and a bed," Martin said.

"Is very kind."

"Where did you fall in the water?" Tom asked.

"Some place," the girl said.

"Flaxham St. Giles, by the mill," Martin put in.

"Where's your home?"

She hunched her small square shoulders. "Anywhere. Everywhere. I am on the roads and I make my living . . . Oh!" She dropped her knife and turned to Martin and said in the most heartbroken way, "My tambourine. I have lost my tambourine."

"Don't fret about that. We'll see about it in the morning. And if the worst comes to the worst, we'll get you a new one."

"Is very kind."

Pert Tom, who had travelled the roads himself, began to ask her questions about this person and that—a stilt-walker, a tumbler called Boneless, a man who swallowed knives. Sometimes she would say, "Yes, I know him," or, "He was at York last summer," but when he pressed for details her answers were vague and unsatisfactory.

"Mostly I am alone. It is better so," she said.

"And if you'd just escaped drowning by a hairsbreadth, Tom, probably some things would slip your memory," Martin said.

"Now somebody once towd me that when you drowned you see your whole life spread out like a picture. I allust wondered if that was true. Is it?" Tom asked.

"I do not know. I saw only a hawthorn tree. So pretty, green and white in the sun. I think to myself: Is Heaven, after all. Then here I am, being slapped in the face, very wet and cold. Sir," she turned to Martin, "I do not wish you to think me ungrateful, but I was . . . Oh well, it is over now."

When she said that Martin looked at her with a sudden, sharp interest, such a look as I'd never seen him turn on anyone, not even his Kate. You'd look that way, maybe, if you were in foreign parts across the sea and suddenly heard somebody speak in your own tongue.

He stopped eating and seemed as though he was going to say something, but he didn't; the habit of easy talk had gone from him in these last years.

I thought over the words again, and couldn't find anything in them. This was June, the hawthorns would be in flower, and most likely the last thing she saw when she fell in the water was just such a green and white tree. And if it wasn't the words she said, it must have been her looks that suddenly made him come to life that way. So then I took another look at her.

I know that men and women see things differently, and I know that I was already against her, but even so she had no beauty, no prettiness. Her face was too thin, all mouth and eyes, and the eyes not set in right. Or at least it looked so. It looked as though her cheeks had been pushed up, leaving hollows where flesh should have been and a heap of flesh up under the eyes, shoving them out of shape. Her skin was all over alike, the colour of porridge. Her mouth, I grant, was as red as a berry. I looked at this face and I remembered what I'd seen of the almost breastless, unfemale body, and I shuddered as I sat there.

Pert Tom, as soon as he had supped, got up and went off for what he called his "last breath of air." That meant Dummy's daughter, not the crooked one, the younger, with the red hair, a very forward little wench, bound for a bad end.

Martin sat on at the table, and again looked as though he was going to say something, and finally did.

"Agnes will look after you. Good night," was what he got out. Then he went to his room and we two were left.

I didn't want her to help me clear the table. I knew that if she lifted the loaf and put it in the crock, I should not want to eat another slice of it. I didn't want her to touch anything; and that puzzled me, life had long ago knocked any fancifulness out of me. But there it was.

I said, "The bed's up there," and I pointed. "And the privy is outside, sharp to the left."

She went out and came in again and climbed the little ladder. I noticed that her toes curled round the staves, like fingers, and that seemed so unnatural that it gave me a shuddering grue once more. Her wet clothes lay on the floor, she'd never thought to hang them out to dry. I did that, because I didn't want her to have the excuse for waiting for them in the morning. For a little while they smelt of wet stuff drying, and then they smelt of wild thyme. The scent reminded me of the sheep run at Horringer, where I had lived as a girl.

In the morning she came down and picked up her clothes and in a minute was down again, wearing them.

"A comb," she said. "Could you lend me? That I lost too."

I had a comb, a good one, not a snaggy-toothed wooden one, a fine bone comb that Martin had bought for me one day when a pedlar came to the door. I handed it to her unwillingly, thinking: Another thing spoilt, I shall never really like it again. She ran it through her hair, which had dried out, black and glossy as a blackbird's wing, but almost as flat as when it was wet. She didn't plait it or knot it, just left it hanging, and that, for some reason, annoyed me, as well as seeing her with my comb, so I said:

"That skirt of yours isn't decent. Why don't you mend it?"

"I cannot sew."

"Rubbish. Any woman with hands and eyes can sew. What can you do?"

"I can play my tambourine. And I can cook a hedgehog."

"A hedgehog! That's no meat for Christians."

She made no answer, but went and stood by the door, looking out at the morning. I stirred the porridge, set out the bread, and drew the breakfast ale. Martin came in from the yard and stood by her in the doorway.

"Did you sleep well?" he asked her.

"Oh yes. Is so long since I sleep in a bed."

He came in and stood by the board, and I put the porridge bowl before him. He always took his breakfast standing. She stayed by the door. After a spoonful or two he said, "Have you had your breakfast?"

She turned around and leaning against the doorpost laughed.

"Once a day is for eating—with people like me." She smacked her flat stomach with her hand. "Get into bad habits and expect to be fed all the time. No!"

Martin, whose very smile had grown into something painful, actually laughed.

"One indulgence couldn't hurt. Still, please yourself. Now, where do I look for this tambourine? Where exactly did you . . . fall into the water?"

She squinted up her eyes so that they looked more misshapen than ever.

"The name of the place? I do not know. There is a bridge."

"Stone or wood?"

"Stone. Two arches."

"Upriver from Flaxham. That'd be Marly?"

"Perhaps. After the bridge is a place for dipping water and there is my tambourine."

I knew that on this day Martin had planned to go to Hedingham, and that was nowhere near Flaxham or Marly way. Wasting his time, I thought.

"Most like it has been picked up by now," I said.

"I do not think anybody will do that," she said.

"I'll go and have a look. And if I can't find it, you shall have a new one."

"It belonged to my mother and I have just bought it new ribbons."

When he had gone I said to her, "Would it have hurt you to say thank you? Here's a busy man going out of his way, promising you new if he can't find your old—and that is most unlikely. And you can't even thank him!"

The bulges under her eyes lifted, squeezing her eyes as she smiled.

"You should know. You are a woman. If you thank a man, he thinks you are in debt to him and so he looks for payment."

"Not him," I said. "He's the kindest and best-hearted . . . This whole place is built up on his good heart, lame folks and daft ones and people in trouble or disgrace, people nobody else wanted." I thought of Dummy and Peg-Leg and Peter Priest, and a dozen more. Me too.

She said, "People nobody else will want, they are very cheap."

Something in my head went "snap" like an overblown bladder. The shocking part of it was that just for a second I thought: That is *true!* Just as he made that tidy little hut in Squatters Row, out of nothing, out of stuff other people would chuck away or overlook, so he's made all this out of human rubbish. Even Pert Tom's savings had been *used*, and Pert Tom so handled that he daren't bring his baggage into the house.

But that only lasted a second; it was like some of the things you sce when you're very drunk; they seem very real and you're scared. Then they're gone. And that was gone.

I said, "I suppose you will have to wait to see if he finds your tambourine; and if you want to eat midday there'll be food here, but I'd thank you to get out of my kitchen."

She went off, and I began on my day's work, which was preserving gooseberries. Our young bushes were in full fruit that year, and some of Dummy's children had gathered them and picked off the tops and tails. I scalded the jars and packed them in close, got the cloths soaking in the mutton fat for the covers, and more mutton fat melted to pour over. Then Pert Tom, who was a slugabed in the mornings, came ambling in for his breakfast.

"Where's Martin's drowned cat?" he asked.

"Out. I'm busy. I didn't want her hanging round me."

"I reckon you'd better get used to it. I've missed my mark if he don't take up and marry her."   .

"Marry her. Rubbish!" But another overblown bladder had gone "snap" in my head.

"You ask yerself. Take the way he looked at her, promised her a new tambourine if hers was lost—and him so mean he didn't even hev a pair of gloves till you give him a pair for Christmas. You couldn't've missed *that*. If you ask me, she's cut to his measure, all skin and bone and grief, somebody to feel sorry for, just like his other one."

I dished him out the heat-up porridge.

"You knew Kate, then?"

"Kate?"

"His wife."

"This porridge is burnt, tastes awful. Kate, was that her name? I saw her, yes. I saw her go into the hut—like I say, all skin and bone and grief. And now he've got hisself just such another, after waiting so long." He laughed and pushed his porringer away. "Still, maybe she can cook."

"She can," I said tartly. "She can cook a hedgehog."

"A hedgehog? That ain't Christian food," he said, exactly as I had done. "Thass real Romany."

"And what's that?"

"Oh, foreign. Out of Pharaoh's Egypt, some say. There's one or two on the roads, but decent people don't hev nowt to do with them. They're heathen. They don't even lay together like other people, they do it cutting their thumbs and letting the blood mix."

"The tales you tell!"

"I only pass on what I hear tell myself. And of course if she is Romany I shall miss my mark, 'cause she couldn't marry him. They ain't allowed to stay in one place more'n a moon month; if they do they die."

He finished his breakfast and went off, it being Wednesday, to idle away his time looking round the market and sitting in one alehouse after another, listening to and spreading gossip. He didn't come in for dinner, nor did the girl, so I fed those men who were on wages-and-dinner terms, finished my gooseberries, and sat down to rest myself before starting supper. I'd hardly set down before Pert Tom came in, full of ale and something else. I could see before he opened his mouth that he had a fine titbit to tell me.

He looked round the kitchen and up in the loft.

"Is she about?"

"No. You can see for yourself."

He pulled a stool near me.

"Now you listen to this. Know what we've got in the house now? A witch, no less!"

"Rubbish," I said, partly because his tales were so farfetched and partly because, like almost every other old woman who was poor and looked a bit wild, I'd had the word "witch" flung at me in my time. Nevertheless, when he brought out the word I thought: That's it! That accounts for the way I feel about her, not wanting her to handle my things, not wanting to touch her.

"Rubbish away. Only tell me this, where'd Martin say he found her?"

"Flaxham. By the mill."

"Right. And what lay upriver from Flaxham. Maybe you don't know."

"As it happens I do. A place called Marly."

"Right again. Well, Tuesday morning, yestiddy that is, a Marly man heard his dog barking early in the morning; he look out and what do he see but a young woman with long black hair raiding his hens' nest. He see her take two eggs, one she stuck in the front of her dress, the other she kept in her hand. Jest as he was he run out and ask for his eggs back. She say, 'Take it,' and give him the one in her hand. He say she've got another, she say she h'ain't, and he say all the time he can see it bulging out inside her bodice. So he go to take it, as who wouldn't? And she say to him, 'Don't you put your hand on me,' she say, 'if you do you'll be very sorry.' But he don't take no notice, he take the egg instead. And then what happen?"

"His arm dropped off at the shoulder."

"You're a funny owd crone, ain't you? No, what happen is that he go out to the hayfield and afore he've been there a quarter hour somebody unhandy with a sickle cut off two fingers for him. Now thass no good saying 'Rubbish,' the man that towd me had jest brought the poor man to the Abbey Infirmary; they'd stopped the bleeding with hot tar, but he was swelling up cruel. Only, here's the point to this tale. Everybody in Marly turned out to chase the witch, and by the bridge they found her. They tied her skirt round her knees and chucked her in to see do she sink or swim. And she swum! Straight downriver towards Flaxham, this chap say, sailing like a swan. Now do you believe me?"

I did. It all fitted in, even to her saying that nobody would have picked up her tambourine from the river bank. Of course not. Nobody would want to touch her gear. Just as, in my unknowing way, I hadn't wanted to touch anything she'd handled.

"Yes. For once I do," I said. "We must tell Martin."

"I can't wait to see his face. Fancy him swallowing that yarn about using the water for a looking . . ."

He broke off and turned his head sharply and looked towards the door. I saw his colour change and he crossed himself openly. I turned, too, and there she was, leaning against the doorpost and holding something in her hands. I slipped one thumb over the other in the shape of the Cross, under cover of the table.

She said, "To wagging tongues things sometimes happen, too." As she spoke she walked in and laid what she held on the table. It looked like a ball of clay, about the size of your head, loosely covered with dock leaves.

I've seen some frightened people, but seldom anybody worse scared than Pert Tom. He jumped up and blurted out, stammering and blinking, "I shan't say anything. I shan't mention it," and he hurried into his room, where, I knew, he would ask his St. Ursula to protect him.

The girl said to me, "You cross your thumbs, but you will tell Martin what you hear?"

"If my tongue still wags, yes. I'm so old that what happens to me doesn't matter any more."

She sat down by the table and folded her arms.

"Is all nonsense, of course. Alone, on the road, as I am most times, a woman must take care. The tale is a lie. Partly. Was Monday evening, not Tuesday morning; and there was no egg. You understand me. No egg. Me, looking for sleeping place, and the man, like all men. You should know, once a man has his hand *here*, who is safe? So his fingers are chopped. Every day, some place, fingers are chopped." She leaned sideways, still with her arms folded, and laughed. "If I could say a thing and make it *be*, I am not wasting my time chopping fingers. No. I would say: Let me dance like my mother! Oh, if that could be!" She sat up straight again and threw back her head, and for a moment in the stuffy kitchen it seemed as though the wind blew on her face.

I was old, and since I had come to live at the Old Vine I'd had a quiet life, nothing much to think about except whether to serve beef or mutton. So now, with so much, all at once, all strange and different, I was confused. Later, I thought, later, in the quiet of my bed, I'll think it all over. Just for the moment I wanted something real and firm to seize upon. And there was this bundle on the table.

"What is that?"

"Is a hedgehog. Is not food for Christians you say, so I will show you."

"Oh no. You're cooking no hedgehogs here. Not in my pots."

"He is needing no pot. He has his own. See." She picked up the bundle and stripped off the dock leaves. "We bury him, so, in the hot ash, and he makes his own pot. When he is ready we crack him and his prickles all come away with the pot."

She buried the thing at the fire's edge, pushed it inwards a little, and pulled a log over it. As she straightened up, Martin, back much earlier than usual, walked in, holding the tambourine.

"Here you are," he said.

She swooped forward and took it from him, the bells jingled and jangled, the ribbons, red and yellow and blue, green and purple and pink, just like the stripes of her ragged skirt, fluttered and shook.

"Oh," she said, "is so *so* kind! My tambourine." She drummed on it lightly with the fingers. "Not spoilt. I was afraid, out on the grass . . . Is good. Now, after supper, I will dance for you."

Pert Tom had to be called to supper, and came out like a dog with a bad conscience. Ordinarily after market day he would chatter on, and Martin would grunt and show little interest until Tom told of some mishap that had befallen some Baildon man, and then he would look up and grunt in another tone. But tonight Tom was silent, every now and again looking at the girl and, if he happened to catch her eye, shake his head a little and make a secret face, trying to reassure her that his tongue would never wag.

Presently Martin said, "What's the matter, Tom? No gossip going round today?"

"Not a thing. Not a thing," Tom said and bent over his food. He was eating what I had cooked, but Martin was eating the hedgehog.

She'd cracked off the clay, and I admit that the meat left inside looked clean enough and smelt very tasty; but I couldn't bring myself to try it, and Tom was too scared.

Martin said, "I will. Come to think of it, if nobody had ever tried anything new there'd be precious little to eat."

As he ate he praised it, and I tried not to mind or be jealous. After all, I longed and prayed that something would happen to make him shake off the dead past and come alive again, and if it took a wild thing out of the woods with a tambourine and a hedgehog to do it, who was I to complain? I could only hope that she would rouse him, make him feel that there was something left in life besides hard work and making money, and then go off and leave him to take up with a decent woman.

All through supper she sat, looking at the tambourine and now and again touching it. As soon as the meal was over she jumped up and asked Tom and Martin to move the table. They began to push it towards the hearth, but she said:

"No, no. The other way. Is better the light behind me."

When the space was cleared and we were gathered at the other end, she walked down towards the fire, keeping close to the wall and sidling along. Then she stood still, like a cat about to make a spring. And then, with a shake of the tambourine and a little hoarse cry, she leaped out into the centre of the space and began to dance.

I've seen many dancing girls in my day. In the old times, in Squatters Row, in a good summer I've known as many as four be there all at once, and late at night they'd dance, not for pay, but to outdo each other. Some were good and some were bad, but the best of them *was* only a girl dancing when all was said and done. This was something different. Dancing she really could cast a spell. What but magic could make that ragged gaudy old skirt shake out into blurred soft colours like a rainbow or the sunlight on the spray over a weir? How else could she move so that it was all movement, a bird in flight, a deer leaping, a tree swaying in the wind? The music was magic too, for a tambourine has but two sounds, the thrum on the skin and the jingle of the bells; in her hands it made real music in which there was the rush of the wind, the birds' calling, even the solemn chant of the Church.

As long as it lasted you could only sit and stare and wonder. Even I, an old woman, with all my fires quenched, could feel again the stir and the ache, not in the flesh, or for it, but for something more, that something which, when you are young, you think lies round the next corner, and when you are old you know you missed because it never could be there. Here, just for once, in the homely kitchen, against the light of the dying fire, it all was held out for us.

When she stopped it was like waking from a dream in which you are warm and full-fed, to find yourself cold and hungry again. We all three let out our breath in a great sigh.

She went and stood by the wall, breathing quickly and lightly. Then I could move my eyes. And just for once I saw Martin's stern thin face and Pert Tom's fat stupid one wearing the same look of naked lust.

The girl spoke first.

"You like?" She lowered the hand which held the tambourine and it gave a little tinkle, like the echo of the question. She dropped against the wall, hunching her shoulders.

"By my mother I dance like a pig. When my mother danced, when she ceased, men wept with the pain of it."

Pert Tom got up and blundered out of the house, leaving the door open; the cool air, faintly scented with hay, flowed in.

All very well for him, I thought; he can go and find his red-haired baggage; Martin has his empty room, with tally sticks for company.

But Martin stood up and said, "You know, you've never told us your name."

"Is Magda."

"Magda." He repeated the name which was as strange as everything else about her, as though it pleased him. He said, "We could do with a breath of air, too." He went towards the door, and it seemed to me that he moved more lightly, more freely, leaning less to his limp than usual. She followed him, I thought unwillingly.

II

That evening they weren't out an hour, all told. I was just in bed when they came in quietly, said good night, and went to their separate beds. I thought to myself: Well, that's over; he's had his will of her and proved to himself that he can so far forget Kate as to go with another woman, and now if she'll just take herself off, everything will be all right.

In the morning, quite early she did go off, with her tambourine; but she was back, just before supper.

"So you've come back," I said.

"You think I will not?" She squinted her eyes at me. "Martin, he is the master here, is it not? He says I am welcome. Tonight I shall dance again."

"Dancing! That's all you think about."

"Yes and yes and yes. I have danced today. Look." She held out her long hand and showed me some coins in its palm. "I am not needing it, no supper to pay for. You can have it." She walked up to me and tried to put the money in my hand. I backed as though she had offered me something red-hot.

"I don't want your money. Save it and buy yourself a shift!"

She surprised me by giving one of the deepest, heaviest sighs I ever heard a human being give, though I'd heard the like from donkeys, already overladen when something else was added to their load.

"A shift, a petticoat, and shoes. And every night the certain supper and the bed. It is much."

"What are you talking about?"

"Things to *have*. Me, I have wanted only to *be*."

"Be what?"

"Such good dancer as my mother."

I said, almost against my will, "I fail to see how she could have been better than you were last night. I've seen a lot of dancers in my time, but I never saw anybody dance like you."

Something lit up in her face; she flung herself at me and would have hugged me, but again I backed away, this time almost into the fire.

"Don't," I said.

"You are not liking to be touched. Me, too, but with men only."

"Then you go the wrong way about," I said. "Any man, watching you dance, is bound to want to get his hands on you."

"But I am not dancing for men to desire me. I am not dancing to be paid. Enough for supper and new ribbons for my tambourine sometimes. And now a new comb."

"Then why do you do it?"

"Because . . ." She paused, smiled, shook her head. "There is no because. To dance I am born, so I dance."

"To me that sounds daft."

"Must everything be because? There is a poppy, very red, beside the road for just one day. Because? Is a red poppy. No good for eating. You pluck him, he falls to pieces. Is enough for a poppy just to *be* a red poppy. And so with me."

I couldn't find an answer except—poppies aren't people and people aren't poppies—and that, because it sounded quite as daft as anything she had said, I wouldn't say.

That evening I didn't stay to see her dance. I went and had a little gossip with Peg-Leg. We spoke of this and that, and of the girl who'd come into the house, and I mentioned what Pert Tom had said about Martin being likely to marry her.

"He might at that," Peg-Leg said. "Once I sailed with a man that had a monkey; he was more set on that monkey than most men are on their wives. Then it died and his heart broke. A month or two after we sailed into Tangier where there was plenty monkeys, cheap. I said to him, 'Whyn't you get yourself a new monkey?' He turned white as a sheet and he said, 'I'll never have another monkey as long as I live.' But . . ." Peg-Leg paused and wagged a finger at me. "We went into Naples and there on the quay was a cat, terrible looking, bones sticking out and mangy all over. He took to that, and within a week was as fond of it as he had been of his monkey. See? We did no good with Jennie and Kitty, they was decent, home-keeping little bodies, they just called his Kate to mind. This, by all accounts, is quite another pair of shoes."

"What do you know of her, barring what I've told you?"

"I seen her," he said simply. "And I was told she was dancing and prancing and shaking a tambourine in the market place today. Can you see Kate doing that?"

"I wouldn't mind," I said, "if I thought she'd make him happy."

"I don't reckon," Peg-Leg said slowly, "that men look to women to make them *happy*. Martin had Kate and they got on better than most, but when they wouldn't have him in the Guild, and then, later on, you remember when he broke his leg and Webster sacked him—you couldn't say he was *happy*, could you? Holy Mother, he was miserable as sin." He broke off and rapped his wooden leg with his knuckles. "Meaning no offence, Agnes, you having been a woman once, women set theirselves a bit too high. Could somebody come along to me and ask which would I rather, the Queen of Sheba in my bed, or my leg back and be at sea again, I know which I'd say."

"Ah, that is because you're old."

"Old! God's blood, how old do you think I am? I'm forty. I'd just turned twenty-four when I was beached."

I'd always thought of him as being an old man.

"Don't you go fretting yourself over Martin," he said. "He's got his business. All he needs now is a boy to bring up in the trade, and he can as easy get that out of a slut as out of a mim little wench that couldn't say boo to a goose."

That at least was true, and I felt my heart lighten a bit.

"Maybe I'd better start fretting about myself for a change," I said. "Peg-Leg, if Martin should marry her, I couldn't stay in the house. The other night she brought in a hedgehog, and I said she wasn't cooking it in *my* pots. They'll be *her* pots. Everything will be hers, to use and handle. I couldn't bear it. Could I come and turn in with you for a bit?"

"I reckon so." He looked round the snug little hut. "Since I took up work again, I've let my mending go." Like all sailors he'd been handy with a needle. "You could stitch me up. And it'd be nice to find the fire going when I got home. You'd have to bring your own bed."

So I'd found myself a hole to run to if the moment of need should come.

It came, three or four days later, when Martin said to me, in his abrupt way, "I'm going to marry Magda."

"I hope you'll be happy," I said; and I meant it. "There's one thing you should know, Martin—or maybe she told you. . . ."

"What?"

"They say she's a witch, and was being swum that day you found her."

"I knew that. As soon as I'd choked the water out of her I cut the cord. I'd seen one swum before."

"And you don't mind?"

"I don't care what she is. She's the only woman . . . Who told you it was being said?"

"Pert Tom."

"You can tell him to keep his mouth shut."

"Oh, she did that, threatened to make his tongue drop out or something."

Martin laughed. I thought to myself: Peg-Leg can say what he likes, a woman can make a man happy or miserable; already Martin is a different man.

"There's one other thing. I told you some time back this was all getting too much for me. You remember? I think now would be the time for me to go. When's the wedding to be?"

"This day three weeks."

"Well, now, there's Dummy's Mary. She's crooked, but she's as strong as a donkey for all that, and she often hangs around watching me work and helping a bit. If I got her in and showed her how things should be, then there'd be a new mistress and a new maid, and that is the best way."

"Maybe. Where'd you go?"

"I should go and look after Peg-Leg."

"I always meant you to end your days by my fire, with your feet under my table, Agnes. But then I never thought . . ."

"But for you Peg-Leg wouldn't have a roof or a fire, so it comes to much the same thing."

"In a way, I suppose. And we'd send your food across."

Stuff she'd have clawed over.

"I'd sooner manage on my own."

"Please yourself. You can have what money you want."

"That's kind. And any day I feel up to it, I'll go in the shed and pick wool for a spell to help earn . . ."

He gave me a very black look and said, "If you think that's easy!" He swung on his heel and limped away. I thought for a moment that he had seen through my excuse for leaving and was annoyed, yet he hadn't been earlier when I said I was going. It took me a moment or two to realise that Kate had picked wool at Webster's, and this was no moment to remind him of her.

Pert Tom had his excuse for getting out all ready to his hand. All these years he'd held onto his bear and been fairly regular about feeding it and putting it through its tricks. Once, when he was grumbling about what the animal cost to keep, I asked him why he didn't sell it.

"Easy come, easy go," he said, "and maybe one of these days Martin'll bite off more than he can chew. First he hev a forge, then hev a row of stables, then he hev a wool business. Grant he've been lucky, but build a thing too high and it'll topple over. If it do, then out on the road we go, Owd Muscovy and me, and no worse off than we was."

"Except that you'd have lost your savings." We'd been given to understand that it was Pert Tom's money that had started the business in the first place.

Pert Tom laughed. "Ah yes, them savings! Well, they wasn't all that much, and I've had years of soft living. And shall do, till Martin overreach hisself."

"If you think he's overreaching himself, you should warn him. You're supposed to be his partner."

"I hate wasting me breath," he said. But he had held onto the bear; and when he heard about the marriage being so near he said to Martin, "I allust promised meself one more summer on the road, and if I don't go soon I shall be too owd. And you'll like the place to yourselves to start off with."

To me he said, "I give it a month, but a month alongside her is more'n I can manage. Half the time I'm frit of her and the other half I'm itching arter her, and I don't know which is worst."

"What'll you do if it lasts more than a month?"

"It can't. I towd you, they can't stay in one place more'n a month without sickening. I shall be back in five-six weeks, according to the weather, and you'll see, she'll be gone."

"Daft talk," I said. "In five-six weeks she may be three weeks gone in another fashion. I surely hope so."

He didn't even stay for the wedding, so he missed the feast Martin gave to everybody on the place. He had an ox roasted in the yard, and there was all the ale we could drink and plenty over. Even

Martin, who'd never, in all the time I'd known him, taken a drop too much, was tipsy as soon as anyone.

Magda, for the wedding, had a dress, very costly, of crimson silk so dark it was almost black, she had shoes on her feet and her hair knotted up and fastened with a pair of silver pins. That way, she looked ordinary and decent, her skin very sallow between the dark of the dress and the dark of her hair; and she had none of a bride's happiness. She looked so downcast that I wondered if the shoes were causing her pain.

We put them to bed in proper style, and I myself put the salt and the handful of barley at the four corners, to make sure that they would be fruitful.

Peg-Leg was easygoing and I was comfortable enough with him, but for me everything seemed out of joint. I missed seeing Martin and seeing to him, feeling as mothers do when their sons marry and move away. I got into the habit of waiting about the yard just to catch a glimpse of him, judging from the way he looked and the way he walked whether things were going well. One morning, not long after they were married, he came out of the house and went towards the stables whistling, and I could have cried with joy. Immediately after I could have cried with rage at myself for letting such a daft fancy put me out of the house and out of his life. One day there'd be a baby there, his baby, and I should have no part in it. I was like a woman who, hungry as she may be, can't go to her own bread crock because a spider is sitting beside it.

Dummy's Mary was so grateful to me for getting her the job, and training her to it, that she was like a dog; she often used to come round to have a bit of a gossip and ask my advice on this and that. She told me that the mistress did nothing in the house at all, still ate only once a day, and spent hours in Tom's empty room, playing the tambourine and dancing, all by herself. Martin had put his foot down about her dancing in the town and threatened, if she disobeyed him, to take away her tambourine.

"He should stop her dancing altogether," I said, when Mary told me this, "rattling her insides about that fashion, how can she hope to breed?"

Another time, a little later, Mary reported that the mistress had a cough, which she said was because she was indoors so much.

"She's not hobbled or chained," I said. "She could do a bit in the garden. The lavender isn't even cut this year yet, and the pea haulms yellowing where they stand. And couldn't she walk into market, like any other housewife?"

The year moved on and it was Michaelmas. Pert Tom had been away longer than he'd planned, because, I suppose, the good weather had lasted. I looked forward to his coming home, partly because I wondered what he would do, and partly because I wanted to tease him about being so know-all about Romanys and their not being able to stay anywhere more than a month.

October was two days old when, one afternoon, coming out of the woolshed, where I'd been picking (which is hard work and made me think of Kate, who used to do it all day long and with two children to mind), I saw Tom just shoving his bear into its shed.

"So you're back," I said.

"So I am, fancy you noticing," he said sourly, and kicked the bear to move it over.

"And she's still there. Using your room to dance in, so I hear."

"If I want me room back, I shall hev it. Remember how I got this?" He turned his face so that the scar the burn had left on his cheek showed up in the light.

"You'd not speak of that and remind him, just when he's begun to be happy again!"

"Why not? He was the one said we was to live together the rest of our lives. He was the one said no women in the house when I wanted to bed Joan in comfort. I'll remind him all right. I'll remind him of a lot of things."

I drew a bow in the dark.

"While you're about it, remind him how your old bear was burnt, too, helping with the brave rescue."

"What d'you know about that?"

"More than you think. A lot more than you think."

Where exactly I'd hit him I couldn't see, but somewhere, for, though he scowled he said, "I don't want to go dragging up owd things. Nor I don't want to go back on the roads. I've got soft and I'm too owd to lay out arter Michaelmas. Where're you living?"

"With Peg-Leg—and a right tight fit it is."

"Well, I shall see what Martin hev to say. Not that I hanker to be under the same roof with her, but this is my home, arter all."

So off he went, and that very evening when Peg-Leg came home he told me that he and several other men had been taken off their different jobs and set to build again.

"Starting tomorrow, digging holes for the posts. A rare fine big room this is to be, too; twenty feet by twenty and ten high. He talk of putting in a window, glassed."

"Just for Pert Tom?"

"No. For Mistress Reed. He had a special word for it. Ah, I got it, a solar he called it."

I tried to imagine such a large room and couldn't see where it could be on such a little house, not without blocking up a door or a window of what was there already. Unless he built it on the forge side.

"Is he aiming to move the forge then?"

"No. The other side."

"That'd block the way the ponies come in from the road to the yard."

"They're leaving that just as it is and building across the other side of it."

"Then there'll be two separate houses."

"No. Martin reckoned to roof over the way the ponies go in and leave that as a passageway. Then folks can get from the kitchen door to the . . . the solar, just stepping across the passage."

For the next six or seven weeks I used to go along every day and watch the work going forward. Apart from the big houses at Horringer where my father was shepherd, and Ockley where my husband was game warden, so of course I never was in them, only saw them from outside, I never had seen such a building. Even the floor was solid oak, every plank about eighteen inches wide and laid as level as a table. And they put in a window, like Peg-Leg said, not flat in the wall, but bowed out, right over the garden I'd made, so it only just missed my lavender bush. It was all made up of little panes of glass, greenish, about as big as the palm of my hand. All that, just for a woman to dance in!

I now had another spy inside the house, as it were. Pert Tom, who had often enough grumbled about my cooking, more to annoy me than because he had any cause, would come slouching round once or twice a week, and, without actually asking, would say something smelt tasty, and complain of Mary's cooking, and I'd give him a piece of whatever was going and he'd sit down and talk. He seemed to have lost most of his fear of Magda and to get along with her very well, "what little I see of her," he said. "I never hang around when she take that tambourine in hand, because thass the only time she's anyway tempting." He spoke as though, apart from her dancing and her lack of interest in the kitchen, Magda was ordinary enough and life in the house pretty smooth-running.

Once, a little before Christmas, he spoke of her having a cough and brewing up a cure for it; it smelt terrible, he said.

Then, even nearer Christmas, Mary came along one evening and begged me to go in and make the plum pudding.

"All them costly things," she said. "If owt went wrong and they was wasted, that would be a pity. 'Tain't like spoiling a pot of porridge, is it?"

I said craftily, "I'll come and help you, if we can do it some time when the mistress isn't about—then you can take the credit for it, you see. You wouldn't want her to know, would you?"

"She's in the solar every afternoon now."

"All right then. Now mind this . . ." I told her that she was to scrub the table, wash the bowl, the spoon, and the big iron pot, and scald the pudding cloth. "Never mind if they are all clean; it's a kind of magic rule, for making plum pudding everything must be washed afresh."

Even if I hadn't had this hatred of handling anything after those long thin hands had been on it, that would have been a wise order. Nothing in the kitchen was as I left it, everything was greasy and smeared and in the wrong place. I scolded Mary—not too much, for she had been brought up like a pig and only had three weeks' training—but I scolded myself most harshly for running away on account of a fancy. I should have stayed, I told myself. I'd come back, I told myself all the time I was chopping the suet; I'd humble myself to Martin, tell him I wasn't comfortable with Peg-Leg and beg him to take me back. I'd force myself to get over this stupid feeling; if Pert Tom could live in the house with her, so could I.

We had the flour and the suet and the eggs and the fine fat raisins all ready.

"We want a pinch of spice," I said to Mary. "Where do *you* keep the spice box? I always had it on the shelf here."

"I think it's in the cupboard."

"God bless you, girl, don't you *know*?" I exclaimed, and glared at her as she went to the cupboard.

Inside it was all of a jumble, in which she ferreted about like a blind woman, while I clucked my tongue, making the most of my impatience. She reached up to the top shelf and as she did so a little bunch of dried-up herbage fell out, she grabbed at it and missed it and it dropped near me. I picked it up, smelt it, and said sharply:

"Mary! Leave hunting that spice box and come here. What is this?"

And I thought: Jesus have mercy, if a poor ugly crooked girl like that can get into trouble! I kept my eye hard on her, but she neither blushed nor blenched.

"That? Oh, thass Mistress's stuff for her cough."

"Her cough! But this . . . How often does she take it?"

"I don't rightly know. From time to time she'll pour water on and drink it when it's soaked."

"I see. Best put it back. Then if you look behind that crock of mouldy dripping, you'll find your spice box."

She brought it to me, saying with a false little smile, like a dog in disgrace wagging its tail too fast, "You do hev good eyes, Agnes."

"Too good," I said.

We went on making the pudding, but my mind was on other things; the feeling that I must come back here and set things right for Martin's sake; the memory of that bunch of dried stuff with the faded flowers that had been pink and the pale rounded leaves with their pointed ends.

I was on my feet, the better to give the mixture the good sturdy whack that it needed, and saying, "Like this, see. Smack it about as though you were beating a bed," and just about to hand the spoon to Mary when the kitchen door opened and Magda walked in. First I was thankful that I was on my feet so I didn't have to stand up to acknowledge she was mistress, and second all my determination to come back and see Martin comfortable just ran away like water down a gutter.

She said, "Hullo, Agnes," as carelessly as though she'd seen me the day before. No surprise, no interest that I should be there, in her greasy, untidy kitchen, making her plum pudding for Christmas. I just gave her a nod of my head and turned to Mary.

"Now to do the thing properly," I said, "we have to have a chunk of wood, borrowed from a friend, to lay on the fire to start up the boiling. Go along to Peg-Leg's—there's nobody there but you must knock on the door and say, 'Can I borrow a log to cook my plum pudding?' You'll find some logs there, choose the biggest and bring it back."

Mary went off. I'd made the thing up on the spur of the moment, but it fitted, I thought, Christmas being the friendly season.

Magda was going towards Martin's room, now their bedroom, but I stopped her.

"I want to ask you something."

She turned back and said, "Yes." And at that moment the fright came on me. All those months ago, when Pert Tom had said she was a witch and I'd crossed my thumbs and thought that was why I didn't want any doing with her, I hadn't been really frightened. That is true. She'd threatened the tongue that wagged about how she got in the river, yet I had told Martin. I'd never been really scared. Now, all of a sudden I was. My breath seemed to catch. Still I said it.

"That stuff you take for your cough, every now and then. Do you know what that is?"

"Is a wildflower. Good for the cough."

She'd turned back and now stood so that the table was between us, and we faced each other as though we were fighting a duel or playing some gambling game.

"I never heard it was good for coughs. It has another virtue. . . ." Then I thought: That slipped out because you get used to speaking of the virtues of herbs, in this case it has no virtue. It'd be a virtue if she was a maid betrayed, or the down-burdened mother of a huge family. . . . I shouldn't have said "virtue." And of course I shouldn't, because she just said:

"So? Is nice to know!" and went sauntering into the bedroom.

I was so angry that I couldn't breathe. My heart came jumping up into my throat, beating like a hammer, bells rang in my ears, and for a moment I couldn't see except for sparks all shimmering against blackness.

I sat down and wrestled with my breath. I would breathe, pull it in, hold it, let it out. I could hear myself making a noise like a blacksmith's bellows.

Then there was Mary, so quick for all she was lopsided, back, lugging a great log.

"What do we do next, Agnes?"

And I managed to tell her, calmly, how to put the pudding into the cloth, leaving plenty of room for it to swell. And she did it. All the time there was no sound from the inner room.

It was growing dark.

"One more thing, Mary," I said. "Take the scissors and cut about an inch off the lavender bush. That has to boil in the water."

As soon as she had gone, I took the bunch of pennyroyal from the cupboard and dropped it into the heart of the fire.

III

I thought the matter over, by night as well as by day, for what remained of the time till Christmas. I felt it was my duty to tell Martin what his wife was up to, and yet I dreaded to upset him. I didn't want to make *too* much of it. There again, I thought, if I'd had any pluck at all, I should have been in the house, and seeing him often, able to drop a hint. However, my chance came, for this Christmas was to be a real merry one of the old-fashioned sort. Martin had a pig killed and roasted whole, and we all had our Christmas dinner on the big wool floor which had been three-quarters cleared. As at the wedding there was ale for everybody, and we sang all the old Christmas songs about the Three Wise Men and the Star of Bethlehem, and about the Holly and the Ivy.

Peg-Leg, like all sailors, was handy with his knife and could whittle any shape you asked; and I'd asked him to do a Baby, and a donkey and a cow about the size so that a small saltbox could be a manger for them. I put a wisp of straw in the box, laid the Baby on it, put the donkey on one side and the cow on the other, and set them all on a board to decorate the table at the end where Martin sat. I'd praised Peg-Leg's whittling and left it at that, and then, on the Christmas morning, when we stood together watching the pig turning on the spit over the fire in the forge, I did another bit of flattering.

"Peg-Leg," I said, "somebody ought to thank Martin for all this, and you're the one. If it's left to Peter Priest, it'll be all long words and no heart to it, and Pert Tom'll be stuttering drunk before the time comes. You're the one."

"Aye," he said, "I reckon I could stand up and say thanks for us all."

"And best wishes. I tell you what, Peg-Leg, say that while you're about it you'll wish that next year there'll be another baby at the table. That'll draw everybody's attention to yours."

"And thass a good wish, too," he said.

So all I had to do was to wait till Peg-Leg stood up and clapped his hands for silence and started to speak. Then I went and got as near Martin as I could, a little behind, so my mouth was close to his ear, and when Peg-Leg said about the baby, I muttered to myself, as any old woman of my age is entitled to do:

"And so there would be if she didn't keep swilling down that cough mixture!"

He heard, I saw him jump. He said, "What was that?" pretty sharp.

"What was what?"

"What did you say?"

"Did I speak? I reckon I was talking to myself," I said and wandered off.

I really did think to myself that that hint was dropped as well as ever a hint was. And it was noticed. It wasn't long after Christmas, the real cold weather was just beginning, when Dummy's Mary came along with some tale about the Master coming into the kitchen just as the Mistress was brewing her medicine and taking it and pouring it out at the back door.

"Thass all froze now, as hard and smooth as glass," she ended.

"Take a shovelful of ashes and put over it then, for Holy Mary's sake," I said. "We don't want anybody breaking a leg."

After that I just sat back and waited. The cold weather ended, the days pulled out, morning and evening, a few birds began to sing and even fly about with bits of straw in their bills, and it was spring again.

I stood one morning, where I usually did, and watched Martin mount and ride off somewhere. I remembered thinking that, badly as Mary managed in one way, she kept him fed and tidy looking. He did look just as usual. I stood there for a bit, enjoying the air, and along came Pert Tom to give Owd Muscovy his breakfast.

"Well," he said, "if you left on account of her, you can move back. Reckon I was right after all. She's up and quit!"

I had another of those turns when I couldn't breathe or see; I had to lean against the wall to keep myself from falling. He was saying something, but the ringing in my ears was so loud I couldn't hear what it was. I did my careful breathing, in, hold it, out, for a time or two and at last I could speak.

"What do you mean, up and quit? When, why?"

"I was telling you. You gone deaf? She took off yesterday morning and ain't been seen since. I reckon I miscalculated. That must be a *year*, not a month they can't stay in one place."

"Oh, stop that jabber! What about Martin? How's he taking it? Was he off just now, looking for her?"

"Not him. He's off to Lavenham. Know what he said, last night, when he come in and found her gone? He said, 'Well, you can't keep a lark in a cage, leave alone make a broody hen of it.' Then he set down and et his supper. If you ask me he've had a bellyful of her and is as glad to see her gone as I am. You'll come back now, eh, Agnes, and cook us some decent grub?"

My mind was elsewhere but my tongue answered him.

"You always used to grumble about my cooking."

"That was afore I tried Mary's!"

"I'll see. Most like she'll come back. She's like you, born to the road; this first spell of fine weather set her foot itching."

Maybe that was the way Martin looked at it. Maybe that was why he had eaten his supper and been so unconcerned.

But that wasn't true. He must have known she had gone for good, for that evening Mary came along, her eyes popping, to tell me that the Master, the minute he was home from Lavenham, had told her to take everything that belonged to the Mistress and put it on the fire in the forge.

"There was that lovely dress she had for the wedding, and the tawny woollen she had for the cold weather, and her shoes and everything, even the pins for her hair. And there was Tim, standing by with the bellows and the flames shooting up, you never see such flames, Agnes."

Oddly enough, I didn't picture the flames; I just saw her, going off in the old red bodice and striped skirt, carrying her tambourine, and her hair hanging. "There is no because. To dance I am born, so I dance." I thought of that. And I thought of Martin's remark about the lark and the cage. That showed understanding, and was a comfort to me, because a blow that you can understand never hurts so much as one which puzzles you. I also thought of Peg-Leg's words about women overrating themselves; this very morning Martin had gone off about his business in Lavenham. He'd survived a worse knock, he'd survive this. Some decent food and a clean bright kitchen, if they didn't help, wouldn't hurt.

I said, "So now there's no mistress in the house. It was bad enough when there was. I shall come along tomorrow morning, Mary, my girl, and put you through your paces."

She looked pleased.

So there we were, in well under a year, back just where we were. My only regret was that there was no baby. Nor would be now. Martin, grown even more silent, never thought about anything but work and business.

The big fine room across the passage was never used. I went in now and again to let in the air and watch Mary wipe away the dust. It was a sad room. I'd go in and think what a waste, his building this just for her to dance in; and I'd end by thinking I could see her dancing.

Amongst us her name was never mentioned, and for all the mark she had left on the place she might never have come at all.

IV

That was the summer when Martin began to speak of buying a ship of his own to carry his wool overseas. It wasn't until well on into November, however, that he heard of a likely vessel for sale and rode off down to Bywater to view it. It was bad travelling weather, and hardly light all day long, so the trip would take four days at least, and his last words to me were not to worry if he was away longer.

I took the opportunity to make brawn, and on the third night turned one out of its mould to see what it was like. We had it for supper, and very good it was. When Mary went to set what was left away for next day, I said:

"Look, you were a good girl and worked hard on that brawn, you can take that piece along to your mother and show her what a clever girl you are."

Pert Tom and I drew up to the fire. He was a bit mopish just then, because Dummy's Joan had taken up with one of the young smiths in the forge and he hadn't yet found himself another hussy. Looking at him, across the hearth, I thought he wouldn't find it so easy this time, and the next harder still, until in the end he'd just be that figure of fun—an old lecher.

We spoke about this and that, and mentioned Martin and the ship, wondering if he'd struck the deal.

"If he don't this time, he will the next. He'll get whatever he's set his mind on. And arter the ship he'll be hankering for a sheep run, so that from hoof to loom ain't nobody making a penny 'cept him."

"Well, what's wrong with that?"

"Did I *say* owt was wrong? You take me up so sharp. I shall go to my bed."

He went off, peevishly, and I shut my eyes and dropped into a little cat-nap, the way old folks do. It was the door opening and a rush of cold air coming in that woke me. Waking that way, neither your eyes nor your wits work well for a minute, and when I looked towards the door and saw a bent-over woman's figure with a bit of grey woollen over the head and upper part of it, I *saw* Mary, and I spoke to her, pretty gruff.

"Don't stand there, letting in the cold." I was glad to see that, though she'd run off just as she was, she'd had the sense to borrow a bit of wrapping to come home with.

Then, before my eyes, the hunched-over figure straightened out and it wasn't Mary, it was Magda. It was Martin's wife, come back. She straightened herself and at the same moment reached out her arm and pulled the door shut. The bit of grey stuff fell back off her head and showed the short stiff spikes of her clipped hair, and the thin face, always hollowed, now like a skull covered with skin, and the queer-shaped eyes sunk back in dark circles.

She stood there, leaning back against the doorpost, just as she had leaned that sunny morning and laughed and slapped her flat belly and said that to eat more than once a day was to get into a bad habit. She looked, now, as though she hadn't eaten once a week.

I had no scrap of pity. Only anger that she should have gone off on a spring morning and dared to come back, with the belly-cramp of hunger on her, as soon as winter set in. I was so glad that he wasn't there, with that soft heart of his, under the hard shell, and I was thinking of things to say, harsh enough, scornful enough to drive her away, when she said:

"Martin. He is not here?"

That brought the words into my mouth.

"No, he isn't. But if he was he'd say what I do. Be off. You went away of your own accord and hurt him sore. He's done with you. You aren't wanted here. Be off. Back where you came from."

She laughed; at least her lips curled back from the teeth that now seemed to be too many in her mouth, and a sound, like laughter, but with pain in it, came out of her.

"You mistake. I am not come to beg. I come to bring something."

"Your love and loyalty in return for a full belly! He saved you from drowning and what thanks did he get? He's away. He'll be away for a week. Nobody here cares about you. Go on. Get out."

It was November, and in November nobody has food to give away. I knew the signs. In twenty-four hours, without food and shelter, she would be dead. It was cold outside and she was starving. I wondered whether, breathless and clumsy as I was, I had the strength to throw her out. As I was wondering she bent over again, put her hand on her knees and braced herself, with a shudder, and the grey woollen, very slowly, slid down, down to the floor.

Then I saw; then I knew.

There is something almost uncanny about having plied a craft for many years; there can come a time when the plying of that craft can become all that matters. You are nothing, you cease to be, except as the tool with which the job is done. You don't even *think*. I didn't think then: This is Martin's child, that he wanted and I wanted. I didn't think: This is the woman whose touch, for me, would have made a bit of bread uneatable.

There was no thinking. There was a woman, in labour, pretty far gone in labour, two good strong pains in four minutes, and there was Agnes, the midwife, who could ply her craft drunk or sober.

I wasn't even the swollen-legged old shuffler that lately I had been. I was across the kitchen and I had her by the arm and onto my own bed in the blink of an eye.

"When did you start?" I asked, as I'd asked a hundred times before.

"This morning. Early. In Sudbury. I think this baby will be born in a ditch. Like me."

"Twenty miles. You walked twenty miles? Like this."

"Is good to walk, I understand. Good, eh? How bad then is bad? Aagh!"

I remembered, without the least distaste, that lean sinewy body.

And I said, with far more truth than I had ever said the words before, "You'll have no bother."

Then I remembered that hollow, starving look. I turned aside and pulled the pot of broth into the heat. It was part of the liquid in which the trotters and cheekbones for the brawn had boiled, good and strengthening. It was warm already and it began to bubble. I poured some into a cup and gave it to her.

As she sipped, I, Agnes the midwife, did what she always did, talked, tried to keep their minds off, tried to make out that this that was happening wasn't the end of the world.

"What happened to your hair?"

"Is sold. My tambourine also. Like this I cannot dance."

Another pain gripped her and the cup wobbled in her hand. I steadied it.

"Why did you leave it so late?"

"To come? Oh, many reasons. Is all a disaster. I go from here to find the wise woman. She is in York, and when I am come to York she is in Chester. And so it goes on. Then too late, or she is not wise enough."

I swear that it was Agnes the midwife, not Agnes, Martin's friend, who asked the next question.

"You tried to get rid of the baby?" It mattered, it meant upside down, feet first, sideways on.

"But of course. To a dancer a baby is ruin. Always I am hearing from my mother how good she is, until I come to ruin her. Aagh!"

She writhed and bit her lip. I took the cup from her; turned away, laid out my scissors and twine. You never made any show of them, but they had to be handy.

"So you've come from Chester?"

"From Chester. And not easy. My hair is sold, and my tambourine. I am to beg and to beg is slow. Too many people will say, 'You wish to eat you shall work.' So here I wash clothes and here I beat flax and here I cut nettles and so goes the time. But I am coming. Then, one day I steal. Bread. And I am not quick." Something that started out to be a smile turned into a grimace. She waited, drew breath, and went on. "Are most kind, these people. For stealing bread is a whipping or to stand in the pillory, but these are not suited to my condition. So I am locked in prison forty days. But still they are kind and they say poor baby to be born in such place and I am let to go." She turned her head from side to side on my pillow, and I saw the sweat spring out on lip and brow. Not long now. I took a cloth and wiped her face, as gently as I ever wiped any woman's. At the next twinge she muttered some words in a language I did not know.

"We're nearly there," I said, "it'll all be over in a minute or two."

At that moment Mary came in and stood goggling. I told her to get out fresh candles, "and the pepperpot," I added in a lower voice. I didn't expect any trouble, but it was as well to be prepared. I then sent her to her bed. I'd always hated to be watched at work.

A little time—more than I'd expected—went by. Magda was plucky; she bit her lip; she muttered the strange words; she moaned. Once she screamed.

"That's right," I said, "don't bottle it up. Scream all you want to."

I had forgotten Pert Tom, who, the next minute, opened his door a cautious crack and asked, "What's going on?"

He held his door ready to slam it to at once. (In the morning he said he thought maybe thieves had broken in and were clouting me; and I said, "If so you were ready with another brave rescue, weren't you?")

"Nothing for you to worry with," I told him. "Go back in and shut the door."

The next pang was weaker, and the next weaker still. She was young and sinewy, but she hadn't been looked after well and had come to the job exhausted and weak with hunger. Dallying at this point could be fatal. So I took the pepperpot, shook some into my palm, and held it under her nose. She gave a mighty sneeze and it was done.

The moment I had Martin's son by the heels, Agnes the midwife, spry, knowledgeable, intent only on the job, cleared off and left me.

First I had a good look at the baby. If Magda's own brew or the wise woman's muck had marked or marred him, I knew what to do; I wasn't having Martin saddled with something crippled or wrong in the head. So far as I could see, though, he was perfect, thin but healthy, and his first cry was real lusty. Then I paid particular attention to his face. There is a moment—and any midwife will bear me out on this—just one moment, when all the newly born bear the stamp of the man who made them. They may lose it and never have it again, but they all, boy and girl alike, come into the world looking like their father will look when he is an old man. Magda's baby was Martin at sixty, bald and wrinkled. Happiness flowed into my heart. Here it was, the boy he wanted, the boy I had wanted for him.

I knew that what I should do was to call Mary down, hand the child to her, and busy myself with the mother. I thought about it, knowing exactly what Agnes the midwife would do. I knew I couldn't do it. That old, shuddering loathing was back on me now: her precious load delivered, she had become once more the woman from whose lightest touch I had shrunk. But that was not all. I had no need to touch her. I could have called Mary and told her what to do.

The truth was, I wanted her to die. I thought how happy we could be now. What life was left to me I could devote to bringing up the baby. But not if she stayed. And she would. She spoke of a baby being ruin to a dancer. Besides, any woman, however wild, is settled by motherhood. Martin would be so pleased with the child that there'd be no question of forgiving her wandering off, it would just be forgotten; she'd be reinstated, more than ever mistress of the house, and I should be back with Peg-Leg.

Oh, I know that women do die in childbed, every day, every night, but not without a fight, not until every measure has been tried. Agnes the midwife had had many a hand-to-hand fight with death, and knew all the tricks.

I, I did nothing. I sat down with the child in my lap and saw to him, while behind me on the bed the Romany blood, the witch's blood, the woman's lifeblood soaked away.

Interval

Of Martin's ventures the Baildon people had said, "Ah, the bigger you blow a bladder, the louder the bang," and, "The higher a kite flies the farther it has to come down." As year followed year they waited for him to overreach himself, for the bladder to burst, the kite to fall. Nobody but Martin himself knew how often their ghoulish hopes had come near to being fulfilled. And he himself could not have said what it was that drove him, time and again, to take another risk, exchanging a certain, comfortable security for a touch-and-go chance. He just knew that he must go on and on.

Most of his ventures had an element of makeshift about them.

He went into the yard one morning, beckoned to Peg-Leg who was in the stables, and asked brusquely, "What sort of sailor *are* you? Could you take a ship from Bywater to Calais, or Amsterdam?"

"If she was sound, I could sail a ship to Constantinople and back."

"The one I have my eye on is old, but she's sound. How d'you know that you could?"

"It weren't my head that clumsy barber-surgeon cut off, you know," Peg-Leg said in an offended voice. "I'd done eleven years with the best sailing man ever breathed, devil in sea-boots though he was. And what you've learned at the rope's end you tend to remember."

"If I buy this ship, with all I've got tied up there," he nodded towards the woolshed, "I couldn't, straight-away, offer a hired captain enough to keep him honest. I've been over, I've seen all their tricks. Good wool marketed at half price, cash in their pockets and written off washed overboard or some such. One deal like that just now could be ruin. But a couple of honest trips, Peg-Leg, would see me clear, and after that you should have a share, a good share, one in forty of the whole cargo."

"You mean *me* be captain?"

"What d'you think I'm talking about?"

"Mother of God, I'd do it for nothing. I'd pay you to let me—if I had the wherewithal. I trudged, soon's I got this wooden leg fixed, I trudged from Bywater to Hull . . . Dunwich, Lowestoft, Yarmouth, Lynn, all the way to Hull. I begged for any job, just to be at sea again. Always the same answer: We can get plenty chaps with two sound legs."

If Martin remembered the time when he had been in a similar case, he gave no sign.

"It'd mean staying sober."

"I'm sober afloat. Sailors ashore . . . well, they make up for lost time. And beached like I was, in my prime. What other comfort was there? Look at Owd Agnes."

"Agnes?"

"Yes. Rolling drunk every time she had the money. Can't you remember? She steadied up as soon as she had a kitchen. I could steady up if I had a ship. You say you got your eye on one. How's she named?"

"*Mermaid.*"

Peg-Leg rubbed his nose. "I knew one by that name once, but that's a common name. Where do she lay?"

"Down at Bywater."

"Then s'pose we went down there . . . Is she manned?"

"More or less. The man that owned her was master; he's sick, he wants to sell, but the crew is ready to sign on with whoever buys her."

"They would be, ready and anxious. Then s'pose we go and go aboard, and you tell me where you want to steer for and I'll land you there."

"Yes," Martin said, "I think you will, Peg-Leg."

"I got a name," Peg-Leg said. "And it's Bowyer. Jacob Bowyer." He turned away to prop the pitchfork he had been holding against the stable wall. "Captain Bowyer," he said softly to himself, "Captain Bowyer of the *Mermaid.*"

The next sudden promotion from common yard hand to a post of responsibility was made when Richard was six years old, and concerned the unfrocked priest who had joined Martin's gang of workmen when the house was being built and the land cleared, and who had stayed on and had lately been working as a pack-whacker. He had a hut in the new Squatters Row behind the stables; it was set a little apart from the others, and he lived alone, aloof of manner, surly of temper.

One evening Martin surprised him by inviting him into the house and taking him into his own room, where upon the table a piece of virgin parchment, two newly cut quills, and an inkhorn were laid out.

"I take it you can write, Peter," Martin said.

"It's not a thing one forgets entirely."

"Sit down then." Peter did so and picked up one quill, rejected it, took the other, and said, "Who cut this? He was no scribe!"

"Cut it to suit yourself," said Martin, handing him a knife. Although he had cut the quills himself the criticism pleased him.

"What do you want me to write?"

"This. This is a deed of grant, made to one Martin and the heirs of his body, in perpetuity, of all the property and messuage known as . . ." He paused and the pen caught up with him.

Peter Priest looked up and asked, "What is this? A forgery?"

Still unoffended, Martin said, "No. A test."

He rose and went to the heavy chest that stood beside his bed and took out another parchment, one with a dangling seal. He took Peter's writing, and, scowling heavily, compared the two.

"There is a fault," he said at last. "You have spelt my name with an *e*."

"*E* or *i*, both are correct. It is a matter of opinion, not a fault," Peter Priest remarked coldly.

"Otherwise it is well done. How is your reckoning?"

"By tally or mentally?"

"In your head, the answer then written down."

"In Roman figuring or Arabic?"

"Both."

"Try me."

Martin went to his bed and from there dictated four problems in arithmetic, laying out, behind the priest's back, the answers as he made them by tally.

"Read me your makings."

All but one of the answers fitted, and in that one, when they reworked it, the error was Martin's.

By this time the possible purpose of the test had occurred to

Peter Priest; the accounts and records of the business had outrun Martin's ability to deal with them; so he, Peter Priest, was to be taken off the road and installed as clerk. The prospect was pleasing; how infinitely preferable to sit indoors, plying his real craft once more, instead of being on the roads in all weathers, handling greasy bales of wools, urging—sometimes having to pull for sheer force— pack ponies through the mire.

"You see," Martin said, "my way is slow and cumbersome, and can be wrong. That is why . . ."

He came round the table and sat down, facing Peter.

Why, Peter wondered, is he so cursed slow stating his business.

Martin was slow, partly because any but the briefest speech now came hard to him, partly because speaking of Richard brought the child to mind, and roused, as his actual presence did, many conflicting emotions. He delighted in the boy and loved him dearly, but he was an ever-present reminder, not of Magda, but of the two other little boys, especially Stephen. To be troubled by this, not to enjoy his fatherhood to the full, was he knew absurd, but he had felt from the beginning, from the day when he had come home and found the baby there, that in some way Richard was a usurper. For a long time even to watch the child being fed, and then later feeding himself, had been both a pleasure and a pain. Stephen, his firstborn, had lived on water gruel, on stale bread thinly smeared with fat, and had spent his days on the stinking wool floor, and finally died because his father was trying to save the miserable hut which was all the home he had. Richard fed on the fat of the land, enjoyed Old Agnes' whole doting attention. Stephen had been a very good, quiet little boy; Richard was naughty and wilful. The whole thing was in such sharp contrast that comparisons forced themselves upon Martin many times every day.

At the same time, simply because he felt this way, he also felt guilty. It wasn't Richard's fault that he had been born after the tide of luck had turned. So, each time that the affection which should have streamed out, full and free, towards the new child suffered the inevitable check and recession, Martin would, by some act of indulgence, endeavour to make up to the boy. He could deny him nothing; he could never punish him lest, into the punishment, should go some of this unjust resentment because Richard was Richard, not Stephen.

It had all mattered less, been more easily smoothed over, while

Old Agnes lived. Doubtless, in her time, Richard had been naughty, ungovernable, wild, but she had never complained; she had acted as a buffer, explaining, excusing, saying, "He is very young. He will learn," saying, "For myself I like a lad to show a bit of spirit." Once, jerked out of silence by her ridiculous attempt to defend some particularly prankish behaviour, Martin had snapped out:

"Stephen was never like that."

And Agnes had made—for Martin—the most terrible answer possible.

"Ah, there's the difference between the colt fed corn and the colt fed grass. You can't expect them to act the same."

Agnes had died when Richard was four, and within a week Dummy's Mary was crying and saying she couldn't manage the housework and Richard; he didn't come when she called him and when she picked him up he kicked her. The answer to that had been a strong, active young woman named Nancy, whose sole duty was to see to the child. She had had one of her own, illegitimate, which had died at the age of two. Martin, engaging her, had cherished the secret hope that her heart might share, with his, the defence of memory, that she might be a little less doting and lenient than Old Agnes who had never had a child of her own. If Nancy arrived thus armed, she was disarmed almost immediately. Richard was a remarkably handsome little boy, so charming when allowed his way, so disagreeable when crossed, that anyone crossing him was almost bound to feel that the change of mood was in some way his or her fault, not the child's. In a very short time Nancy, too, was enslaved. And so had happened the stupid, inexcusable incident with the bear.

Richard was almost six, and ever since he could toddle he had seen Uncle Tom go to the shed where Owd Muscovy lived, open the door, and place food within the bear's reach. The muzzle, no longer needed, hung on a peg in the wall, and the chain, attached to the bear's collar at one end, was hooked at the other over a strong nail driven slantwise into the wall of the shed.

Pert Tom, after that one summer on the road during Magda's brief rule as mistress of the Old Vine, had grown slack and old. Dummy's Joan's leaving him had, as Agnes expected, been a turning point in his life. It, or rather the difficulty he had found in replacing the young hussy, had loosened his mainspring. But he had kept his bear. And when Richard was five, at Christmastime, he had actually brought Owd Muscovy out on to the wool floor and put him through his tricks.

Richard watched, entranced.

"Uncle Tom, let me blow the whistle and make the bear dance."

"He wouldn't do it for you," said Pert Tom, who was the only person who ever treated Richard as an ordinary human being, an equal.

"Why not?"

"You ain't his master."

"Let me try."

"Get outa the way," said Tom.

Shortly after that Christmas, Richard began asking Martin for a whistle, and Martin remembered another little boy who had never asked for anything, had his pang of guilt, and provided the whistle.

The thing in itself was enough for Richard for a long time. He blew and a shrill level noise emerged. By accident he put a finger over one of the holes and a different noise resulted. Bit by bit, untaught, by a process of trial and error he learned to play a tune, one of those sung in the woolshed at Christmas, "The Holly and the Ivy." Once he could do that, he plagued Uncle Tom to teach him *his* tunes. Tom said, "One day" and "Sometime" and "Don't bother me now," but in the end he succumbed and after an hour or two with the child, said to Martin:

"He've got a true ear, and come to the point he's teachable. He'd got 'Gathering Pescods' and 'Granny's Bonnet' in nearly no time at all. If I'd had him on the road, with Owd Muscovy, I'd hev made a fortune."

The two tunes were all Richard wanted to learn. He played them over and over until he was sure, and when he was he set out to test them on Owd Muscovy.

The shed was never locked for the simple reason that no one except Pert Tom was ever likely to open it. Except for that one Christmas outing, the door had never opened except when the bear was fed or the shed cleaned, and when Richard opened it the bear ambled forward, expecting to be fed. Richard pushed past and went to where the extreme end of the chain was hooked over the slanting nail. Even on tiptoe he could not reach it, so he turned back, and, exerting all his strength, pressed the hook which held the other end of the chain to a ring in the bear's collar. The chain fell free,

into the soiled straw on the floor, and Richard realised that now he
had no means of leading the animal up to the kitchen door as he
intended, to cry, "Come and watch, Uncle Tom," and demonstrate
his disproof of the old man's statement, "He wouldn't do it for
you." But he was undismayed; so long as the bear stayed on all
fours—which he would do until the whistle sounded—his collar
was within reach of Richard's hand; he could be hauled along by
the collar.

Owd Muscovy had never before, since his remote forgotten cub
days, been free of both chain and muzzle at the same time. Without
them he felt, not liberated, but strangely vulnerable. Children he
knew and hated, they tweaked and pinched and poked. Against
them Pert Tom was his defence, and now here he was, stripped of
his appurtenances, at close quarters with a child, and no Pert Tom
in sight. When Richard attempted to take his collar, he backed
away nervously but with a warning growl, and when Richard hung
on, tugging determinedly, it was nervousness rather than vice that
made him bite. His teeth closed on the child's forearm and, through
the sound woollen stuff of his sleeve, inflicted only two incised
wounds. But the blood sprang and the yell which Richard let out
was a yell of pain as well as wrath. He loosed his hold on the bear's
collar and ran to find Nancy. Owd Muscovy made no move to
pursue him, nor, though the door stood open, did he immediately
leave the shed; he emerged a little later, just as one of the pack
teams was coming into the yard. The ponies, though weary, were
capable of being thrown into a stampede, one of the pack-whackers
was caught between a frightened pony and a wall and had his
ribs crushed, and added his cries to the general pandemonium.
Dummy's eldest boy was in the loft, pushing hay over the edge of
it into the mangers, ready for the incoming team; he heard the
shouts and the cries. "The Bear," "The Bear's on the rampage,"
and, with a heroism never given its rightful due, jumped into the
manger, fork in hand, jumped from the manger to the stable floor,
and ran out into the yard, where Owd Muscovy, by this time in a
state of panic, had risen on to his hind legs and was doing his
dance in an attempt to placate. Dummy's Jack charged and drove
the pitchfork home into the hairy chest thus exposed; one prong
must have penetrated to the heart, for within a few minutes Owd
Muscovy was dead.

If Richard could have controlled his temper and his tongue, he would have emerged blameless, a victim of the escaped bear, like the clawed pack pony and the man with the crushed ribs; but, his wound smeared with tar and his pain deadened by a dose of laudanum, he was furious to hear that Owd Muscovy was dead.

"Now he'll never dance for me. And me going to all the trouble to learn the right tunes."

Pert Tom, inconsolable at the loss of his bear, which he had hated, exploited, cherished, and loved, all at once, said, "You! Thass it. You let him out, you little hellion!"

Martin said, "Tom. Mind your tongue!"

"Bugger my tongue! You let him out, didn't you? You opened the shed door."

"Bugger my tongue," said Richard, enjoying the sound of a new, attractive phrase. "I wanted him to dance for me, but he bit me instead."

"There you are," said Pert Tom. "Straight from his own mouth. He opened that door. So Owd Muscovy, the one thing I ever owned, is dead, just a lump of stinking carrion. Go on, sit there making your goddamn faces at me. Look what you've got, a great flourishing business, ships on the sea, and who knows what. Where'd it all come from? Something so dark and dishonest you never could say where. Had to pretend it was my savings. My bitch had to be bedded here and there, out on the hard ground mostly, yours gets a wedding and is called Mistress, and finely she served you. But you get this . . ." he flung his hand in Richard's direction, "and he go and let out my bear. So he's dead, my Owd Muscovy."

"Nancy, take Richard to bed," Martin said.

"I don't want to go to bed."

"You see," said Pert Tom. "Thass like the Bible say: 'If these things be done in the green leaf, what shall be done in the dry?' You see how he hev the upper hand of everybody here. You mind what his mother was. You're making a fine rod for your own back, and I only hope I live to see it beat you."

And so, in the end, Martin had realised that Richard must be tamed. And so, here he was, having put Peter Priest through his paces, saying, "What I want is for you to teach my boy."

Peter Priest's vision of a quiet, clerkly life vanished, leaving behind it a sense of loss so sharp that it hurt.

He said sourly, "I couldn't teach him. Nobody could. To teach a child you must be his master."

"That," said Martin, "is what you would be."

"And the first time I punished, or even chided him, he would run to you, wailing, and you would turn yourself inside out to make things right for him." He rose from his seat. "Thank you, no! Three hundred days a year in this part of the country the wind blows from the east, but I would rather walk into the teeth of it, running the ponies who can be beaten if needs be."

"Richard can be beaten—if needs be, but not over the head."

"Beaten. The young Master of the Old Vine?"

"How else could he learn?"

"How else indeed? Well, well. Even you, at last, come to the end of your indulgence and hand over! What do you wish him to learn?"

"To read what is written and write what can be read. To reckon, as you now did, in his head, and write down his reckonings in figures Roman or Arabic." Without intending it, his voice, as he said those words, took on a sardonic note.

"You see," said Peter Priest, "already you are against me. And what the parent is against how shall the child learn? The figuring, Roman or Arabic, are not terms of mockery, as you in your ignorance make them sound. I can slave out my guts teaching him, and you, with a few mocking words over the supper dish, can undo all I have taught him. I will stick to the ponies. You send him to school. From school he can't come running to cry and show his stripes."

Martin said, with a black look, "Sit down. Stick to the ponies, you say. Whose? Not mine. I can go to the town gates tomorrow morning and find a dozen pack-whackers. And, maybe not tomorrow morning, but some morning not so far away, I can find Richard a teacher. You have your choice, teach him, or take your foot in your hand and leave the Old Vine. If you teach him, I promise that, so long as you do not hit him over the head, what you do will be right with me."

"Why so shrewd about hitting over the head?"

"Once, long ago, when I was young, I had some lessons. And to be hit on the head made me more stupid."

"What would you pay me?"

"Twice your present wage. And you would live in the house, in comfort. I planned to build two rooms above the solar." He remembered the way in which Peter had asked about the figuring and added solemnly, "Meanwhile, you would have time to renew your learning and get the dirt out of your hands. Also you should have some garment more suited to your new position."

Peter Priest gave him a look of unadulterated hatred and said, "That could be seen to."

From that day onwards Peter Priest did no manual work at all; he would not even help with the building of the new rooms above the solar or the stairway that led up to them. He told Martin, arrogantly, that he would need books, and to buy books cost money. Martin asked how much he required, and Peter named a sum which made Martin gasp.

"By that reckoning a book costs as much as a pack pony."

"Why not? Ponies breed their young. A new book may mean a year's hard work for a scribe."

"The priest who once taught me carried his learning in his head," Martin protested, less from meanness than from his dislike of Peter Priest's tone.

"And he taught you so well that, when it comes to passing on what you learned, you hire another man to do it for you."

"Buy what you need," Martin said.

On the day when lessons were to start he was careful to be absent; he would be away four days, he said. Nancy had her instructions, and at the given time called Richard in from the yard, smoothed his hair with her hand, gave him a handful of currants, and told him to go up the new stairs to Peter Priest's room.

"What for?"

"You'll see when you get there, my poor lamb."

Munching the currants and licking his fingers, Richard marched up the stairs. The door of Peter's room stood open and just by the window was a table spread with unfamiliar objects. Peter had sent for him to show him something, just as the men about the yard would call and say, "Master Richard, look, I've found a young owl," or, "Master Richard, Peg's dropped her foal, like to see it?"

Richard walked over to the table without noticing that behind him Peter closed the door and shot the top bolt.

"What's this?" he demanded.

"Don't touch anything. Come here and wash your hands. And in future always come to me with clean hands."

Richard looked at the bowl of water.

"Nancy washed me this morning."

"Nancy washed me this morning," repeated Peter in a cruel mockery of the childish treble voice. "A great boy almost seven years old. Wash your hands and dry them thoroughly."

"I shan't. I didn't come here to wash!" He swung round and made for the door.

"You come here to take lessons. And the very first lesson is unquestioning obedience."

"Open this door," yelled Richard, having found the door bolted and the bolt just out of reach. "Peter, do you hear me? *Open this door!*"

Peter Priest walked up behind him, encircled him with his left arm, hoisted him from his feet, and brought his right hand down on the little backside thus exposed, once, twice, thrice, with a will.

"That," he said calmly, "is for saying 'shan't' to me."

Richard roared from pain and insult.

"Stop that. Stop it at once," said Peter Priest and shook him, until from sheer breathlessness he hushed the noise.

"Now come here and sit down." He pushed the boy towards the table and down into a chair. Richard jumped up at once.

"I don't want to. I'm going to Nancy. She's making me some gingerbread men and I . . ."

"You will have no gingerbread men, nor any other goody, until you know your letters, so you'd better listen carefully."

When he could repeat all the letters of the alphabet without prompting and recognise ten of them without hesitation, Peter Priest said, "That will do for today," and opened the door and let him go.

For today! There would never be another day like this! Never again would he enter old Peter Priest's horrible room.

Next morning, well before lesson time, he went towards the stables, intending to take his pony and be miles away before Nancy could even wonder where he was.

Peter was waiting for him in the dim stable.

"I anticipated some such trick," he said, and took Richard, not by the hand, or the arm, but by the ear. It really hurt, and, pulling away, jumping about, and trying to kick at Peter's shins only made it hurt worse.

Upstairs in the hated room, Peter Priest said, "I am now going to beat you for putting me to so much bother. You will have six stripes today. Tomorrow, if you repeat this idiotic performance, it will be eight and the next day ten."

He laid on the stripes dispassionately, enough to hurt, not hard enough to cause injury, and then, putting aside the little cane, asked in a conversational tone, "I wonder how much you remember of yesterday's lesson. Let us see."

Richard, snuffling, said, "You just *wait* till my father comes home!"

"We will wait. Meanwhile, let us see how much you remember."

When Martin rode into the yard Richard was waiting for him, and he was hardly out of the saddle before the tale of woe began. The child had already witnessed the collapse of one small world. Mary and Nancy, though they petted him and spoke pityingly, had put up no real defence against Peter, and Peter had managed at every turn to outwit him. Even when he had rushed straight out the house before breakfast and hidden himself at the very back of the woolshed, Peter had found him—and that was ten strokes with the cane. The one thing that had sustained him was the certainty that when his father came home and heard of all this mistreatment, he would take full vengeance.

His father actually asked only one question, "Were you beaten over the head?"

"Why, no. He beat me here," said Richard, rubbing his sore seat.

"Then," said Martin, "he was only doing what I told him."

Quite slowly—because this could not be taken in all at once—the rest of the world began to quiver and crumble.

"You mean you *told* old Peter Priest to beat me, and lock me in and not let me have any gingerbread?"

Martin looked at the angry, handsome little face. Going on for seven years old; and if Stephen had lived to that age no doubt he'd have been picking wool alongside Kate and never have known what gingerbread tasted of.

Stiffened by that thought, he said, "Yes. He only did those things because you were naughty and disobedient, and would not learn."

So, there lay the world in ruin.

Slowly Richard said, "But I did learn. I know my alphabet, backwards and forwards, and when Peter draws the letters I can name them. Tomorrow I am going to draw them, too."

Martin's mind had done its familiar *volte face*, remember Stephen, feel guilty, pet Richard.

"There's my good boy," he said heartily. "And now come and see what I've brought you."

Never again, as long as he was in the schoolroom, did Richard give Peter Priest cause for anything but the mildest verbal rebuke. This fact Peter attributed—not without reason—to his own first firm handling. Richard became a good scholar, a little too studious indeed for Martin's liking.

Youthful resilience survived the shock of those four horrible days, but deep down the damage remained. The spoilt, arrogant little boy grew into a youth more than averagely handsome, talented, charming, a little too eager to please, more than a little lacking in self-confidence. The lack was not obvious and did not show itself in any physical way of slouch or stutter. Transmitting Martin's orders, his voice had the almost genuine ring of authority. He knew the business thoroughly and before he was twenty had made several visits to the wool-buying centres of the Low Countries. Yet even Martin could never deceive himself into thinking that the boy's heart was in the business. It was difficult to say where it did lie, with his books and his lute, perhaps.

The solar was furnished and in use now, Richard spent his evenings there and Martin tried to, but somehow he could never settle there for long, he'd get up and make some excuse for going into the yard or to the office, or even to bed. And as he retreated he would sometimes think that Richard's lute-playing in the big room sounded lonely. What the boy needed, of course, was a wife.

Not—and this thought always followed hard on the other—not a Baildon girl, Martin hoped; there were, after all, plenty of other places to choose from; and he would devise a trip for Richard, to Colchester, to Kelvedon, overseas again. And when the boy came home Martin's "Well, how did things go?" held an interest not entirely concerned with the business that had been the reason for the journey. Richard never had anything except business to report upon.

Presently he was twenty-four, and sometime during the following spring Martin spoke the words outright.

"Don't you think it's time you thought about getting married?"

Then, though neither of them saw it, the flaw in his confidence showed itself. Richard smiled his charming, rather secret smile and said, "I think I shall never marry. You see, I know the girl I want, and her parents would never allow her to marry me."

Everything tough and aggressive in the elder man rose to that challenge.

"We'll see about that," he said. "Who is she?"

Part Three

ANNE BLANCHFLEUR'S TALE

I

On the morning when the whole course of my life changed, Mother and I were in our hall, busily contriving to make a new dress for me out of one of her old ones. In its day it had been a fine garment, but its day was long past. There were many threadbare places and the colours had faded. Our task was made the more difficult by the fact that, at sixteen, I already topped Mother by half a head.

"But there is a hem," Mother said, with her eternal optimism. "We'll let it down and hang it in the sun and it'll fade all over alike, I have no doubt."

The hem came down, showing the stuff in its original colours, green and crimson, in a sprawling, all-over pattern. Elsewhere the green had rusted, the crimson had faded until they were almost alike.

Mother saw me look glumly at it and said, "So long as you are tidy the *shabbier* you are the better. Your Aunt Astallon will take pity on you, I trust, and buy you a new gown."

Only by biting my lip hard could I hold back the sharp retort, words no girl should speak to her mother, especially one so kind and indulgent as mine. My Aunt Astallon was as likely to give me a new gown as she was to jump in the river, or walk out barefoot in the snow. But my mother had lived on hope—and hope alone—for so long that she could no longer distinguish between the likely and the unlikely. My father, though less resolutely cheerful, was well-nigh as feckless, and the wonder was, not that we should have fallen so low, as that we should, somehow, have managed as well as we did.

While I bit my lip and scowled we heard a horseman ride into the yard. Minsham Old Hall, as our place was called, was very old, built for defence, not for living in, and the only windows were set high in the walls and narrow. Mother had to hop on a stool to look out.

"I declare," she said, "it's Martin Reed again! What can he be wanting now?"

"The same as last time—his money," I said; and I intended no joke. Mother laughed, however.

"Poor silly man," she said; and hopped down and picked up the dress and gave it a shake.

Master Reed was the man who owned the sheep run near us. Once all the acres had gone with the Old Hall, but they had been sold away, years before we went to live in the house. Our few acres and Master Reed's sheep run were quite separate, and to reach his part and his shepherd's hut he had no need to come into our yard. For a long time after we moved into the house he was just a name to us, and then one day he had come, walking quickly for all that he limped, and asked Mother if she would, as a favour, heat a tar bucket for him. The shepherd he had then was ill or idle or runaway—I never bothered to hear the whole of it—and he'd come out to find several of his sheep flyblown. He'd found the tar bucket in the fence which was nearer our house than to the shepherd's hut and had run to ask Mother to lend him her fire for ten minutes.

Mother, of course, had been obliging, and while the tar warmed and he stirred it, she had stood by him talking about sheep. Mother could talk about almost everything, she'd had such a crowded life, moving about from place to place and always taking interest. She'd learned quite a lot about sheep when she was staying with her Uncle Bowdegrave at Abhurst in Kent, where the sheep were quite different from those in Suffolk, she said.

Stirring away at his tar, Master Reed shot her a look and said, "That's right, ma'am; shorter legs and blunter heads."

Then, his tar melted, he picked up his bucket and hurried away with the briefest of thanks.

But about three days later, when I was alone in the house, my father and mother having been asked to dine with the Fennels at Ockley, Master Reed came to our door and handed in a bundle of cloth, very fine, blue in colour. He said, and I remembered the exact words to tell Mother:

"I don't like to be in debt. I borrowed your fire the other day. I hope this will be accepted as payment."

There was someone with him, sitting astride one horse and holding the other. I gave him no heed. To Master Reed I said, "But I am sure my mother would not wish for payment for so small a thing."

But he pushed the blue cloth towards me, and I remembered that my brother Godfrey—at that moment milking the cow—was being fitted out to go to our cousin Fortescue. So I made my curtsey and said:

"I thank you kindly, and so will my mother, though there was no need." But, handling the good cloth, I thought it would make a fine cloak for Godfrey. I had already started my round of visits to great houses and rich relatives and knew how important clothes could be.

The blue cloth made Godfrey a cloak, but three years later, when he must cease to be a page and become a squire, he needed another and more expensive outfit. And it was then that it occurred to my parents to ask Master Reed for a loan.

In fairness to my father I must say that when he borrowed he did have expectations. (Expectations have been our downfall.) Father's Uncle Dawnay was, at that moment, on his deathbed, and so far as we knew Father was his only kin. However, Uncle Dawnay, who had been a jovial sinner all his life, became frightened on his deathbed and willed everything he had to a Chantry, where Masses are being said for his soul to this day. (Mother, when she heard the sad news, said, "But I'd have prayed for him, night and day without ceasing if he'd left the money to us!" Then she'd laughed and added, "Of course I shouldn't, I should have been too busy spending it!")

Our debt to Master Reed was never paid, and on the May morning when he rode into our yard it was over three years old.

Our windows were not glazed—and never would be—so presently we could hear my father's hearty booming voice greeting the woolmaster, and Master Reed's gruff tones. We could hear the two voices, but not the words. Mother listened for a moment, her head on one side, then she said happily:

"They don't *sound* cross. We'd better try this on. An empty dress hangs longer than a full one."

I put on the dress and she walked all round me, looking at it critically.

"Oh dear, you need every inch of the hem down. We shall have to face up the inside. What with, I wonder? Something the same weight or it won't hang right." Then, to cheer herself, "We could *dag* the sleeves, Anne. Dagging is very fashionable, and it would cut away some of that worn edge."

You would have thought that the remaking of that old gown was the only thing in the world that mattered. With the wool-man in the yard, demanding his just due.

Presently we heard the horse trot away, and after a minute Father came in. He had his favourite hawk, Jess, on his wrist and he stroked her as he went towards her perch, transferred her onto it, and fastened the chain. Then he pulled off his glove and stood slapping it against his leg and looking at me as though he had never seen me before. I imagined it was the effect of the dress and hoped that perhaps it was not as ill-becoming as I had feared. Then he said:

"I want a word with your mother." I gathered up the long dress and went to the stairs. They ran up alongside the wall and were made of stone and had no handrail. At the top was a gallery, with the floor so rotted that you had to mind where you trod, and behind the gallery one big room had been partitioned into three. I couldn't hurry, and before I reached the room which I shared with my sister Isabel I heard Father say:

"That fellow Reed has just made me an amazing proposition." I was curious to know what it was, so I just stepped out of sight, leaving the door wide, and listened. ". . . wants Anne for his son, Richard. He's prepared to make a substantial settlement and cancel the debt."

Mother gave a sort of yelp; there is no other word for it. She sounded just like a dog that has had its paw trodden on.

"The saucy upstart! I trust you sent him off with a flea in his ear."

"Why, no. I said I'd think it over. Talk it over with you." She must have scowled, for he asked, in a surprised way, "You mislike the idea?"

"Mislike? Mislike? He must be mad to have thought of it. And you must be mad to have carried it to me. We've come low, Mary pity us! But not so low as that." Her words began to come out jerkily, and I knew she was throwing her arms about as she did when excited. "Look where you will, through the length and breadth of the land, and you won't find a girl with better blood in her veins. On both sides. Blanchfleur, Bowdegrave, Astallon,

Dawnay, Fortescue. *And,* don't forget my grandmother of Ramsey, Royal Saxon. And you'd put my daughter to bed with the wool-master's son. You should be ashamed."

"I didn't bed them. I only said I'd think it over."

"These jumped-up merchants with their new money, they think they can buy anything. If you wish to please me, Blanchfleur, get on your horse and ride after him and tell him my daughter is not for sale."

"I should never catch him," Father said truthfully. "Besides, perhaps Anne . . ."

"You are crazed," Mother said. "Since when have wenches ordered their affairs or been asked for an opinion. Up and after him. Tell him to buy his great silly son a wife where he buys his fleeces. My daughter is not for sale."

She had fallen in love with that phrase.

"The man spoke modestly and not in huckstering fashion. He said he knew the difference in their estates. I don't think he was in full favour . . . but the boy saw Anne once and fell in love."

"Fell in love," Mother repeated with great scorn. "The wool merchants now must fall in love—aping their betters. What next? They'll be riding in tourneys, I suppose."

"Wool merchants have been knighted. . . ."

"That's enough," Mother said. "Will you ride after him and give him his answer or must I?"

"You never even heard his offer," Father said. But the words were a requiem for something dead and done with, not a renewal of live argument. In a minute he would be on his old horse, and, though it might be suppertime before he reached Baildon, when he got there he would give the answer that Mother sent.

I rushed out on to the gallery and cried, "Wait."

They stared up at me. I went halfway down the stairs and stopped. Standing high made me feel bolder.

"He sets some value on me, which is more than anyone else does," I said.

"I should box your ears," Mother said. "Listening in corners! And what do you know about values? You have never had a chance. You're only just sixteen. . . ."

"And I've been on offer for *years.* Who is her father? Good! Who was her mother? Good again! *What is her dower?* How many times have I been passed over for some snippet with teeth like a rabbit's and two good manors? I'm sick of it. And another aunt saying I spoke when I should have been silent, or looked up when I should have looked down. Blaming me for what I can't help."

Every one of the shames and humiliations that I had suffered in four years came back, as burning and hurtful as in the moment when they happened. Rage made me feel as though I were drunken.

"It is the same with Godfrey," I declared. "Why wasn't he knighted when he'd served his three years? For one reason only. A knight needs equipment, and you couldn't and Uncle Fortescue wouldn't lay out the cost. He'll spend his life polishing other men's mail and waiting, just as you would have me wait for something that never comes. And I will wait no more, I will marry the woolman's son."

"I will box your ears. You are out of your mind. That a daughter of mine . . ."

"Yes," I said. I could feel the sneer curl my mouth as I thrust out one foot and held it clear of the stair. "Saxon royal blood in my veins! And what on my feet?"

It was a little unjust. For my last visit—to my Aunt Bowdegrave—I had been provided with shoes, but I had outgrown them and passed them on to Isabel. For my forthcoming visit to Aunt Astallon I have no doubt Mother would have procured me some shoes, somehow, from somewhere, but at the moment I had a peasant's footwear, a roughly shaped wooden sole, with cloth nailed around it and tied in a bundle round the ankle.

"They are only makeshift," Mother said.

"Our whole lives are makeshift, and pretence, and believing what isn't true."

As soon as I said that I was smitten with compunction. With their faces tilted up towards me and wearing such shocked helpless expressions, my parents looked like two children, who had been playing happily that they kept house, and a grownup had come along and kicked over their make-believe furniture and said that the game was silly and unreal.

Father shifted his eyes and looked at Mother, waiting for her to strike, as it were, the next note in the tune. Every time I came back home—my eye made sharp by absence—I noticed that her ascendancy had increased; his movements, speech, and impulses were all slowing down, she was just as quick and positive and vehement as ever. This morning though, for once, she was at a loss, and looked as though she might cry. Upset by that, Father lashed himself into a rage and shouted at me.

"You're overripe, my girl; that's what ails you. You're ready for a roll in the hay with the pig-man." Whether he intended to or not he had forestalled Mother's tears. She rounded on him.

"Pig-man indeed. What a thing to say to your own daughter. Didn't her Aunt Bowdegrave complain of her prudery? And quite right too. A maid should be modest."

I said, "I shall marry the wool-man's son, who has made me an honest offer, or I shall go to the one aunt I have not yet visited— my aunt at Ramsey, and be a nun."

I then turned on the stair and made to go up, but I had forgotten the long gown, caught my foot in it, and fell to my knees.

From the hall below Mother wailed, "Saints have mercy. Nothing is more unlucky than to fall upstairs."

Where, I wonder, did that superstition have its origin? I can see that to spill salt, or to break a looking glass is in itself a misfortune, since both are valuable, and the glass at least hard to replace. But to fall upstairs . . .

Anyway, I had more important matters to think about. I had held over my parents the only threat that a girl could hold; from any other decision they could beat me off, by argument or force if needs be, but once a girl had declared her intention of taking the veil they would be hardy parents indeed who tried to stop her. My great fear, when I came to think things over, was that my parents might take me at my word, steadfastly refuse to let me get married, and so force me into the convent. Little as I liked my present way of life, I should like that of a religious less, especially at Ramsey, where my aunt, the Abbess, was very strict in keeping to the rules of the order. I had seen her once, at a wedding, and even on such an occasion when most nuns disregarded all the rules, she held to her habit, wore no jewels, ate sparingly. To be a nun at Ramsey was to be a nun indeed.

I began to wish I had never spoken those rash words; yet, when, some hours later, Mother climbed the stairs and came and sat on my bed and asked did I really mean what I had said, I replied with a firmness that astonished myself.

"Yes. The wool-man's son is the only one who has ever made me a serious offer of marriage; I suspect he is the only one who ever will. Unless I take it, I shall go to Ramsey."

"In which case," she said, pulling a sorry face, "we should see you seldom or never. Baildon is within reach, even with such poor horses as we can afford."

I said nothing.

"Anne, to please me, try once more. Go to your Aunt Astallon—it will be different this time; her own girls are married and gone. She could give you more mind. And you're prettier, you grow prettier every day. You have everything, except a dower. You'll make a good match, yet."

I stayed silent. And at last she said, "Oh, if only things had been different. . . ."

Upon that I almost broke down, thinking what her life had been. My father was the youngest son of a youngest son of a great family; he had, therefore, connections, ambitions, and military obligations without anything to support or forward them. His one hope was to have married an heiress, instead he married my mother who was, if anything, even more highly connected, but one of several daughters and but modestly dowered. For years, however, the insecurity of his position had not been evident; he was a good man in the lists in time of peace, a good soldier in time of war. Trailing his family after him, as a kite drags its tail, he had moved from castle to castle, from great manor to great manor, riding in tourneys, supporting this lord and that in their petty squabbles, making war on the Scots, and on the Welsh, cheerful good company always, Sir Godfrey Blanchfleur, most admirable knight-errant. Mother had borne seven children and four had died before she had a bed to call her own. We had all been born in different places, grand, high-sounding places, Beauclaire, Abhurst, Rivington, even Windsor, but Godfrey was thirteen, I was nine, and Isabel was three before we had a settled home, and that came about by accident.

Father was unhorsed in a tournament at Winchester, and fell on his head, denting his helmet so that it could not be removed in the usual way. They say that he was unhurt, rose unaided, and walked from the tourney ground to a forge where an unhandy smith, in hammering off the helm, damaged his skull. He lay like the dead for four days and when he finally rose from his bed his days as a fighting man were done. His left arm and leg, though whole and uninjured, had lost power, were weak and heavy; and he was slow, even in his speech.

He was no whit less cheerful, quite confident that somebody

would arrange something for him. And somebody did. One of my mother's Bowdegrave cousins owned Minsham Old Hall and the few poor acres that had been left when the rest were sold for a sheep run. The house had stood empty for some time and was so old-fashioned and comfortless that nobody wanted it.

The sad thing was that there was just enough land to have supported us, had it been properly handled; and my brother Godfrey, most sternly sensible always, would have *tried*. The life we had led, flitting from place to place, had aged him; he belonged nowhere and had found his own company, often with working people who at thirteen are men. He would have looked after cows and pigs and tilled the few acres. But no! He must follow the pattern, go to be a page, then a squire, and finally a knight. I have no doubt that his life had been as full of humiliation as mine.

I had started my round at the age of twelve, going from cousin to aunt, from aunt to cousin-by-marriage, to learn manners, to learn dancing, to learn to play the lute, to learn to embroider. One day one of my powerful rich relatives was supposed to take a rich young man by the ear and say, "Marry this girl." But there was no man so rich that he did not look for a bride with a dowry. And also there was, at that time, a curious dying out in the old families, so that in many of them there were no sons, only daughters who thus became great heiresses. Once, at Beauclaire—I remember this so sharply—there was a little creature, Catharine Montsorrel, so ugly, so mis-shapen that I pitied her. But somewhere near Chester a man could get on a good horse and ride for three days around the boundaries of one of her properties, and out by the Welsh marches another man, on another good horse, could ride for six days. So she got married from Beauclaire and I did not. My failure was, in a way, the failure of the relative with whom I had stayed, and of course excuses must be made. I was sent home with the report that I had two fatal defects, a sharp tongue and a prim manner.

I will say for my mother that she never took these things seriously as most women would. Many another girl, sent home with such a character, would have been scolded, beaten, had the shame of her failure rubbed into her every day.

So now looking back, all in a moment, over Mother's life, and mine, so far, I felt kindly and weak towards her.

"If things had been different, they would have *been* different," I said. "But they are as they are. This man Reed is well-to-do and we owe him money. He said he would cancel the debt. That in itself is a thing to consider."

Mother clenched her little fist—she had beautiful, delicate hands which no amount of work could spoil—and beat upon the bed.

"You are not," she said fiercely, "to think of that. I said to your father . . . but for the debt he would never have dared. . . . You don't know the world, Anne. Poor we have been, but you have never been brought face to face—I mean to talk to, to be with—any man who hadn't . . . who wasn't . . ." She broke off, threw her hands about. "Chivalry," she said, snatching at the word like a drowning man at the straw in the proverb. "To know what good manners are—even if he doesn't always exercise them—that is the mark of a gentleman."

"Uncle Fortescue once dragged my aunt upstairs by the hair of her head, in the sight of all, and broke the jaw of the young squire who protested," I said quietly, as though speaking to myself. Mother blushed her quick bright blush.

"There was reason for that."

"Unmannerly just the same."

"That may be. But," said Mother, wagging a finger at me, "I'll warrant that none in that hall knew *why*, his real reason, I mean. And there is just the difference. He might pull her hair, but he did not besmirch her name as a common man in a rage would have done."

"I shall be careful," I said, getting back to the point, "to behave in such a manner as to give my common man, as you call him, no occasion either to pull my hair or besmirch my name."

"Marriage lasts a long time," said Mother dryly. "Suppose you never grow to like him, or tire of him, and he of you. Then where would you turn? To some blabbermouth apprentice who would boast when he was pot-valiant? Oh," she said, jumping from the bed and beginning to wave her arms, "these are not things to say to a young maid, yet they must be said. In a proper household such things are understood, arranged, there is constant change, comings and goings, blind eyes turned, allowances made."

"And ladies dragged upstairs by their hair."

Mother, like a skilled fencer, ceased her pressure at that point, and attacked from another angle.

"I can't see you as a nun at Ramsey. You may expect no favour from your aunt, if anything she will be harder on you than on the others out of her wish to be fair. You love your comforts, and are greedy, and vain. You have no vocation, which alone could make such a life bearable."

She had put into words what I had been thinking, and inwardly I wavered. But I said, "Add to my failings that I am proud. I cannot go to my Aunt Astallon again, and be looked over and passed by; and have them say, 'Let me see, how old are you now?' and have them nod and pull their mouths down. At least at Ramsey I should have no cause for shame."

"There's another thing," said Mother, flitting like a butterfly. "Think how it will sound, to send to all the family and say that you are to marry the son of a wool-man. Is that not shaming?"

"Not in the same way. Besides, why should they be told? Except when one of us is being foisted off on them they forget that we exist. We might starve to death for all they care. They're afraid to visit us for fear their hearts should be wrung. Aunt Astallon went to Walsingham, missing us by four miles, did she turn aside? No, she rode on and lodged at Sudbury. Uncle Bowdegrave visits Rushbrooke every year, when did he ever give a sign of being within riding distance?"

These were truths, facts, which my parents had steadily refused to recognise. Now, confronted with them, Mother seemed to shrink a little.

"Anne," she said, "you're very hard."

But it wasn't true. Seeing my point pierce her last defence, I was filled with pity and weakness. I really longed to cry out that I had not meant what I said, that I would go to my Aunt Astallon and try once more. But something held back the words. I was sick of pretending.

"I shall tell your father that you are set in your mind," Mother said.

Father, always three-quarters in favour of the match, rode off to Baildon to tell Master Reed his offer was being considered, but that, before any conclusion was reached, Mother wished to inspect the young man. Master Reed invited them both to supper. So the hem of the green and crimson gown had to be stitched back into place and the seams let out instead of taken in. Wearing it, and a very wide wired head-veil, she went off to Baildon and came back in a very curious state of mind.

I asked her the one question which troubled me most.

"Is he surly, like his father?"

Mother lifted off the headdress and ran her hands through her hair.

"He's not in the least like his father." To me that was pleasant news, but she said it regretfully.

My father fumbled in his pouch and brought out a little lump of pink, undercooked meat and offered it to Jess on her stand.

"If you married that boy, you'd have a very comfortable home," he said.

"If?" I asked.

Mother said sharply, "My mind is not yet decided. And when it is I shall take my time telling them so. *I'm* not one to fall on my face at the sight of a few silver cups, a glass window, and a great tapestry that still smells of the loom."

"It was well meant," Father said. "They wanted us to see that . . ." He cast a look about our comfortless hall and grinned. "Four main dishes, then gooseberries in a glazed coffer, and a syllabub that you could have turned upside down without spilling, it was so well whipped."

"I was ashamed of *you*," said Mother, "pocketing a piece as though you feared to be hungry on the way home!"

"I told the boy—what's his name, Richard—that it was for my hawk. He was knowledgeable, though he has never handled a bird. Said he had read a book."

"What did *you* think of him, Father?"

"A modest, amiable young man. And if he was some poor knight's son that had gone into the wine trade, your mother would think so too."

I suspected that they had argued all the way home.

"There's a difference between trading in wine and handling dirty old fleeces," Mother said.

"But the man was at pains to point out that the boy never soiled his hands. . . ."

"That I can well believe!" It was plain to me that something had happened to upset her and bring her to the brink of deciding against the match after all.

Presently Father went outside and I signed to Isabel to go to bed, which she did reluctantly. As soon as we were alone Mother got up and went over to the livery cupboard and began banging about in it. Our livery cupboard was never well provided at any time, and she couldn't be hungry, having come straight from a supper of four main courses, pie, and syllabub, so I could only guess that she wanted to keep her back to me. But why? After a minute I could bear it no more.

"You didn't like Richard Reed?"

"There's nothing about him to like or dislike. Truly, Anne, I'd be more at ease if you were . . . if it was a question of marrying the father, old as he is."

"Why?"

"He's a man. There's something about him. You could see that he was being civil, for the boy's sake; he wanted us to take to the idea and know you'd be . . . well looked after. But in his heart, he didn't care; he thinks he's doing *us* a favour!" This, which she should have mentioned with irritated scorn, she brought out as though it were admirable. "The boy's grown up in his shadow, pampered, made much of, never had to shift for himself. You'd have the upper hand of him in no time."

I thought what an astonishing thing to say—in that *complaining* manner!

"Would that be so bad?"

She flung something into the cupboard and turned round.

"Yes. No woman can be happy with a man she can master."

I suppose what I thought showed plain on my face.

"Ah, but we weren't always this way," she cried. "Not this way at all. Why, I've sat amongst the other women and looked down as Blanchfleur rode by, and he'd look up and I'd go hot and cold and almost choke with pride because I belonged to him and he was the strongest, boldest . . ." She gave a little shiver and hugged herself with her arms. "You were nearly born on the road. We were at Rivington and he said, 'I'm off to Beauclaire in the morning.' Just like that, and I knew I'd be in the straw next day or the one after, and I knew that if I let him go alone there were plenty at Beauclaire that would be glad to see him ride in by himself. So I said, 'I'm coming too.' And he said, 'D'you think you'll hold together so far?' And I said, 'I shall hold together so long as I have to.' And I did. And he liked me the better for it. That was the time Lady Warwick threw him her glove—but he wore mine for all to see."

There was something—even after all those years—so triumphant in her voice that it made me feel as I sometimes did when trumpets blew. She spoke of what I understood; I had so often sat in the humble back seats of the Ladies' Gallery and watched the knights ride by, saluting the ladies who threw them favours. I'd dreamed of one day having a knight of my own. . . .

I put that thought away.

"Richard has been under his father's thumb," I said. "You shouldn't judge from one visit."

"It isn't in any way what I want for you, or what you should have. Anne, if you'll try once more. I'll persuade your father to sell Jess and you shall have a brand-new gown."

"I will marry Richard Reed and have two new gowns."

How long these arguments and this indecision would have lasted I do not know. My Uncle Bowdegrave, staying at Rushbrooke, helped to clinch the matter, by, for once, remembering his poor relatives and sending us a haunch of venison.

Mother looked at it calculatingly and said, "Now, if we were proceeding with this business, we could ask the Reeds to supper. It won't keep, so we must make up our minds."

"You know mine," I said.

"And mine." That was Father, speaking quite firmly.

"Well, only the Virgin knows when next I shall have meat in the house for five people. I think you're being a stubborn, hasty, foolish girl and I only hope you won't live to regret it."

So she capitulated and Richard and I met.

I I

Within a few minutes of our meeting I was certain that Mother's slighting remarks about Richard were due to prejudice, and perhaps a little to jealousy. He was such a very handsome young man, and so elegant, with a charming smile and the nicest manners in the world. I think my heart went out to him at once, just as I thought that if only he'd had breeding *how* Mother would have praised him, and said I was lucky. And what is breeding after all, largely a matter of money and land and staying in one place long enough to establish a name and a family; or pleasing the King and getting some honour conferred on you. I'll warrant that if Richard could have gone to Westminster, calling himself by some Norman French name and played his lute, he would have pleased the King so much that he would have been knighted straight-away.

Old Master Reed was lame of one leg and had grown crooked, as well as solid with the years; his face was weathered and deeply lined, he looked as though he had been too busy all his life to take much pleasure in anything. Beside his father Richard looked like a young larch side by side with a gnarled old oak.

The supper party was much easier and merrier than I had expected, largely, I think, because Father, when Mother was worrying about having only the one dish, had said, "There are times when wine counts for more than food."

"This is one of them—and we have no wine."

"I'll ride over to Ockley and borrow some."

"Don't say for what reason. Nothing is settled yet."

Sir Stephen Fennel, bless his heart, gave Father some good Rhenish, which made everyone cheerful and unembarrassed; even Mother so far relented as to behave as if Richard were a very eligible suitor who must be charmed. After supper she bade me fetch my lute and play a little. A little is what I played, just as I danced a little, played Nobbin a little, embroidered a little. I had no ear and no talent, but I had mastered four or five pleasing little tunes.

While I played Richard watched me, and I could see that he loved me. I remembered something I had forgotten—Father saying some words about Richard having seen me and would look at no other girl. That had a smack of romance to it, like a minstrel's tales, and as I played I looked back at him under my lashes. Presently he rose and crossed the hall and sat down by my feet, and at the end of my last tune took the lute from me and said:

"Allow me now to play for you, Mistress Anne."

I had never, anywhere, heard anyone play like that. It wasn't just music, it was something more, like being under a spell, so that when it ended you sighed and your spirit settled back into your body again, a little painfully. You could have loved him just for the way he played the lute.

He ended his special music and gave us back our souls and then said, "Now, the tune that everyone knows. Will you sing?"

He struck up "The Pleasant Month of May," and we all began to sing. Under cover of it, Richard said to me, "I saw you once. I thought you were the most lovely lady in the world. Will they let you marry me?"

"They must. They shall. Or I will be a nun."

Afterwards, when more of the wine was being served with some little saffron cakes, Mother came to me and said, "Well. Are you still of the same mind? The old man is pestering your father for an answer."

I could hardly speak for the fullness of my heart. I had made my choice in a blind rage against the way the world had used me, and I had picked this jewel.

After that it was settled, and Mother began seizing every opportunity to send messages to every branch of the family. I could imagine, in all those distant places, relatives of all degrees putting their heads together and agreeing that at last my parents had come to their senses and done something suitable to their estate. In their relief they all sent me gifts of great generosity. Ironically, Mother's remark about my Aunt Astallon giving me a new gown proved to be prophecy, for she sent me enough of the best French velvet for a wedding dress; that inclined me to think that she had been dreading my next visit almost as much as I did. With the gifts came excuses for not making the journeys to bring the families to the wedding, and that was just as well; but the Fortescue cousin in whose household my brother Godfrey languished gave him permission to ride home—hoping no doubt that the wool chandler had a daughter. When Godfrey did arrive, he was leading a pretty grey palfrey, my present from that branch of the family.

The Reeds had no relatives at all, and Master Reed, talking over the wedding with Mother, said that he wanted nobody from Baildon at his son's wedding. But he professed himself willing to provide a feast, so the few guests we had—mainly friends of Father's, who came to see what the poor fellow could find to spread on his board—were vastly and pleasantly surprised.

Martin wore mulberry-coloured velvet, the tunic edged with fur, and the one thing that marred my day was to hear two old men, hawking friends of Father's, muttering about it.

"In my young days nobody less than a knight could wear miniver; and if he tried to it was ripped off and sold for the benefit of the poor."

"Times change."

"So they do, and not for the better."

I hated them for thinking the old days, when someone like Richard mustn't wear miniver fur even if he could afford it, were better than these more enlightened times.

After the feasting was done, Richard, his father, and I rode to Baildon. I was thankful that owing to our circumstances there could be no public bedding. During my various visits to my relatives I had assisted at these grossly indecent rites, and I knew that I should find them agonisingly embarrassing. Yet, when we reached the house which I had never yet seen, and stood uneasily in a small solar, most elegantly furnished, and drank a last stoup of wine from the silver cups which Mother had mentioned, I realised that the public bedding ceremony does serve a purpose. The lewd talk, the thrusting of fertility emblems upon the bride, all the jokes and the laughter and the ducking away from those who try to undress the newly married couple, help to break down the reserve between them, and once they are in bed, with the curtains closed, half the work is done.

If even Master Reed had been a little drunken and hearty and slapped Richard on the back and said, as I have heard fathers say, "Well, boy—to your work!" that would have helped. But he only looked at us, rather sadly, I thought, and raised his cup and said:

"I wish you happy." And when he had drunk his wine he went away; and we were two strangers, left alone.

Then Richard said, as though I were a visitor who had come a great distance, "I expect you are tired. Come."

He did take my hand, however, as we climbed the stairs, and still holding it he led me into a room far more comfortable than any I had ever slept in, for even at Beauclaire, being young and a poor relation, I had always shared one of the worst rooms. He pulled on my hand a little, so that we stood close, and he put his face to mine. We were cheek to cheek.

"You belong to me. I never dreamed it could happen." There was a kind of exultation in his voice, but awe as well. I realised that he was as nervous as I was myself.

"I belong to you and you belong to me," I said. "Are you happy?"

"So happy that I am frightened."

I thought that a strange thing to say, but very touching, too. I put up my hand and pressed it against the other side of his head, forcing our faces closer.

"There is nothing to be frightened about. And if there were, it is I who should be frightened." I said that rallyingly.

He said, almost in a whisper, "I would never do anything to hurt you. Never."

Was it, I wonder, the fear of hurting me that made him fail? He loved me, I loved him, we were both sound and young. . . . But it was no good.

It was an odd circumstance that I, who at Minsham had been so clear-sighted, so contemptuous of all pretence, should change my nature with my name, and wholeheartedly begin to play a game of make-believe. I had not realised that I was so truly the daughter of my parents; here was I, pretending that all was well, pretending that I was a properly married woman, just as Mother always pretended that some day something would happen to restore our fortunes, and Father pretended he was a landed gentleman. I discovered another thing about myself, too, I was hotly passionate. There were times when I felt that out of my own eagerness I could *make* it happen. This time! This time! I would think. Now! Now! Poor Richard, groaning and sweating, as puzzled as I was myself, would eventually fall asleep, and then I would cry, softly, secretly, and rather ashamed. I would accuse myself of being ungrateful, too; for apart from this one thing my new life was wonderful, better than I had ever imagined life could be.

The sheer comfort we enjoyed was a lasting joy and an amazement. People might laugh and sneer about merchants and their new money; they knew how to live, how to build, and how to furnish. There was more warmth and softness at the Old Vine than in Abhurst, Beauclaire, and Rivington rolled into one. As for Minsham Old Hall, I was soon wondering how I had endured the stone floor, the unglazed windows, the draughts that stirred your hair even as you sat by the hearth.

The Old Vine was really two houses, divided by a wide cobbled passage which was entered by a doorway, big enough and high enough, when it was fully open, to allow a pack pony, loaded, to trot in. On the right of this passage was that part of the house which Master Reed had built first and lived in when he was starting his business. Richard took me over it and showed me how it had been. His father had had one room, his Uncle Tom the other, and there had been a kitchen for cooking and that was all. After some years, rooms had been built above all these apartments. One of them had been the room in which Richard had learned his lessons, he said.

Because I loved him, everything about him, back to when he was very young, was interesting to me, and when he pointed to the door and told me that, I was interested to see the room.

"The servants sleep there now. You don't want to look in there," he said.

"I think you hated your lessons," I said teasingly.

"No. After a week I liked my lessons, but I hated my master. Sometimes even now, I dream . . ."

"Oh, so do I. My Aunt Bowdegrave, teaching me to dance, and saying I had two left feet and would never find a husband . . ." I cut that off sharply and said, "I was ten years old." Something that I could never find a name for had made me withhold from Richard all the story of my humiliating youth. I wanted him to desire me, so I must always seem to have been desired. "Little she knew!" I said gaily.

"In those days I used to sleep here," Richard said, moving to the other door. "When Father made the office downstairs, Uncle Tom moved up. He's not my real uncle, but I still call him that. He was Father's partner once. He's bedridden now and a bit . . ." He tapped his head and made a face. "But if you'd like to see him."

"I want to see everything."

Richard opened the door and said, "Uncle Tom. I've brought you a visitor."

The old man in the bed must once have been big and stout, he had shrunken and the flesh hung on his bones in heavy folds. There was a musty, old-man smell in the room, and, added to it, another, even less pleasant, which, as I moved towards the bed, I knew came from a great, badly cured bearskin which lay across the foot of the bed.

Uncle Tom's eyes were bleary and his stare vague at first, but when I was near enough, something quickened in them and he grinned. I'd seen his like before, hobbling old dotards until they catch you behind the screen or in a lonely passage.

"A pretty one, too. Cure for sore eyes, you are, little mistress."

"Thank you," I said; and smiled and for fun bobbed him a curtsey.

"Aye, and better still, saucy."

"Anne is my wife," Richard said, a trifle stiffly I thought.

"Your wife, eh?" That seemed to take a little while to sink in. Then he said, "You're Lucky Dick; allust hev bin. Right from the first. Like your dad. Well . . ." He looked me up and down, and I had a sudden, disconcerting certainty that he knew about us. This going over the house took place on my second or third day there, and the thing was, naturally, still raw and tender, in the forefront of my mind. "See you do right by her," Uncle Tom said. "Make the most of your chance while you can. You shrivel and dry up afore you know where you are."

Richard took hold of my elbow and said, "Come along."

That was the old part of the house.

On the other side of the central passage the rooms were larger and higher. There was the solar, with the window which looked out into a garden, with a plot for herbs, and some fruit trees, and roses. Behind the solar was a dining hall, where, every day, at dinner and supper, we and several of the workmen and apprentices sat down together. Except that it lacked a dais, it was like the hall of a great house. Richard, his father, and I sat at a solid oak table which was never moved; the rest had trestles and boards which could be set up or taken down according to the number of places required. The food served here was good and plentiful and to me delicious; but there were always other dishes, cakes, fruits, and sweetmeats, in the livery cupboard of the solar.

Above the solar and dining hall were the bedrooms of the family.

Across the yard were stables and lofts, the sheds where wool was stored, the "floors" where the fleeces were picked over. There was a smithy, a cow byre, a pigsty and a hen roost, a round house for pigeons, and a pond. Thirty years ago, Richard said, when his father had started, there had been nothing at all, just a field full of old vine stumps. It seemed to me a lot to have built up and set working in thirty years, but that was not all; Master Reed had two ships on the sea, a warehouse in Amsterdam, and, of course, the sheep run at Minsham. He would have been justified in being very proud of his achievement, but I never saw him give any sign of being so. Except that he loved Richard, was kind to me, and apparently faithful to his old partner, he showed very few signs of any emotions; he was never angry, he never laughed, he never seemed to be in a hurry, and he was never ill. Richard said that he was a strict, but just employer. It took me a little time to learn that his settled scowl and silence and sombre looks were not due to ill-humour, and I was always disproportionately pleased if I could coax a smile from him. I often felt a little sorry for him; he worked so hard, every day, from dawn to dusk, just, it seemed, for the sake of working; rather like an old horse at a millwheel or a well, which will go round and round, plodding at the same pace, whether it is being driven or not.

You might have imagined that a man who set such high store by work would have been a hard taskmaster to his son. Nothing was farther from the truth. Mother had said that Richard was under his father's thumb, but it was a most gentle, kindly thumb. "Leave that to me, boy," or "I'll see to it," were words constantly on his lips.

All through that first autumn of my married life, Richard and I just frivolled the time away. We took long rides, went to Bywater—where I saw the sea for the first time—and to Walsingham, and Colchester, Lavenham, Melford, Sudbury, and Clare. Summer died slowly that year, and in the fine warm weather the roads were busy with pilgrims and merchants and the people who made their living by amusing them. These last, the minstrels and tumblers and jugglers, had a fascination for Richard; he would watch them for hours, even make a special journey in the hope of catching up with some particularly pleasing performer again, and seemed actually to envy them. Once he said:

"Not to be tied to any place . . . don't you think that would be pleasant. I've often thought that I should like to take my lute and just set out."

"You play well enough. But it must be a hard life, especially in winter. And not being tied to any place means not belonging anywhere. I know. I spent my childhood moving from place to place. I hated it. I always had to leave something behind." I told him how, once, at Rivington, I had almost tamed a wild cat out of the woods; he was so pretty, striped tawny and grey, with tawny eyes. We must have stayed there for some time, because I had got him to the point where he would come when I called—if I waited long enough—and take meat from my hand, though he never would let me stroke him. At another place I had made a little garden; I'd planted gillyflower seeds and meant to make some gillyflower water and scent myself all over. We moved on when the little green plants were two inches high.

"Poor Anne," Richard said. "You've always wanted to settle. I've always wanted to get away."

"From what?"

"Ah. That I can't tell you. It's something that comes over me. I

sit at the table sometimes and think here we are and here we shall
be next year and next and next, and I feel as though I were stifling.
Then I think: If only I could take my lute and go, gather a crowd
and play and *play*."

For a moment he looked unlike himself, wild, altered, as though
the wind were blowing through him, as though he could hear the
music he dreamed of making. I felt left out, left behind.

"It's silly. I should hate it really, sleeping in a ditch or under a
haystack."

"And rough company. And not enough to eat."

One place where we rode often, was of course, Minsham. Mother,
on my first visit, had contented herself with asking was all well with
me, and I told her everything was wonderfully well. The second
and third time she asked no questions, but on the fourth, I remember it well, it was in October, and Richard had gone out to join
Father and Isabel in beating the walnut tree, Mother said:

"You've not quickened yet?"

"Two months . . . no three . . . Three months is not long."

"No," she said. "No"; but her voice said the opposite. "But you
should lose no time. You know what they say, and truly: For every
year over sixteen there's an hour's labour with the first. You were
sixteen last February. I bore my first a few weeks after my sixteenth
birthday—they say women forget, but I remember it to this day, and
I would not have you go through that *and* the extra hour. Get your
first with all possible speed—the rest comes easy."

"It's not a thing I can order."

"You shouldn't ride so much. We are pleased to see you. . . .
But unless compelled no married woman should set foot in stirrup
for a year. It's like junket—it will never set if you keep stirring."

That evening, riding home, I was thoughtful. Once, on one of my
visits, I had been present at a birth. One of my Aunt Astallon's
attendants had had a clandestine love affair and had, up to the last
moment, concealed her state, wearing a heavily pleated houppe-
lande and joking about getting so fat. In the night, in the dormitory
where six of us lay, her hour had come upon her, and nine hours
later she was delivered. I could hear her screams still. And she was
. . . how old? Getting on. Twenty-five perhaps. Yes, it worked out.

In the night, in the bed I said, "Are you afraid of hurting me? Is that it? Darling, pain now will spare me later. Hurt me. I want to be hurt."

But we ended, as we always had, with me comforting him, pretending, pretending. Never mind. Next time. All will be well.

I still rode—though the days drew in; but I made excuses not to ride Minsham way, and I did not have to face Mother again until Christmas, when, at Master Reed's invitation, she and Father and Isabel rode in to keep the feast with us. They stayed four days, and we had a right merry time, and I managed never to be alone with Mother long enough for her to ask me awkward questions. However, my father, who had remembered his first conversation with Richard—about hawks and hawking—had procured for him, as a Christmas gift, a young eyas tiercel which was to be trained, and eventually flown at Minsham.

"A lot of riding for you," Father said. "Because if you want him to answer your whistle, you must give him his beef as often as possible and whistle as you do it."

Mother gave me what she no doubt thought was a subtle, sly look, a grimace that would have been noticeable a street's width away. I nodded to show that I understood.

So the new year opened for me with a most embarrassing problem. Richard was riding out to Minsham twice a week, and always expected me, unless the weather was very foul, to go with him. And if I did, Mother would accuse me of stirring the junket. Under the strain of making silly excuses, either to one or the other, I became bad-tempered. His lute first, now his hawk I'd think to myself, he really never wanted a wife at all!

Once that thought had entered my head, I never completely got rid of it again. Richard had told me how he had first seen me—at the time when his father brought the blue cloth; how he had fallen in love with me then and dreamed of me ever since. When I heard that story first I thought it was romantic, now, looking at it in the light of later knowledge, I had a suspicion that perhaps he would have been content to let it *stay* a dream, just as he was content to dream about that other unlikely thing, being a wandering minstrel. He liked the idea of being in love, he liked my company, perhaps (may God forgive me the unkindness of this thought) the knowledge of my better birth and station added to the romantic idea;

what he didn't want, and had no need of, was a real flesh-and-blood woman in his bed.

I rode out with him once during January at the time of the month when even Mother could not complain of my being in the saddle. Then, despite all his pleadings, I made excuses until the next time the moon ruled my blood. That time, as she greeted me, Mother said, "What, again!"

The ill-humour into which this remark threw me was not improved by the tone of her conversation throughout my visit. Had I been eating green apples? Where, I retorted, would I find green apples in February? Don't sit on grass. Lately, I snapped, there had been little temptation to do so.

"You are so irritable," she said, "that I wonder if you are not already pregnant and deceiving me. Is that so?"

I was tempted to nod and so end it, but I had no wish to complicate matters even more, so I shook my head. She then went on to tell me two more helpful things. I should steep a pound of red meat in water, let it soak overnight, then squeeze it and drink the juice. And I should borrow a shift or a petticoat from a woman lately brought to bed, wear it without washing it for a month, then return it to her with a present of a new garment, red in colour.

"What an old wives' tale!" I said.

"Old wives are usually mothers and their tales should be heeded," she replied.

That afternoon, as we rode home, it began to rain, and as soon as we arrived we went up to our room to throw off our wet clothes. Flinging my soaked hood on the floor, I said angrily, "It'll be a long time before I go to Minsham again!"

"Why, sweetheart? I thought you liked to go."

Suddenly everything boiled up in me.

"How can you be so stupid and blind," I shouted at him. Then I began to cry, and mixed up with the sobs and the blubberings it all came out, Mother's questions and admonitions, my evasions and pretences, my suspicions that he wanted a sweetheart but not a wife, everything, everything.

I had flung myself down on the bed, burrowing my face into the pillow, and when I had said *everything* I knew that I had said too much. I lifted my head a little and looked at him. I was frightened. He had the wild look on him and had gone as white as chalk. Now

I had thrown away what I had had, a loving and pleasant companion, I thought.

He said, "I'll show you."

And there, amongst the wet clothes and the messed bedclothes, in the fading light of the February afternoon, I lost my virginity at last.

III

Now for me no more riding horseback; no green apples; no sitting on grass; retching and revolted, I gulped down pints of red meat juice, and when, early in June, one of the workmen's wives in the huts beyond the stables was brought to bed I borrowed her filthy petticoat and wore it, flea-ridden as it was and returned it, in July with a fine red woolsey cloak. It all availed me nothing; the August moon ruled me, this year as last.

All this was my private concern. Around me things moved on. Master Reed had taken another stride forward, and was building again. His new notion was to bring over some Flemish weavers to ply their craft in Baildon.

The Flemings were, at this time, an unhappy people, subject to this rule and that as the fortune of war decided. Richard had told me how, on one of his visits to the Low Countries, he had seen between three and four hundred people, men, women, and children, being herded along the roads, like animals being taken to market. Their ruler of the moment, the Emperor, or the King of France or the Duke of Burgundy—I was never clear on that point —had decided that one town was too full of people and another too empty, so they were arbitrarily chosen and made to move.

With such circumstances prevailing in their home country, Flemings were always willing to take service elsewhere. The best hired mercenaries were always Flemings, *routiers*, they were called. And the best craftsmen, the weavers, were unsettled too. Master Reed, who at set intervals made the voyage in one of his ships and visited his warehouse in Amsterdam, had engaged eight skilled men to come to Baildon and ply their craft.

A new building was reared, running out at an angle from the main house. The upper floor, very stoutly built to sustain the weight and thud of the looms, was to be the weaving shed; below it the weavers, all single young men, were to live. The weaving shed was a unique structure in that its walls were almost all window. The glass was very costly, but Master Reed was sure that within four years he would have reimbursed himself. There would be no duty to pay on the home-woven stuff, and he reckoned that he could sell it so cheaply that he would undercut everybody else.

"I began," he said once, "by doing smith work cheap. Then I offered cheap stabling. And when I went into the wool trade I was still cheap; I gave a little more for the raw fleeces and sold the baled wool for a little less. Now I hope to sell good cloth, *cheap*."

I think that was the longest speech I had ever heard him make.

The building was finished and the Flemings arrived in June— while I was wearing that horrible petticoat and trying to scratch myself without being noticed. And all through July and August, Master Reed and Richard were dealing with the problem of language. Master Reed had learned enough to make himself understood in Amsterdam; Richard knew rather more, he had been inland as far as Bruges and being young had a more pliable mind. But the Flemings were difficult; they worked very well and needed little instruction or guidance so long as they were at their looms, trouble began when they took their feet from the treadles. They made straight for the town then, and in the town they were foreigners, everything they did suspect and resented; this they could not, or would not understand, so fights took place for the most trivial reasons, or for no reason at all. They were woman-hungry, and since no respectable females would have anything to do with them they fell into the hands of whores and harpies who cheated and robbed them. It would all have been different and easier had Master Reed been popular in Baildon; but just as he hated all the townspeople, they hated him and took pleasure in dealing him a knock through the foreigners he had imported. Once they were all inside the town wall when the gates were locked for the night and then arrested for being vagrants. By the end of August, Master Reed was talking of finding someone capable of speaking to them in their own tongue and of controlling them.

"Some old *routier*," Richard said, "with a good hard hand. They'd understand that."

"And where would you find one, except on the road, a broken-down ne'er-do-well?" Master Reed said.

Anxious to be helpful, I said to Richard, "My father might know of one, or my brother. Mention it next time you are at Minsham."

He still rode out there two or three times a week, and I always sent a present of some kind, with some kind of excuse—we'd killed a pig and were glutted with pork, or this was a cake I'd made myself, or this was one of the first pieces of cloth from the Baildon loom. I did not go myself. Now that all was well between Richard and me I could send a downright frank message—"Tell Mother to remember the junket," I could say. And he could laugh.

Halfway through September he came back from Minsham with two pieces of news. One was that Isabel was to go to stay with Aunt Astallon, and the other was that as soon as she had gone Mother was coming to see me; she intended to stay two nights in Baildon at least.

"Is Father coming too?"

"No. Your mother only. She said she had business to do."

I sighed. What her business might be I could not guess; one thing was sure, she would find time to go into mine. Still, I braced myself. I was no longer playing at being married. Richard and I were *married* and in that assurance I felt I could face her.

She arrived riding the better horse of the two, the one Father usually rode, and when I had greeted her I asked, "What happened to Mag?"

"I'm going farther afield," she said mysteriously. "I was on my knees the other night, with my rosary in my hands, and the blessed Virgin herself put a thought into my mind."

I had a feeling that this concerned me, so I said, with levity, "That poor old Mag should be put to pasture?"

Dear Mother; she laughed.

"No. That we should go to St. Edmundsbury."

"What for?"

"Anne, you have now been married for more than a year. And you've been a good girl and followed my instructions. The time has come when nothing but a visit to St. Petronella can help us."

"St. Petronella. I never heard of her."

"Nor I, until I consulted the priest. Now there's a thing you never thought to do, I'll warrant." She looked at me gaily. "St. Petronella is the one for us. And how fortunate that she is so near."

We had the solar to ourselves; and while Mother refreshed herself she told me all that she had learned from the priest.

St. Petronella, in her lifetime, had been a fish-gutter at Talmont in France, and in a quarrel with a fellow-worker had been so slashed about the face that no man could look on her without a shudder. So her longing for children was never gratified, and when, after a long and holy life, she died and was beatified she gave special notice to the prayers of barren women.

About a hundred years before I was born a Franciscan friar found his way to St. Edmundsbury and was concerned by the number of lepers living in destitution outside the town. He wished to help them, but had no money, nothing but faith and his own resourcefulness. He made a Cross of elmwood and carried it, preaching and begging as he went, all the way to Le Mans where he laid it on St. Petronella's shrine amongst all the glittering votive and thanks-offering that covered it. He prayed that some virtue might pass into the wood. Then he carried it back and announced that virtue *had* passed into it. He set it up under an arch of rough stones and it had become a place of pilgrimage for childless women. As long as he lived he used the income of the shrine for the relief of lepers, and when he died the Abbey took over the shrine and built a little house for the lepers.

All this Mother told me as she drank some ale and ate cake in the solar. I listened and thanked her for her interest and concern for me. Once I had resented her questions and advice, but now it was different. Nevertheless, when she said:

"We'll go there, together, tomorrow," I protested.

"What excuse can we give?"

"Why excuse. You can give your real reason."

"It is a matter that is never mentioned, not even between Richard and me. As for his father . . ."

"Nonsense! To not mention a thing is not to say it does not exist. I'll warrant that Richard and his father have watched you with eyes as keen as mine, and been as greatly disappointed."

"Oh dear," I said.

"Never mind, we are doing all that we can. And the priest assured me that the Saint has worked some wondrous miracles."

I announced—brusquely because I was embarrassed—that on the morrow Mother and I intended to ride to St. Edmundsbury. Richard put out his hand and squeezed mine, understandingly. Master Reed looked at me sombrely out of his sad eyes and presently, when we chanced to be alone for a moment, said to me:

"Anne, I know the purpose of your journey, and I wish you well. But . . ." He hesitated and then said jerkily, the words coming out of him in a rush, "Don't count too much upon it. Miracles . . ." He paused again and looked down at his lame leg and the thick-soled shoe. "They work in a queer twisted way," he said. "And I can't for the life of me see how what you're wanting could be other than straightforward. And I don't believe they can be that way. Miracles, I mean." He touched my shoulder and said, "Perhaps your faith is greater."

Next morning we set out, Mother and I, with a man to escort us. Richard wanted to come, but that I did not favour, why I could not say. I would not have taken the man, but Master Reed insisted; he was shocked to learn that Mother had ridden in from Minsham alone. His view of the open road was the view of the man who transports stuff of value from place to place and must ever be on guard against robbers.

There was no need to inquire the way to the shrine. Long before we reached it we found ourselves in the centre of a kind of fair, a fair devoted to the exploitation of childless women. It was so shameless that I wonder the Abbey allowed it. There were people selling charms, all guaranteed to bring fecundity; cakes made in the shape of babies; trinkets of bone or wood or stone, even of coral and ivory, all in the shape of babies. There were strings and strings of blue beads—blue being the Virgin's own colour and thus associated with motherhood. There were slatternly women with great broods of children—borrowed or hired, I suspect, lining the road and screaming that they would sell, for a penny, the secret of their fruitfulness. "Twopence, lady, and I'll put the good wish on you!" "Threepence, lady, and you shall be in pod by Michaelmas." I was ashamed and drew my veil close, and even Mother said:

"They overdo it somewhat."

Monks are cunning. After all that brash huckstering along the road, with the constant demand for pence breeding disbelief until you were ready to think of St. Petronella as just another fraud, out to rob you, you rode through a gateway where only petitioners and their attendants were allowed to pass. Inside was a kind of inn; rails to which horses could be hitched, a stone trough full of water, benches and tables where people could refresh themselves. The whole place was shaded by chestnut trees, from which, on this day, the great yellow fans of dead leaves fluttered gently and quietly to the ground.

On the far side of this enclosure was a gate in the wall. Through this the petitioner must go alone. The path beyond was paved and bordered on each side by a green hedge, neatly clipped, very thick, and an inch or two taller than a man. The path wound in curves so that at no time could I see more than a step or two ahead. I have never felt more lonely, more isolated from all other human beings. The contrast after the bustle and hurly-burly outside was complete. When I rounded the last curve there was the plain wooden Cross, under the rough stone arch, just as the Franciscan had set it up, more than a hundred years ago.

Offerings to this shrine were always in money—used for the relief of lepers and other purposes—so the shrine was quite bare, without even a flower. It was humble, and touching, and in some strange way far more believable and impressive than any other shrine I had ever seen. I went down on my knees and prayed that St. Petronella would use her influence, and intercede for me and give me a baby. Here, alone, in the quiet before this simple Cross, I could acknowledge the need which hitherto I had hidden even from myself. I thought about holding a baby in my arms, feeding it at my breast.

We rode home, and that evening at supper there was a new face halfway down the first trestle table; and because Mother was staying with us and sat at my usual place, I had a good view of the newcomer.

It is hard for me to describe this man, Denys the Routier, or Denys Rootyer as he came to be called. The most immediately noticeable thing about him was that he had only one eye; over the empty socket on the other side he wore a black leather patch, kept in position by a black string tied at the back of his head. His hair, roughly cut and inclined to be curly, was a pale sandy colour, many shades lighter than his weatherbeaten skin; his one eye was brightly blue.

I was looking at him with interest because he was a stranger, and because of the black patch, when he turned his glance on me and immediately something happened inside me, as though something had given way and all my vitals had slipped. It was not unlike the first onset of sickness and I pressed my hand to my mouth and thought: Holy Mother! The miracle has happened and I have quickened. I looked at my plate, and although the dish was to my liking, specially made in honour of Mother, I knew that I could not take another mouthful.

Richard said, "The journey was too much for you. Come to bed. When you are rested I will bring you your supper."

"Fetch some wine; that will revive both our travellers," Master Reed said. So the wine came and I sat there holding the cup in my hands and turning it about, not daring to drink until my inside settled.

Mother and I answered questions about the journey.

Presently I said, "I see we have a new man."

"Ah yes." Master Reed turned to Mother and said, "Please tell Sir Godfrey that I am grateful and obliged to him for his good offices in finding so suitable a man."

"Oh, did Blanchfleur remember? He grows more and more forgetful these days." She smiled as though describing a child's vagary. "Still, he would remember a thing like that better than any simple errand I set him. Which is the new man?" She craned her neck.

"The one with the patch over his eye," Richard said. "A good stout fellow, is he not?"

I looked again and saw that everyone else at the board was suddenly diminished. The weavers were always somewhat pale, inclined to fleshiness—that was a mark of their trade—but they were not all weavers at the table. I glanced to right and left; Master Reed looked thick and shapeless, Richard too fine-drawn, a pretty boy.

I told myself that it was because the new man wore no collar, his dark, creased neck rose out of a collarless leather jerkin which fitted close to his wide flat shoulders, and so he looked all of a piece, stripped of all non-essentials, ready for action.

Mother was rippling on about *routiers*; their high reputation for loyalty and courage, despite being mercenaries.

"But that is why," she explained. "Nobles and knights are forever changing their causes for this reason and that, *routiers* fight for pay and stick with the man who pays them." She lowered her voice a little. "You must look to your maids, Master Reed; these old soldiers have a way with women."

"Not old soldiers only," he said dryly. "I always choose old serving wenches."

"Very wise."

I said, "I think I will go to bed now."

When I had been there a little while Richard came softly in, bringing more wine and some food.

"Are you asleep?"

"No."

"Could you eat now?"

"No. I thank you all the same."

He put the things down and came and sat on the side of the bed.

"What really happened today?"

"Nothing really. . . ." I told him a little more about the way I had felt by the bare, humble little shrine. Then I put my hands on either side of his face and said, "I love you, I love you, I love you. You know that, don't you?"

"Could I ever doubt it? I love you too."

Words, true words; but I need something more.

"Come in the bed with me, now."

He came to me eagerly, tenderly. He gave me all that he had. But afterwards, in the dark, I lay alone again, and a voice, within my head, yet distant as a star, asked, "Is this all?" I closed my mind to it, pushing against it, as one might push a door against an intruder. But it tried again; it asked, "How would this be, if done with the man with one eye?"

IV

Madness, we know, takes many forms; and this was mine. I never for one instant ceased to love Richard. There never was a moment, mad as I was, when to have saved Richard a pang of toothache I would not gladly have seen Denys the Routier hanged, drawn, and quartered. By all that is holy, I swear that that is true. The lust I felt for him was like a poison, swallowed unwittingly, doing its damage, taking possession of the whole sound body.

With Mother gone home I was back at my old place at the table, and could see him clearly only when he leaned forward or the man sitting next him leaned back. And after the first few days he was never there for the midday dinner and not to be counted upon at suppertime. In no time at all, talking to the Flemings in their own tongue, he had put the fear of God into them, and Master Reed, never one to waste anything, had begun to send him with the pack ponies as a kind of guard. So I never knew, when I entered the dining hall, whether his place would be filled or empty, and every evening, every evening for weeks, I vowed that this time I would not look. But I always did, sooner or later; and if his place was empty a kind of greyness would come over everything, my food would be tasteless. . . . Tomorrow, how many hours? Or perhaps, a long journey, the day after tomorrow. . . . It was like walking down a dark stone passage with a light at the far end. No, not a light, a dancing will-o'-the-wisp. For when the moment came and I looked and there he was, what then?

Oh, then, at some moment during the meal that one blue eye would look at me, and my inside would turn its now pleasurable somersault; the candlelight would brighten, the fire behind me throw out more heat, and I would know a moment of what I can only call timelessness. In that moment all kinds of things would rush together, reminding me of small pleasures I had known in the past and promising me a great pleasure to come—there'd be the cool scent of primroses, the warm scent of roses, the sound of trumpets, the feel of my Aunt Astallon's silk gown, the taste of strawberries, the colours of a sunset—all mixed up in one mad moment, meaning nothing, meaning everything. How can I explain it? It was as though every pleasant thing that I had ever felt in the past was a separate string to a lute, and his glance was the running of a hand over those strings, so that they all cried out together, in no tunable pattern.

I never spoke to him, never had occasion to go near him until one morning in the spring. It was March, I remember seeing the daffodils breaking yellow in the garden close, under the apple trees. Richard was riding out to Minsham, and I said I would go too. St. Petronella had failed me yet again, and I had spent the whole winter cooped in the house.

Martin's horse and my palfrey stood awaiting us, and nearby a string of pack ponies, laden with the new Baildon cloth, were lining up for the first stage of their journey to London. Denys stood with them. He came forward—one of Martin Reed's servants, civil, obliging—and helped me to mount. When he touched me my bones melted. In the two seconds before I was in the saddle it was all said. "I am yours, take me," my flesh said to his; and his said, "Would that I could."

"You look so pale," Martin said, turning his horse beside me. "Are you sure you should ride?"

"You know that it is only when I am pale with such good reason that I dare face my mother," I said crossly. And all the way to Minsham I thought about Denys. We would make a child, I thought, the moment we came together. We could defy the moon, the pale moon with its fluxes. . . .

After that I suppose it was merely a question of awaiting an opportunity.

April passed and May. I had grown thin, which was not becoming to me. One day, looking in the glass, I was horrified to see that after all I had inherited the Blanchfleur nose and would one day look exactly like an aunt I detested. Richard and his father put down my lack of appetite and uncertain temper to disappointment and were kinder than ever to me, which, because it made me feel ashamed, made matters worse.

June was always a busy month, with the new-cut fleeces pouring in from miles around, and often Richard would rise early, leaving me to slugabed. One morning he did so, and when I did go down I looked into the office, but he wasn't there, which was nothing unusual. Dinnertime came and the oak table was set with two places only.

"Where's Richard?" I asked.

"Gone to Bywater. We had word early this morning that *Sea Maid* had run into another ship and was damaged. He rode down to see what the damage was. He'll be back tomorrow." He set about his meal and then stopped. "I'm off myself to Kelvedon this minute. You'll be alone in the new part. Would you like Nancy or Meg to move over?"

"For fear of what?"

"Whatever it is women fear. Ghosties and goblins?" He gave me his painful, rare smile.

"Anything a kitchen wench could save me from I do not fear," I said.

Yet I had no intention of taking Denys into Richard's bed. I had no intention of doing anything. I did not even go into the hall for supper, to sit there alone, displaying my solitariness. I stayed close in the solar, thinking that he would think that I also had gone away. From the solar I went into the garden.

Every rose had its heart wide open; the languor of a summer evening weighed heavy on every leaf. I walked, lingered, walked on, unable to draw a full breath, my heart was so shaken.

Presently, between the rosebushes old Nancy came hobbling on her flat feet.

"Mistress," she began as soon as she saw me, "there's that Denys Rootyer at the back door. He say Master went off and never give him his orders for tomorrow. He say he ought to talk to you."

"Oh," I said, and struggled with my breath. Surely she must notice and wonder. "No orders were left with me. I know nothing."

"He seem to hev something in his mind. He just want somebody to say go ahead like. There ain't nobody else but you."

"I'll see him."

"Out here? Then you should hev a shawl. The dew's falling."

"Give him the shawl. That will save you a few steps."

" 'Tain't everybody'd be thoughtful of an owd woman's feet," she said, pleased. "I give you good night, mistress."

Thinking no evil, thinking only of her bed, she plodded away. And presently, with his light, firm, soldier's tread, carrying my shawl over his arm, Denys came through the roses.

V

There followed some days during which, with a sense of bewilderment, I thought of Mother's words. I'd sit at the table and look at Richard, whom I loved, and then at Denys, whom I did not love, and I knew which of them gave me that feeling of triumph, of pride that had sounded in Mother's voice when she spoke of Father. How I envied her—and any other woman who could have that feeling lawfully, together *with* love. Those were days when I had only to see his great brown hand close on a piece of bread in the trencher to feel its touch on me again and wonder how, through all the years of my life, I could manage with what I had.

Those days were soon over. The July moon was a horned crescent, was a silver-gilt plate, grew gibbous and copper-coloured. It drew no response from my blood. To myself I said: I was right; I knew this would happen. To the others I said nothing. I waited until one morning towards the end of August, as soon as I set foot to the floor, I was deathly sick. Then I said to Richard:

"I think I am with child." And presently I was sure enough to send a message to my mother.

There was, naturally, great rejoicing. Even Master Reed threw off his melancholy air, and Richard's pride and pleasure cut me to the heart. I had other troubles too. One was shame and one was fear.

Now that the work was done and my womb was filling, all the lust went out of me, and all the madness, and I could see Denys for what he was—a great hunk of man flesh, a common hired soldier to whom I, Anne Blanchfleur, had submitted! There was the shame.

The fear lay in the thought that children tended to look like their parents. Suppose my child were born with that pale sandy hair and only one eye. How could I ever have been so crazy as not to have thought of that?

I studied Richard and his father. At a first glance they were unlike, Richard was much darker, much more lightly built, but the way the hair grew off their foreheads was the same, and they both had crooked little fingers on their left hands. True, Master Reed was lame and Richard had two good straight legs, but there were two schools of thought about such things. Some people held that anything that had happened to a man or woman by accident during his or her lifetime was not passed on to the offspring; other people claimed that anything that happened, even to having been frightened by a mouse, could leave a mark upon the child.

Mother rode in to see me and we had a long talk, all about such mysteries; I encouraged her and then wished I had not. She had a story of a pregnant woman who had longed for strawberries in December and who bore a child with a red strawberry mark on its left cheek.

"Whatever you long for, no matter how silly it sounds, speak out, Anne. Make them get it for you if possible."

I thought: I wonder how you would look if I told you that the one thing I long for is the assurance that a one-eyed man's child will not be born with one eye.

All this uneasiness of mind took its toll of my body. I think I suffered everything a pregnant woman can. They say that if you are sick at six weeks, at six months you'll be lively. They say that cramps beforehand are a sign of easy labour, you've had so much of your grue. They say that if your legs swell your face does not. I broke every one of the rules. I was sick at six weeks, and even sicker at six months; I had cramp; my face swelled to the size of a bladder and my legs swelled till they were as big as my waist ordinarily was; and in the end I was in labour for two days and three nights.

Before the end I had my story ready. If I gave birth to a child with one eye I was going to say that on the night when Richard and his father were both away, Denys made an excuse to come to me in the garden, and there raped me. Old Nancy would bear me out about the excuse, I was in the garden, innocent as a lamb, and he did make that opportunity to seek me out. Richard and his father would ask one dangerous question: Why had I not complained? To that I had a silly sentimental answer, silly enough to sound true. My father had found Denys for Master Reed, and I didn't want him to think that Father had sent him a rogue.

My last sensible thought was of my story and how, if needs be, I must stick to it. Then my agony began; and presently I didn't care if the child were born with one eye or four, if only it would be born. I saw Mother and screamed to her, "Help me!" and with tears on her face she said, "You must be brave. You must help yourself. None other can."

I tried to be brave. I told myself that I was the daughter of one of the boldest knights that ever rode in tourney, and of a woman who had set out to ride from Rivington to Beauclaire, risking being brought to bed in a ditch. But it went on too long. In the end I was screaming like a trapped hare and I went on screaming until I had no voice left and could only make harsh, weak cries. The pain abated and I floated away, and was walking towards St. Petronella's shrine, but the solid green hedges were all covered with open-hearted roses, drenching the air with scent. Just before the shrine Richard waited for me, but as I went near he turned into Denys, holding a dark cloak with which he smothered me. I fought against the weight of it and struggled up into the air and light again. The priest was in the room.

I thought: I am dying. I wanted to say: I have a great sin to confess; I have committed adultery. Had we been alone I might have said it, but beyond the circle of the candlelight I saw other people—Mother, another woman, several . . . Richard will hear about it, I thought, and be hurt, and not revere my memory. No, sooner I would die unshriven and go to Hell.

Hell was the Long Gallery at Abhurst, brightly lighted so that there was no shadow into which one could retire. I stood alone and watched four or five young men crowd about Catharine Montsorrel. My Aunt Bowdegrave came and stood by me, showing her yellow teeth and saying that with my sharp tongue and prim manner I should never find a husband.

From there I slipped into a bottomless pit of darkness and lay there until someone above reached down with a grappling iron and hooked it into my body and hauled me up, screaming and struggling, and with each struggle the iron bit deeper into me, I was being cut in two. When I was severed what remained fell down upon the bed and the pain was over. I could hear a bustling and a soft clucking of tongues. Then I opened my eyes, and there was Mother, holding a baby, and the midwife with another.

"Twins," Mother said. "Boy and girl."

Twins were freaks; nobody expected them to be quite ordinary; if one, or both, lacked an eye, or even a limb, it would be no wonder. Holy Mother of God, you have dealt with me more gently than I deserve.

"Are they whole?" I whispered.

"Whole? They are beautiful."

Twins, Mother and the midwife agreed, are ordinarily smaller than other babies, but Walter and Maude were each as large as any single child; from this, and the abundance of hair on each of their heads, Mother deduced that I had carried them overlong and muddled my dates.

"Young women are so careless," she grumbled. "You told me March, and if they'd been born when they should, I might not have got to you in time."

They were not a bit like one another once the red, crumpled, newborn look had worn off. They were both born with black hair, but they shed it in the first weeks, and Walter's grew black again, Maude's reddish gold.

"The wrong way about," Mother said. "The boy should favour you, and the girl her father. As often happens."

"To our cost. My Blanchfleur nose! I would sooner have had yours."

Such trivial, cosy little conversations seemed to underline my sense of safety; as though I had forded a dangerous stream, been almost swept away, but struggled to safety and now could afford to talk about currents, deep waters, lost footholds. I was safe. I was lucky. I now had everything.

In a month I was up and about, fully restored to health, and, miracle of miracles, my waist was its normal size, I knew that by my dresses; my nose, now that the flesh was back on my face, took its proper place again, and I knew that I was prettier than ever.

There being two babies to feed, we were forced to engage a wet nurse—a thing not common in households of our degree, however rich—and when I proved to be a poor milch cow, while she had enough for four, she took on all that duty, and I was free to enjoy the summer and go riding with Richard again.

It was he who suggested that we should ride to St. Petronella's shrine and take a further present to show our gratitude. Something, and to this day I do not know exactly what it was, made me demur.

"I don't think that is customary. Women only go there to *ask*."

"Then it's time somebody had manners enough to go and say thank you," he said, smiling.

I smiled too.

"I believe you have never been to St. Edmundsbury."

"That is so. We'll go, shall we?"

"You have to ride through the rowdiest kind of fair."

"I shall be with you. And this time you can look down your nose at all the spellbinders. I warrant none of *them* bore *two*, weighing a full stone between them."

To settle an argument between Mother and the midwife, Master Reed had carried the babies out and weighed them in the wool scales.

Having no argument, no reason for not riding that way, except a vague and mysterious feeling that it would be wiser not to, I gave way, and we set off on a fine warm morning.

Richard enjoyed himself enormously, especially when we reached the stalls. I was newly puzzled how anyone so gentle and fastidious and dignified should seem so much at ease in such surroundings. He bought gingerbread babies and charms of every kind, and a long string of blue beads which he slipped over my head, tangling it in my veil. Even the shaggy old harridan who so brazenly shouted "in pod"—only now she had changed her cry to "in pod by Lammas"

—did not disgust him. He gave her fourpence and laughed when she promised us four lusty sons.

"Old fraud," he said as we moved on, "none of that gaggle of brats is hers, I'll warrant."

"Then why encourage her?"

"She must live. There's something about people who try to wring a living out of the world, with nothing but a slick tongue or a penny whistle, that appeals to me."

"I know. You might have been born at a fair, you seem so much at home."

"Then I could have played my lute."

"And dreamed of being the only son of a prosperous wool merchant, no doubt."

"No doubt at all."

We rode on and entered the enclosure. Richard slipped a gold piece into my hand, and I gave it to the monk by the inner gate. I set off briskly down the path, feeling the delight of moving freely and lightly again, and thinking that I had only to kneel and offer a few words of thanksgiving. But as I rounded one curve and then the next I found myself walking more and more slowly, while the distaste I felt for this apparently simple errand grew until it was terror. The day seemed to darken, and when I looked up at the sky I saw that a great purple cloud had reared up from the west and engulfed the sun.

I stood still and thought: I don't *have* to go any farther, no one will know. Stand here and count up to a hundred, twice, slowly. But that would be cowardly, and later I should despise myself. All my life I had heard a high price set on courage, and cowardice spoken of as rather worse than sin, and when I was a child, with my full share of childish fears, I had always schooled myself to overcome them. Now to be frightened of nothing, that was ridiculous. So I set myself in motion; walked on and reached the shrine which was in all respects just as before.

I went down on my knees and suddenly could think of nothing except the words Master Reed had said to me just before my first visit here. "Miracles . . . they work in a queer twisted way, and I can't for the life of me see how what you're wanting could be other than straightforward." But I could see, with sudden, clear sight, how my miracle had come about in, as he said, a queer, twisted way. Doubly twisted. First my madness, and then the fact that neither child bore any mark of its paternity. For let Mother say what she would about weight and crops of hair and muddled dates, I *knew*.

No doubt St. Petronella has been passionately thanked, even if the grateful petitioners did not make a journey to her shrine to do it, but she surely never was thanked, so passionately, so much from the heart, as I thanked her in that moment when I understood the extent of her miracle.

I went back to Richard and suggested that we should wait for a little, since that cloud threatened rain. We sat under the chestnut trees and ate and drank, and still the rain held off, and at last he said, "In summer it often clouds over without a drop falling." So we set off. When we were on the open road, far from any house, there was a fearful clap of thunder, and the heavens opened and down came the rain, mingled with hailstones as large as the blue beads I was wearing. I suggested sheltering under some trees nearby, but Richard said they were elms, dangerous at any time and doubly so in a storm, so we rode on, soon drenched and then shivering, for the day had turned cold as the hail fell.

Next day Richard was feverish and stayed in bed, hot and cold by turns, and coughing now and then. I made linseed poultices for his chest and rubbed him well with neat's-foot oil and beat honey and vinegar together for him to swallow, but the cough grew worse, and after the third night, when he had kept all our side of the house, save the babies, awake with it, Master Reed sent for the doctor. He had several remedies to try—one, the nature of which I concealed from Richard—was the liquor in which snails had been boiled, but nothing did any service until one morning he came along with a little horn full of a greenish-grey powder. One pinch of it, as much as one could take between finger and thumb, was to be dropped on top of a cup of warm milk or wine; just the one pinch and the dose was not to be repeated in less than twelve hours.

"It is," the doctor said, "a sovereign remedy, but it is also a powerful poison; taken in quantity, or too often, it could be fatal."

"I alone will administer it, and I will be very careful."

That night he slept, and sleep is itself a healer. In the morning his fever was lessened, his skin moist and cool to the touch. During the day the cough returned, but less violently, and so day by day he made progress. In most ways he was an easy patient, grateful and cheerful, but being held to the one room irked him; his only complaint was that the walls seemed to be closing in. We pushed the bed close to the window and propped him up so that he could look out and see the sky. And as soon as he was well enough—about three weeks after our unfortunate journey—he came down, leaning on his father's arm, into the solar.

That was a happy day, and as soon as he was settled in the window seat, overlooking the garden, I got out my sewing which I had neglected lately. I was making Mother a winter cloak, of our own Baildon cloth, the cloth which was to become so famous that men would speak of "my Baildon breeches," and women say, "I will wear my Baildon." The cloth itself was dove grey, there was an interlining of shredded-out lambs' wool, and a lining of red silk, the two last quilted together. It had a hood which could be pulled over the head or thrown back. It was, in fact, such a garment as Mother had never owned. Master Reed, immediately after our marriage, had done a generous thing, hired, for some absurdly high price, several of the acres which went with the house, to add to his sheep run, but none of the extra money found its way into Mother's wardrobe. Isabel went out into the world better equipped, and Mag, the old horse, had been replaced.

I was stitching away, when Richard said, "That is for your mother's birthday, isn't it?"

"Yes. The day after tomorrow and I still have this much of the lining to fix, and then the hood to stitch on." I held it out and showed him.

"It'll be ready. And I shall be ready to ride out and take it."

"I should no more dream of letting you ride out to Minsham the day after tomorrow than I should dream of . . . well . . . of throwing myself into the river."

"But I'm better."

"You're downstairs today for the first time. A fortnight hence will be time enough to talk about mounting a horse."

"I want to see Jason." That was his hawk.

"Then you must want," I said, stitching away.

"Uncle Tom once warned me that all high-nosed women were masterful and domineering!"

"How strange. Somebody once warned me that all black-haired men were obstinate and unreasonable."

He laughed and coughed.

"You sound like riding abroad the day after tomorrow."

"I shall."

"Then you'll go alone. I will not lend my countenance to such a thing."

Just then Master Reed entered the solar and Richard appealed to him to decide.

"You would be more than foolish. Just to visit a hawk."

"But Anne will want to see her mother."

"So she shall. Clement can ride with her and take out the tar and spend his day helping the shepherd."

Mother's birthday dawned clear and bright, and Richard woke feeling so much better that I had to repeat my threat that if he rode I would stay at home. His improvement and the fair morning sent my spirits soaring.

When I was ready to leave Master Reed came into the yard with me, carrying a small cask of wine.

"For your mother, with good wishes," he said, and muttered something about it being a balance for the tar barrel.

There in the yard stood a big brown horse, and my palfrey, and standing between them Denys.

I know my step faltered, for Master Reed said, "Forgotten something?"

I shook my head and went forward, wondering whether I could at this last moment say that I felt ill. A coward's trick, and disappointing for Mother. And perhaps, after all, Denys was only holding the horses; it was Clement—who understood sheep—who was supposed to spend the day at Minsham with the shepherd. I stood, all confused and uncertain, sweat breaking out on my forehead and upper lip and the palms of my hands, while the two men slung the wine cask.

There was still time to droop and dwindle and pretend a sudden pain. But I said to myself: Courage, courage.

Master Reed turned to me and said, "Up you get," and helped me into the saddle. I rode out through the covered way first and, once out of the gate, drove in my heel. My palfrey had never once been underfed or overburdened, or hard pressed, and during Richard's illness had stood in the stable cramming corn. "Let's see what you can do today," I said in its ear.

It did well. The road, heavy from the recent rainy spell, was in our favour; the brown horse was bigger, but Denys weighed all of twelve stone, and there were the two casks.

For eight of the ten miles I stayed ahead, then my beast slackened pace, and nothing I could do could make it recover speed. Out of nowhere there came to me the rhyme which Father had said to us, jogging us on his knee.

"This is the way the ladies ride, trippety, trip, trippety, trip. This is the way the farmers ride, bumpitty, thud, bumpitty, thud." And in the end, I thought, bumpitty thud will always catch up with trippety trip. How I longed for the horse in the end of the rhyme, "This is the way the gentlemen ride, gallop and trot, gallop and trot."

Denys came level with me and snatched at my rein.

"Did the brute bolt?" He pulled the rein savagely, so that my palfrey's head was wrenched round and we stood sideways across the road.

"Don't do that. I set the pace. I am anxious to arrive."

He said, and I shall always remember the curious simplicity and innocence that there was both in his voice and in his eye, "I wanted to talk to you. It's been a whole year, with never so much as a word."

I said nothing.

"This was our chance to fix something; to meet; to get together again," he said, as though explaining something to a stupid child. "I've been wanting you so badly, I wonder I haven't done something desperate, all these months. I wonder you never tried . . ."

He had no suspicion of the way I felt. I'd swung my horse about again so that it was facing the right way, and he brought his alongside, and put out his arm to touch me, but the tar barrel prevented him coming close enough.

"Come on, get down," he said in a thick, amorous voice.

I thought the quickest cut would be best. He had dropped my rein, so I set my palfrey going, and he came level, and I said, "What happened last June twelvemonth happened because I was mad. It must never happen again."

"Oh, come! What was so mad about it? And what harm did we do? I'd lay a year's pay you never had it so good—and nor did I. Things being so cursed difficult I tried to put you out of my mind, but I never could. And you'd say the same if you weren't trying to play coy with me. There's no need for that . . . and no time."

"I mean what I say. It's finished. Over and done with."

"It'll all come back. Women are often that way, after childbed. You'll see. This evening, eh? On our way back."

"Not then, or any other time," I said, trying to get another spurt of speed out of my horse.

He seemed genuinely puzzled. "What's got into you? What've I done? I'm just the same. You were starving for it—oh, I could tell. And I didn't do so badly by you. Two sound brats, with no lung rot."

Anger flared in me, but I mastered it, and said coolly, "You flatter yourself."

"Do I? Bedded for a year with a pretty boy that couldn't father a mouse—a woman like you! Think back to that night on the grass and look what you're missing." He followed this by a remark of such coarseness and familiarity as was not to be tolerated, even if it were deserved.

"At the next bend we shall be in sight of my father's house," I said. "Drop back and ride behind me as a servant should."

He laughed. "That's my lady! Like plums, the higher the sweeter, once you can reach them down." He hit my palfrey a sharp blow and it shot forward.

"That's the way," he cried, "let's ride in in style."

VI

For me the day was ruined. Mother was delighted with the cloak and the wine, pleased to see me, and avid to hear the last smallest detail about Walter and Maude, but I had to make a great effort to chat lightheartedly, and a greater one to do justice to the birthday dinner. I had to ride back to Baildon in Denys' company. The irony of the thought that little more than a year ago no prospect would have pleased me more only served to underline the horror of my present situation.

I have never known a day go so fast.

I gave Jason the gobbet of red meat which Richard had sent him, and listened absent-mindedly while Father explained that these last three weeks, during which Richard had not ridden out to Minsham at all, would make an excellent excuse for the fact that the young hawk would never accept him as his master.

"I've feared it all along," he said in his slow, fumbling way. "Twice a week . . . and let him be the only one ever to take the rufter off. I thought that might just do it. I was wrong and I was afraid the poor fellow would be disappointed, we can lay the blame now on these three weeks."

With some vague idea of handicapping Denys on the return journey I said, "I can't think why you didn't let Richard have his hawk at the Old Vine in the first place. Shall we take it back with us this afternoon? I think that would please him."

"But who at the Old Vine understands falconry? That's just it. A tiercel isn't a lap dog, Anne. Maybe I was foolish . . . but he had shown some slight interest in hawking . . . I told you, that first time. And your mother thought . . ."

"Mother thought *what?*"

"That to get out, out of that office, into the air . . . Oh, I know twice a week isn't much, isn't enough, but it did make an excuse. And, as usual, your Mother was right, wasn't she? So the hawk wasn't wasted, though I daresay Richard will be a bit jealous that I can now handle his bird. Still, nobody can help being ill."

"May I carry Jason back with me this afternoon?"

"No. You can't handle him. . . . Isabel now, if it was Isabel, but you never cared for the sport. And you'd have no place—not so much as a perch. An unhandled hawk, especially one half trained like Jason'd go mad, or pine to death. No. When Richard is better, which God send will be soon, he must come out, and I'll fool them both. I'll stand close to him and whistle my whistle through *his.* We'll manage."

Alone with Mother again, I put on the drooping, dwindling look which I would have been wise to have put on in the yard hours before.

"You warned me about riding, but you had it all wrong. It is now that the jolting hurts me."

She looked concerned. "I thought you looked very wan when you came in. You had a hard time, you know, and it's not so long. Richard ill too, I daresay you've been up and down stairs and having broken nights."

"If my bed were aired," I said, "I would lie here tonight. Denys could tell them that I was just tired."

"The bed hasn't been slept in since Isabel went. But I could air it in an hour."

"Then I'll stay, and gladly."

Mother threw fresh wood on the fire and began to climb the stairs.

"I'll help you," I said.

"You'll do nothing of the sort. I can handle that bed. It isn't like those great fat feather bundles you lie on at Baildon." She laughed. In a few seconds she came out of my old room with the bed—a poor thin thing indeed—folded over into a roll and held in her arms. She came down three stairs, then the inside edge of the roll loosened itself and fell lower than the rest; she stepped into it, as it were, missed her footing, almost righted herself, and could have, had that staircase had a handrail to clutch at, but it hadn't; she clutched at air and fell sideways onto the floor of the hall.

She was up in an instant, before I could get to her.

"Clumsy!" she said, and laughed.

"Are you hurt?"

"Not a bit." She went to the foot of the stairs where the mattress, now fully unfolded, lay, and picked it up and gave it a shake.

"Trip me, would you?" she said. "I'll roast you for that!"

We propped it up before the fire, and the amount of steam which rose from it proved its need for airing. Minsham Old Hall was very damp always, on the hottest day of summer you could write your name on the dewy moisture of the walls.

For supper we ate the remains of the birthday dinner and drank some more of the wine, and now we were truly merry. Denys had gone, with a black look for me over Mother's shoulder when she gave him his instructions at the door. Tomorrow Father was to ride in with me, and once in the house I should be safe. I'd never ride anywhere again until Richard was fit to ride with me.

Getting up from the supper table, Mother clapped her hand to her side and gave a little cry.

"I must have caught myself a clout without knowing it. A bruise, no more." But even her lips had gone white.

She was up in the morning, however, very cheerful, holding herself a mite stiffly and saying that forty-six was a bit old to go turning somersaults.

"I shall ride in myself next Wednesday to see those dear children," she said, as we parted. "Meanwhile, wish Richard good health for me and thank Master Reed for the wine."

I rode back to Baildon, thinking that I had managed very well.

Mother's birthday was on Thursday. I went home on Friday. Richard was better, but still taking his meals apart in the solar. I ate my supper with him, in the golden, slanting rays of the sinking sun. Master Reed, who had supped in the hall as usual, came into the room afterwards, looked into our wine cups, saw them full, and poured his own. Then he said, "Anne, Denys the Routier wants a word with you."

Whether I went red or white I cannot tell; I could only feel my whole face stiffen.

"With me? What about?"

"I don't know. He just asked if he could have a word with you."

I suppose it was my guilty conscience that made me think his manner a trifle more restrained than usual, his eye just a little suspicious . . . no . . . curious.

I turned and hurried, trying not to hurry, out of the solar.

The dining hall, on the eastern side of the house, was already dim and full of shadows. It smelt strongly of rabbit and onion stew, and even in that moment of extremity some part of my mind noted the curious fact that a dish of which one has not partaken always has a stronger odour than one which one has eaten. Richard and I, in the solar, had shared a cold capon.

Old Nancy stood in the doorway between the hall and the kitchen, watching Meg and Jane, helped by the two youngest apprentices, clear the tables. Denys leaned against the doorpost of the outer door, his back to the hall, looking out into the yard. The presence of four other—five other people gave me confidence. I walked towards him and said, "You wanted to speak with me."

He turned quickly, so that in the doorway we faced one another and he took hold of my hand. The action could not be seen by those inside in the hall because the bulk of my body was in their way. He fumbled with my hand for a second and then had me by the little finger, bending it down, pressing hard. There is no simple, quiet, secret action that can cause more sharp pain. Anyone who doubts this should try it on himself. Pressing ruthlessly on my finger he pulled me over the threshold. At the same time he hissed into my ear, "Call back and say your palfrey is lame and you are looking to it."

I leaned back, and, only just able to speak for the pain in my finger, said, "Nancy. Tell Master Richard I have gone out to look to my palfrey. It is lame, it seems."

"Now," he said, with a little more pressure on my finger, "come and look just how lame it is." He dragged me across the yard and to the fence of the pasture. "A pretty trick you played me yesterday. Now listen. Tomorrow is Saturday. In the afternoon they'll all go to their shooting at the Butts. I don't have to go. I've done my soldiering. I shall wait for you in the wool loft, the far end."

I said, and I could hear how thin my voice sounded, "Unless you let go my finger . . . I can give you no mind . . . I shall faint."

He let go then, but he put his arm around me and said, "You bring it on yourself, you're so tricky. It could have been yesterday, you silly little hussy," and he pushed his body against me. "Now it must wait till tomorrow, and I've waited so long. . . ."

"I can't. I can't. Even if I wanted to . . . my husband, his father . . . I can't just walk out of the house."

"Women always have two excuses—church and the dressmaker. Choose which you like, but I'm telling you, you had better come."

He let me go, and stooping tugged up a little tuft of grass with the soil clodded about its roots. He tossed it gently over the fence at my palfrey which was grazing amongst the other horses, a pale shadow amongst the darker ones. It started and moved away, one hoof hardly touching the ground, lame as a tinker's donkey.

"This time I made an excuse. If you fail me tomorrow I shall ask for you again, and again, and every excuse will be shakier than the one before. And I shall talk about you, in alehouses. . . ."

"You'll find yourself in trouble if you boast of rape."

He laughed, it seemed with real pleasure.

"I always knew a devil lurked behind that angel face of yours, my pretty! Rape indeed. Was your dress torn? Did you run screaming? Did you complain? Besides which, once I've set them all asking questions I shall make myself scarce, leaving you to find the answers."

Had I been innocent, I suppose that would hardly have been a threat at all. I remembered how my face had felt when Master Reed brought me Denys' message, I remembered the look I thought he had given me. My best weapon, a clear conscience, was snapped in my hand; I was not equipped to fight.

"I'll come," I said.

"And I'll set your horse to rights." He rested one hand on a post of the fence and vaulted lightly into the meadow.

I turned away and hurried towards the house. Master Reed stood at the back door looking out over the yard. I wondered how long he had been there, and whether, at that distance, he could have seen Denys lay hold of me.

"Anything amiss?" he said.

"My horse is very lame. Denys thinks it picked up a stone. He is dealing with it."

"How handy is he? He might worsen matters. I'd better . . ." He went, with his lurching yet rapid step, towards the pasture.

That night I hardly slept at all. It was easy enough to say: Come to the wool loft . . . two excuses . . . church and the dressmaker. I had never been one of those pious women, forever running to church at odd hours. Because of Master Reed's hatred of Baildon and all its folk, and because, living outside the town boundary we were free to choose, we went to Mass at the tiny church of Flaxham St. Giles, and usually went, the three of us together, to make our Confessions on Saturday, before supper in winter, after it in summer. Richard would think it very strange if I proposed going to church alone on Saturday afternoon. As for my dressmaker—who was a little hunchback—she always came to the house when I needed her; I wasn't even certain of where she lived. She was a relative of one of the pack-whackers, and when I had sewing to be done I simply asked him to ask his Aunt Margit to come.

To people who live more grandly, or more poorly, it may sound incredible that a grown woman should find it so difficult to absent herself, without rousing questions, for an hour on a Saturday afternoon. But always, when I wasn't with the children, I was in the solar, or the kitchen, or the garden, and with Richard just on the move again the whole thing was doubly difficult. If I said I would go and look in on the children, he would say he hadn't seen them lately and would come too; if I said I would see how my palfrey did, ten to one he would say that a stroll in the sun would do him good.

All this I had to worry out in the night, and to think that it wasn't just this Saturday . . . this kind of thing could go on and on.

In the end I pleaded the routine female excuse; I had a headache, I said, due to sleeping badly. That I had slept badly Richard knew was true. I said that after dinner I would go and lie down. Master Reed went into the garden, where some plums on two trees on the south wall should be ready for plucking, and Richard said:

"I shall go and do an hour's work in the office. Father hasn't complained, but the work must be mounting up."

That was better than I had hoped for; he might have offered to come and sit beside me and dabble my head with a vinegar cloth. I went into the children's room, brooded over them for a little while, and then stole out.

The yard was empty and quiet. No work was done at the Old Vine on Saturday afternoons; the young men went to practise their archery at the Butts on the west of the town; those whose age or some infirmity excused sought their own amusements. From the huts which we called Squatters Row, at the back of the stables, I could hear voices and the sound of a fiddle.

I felt extremely large and conspicuous as I made my way to the woolshed, hugging the walls of each building I passed. I told my-self that I had a perfect right to go out and see how my palfrey did. When I was level with the pasture fence I did step out of the buildings' shadow and stand, for a moment, staring. Then I cut back, through the two wool-picking sheds, where the sun cut in in golden, dust-filled rays, and then, at the end, up the ladder and into the wool store.

Denys was waiting for me. He took hold of me and kissed and pawed me for a minute or two like a madman. I pushed him away and said, "Wait. Wait. You want it to be good. . . . You said after childbed women were . . . And it is true. I think that is what ails me and I think a little wine would help." I held out the little leather wine bottle that I had brought.

"You don't need that," he said.

"Oh, I do, I do. Just give me time." I loosed the stopper and tilted the bottle to my lips, pretending to drink. "You know what is wrong with me, don't you? I was in labour two days and three nights. . . . A woman has to be pot-valiant to risk that again."

"You're over the worst. The next lot'll be as easy as shelling peas."

"I'm pot-valiant," I said, wishing to God I were. For when neither flesh nor spirit is desirous this is a sorry, sad business. He didn't think so; and, anxious to pleasure him, I made as good a pretence of sharing his joy as I could.

When he was spent he lolled back against the soft, greasy fleeces and sighed and smiled. After a minute he said, forestalling me by a count of ten, "Is any left in that bottle?"

I reached out and lifted and shook it.

"Not enough for both—but you're welcome to what there is. It heartened me."

"Rubbish. I heartened you. I told you everything would be all right. Didn't I? Didn't I?"

"Yes. And you were right."

He set the bottle to his lips and drank.

"I must go now," I said. "And I must take the bottle. It might be missed."

"Next Saturday. Here."

"Next Saturday. Here," I repeated. He tilted the bottle and then gave it back into my hand. "I had to force you. You see, I knew what was best for you. You're my beauty, my darling, and I don't know how I shall wait the week out. But I will." He burrowed his head into my breast and clutched at me with his hands. In one moment it would all begin again.

"I *must* go . . . or there'll be no next Saturday." He sighed and set me free.

I climbed down the ladder of the wool loft with the words "no next Saturday" still sounding inside my head. By the pasture fence I picked up a young apple that I had left there—how long before, half an hour, an hour? How long had the whole thing taken? I called my palfrey and it came, took the apple, and slobbered over my hand and sleeve.

I went back into the solar where Master Reed was laying plums on a dish.

"I couldn't sleep, so I went out to see how my horse fared. I gave it an apple," I said, "and look what a mess it has made of me. I must go and wash."

No next Saturday, I thought. There will be no next Saturday.

VII

The next day being Sunday, Denys was not looked for and when he was found on Monday nobody could tell which day he had died, until one of the weavers said that he remembered seeing him come into the yard late on Saturday, very drunk. This—though it is unpleasant to think that in cases of felony some of the evidence given may be equally false—most admirably served my purpose, since it prevented the possibility, remote indeed, but lively in my mind at least, of anyone connecting Denys' death with my wandering around on the Saturday afternoon.

"He was probably not as sound as he looked," Master Reed said, and passed on to the matter of replacing him. Until that was done I knew I must be prepared to face hearing Denys' name now and again. I must keep my face smooth and secret, and show enough but not too much interest. Actually even that was spared me, though I would rather have been tested than excused the way I was. What happened was that within half an hour of the discovery of Denys' body, a hind, bumping and bouncing on Father's best horse, came to tell me that Mother was in bed.

"Very sick," he said she was, and anxious to see me.

Richard, who now had great faith in the doctor who had relieved his cough by night if not by day, insisted upon sending for him to ride out with me, but I was too anxious to be off. So he was to follow.

Mother was in bed, and as I set foot on the gallery I could hear the gasping rattle of her breath. Her brow and nose and chin were bone white, her cheeks dark purple with fever. Her eyes, dim with pain, were open, but she did not know me, even when I took her hot dry hand and spoke her name. Father was in the room, looking almost as ill and half crazed.

"What happened?" I asked him.

"Yesterday, no the day before, no, yesterday, she complained of pain in her side. I looked and it was bruised, very black and swollen. I made a poultice, a linseed poultice, and she said it eased her. Then she sickened and cried for you, but she was sensible then. It is only this morning . . ."

Suddenly the deep crisscross wrinkles below his eyes were wet. I envied him being able to cry. My need to cry scorched me. It was my fault that she had her fall, and if she died I'd have killed her as surely as I had killed . . .

"The doctor is riding close behind," I said. "He's . . . very clever. He'll do something."

"I hope to God . . ." Father said.

Mother went on fighting for breath. Every now and then a gobbet of thick yellow stuff, streaked with blood, bubbled from her mouth, and I wiped it away. Once, just after I had thus cleared her lips, she spoke, in a surprisingly bright, vigorous, *young* voice.

"I can hold together as long as I have to," she said, and then went back to that broken-winded breathing.

Father gave a sort of groan. "She said that to me . . . once before. The bravest . . ." he said, "braver than . . ."

And brought this low by her own daughter, a coward.

I thought of her courage, her unquenchable hopefulness which I had so much despised; I thought of her kindness to me every time I came back to Minsham, rejected and in what was tantamount to disgrace. It seemed to me at that moment that the only person on earth whom I truly loved was my mother.

I did not stand idle. All this time I was busy with what might be helpful. Remembering Richard and his cough, I propped her higher, to ease the breathing; I tried to make her drink something hot to wash the thick stuff from her throat; I wiped her face and hands with a cool cloth. Once, when I was doing that, she eyed me and said:

"I'll thank you, my lady, to take back this glove. Blanchfleur has no use for it!"

"Holy Mother of God," Father cried and dropped his head against the wall. "That that should trouble her now!" He banged his grizzled head against the wall several times and then went to the other side of the bed and cried:

"Maude. You know. You must know, there was never any other. Any good tourney man, it was the fashion to pursue him. Whose glove did I carry?"

But Mother had gone back to her fight for breath and minded neither of us.

Then the doctor arrived.

He looked at the bruise, just below her left breast, and said gravely, "Most unfortunate, the heart has been bruised; and the heart governs the melancholy humour. And the melancholy humour, left to run its course, can lead to death. However." He opened his bag and gave me some small objects, the seed cases of some plant, rounded at one end, pointed at the other.

"Make an infusion," he said. "Foxglove is a sovereign remedy for the heart."

But it was difficult to make her drink—as I had already discovered; the battle to breathe was too urgent, too closely pressed; most of the infusion was wasted.

She died just before sunset. The doctor, sadly disappointed by the result of his infusion, had gone; he had other patients waiting, he said, and he had done all he could. He had at last given an opiate, so that Mother seemed to sleep, though the battle for breath went on.

Just before sunset she woke, and returned to her senses. In a very weak fluffy voice she said my name.

"Anne."

"Here I am," I said. And my heart lifted. She knew me, she wasn't going to die. Some of the infusion, that sovereign heart remedy, had gone down and done its work; or the drugged sleep had helped to mend.

"Take good care of Blanchfleur," she whispered. Then her eyelids fluttered, the death rattle sounded in her throat, her mouth fell open, and she was dead.

I would gladly, and this is true, have lain down there on the floor by her bed and died too. On Saturday afternoon I had deliberately killed a man and been no more troubled than if I had crushed a fly which pestered me. But this was different. Remorse, perhaps the most terrible of all feelings, now had me in its mangling jaws. By accident, by a side blow, I had killed somebody who loved me and whom I loved. There is, and of this I am certain, no more terrible knowledge in the whole world. I should carry it with me until I died, and that seemed too much to face. I flung myself down on the floor beside the bed, and sobbed, in that dry, tearless way which brings no healing, and wished that I could die, just to be rid of the burden of guilt.

People don't—unless they are old and nearly ready for death anyway—die from the wishing. Presently I was aware of Father, sobbing and groaning away on his side of the bed. "Take good care of Blanchfleur," had been her last words to me; and taking care surely meant comforting him now. I got up and went round to him and sat on the bed's edge and lifted his head so that it lay in my lap. I tried to speak comforting words about Mother soon being with the Saints in Heaven, about the great reunion of all families which would one day take place there.

But Father was also deep in this business of self-accusation; and unlike me he could accuse himself aloud. He blamed himself for a multitude of faults, ranging from never having made a proper home or clothing her suitably, to having given her cause for jealousy in the old days. On that score, at least, I could comfort him with what I knew was truth. I told him of the talk we had had before my marriage and of the pride and triumph in her voice as she spoke of his wearing her glove and rejecting the great lady's. As I spoke I remembered that during my time of madness I had looked at Denys' flat archer's shoulders and imagined myself sharing Mother's pride. So even that was spoiled and sullied, and my words which made Father feel better made me feel worse.

I turned at last, for relief, to material things. I had not eaten since breakfast, and most likely Father had not even broken his fast. I slipped downstairs in the dusk—seeing, as I did so, Mother's fatal stumble and fall—and looked into the buttery. There was precious little to eat, some bread and three pigeons, ready plucked but uncooked. Another pain stabbed me at the thought that had she felt well yesterday Mother would have cooked those birds. I turned away from them and took up the bread. And then I saw the little cask of wine which Master Reed had sent on Thursday for her birthday. Her birthday!

The wine, I thought, would help down the dry bread; so I drew a jugful, found two cups, cut the bread into slices, and set it all on the table in the hall. Then I lighted three candles, one for the table and one for the head and the foot of the bed, and carrying them went up to the room where Father was waiting.

"I will do what is to be done here, after," I said. "You come now and make shift to eat a little."

Moving like a very old man, he dragged out onto the gallery and at the stairhead looked down and said, "If I'd been half a man, I should have railed in those stairs. I always meant to, but I pretended to be busy with my hawks and other toys."

"It was an accident. Like your own. If you had not your mishap, you would never have been compelled to live here. Do not blame yourself overmuch."

Rather pity yourself, too, I thought. And that applied to me as well. We may make victims of one another but we are ourselves the victims of Fate, also. I had turned to Denys to seek what I could not find elsewhere.

We made some pretence, at first, of dipping our bread in the wine and eating, but we soon put that aside. We emptied the jug and I took a candle and refilled it. Father drank most and most quickly benefited. He began, in his slow bumbling way to talk of the past.

"You say she was proud of me, eh?" he began, and then went on to tell of triumphs here, there, and the other place, of doughty champions met and defeated, of noble horses he had ridden, of presents and compliments he had been given; and all so muddled that sometimes it sounded as though it was the horse which had complimented him and the gift which he had unseated. I thought of the body upstairs on the soiled bed and of what I must presently do, and wished that I could sink into a like soft confusion of mind. So I drank some more, and presently was eased. Father's stories ceased and he began to nod. I said, "Come to bed," and he was so fuddled that on the gallery he began to walk, of habit, towards his own room. I took him by the arm and turned him gently towards the other door, towards the bed upon which I had spent Thursday night. Then he remembered and whimpered a little.

In Mother's room I did what was to be done, all the more easily for being a little blurred in my mind. Then I set fresh candles and drew up a stool, intending to watch all night; but the wine got the better of me and in the end I lay down on the floor and slept.

Interval

I

One day—Lady Blanchfleur having then been in her grave for three months—Martin Reed said to his son, "Have you noticed the change in Anne?"

"I think her grief is easing—a little," Richard said carefully, and, turning his head away, coughed.

"She drinks too much wine," Martin said bluntly. "Last evening, and the one before, she was flown."

"I know. And a good thing too!" Answering his father's astonished look, he added, "If she goes to bed with wine in her she sleeps. Otherwise she wakes, screaming from nightmare, and then cries for hours."

"About her mother's death?"

"They were very close," Richard said. "You and I who never knew a mother's love cannot measure her loss."

"It is a loss many people sustain without resorting to wine—in such quantity."

Richard coloured. "If you grudge so simple a comfort . . ." he began angrily.

"I grudge nothing. You know that. I just do not care to see a woman the worse for—and reeking of—wine."

"What you call worse I call better; and as for the reek, it is my bed she shares."

"I'm not wishing to quarrel," Martin said and left the matter there.

Richard himself was puzzled. Once, in the night, sobbing against his shoulder, Anne had said, "It was my fault. I killed her." He had dragged out of her the story about a bed to be aired which had caused the fall. He had said, at the end of it:

"I can see how you feel, but you must not blame yourself too shrewdly. The bed was to be aired some day for Isabel. It could have happened then."

But she had insisted that it was all her fault. Presently, thinking to comfort her, he said that everybody had to die one day. And that was a mistake, for she flung herself from him and spoke in a wild way about killing and a sin.

"A sin, sweetheart, to wish to spend a night under your father's roof! Come now!"

That night he took a candle and went padding barefoot down the stairs to fetch the wine which seemed to comfort her; and from then on, until Martin mentioned the matter, it had been Richard who would fill her cup, twice, three times, from the livery cupboard in the solar. What harm could it do? She never woke bad-tempered or liverish as those who drank too much sometimes did. The wine eased her grief, just as the grey powder eased his cough in the night. Where was the difference? It was Richard himself who first gave her another and far more potent draught, "to try." It was neither French, Spanish nor Rhenish; it came from the Low Countries, where it was called brandewijn. Half a cup of it was as potent as three of any other kind.

One evening, some weeks after Martin's first protest, he came into the solar to bid Richard and Anne good night. It was almost bedtime and Richard had poured the brandewijn into a cup, given it into Anne's hand, and then, taking his lute, sat down at her feet on a cushion, playing a gentle, soothing tune. One candle was out, the other nearing its end, the fire sunk to a rose-hued glow. It should have been a pleasant, domestic scene, gratifying to the older man, but by some indefinable degree it missed so being and was something else, so that, even before he smelt the liquor, he was irritated; and when he did scent it and knew it for what it was, he spoke more sharply than ever before in Anne's experience.

"Brandewijn!" he said. "That is no drink for a lady."

She said, "How would you know?" Just the four words, with the faintest possible stress on the second, but the whole speech so insolent, so full of hurtful meaning, that for a second he was checked.

Then he said, "I should have said for a respectable married woman."

Richard asked, with a flippancy which annoyed Martin even

more, "Must all pleasure be reserved for the disreputable and the unmarried?"

Anne laughed and reached out her hand and patted Richard's cheek. Trollop! Martin thought suddenly, and then, because that was too harsh a thought, he said, "Maybe you know best. I'm old-fashioned."

From him it was a handsome apology for one word, not even spoken aloud.

He stumped up to bed, and, shedding his clothes, wondered— for he was a just man—why it had slid, that condemning word, so easily into his head? In his cool, undemonstrative way he had been fond of his daughter-in-law. Had been? Was! She was part of his achievement. A knight's daughter. And never, until this evening, when he had blurted out his rebuke, had she by word or deed lain any stress upon the difference in rank. Provoked, she had retorted, as any woman of spirit would. He bore her no grudge for that. And even had he done there was no reason, surely, why his resentment should put that word into his mind. And yet . . . and yet. Even as he accused himself of injustice, he recalled something so fleeting that he had sensed it rather than seen it, something so unlikely that he had pushed it away as nonsense and never thought of it again until now. Three months ago, one evening in the summer, he had stood by the back door of the house and looked out over the yard, towards the fence of the pasture. Anne and Denys Rootyer were standing close together, so close that they might have been touching; if they were they moved apart instantly, just as his eye lighted on them. No, he would never be sure, never admit to himself even, that they had stood closer than needs be. Nor would he admit that there was anything odd in the man's fetching Anne out in the twilight to look at her lame horse; though there again the obvious thing would have been to call a smith.

Why had he remembered it? Why think of it now?

Getting old, and fanciful. Sixty, he thought, and remembered the priest at Rede telling him that at twenty half his life's span had fled. Out in his reckoning there, Martin thought grimly: but for my leg I'm as good as I ever was, good for another twenty years. Unless I go awry in my wits! For suddenly, out of nowhere, another fantastic fancy had slipped into his brain. In June of last year, he and Richard had both been absent from home at the same time, and he'd offered that one of the maids should come across and sleep on this side of the house. What had she replied—that what a servant could save her from would never hurt her. And the twins had been born on St. Joseph's Day, March the nineteenth.

Here, alone in his own bedroom, he felt his face go red and hot, his heart beat so hard that it thudded inside his skull, exactly as though he had been caught out, publicly, in some misdemeanour. *How* was it possible that he should have entertained such a vile, shameful thought long enough to do the reckoning? Where could such a thought have come from, unless direct from the Devil?

He lay down in bed and blew out his candle. When next his business took him to Colchester he would buy Anne some trinket, something pretty and of value, a secret proof of his shame for allowing fantasy a place in his mind, even for a minute.

II

The busy, happy years sped by. With Maude always just one pace ahead, the twins passed through all the fascinating stages of early childhood. When they were six years old an uninformed observer would have taken them for any brother and sister, the girl the elder by a year.

Richard's cough persisted, a little better in summer weather, a little worse in winter; his cheerfulness, his fixed refusal to regard himself as an invalid, screened, even from Martin and Anne, the stark fact that that was what he had become. He had ceased to ride abroad, never for the reason that he was not fit to do so, always because the weather was remarkably inclement, or there was too much work to do in the office, or the errand was something which Martin preferred to do himself. It was Anne who suggested that it was useless for him to ride with her on her regular visits of inspection to Minsham.

"He doesn't know," she said, speaking of her father, "whether we go or not. I only go to see that he is being cared for. I shan't stay an hour."

"I like to come with you. It's such a miserable business."

Sir Godfrey had sunk into apathy, prematurely senile, dirty, careless, almost witless, firm only on one point, he refused to leave his home.

"It's miserable," Anne agreed. "But why should we both suffer? You stay at home and then I shall be happy to return and find you cheerful."

She appeared to see nothing sinister in his acceptance. And when, one day when Maude was five years old and in boisterous play had all but pushed Richard from his feet, Anne said, "Maude, play a little less roughly if you please. Such behaviour is not becoming." The extreme fragility of Richard, which was then for a moment painfully plain, had escaped her.

On her own remorse-ridden grief time had worked its old healing magic and effected an almost complete cure. She no longer needed brandewijn to make her sleep; on Richard's good nights she slept well. Every now and then—often after she had been to Minsham— she would suffer a nightmare and wake, and be comforted by Richard and presently sleep again. But for Maude, Anne would, during the children's first six years of life, have been perfectly happy. As it was, she was like a person who has fallen amongst thistles and afterwards carefully removed every tiny prickle except one, which breaks off and burrows down and cannot be plucked out; it can be ignored most of the time, but is capable, nonetheless, at any accidental pressure, of causing a sharp pain. There were days when Maude was just a little girl, inclined to be headstrong and venturesome, but easily ruled because she was so affectionate. Then a slanting ray of light would strike the child's head where the babyish fairness was giving way to bronze; or someone would remark Maude's size and strength, by comparison with Walter, and Anne would be most sickeningly reminded. The mystery was that Walter gave the appearance of being Richard's son; he had the dark, slender grace, the delicate structure of bone, the slight air of defencelessness which called out all that was maternal in Anne just as surely as something, unnameable, in Maude, called forth dislike. The sense of guilt was thus kept alive, and occasionally exacerbated by a curious look which would cross Martin's face, usually when Anne allowed her resentment to take the form of an oversharp rebuke to the little girl.

"I shall forbid you to play with the yard children if you bring their manners indoors."

"How can you be such a hoyden? Look at your hands, your dress. Anyone would think you were a tinker's child."

Apart from putting in some mild defensive word on the child's behalf, Martin never said anything, but he wore that oddly disconcerting look.

Richard had a warm partiality for his daughter, and one night, in bed, at the end of a day in which Maude had incurred her mother's displeasure, said, "She's exactly like I used to be, at her age."

"You!" Anne sounded startled. "You were never like that, I am sure."

"But I was. I was the naughtiest boy in Suffolk, until Peter Priest took me in hand. Always into mischief. Uncle Tom's bear . . . did I never tell you?"

As usual he had come to bed first and then, a little later, Anne had brought up the cup of milk, into which the pinch of grey powder was sprinkled, and his voice was blurred by drowsiness as he recounted the tale of his misdoings.

Anne remembered the old man, the stuffy room, the malodorous bearskin on the bed. Pert Tom had died during that time when she was too much engrossed by her prolonged virginity to give the event much heed.

Lulled by the drowsiness of Richard's voice, she too fell asleep as soon as the story was done.

She dreamed that she was in the Ladies' Dorter at Beauclaire, helping to dress Maude, aged about sixteen, for the St. Barnabas Tourney. The girl's dress, a crimson and green silk, was beautiful and her headdress was a cloud of gauze. Anne looked at her with satisfaction and pride, thinking that with her looks and her clothes and her dower she was the equal of any young lady there. Then, under her eyes, Maude changed and became Denys. The wide archer's shoulders strained against the silk, the tough-looking red hair lifted the headdress. She said in an appalled whisper, "You can't go into the *Ladies'* Gallery." The dreadful creature said, "I must. You must take me. You can always say that I am your dressmaker!"

She screamed out her protest.

As on a score of similar occasions, Richard stirred and spoke.

"Sweetheart. It's all right. I'm here." His voice was thick and when he had spoken he coughed.

She said, "I'm sorry I woke you. Just another horrible dream."

He did not, as usual, ask should he make a light; nor did he turn in the bed and put his arm about her, comfortingly. He made a coughing sound which ended in a choke, and then there was a gentle bubbling.

Jerked from dream horror to real fear, she said, "Richard."

He did not answer; and it was she who made the light and saw on the pillow the spreading pool of crimson.

III

For a while the shared sorrow brought Martin and Anne closer than they had ever been before; her grief was so intense, so shattering that his half doubt—it had never been more than that—vanished in a wave of shame. They could say, over and over again, how blind they must have been, and then, inconsistently, mention things that they had noticed. They could say that they should have been more careful, and follow that statement immediately by giving instances of how careful they had been.

Under this apparent unity of spirit there gaped, however, a great gulf. Martin, who thirty-five years earlier had cried over Kate, "She never had anything!" could now, in an attempt to comfort Anne, say:

"He had a short life, but he enjoyed it all. He never lacked anything; he had you, Anne, and the children. You must think of that. And think, too, how much better this way than after a lingering illness, knowing that death waits." That was, in truth, his own private dread.

"Oh yes," she said. "That last night, he was laughing, telling me how naughty he had been when he was a . . ." The words "little boy" would not be spoken. It was unbearable to think of a little boy growing into a man, stricken with lung rot and now dead.

The dreadful remorse, the guilt which had assailed her after her mother's death, was now returned, doubled. She remembered how once, during her madness, she had dared to think that his love for her was a dream, like his dream of being a wandering lute-player. She had lived to prove how wrong that thought was. Only a true, firm love could have helped her through the time after her mother's death.

Over and over again she remembered that the last words he ever spoke to her were words of comfort—because she had waked from a dream which only her guilt had made possible. She tore herself to pieces on the spiked thought that if she had not wakened him he might have stayed asleep, flat, and the lifeblood would have remained in him. So she was doubly guilty, twice over the murderer of those whom she had loved, those who had loved her.

One evening, three weeks after Richard's death, Anne and Martin were in the solar. He had forced himself to overcome his dislike of the room in order to keep her company. They had said all the old things and she had broken down again and wept bitterly. She ate almost nothing, he knew, and slept hardly at all. Often, waking from his light old man's slumbers, he had heard her walking about, up and down, up and down in her room.

This evening, at last, she sat down and snatched up a piece of sewing, but she did not work as a woman should. The needle stabbed in and out, like a weapon. Then she would pause, stare wild-eyed at the wall, and stab again.

He watched her. Her looks were all gone. She was worn down to the bone, and her skin was the colour of parchment. He recalled suddenly the pretty, soft-fleshed woman who in this very room had laughed and patted Richard's face with one hand and held a cup of brandewijn in the other.

He got up and limped to the livery cupboard, fumbled about and turned back to her, a cup in either hand.

"Richard," he said, and stopped because the mention of his son's name, like that, was still a pain. "Richard told me that when your mother died, Anne . . . this helped you to sleep. You see, you have the children. You must think of the children."

She had not, since Richard's death, been able to bear the sight or sound of them.

And from some deep, obscure desire for self-punishment she had, for three long weeks, avoided the palliative which, she knew, stood there waiting in the livery cupboard. She had proved its worth and knew that once accepted it could convince her that she was not to blame; that she had done what was best in the circumstances. One drink and she would be thinking of the joy Richard had taken in this proof of his virility; two and she would be making intimate little reckonings, remembering that on the night before he left for Bywater and on the night when he came back, Richard and she had lain together. Only the one night between. And he never knew. I never by word or gesture gave a sign or swerved from my outward allegiance. . . .

She took the cup and presently the feeble voice of her own reason raised a bold loud echo in the cavern of intoxication, calling
that she was not to blame for everything, that circumstances had
played a hand in what had happened, that she also was to be pitied
a little.

Nothing, however, no amount of brandewijn, no amount of rea-
soning could make her look on Maude with anything but a carefully
controlled loathing. She knew that as long as she lived the sight
of her daughter would call to mind that dream, and with it all that
came after. It became her fixed and relentless purpose to get the
child out of the house.

Several times during the next months she mentioned, casually,
the question of Walter's education. Martin was inclined to shuffle
the matter off, there was plenty of time, he said; such matters
needed much consideration.

Once Anne said, "I seem to remember Richard saying that he
started his learning when he was six."

"I had Peter Priest ready to hand at that time," Martin said.
"Also, Richard, to tell the truth, was more unruly than Walter. Walter can wait a year or so."

When next Anne mentioned the matter he said, "I bear it in
mind. I keep my eyes and ears open for a suitable tutor for the boy."

She said, with a tinge of sharpness, "If you wait for another unfrocked priest, you may wait until Walter grows a beard."

"I'm not waiting for that. I'm looking for some clerk who could
help me as well. I'm missing Richard sore on that side of the
business."

The ache in his voice prevented her from speaking on the subject
again for a long time.

The twins had their seventh birthday, and in the winter following
it, on account of a piece of flagrant disobedience, a narrow escape
from death which did give Anne ample reason to say, "That settles
it. Walter must go to school."

"To school?"

"Yes. He needs the company of boys of his own age—and kind.
Also he has some talent for music. The Choir School at the Abbey
is just the place for him."

"Maybe," Martin said a little doubtfully. "If we could spare him."

"We should see him often; and they have holidays." She then
spoke the words to which the months' old discussions about Wal-

ter's future had been a mere preliminary. "As for Maude, I think I shall send her to Beauclaire."

More startled than when she spoke of school for Walter, Martin said, "Where *you* were so unhappy yourself?"

"I was so poor, so ill-equipped. Still, even so, I learned everything that a gentlewoman should know."

"And that has been of use to you?"

"I learned how to conduct myself. I feel it my duty to see that my daughter has like advantages."

He said, "Maude could be dressed and fitted out. She will have a dower . . . but she might . . . suffer in other ways."

"Some pert jackanapes or spiteful girl, saying, 'Do I smell fleeces?' Is that what you mean?"

He nodded, a little angered by her instant perception.

"I'll tell you straight, Anne; I've no mind to see my good money go where it will be despised because I made it."

"No one in their senses would despise it. I said a pert jackanapes or a spiteful girl, didn't I?"

"I'm against it."

"Very well," she said, more meekly than he had expected. "Would you be against her going to the nuns at Clevely for a year or two?"

"Not against; but I see no good reason."

"Don't you? What about Walter? They've always done everything together, in fact in all their pranks Maude is the leader. Don't you think he would be hurt, and justly, if he were sent to school and Maude stayed here to be spoiled?"

"I hadn't thought of it that way. Yes, it might be so. I expect you know best."

"I'm their mother. So will you see about Walter entering the Choir School?"

"I will. There's no great haste, is there? I could bring the matter up when I go to pay my rent."

That ended the conversation abruptly. The rent of one red rose to be paid in June had always been a matter of joking with Richard, who had made, and set to a lively ballad tune, a comical song on the subject, all about a year when poor Master Reed could find only a white rose and was obliged to take it to the dyer's.

The twins had their eighth birthday in March, and in June Martin made application for a place in the Choir School for Walter. Dreading the time when he and Anne would find themselves alone in the house, he was delighted to be told that there would be no vacancy until Easter in the following year.

Making her own inquiries, Anne was much displeased to learn that, except in the case of girls who had lost both parents and were homeless, Clevely Priory did not open its doors to those under twelve years of age. Riding back from Clevely, she made up her mind that, when Walter went into the Choir School, Maude should go to Beauclaire despite anything Master Reed should say.

Part Four

MAUDE REED'S TALE

I

So long as my father was alive, I never noticed that my mother disliked me. We paired off naturally, when Walter sat in Mother's lap I sat on Father's knee; when Mother hugged Walter, Father hugged me, and though, even then, Mother was stricter to me than to Walter that was easily explained; I was much worse behaved.

Father died when Walter and I were six years old, too young to understand or to know what we had lost. Children are very self-centred; the sorrow in the house brushed against us but was soon forgotten. For a little while Mother seemed to want neither of us; then she changed and doted on Walter more fondly than ever. It was then that I noticed that she disliked me. She'd sit on the window seat or the settle and draw Walter to her, put her arm around him, smooth his hair with her fingers, and look at him with love. I would run over to join them, never—I was careful about that—never trying to push between them, trying only to take my place by her other side, hoping that she would put her free arm about me. She never did. She would jump up and busy herself, or push me away, telling me to go wash my hands or comb my hair, or send me to fetch something.

I could make her notice me, but only in a way which did me no good. If I behaved badly enough, she would give her full attention to scolding me; sometimes she beat me. Once, when Walter and I were seven, a very strange thing happened. It was in the winter and the horsepond had frozen solid and Walter and I had played on it for several days, old games which seemed new because we were playing them in the middle of the pond. Then one morning our grandfather came in and said there was a thaw and that we were on no account to set foot on the ice that day. However, Walter had left his hobbyhorse on the ice, and he said to me, "When the ice melts my hobby will fall into the water." He looked at me the way he always did when he wanted me to do something for him. So I went to fetch the hobbyhorse and had it in my hand when the ice bent under me. I shot the hobby across the surface towards where Walter stood, and managed with my two hands to grip the edge of the hole and keep my head free. I yelled, and Walter, yelling, came towards me, and great cracks ran out under his feet; he went down, too, screaming like a pig having its throat cut. Men came running from the wool and weaving sheds, and we were pulled out.

Walter was blue in the face and very sick in his stomach; I was merely wet; so Mother beat me. She said I was bigger, girls should have more sense, and I went onto the ice first. I'd never had a beating like that, and I cried, saying I only went on to fetch Walter's hobbyhorse, but that didn't excuse me.

That night I woke to hear somebody crying and to feel a weight on me. I was frightened until I opened my eyes and saw a candle on the chest and Mother kneeling by my bedside with her arms spread out over me. She looked different, though where the change was I couldn't have said; and she smelt different. Ordinarily she smelt sweet from the little bags of lavender and rosemary that hung and lay amongst her clothes. Tonight she smelt of something sharp and sour. She was crying and saying jerky words, calling me poor Maude and saying she was unfair to me, with many other things which made no sense. I thought she meant that she had been unfair to beat me and not Walter. So I struggled up in the bed and put my arms round her neck and said:

"You didn't hurt me." I would have had a beating every day if it meant that she would put her arms over me and let me hug her. She went on mumbling about being unjust and I said, "I forgive you."

She gave a kind of squeal and pushed me off and jumped up, crying, "Holy Mother of God. That is all I lacked!" Then she went out of the room, walking in a funny way, bumping against the foot of the bed, and against the side of the doorway. She left the candle, and until it went out and I was in the dark I lay and wondered what was wrong in saying, "I forgive you." Perhaps it was a wrong thing for a child to say to her mother.

That must have been it; for next day she disliked me again.

We had another grandfather who lived in the country at Minsham and was too old, or too ill, to ride, so we had never seen him. He had a servant called Jacob, who used to come to the Old Vine every Friday and pick up some provisions and say, "Much as usual," when asked about his master's health. Mother sometimes rode out to visit her father, but as time went on she made more and more excuses not to do so.

One day, however, on a fine summer morning, she said, "You're eight years old now and able to make a longer ride. We'll go to Minsham today and you can meet your Grandfather Blanchfleur and your Uncle Godfrey who is staying there."

Walter and I had ponies which were much more like twins than we were, both brown with paler manes and tails. I called mine Browny; Walter, who was much more fanciful than I was, had named his Robin Hood, out of a story Father had told us.

Minsham Old Hall, we found when we reached it, was shaped like a barn, but built of stone, with very narrow window openings, unglazed. It stood in a yard, with no garden near it, just a tumbledown stable and a piece of pasture.

Inside it was even more desolate, and very cold, despite the sunshine outside and a fire on the wide hearth. In a chair sat an old man with grey hair and a beard, so overgrown that there was nothing else to his face except a loose wet mouth and eyes which had no life in them. I saw Mother brace herself, like she did once when a servant came screaming that there was a mouse in the meal-bag and Mother had to deal with it. She leaned down and kissed the old man, and then said to us:

"This is your Grandfather Blanchfleur."

Walter made his bow and I my curtsey, as we had been taught. Our grandfather seemed to take no notice of us at all, but he mumbled and I caught the word "Maude" quite clearly. I thought he meant me and, intending to be as brave as Mother, I moved forward, prepared to kiss him.

But Mother said, "It is not you he means. Go play in the yard."

As we went out she moved to the foot of the stairs and called up, "Godfrey!"

There was nothing to do or see in the yard; but Walter happened to say, "Grandfather is like Daft Jimmy." That was a poor witless creature who lived in the row of huts behind the stables at the Old Vine; *his* grandfather had been deaf and dumb, we were told, and

Walter and I had invented a game in which we pretended to be thus afflicted and bound to make ourselves understood by signs. We played it now, until we were called in to dinner.

We were then introduced to our Uncle Godfrey, who was very handsome and finely dressed.

He greeted us by name, and very kindly, and—the first person ever to do so—seemed to notice me more than Walter.

"So this is Maude." He looked me over, and smiled, and said something about lovely curly hair. "A real Astallon," he said. "Ralph and his golden Eleanor have managed to breed two little fawn-coloured creatures. Isn't it odd?"

Our grandfather's chair had been turned so that he sat at the head of the table. He ate as we had been forbidden to do, sucking and slobbering at his food and wiping his fingers, now on the cloth and now on the front of his soiled robe. Walter gave me a kick under the table and a meaningful look, like when we played "Dummy." I kicked him back and made faces, trying to say, without words: Yes, and wouldn't we be in disgrace if we did it?

Over our heads the talk went to and fro between Mother and Uncle Godfrey.

He said, "You hated it so much."

"I went to Beauclaire with one pair of shoes. When my feet grew I had to curl up my toes, and they are crooked to this day. You hated being at cousin Fortescue's; you wanted to farm here. Do you remember that? Are you sorry now that you didn't?"

"Not now. You saved me, Anne. You sent me the money so that I could buy my knight's equipment, and I . . ."

Mother interrupted him.

"And that wasn't easy; it wasn't a cause that either of them would have understood or sympathised with, let me tell you. That was my dressmaker's money for two years, and it meant refurbishing old ones, turning and twisting. I say this to show that what I ask you isn't so outrageous."

"I know. I know." He looked about the cold room with its damp grey walls and smoke-blackened rafters. "Here, too, you have taken responsibility, while I, with your good destrier between my knees, rode in tourneys. Nothing that you asked of me in return would be too great."

"You see," Mother said, "when I made the suggestion he rejected it, flat." She put her hand down on the table. "For me to raise it again would . . . You may find this hard to believe, but they have a pride of their own, more stubborn and stiff-necked than ours. When they speak of 'my good money,' that is the same as 'my good name.' I told you what he said. But an invitation from you would allow me to open up the matter again." She looked at Walter and me, and said, "If you have finished, you may go back to play."

We played until we were called in to make our adieus. As we stood there, my Uncle Godfrey looked at the figure in the chair and said, "My God, Anne, what a way to end! I can just remember when he won the King's Cup at Windsor. If you ever pray for me, pray that I never stop a half-fatal blow."

Mother turned the colour of the heaped-up ashes on the hearth. She looked towards the stairs.

"He was all right," she said. "Flying his hawks, riding his old horse. Until Mother . . ." She broke off and shuddered.

My uncle took her by the arm and said, "Poor Anne, you had that too! I was in Poitou. You've borne it all."

"More than you will ever know. But this one thing. You will do it?"

On the way home she set such a pace that Walter and I on our ponies and the servant who attended us on his thickset solid horse had much ado to keep up with her.

Shortly after this visit Walter was told that after Easter in the next year he was going to the Choir School at Baildon. The idea disgusted him; the schoolboys lived monkish lives, slept on hard beds, ate horrible food, washed in cold water.

"I don't want to. Why must I?"

"Because you will be a merchant, with a great business to run. You must learn to read and write and reckon."

"I don't want to be a merchant," Walter said. "I want to be a minstrel . . . you know, walk about from place to place, playing the lute and singing."

Mother said, in a way in which I have never in all my life heard anybody say anything, "You want what, Walter?"

Confidently he repeated his statement. She snatched hold of him and kissed him.

"One day you'll know better. You wouldn't like to be poor. And at the Choir School you will learn all about music."

"Church music," he said. "Not the same thing at all. Besides, it isn't fair that I should go to school and Maude should stay at home."

Mother said, "Maude is not staying at home. When she is twelve she is going to the nuns at Clevely, but in the meantime she has received a very pleasant invitation. She is going to stay with your Uncle Godfrey, at Beauclaire."

For a moment that took the sharpest edge from Walter's dissatisfaction, but he was soon grumbling again. I, he said, should be leading a merry life with ordinary people, while he was shut up with monks. If anyone beat me I should have Uncle Godfrey to complain to, he would have no one.

When the arrangements were first made, "after next Easter" sounded a comfortably long time away; but the months sped past. When the details were fixed and Walter learned that I was to ride into Sussex on Browny, while he must leave Robin Hood at the Old Vine, he flung himself screaming on the floor, shouting that it was unfair. My grandfather came to see what the noise was about and said, in an uncertain manner:

"Anne, is it worth it? Perhaps we were hasty. I heard recently of a young clerk who might serve our purpose."

Mother simply said, "Walter is jealous because Maude is to take her pony. Imagine his state if she were staying at home!" She took Walter by the arm and jerked him to his feet, speaking more firmly than she usually did to him.

"Straight into bed with you, you naughty boy!"

He was still in bed, being given possets and mixtures to bring down his fever, when I left for Beauclaire.

My grandfather, always a man of few words, gave me a broad gold piece, and kissed me.

"I hope you'll be happy. You mustn't mind too much if you find things different there."

Mother came into the yard where one of the men, named Jack, was ready, with my little clothes chest fixed behind his saddle. She kissed me, and for a moment I clung to her, hoping even at this last moment for some sign of love. She loosed herself from me in the old familiar way.

At the end of the covered passage which led from our yard to the highway, I turned and looked back. Mother was staring after us and her face was just like Walter's when I had let him win a game.

Whatever we played at I could always beat him if I tried, but now and then I would hold back and lose deliberately. Then he wore a satisfied look, a look that said, "Well, I managed that!"

I puzzled over it for a long time. Much later, when I learned that Walter never did go to the Choir School, but stayed at home and had his lessons there, I did understand all to well. I saw then exactly what Mother had managed; she had kept the child she loved and got rid of the one she disliked. At the time I could only wonder *why* she looked like that. All the same she had done me, all unwittingly, a good turn. Had she gazed after me with the slightest affection I should have broken down, for I still loved her then. As it was she sent me on my way exercising my head and not my heart, and that, in many of life's turning points, is an excellent thing.

II

We approached Beauclaire from the east, at the end of a sunny afternoon, so that it stood up against the gold and rose of sunset's first display. I thought to myself: But this is a town, not a house; and my homesickness deepened.

A great castle of grey stone stood in the embrace of a wide moat which was spanned by two bridges, one directly in front of us, at the end of the road which we travelled, and the other to the side, at the right. The second bridge linked the castle, which was very old, with the house, much of which had been built within the last sixty or seventy years. The face which the house turned to the road was very handsome and large, but—as I was soon to learn—it was only one small part of the whole. It was built of brick at the bottom and above of timber and plaster, the plaster moulded into patterns. There were many windows and all glassed, but I could see no doorway at all.

We clattered over the drawbridge, through a gateway at its far end, and there turned sharply to the right and through a small deserted courtyard, then over the second bridge and into a larger yard full of bustle, several men mounted, and servants running about. We then passed through an archway and into a stable yard, where I thankfully dismounted.

Almost immediately there appeared a solemn-looking man, by his dress neither gentleman nor servant, to whom the man who had been sent to fetch me said, "I'm back and all's well, Master Sheldon."

Master Sheldon glanced at me as he might have done at any package or parcel that had been conveyed from one place to another, noted that I was all in one piece, and nodded his satisfaction.

"You made good speed," he said.

We should have made better had the servant had his way. I had disliked him from the start; he was one of those—a type then new to me—who are intensely servile when they must be, and make up for it by being insolent when they can. It was plain, at the moment of our meeting, that he despised me on account of my youth, and Jack because he was a plain unliveried servant. The new man wore green with the Astallon badge, a falcon, on his breast.

Jack helped me onto my pony, for the last time, and then dived into his pocket, brought out a little handkerchief, edged with pegged lace, and tucked it into my sleeve.

"It's to be hoped you 'on't need it, my little dear, but if you do you'll know where it is."

He then turned to the Astallon man and said, "You take good care of our little mistress; she've never been from home afore."

That remark, and the thought of parting with Jack, thickened my throat again. The Astallon man merely sniffed and looked down his nose in a way that said plainly he was taking no orders from servants.

I said, "Good-by, Jack. I shall see you at Christmas."

We rode in silence for some time. The man broke it to ask, in a burring voice which made it hard for me to understand his words, "Is that the best pace you can make?"

I thought I had not heard aright; Browny was, for his size, very speedy and he was trotting his best.

"What did you say?" I asked. He repeated the question.

"Yes, it is. Browny is only a pony, as you can see for yourself."

"We'll see," he said, and he lifted his whip and brought it down hard on the pony's rump.

Certainly since the two matched ponies had been given to Walter and me on our fifth birthday, Browny had never been struck like that; Grandfather Reed was softhearted towards all his horses and had given us a little homily about treating the ponies properly;

and I loved Browny who was, anyway, quite willing to run as hard as he could without being beaten. Now, frightened and hurt, he broke into his little short-stepped rocking gallop for a minute or two, and then slowed down to a trot again.

I had a good enough reason of my own for not wanting him whacked into a gallop; I had been in the saddle two days and was very sore. I was only accustomed to taking short rides, or—as on our visit to Minsham—a long one with a rest in between. When Browny galloped, I bumped, and it hurt.

When the man came up to strike the pony a second time I cried, "Don't do that!" But he did, and we bumped forward as before. It happened twice more and Browny began to blow; so next time, just as he began to slow down, I pulled him to a standstill, clapped my hand to my eye, and let out a yell.

"There's a fly in my eye," I said.

The servant, close behind me, said, "Damnation!" and then, coming alongside, "Can't you get it out?"

I made a quick movement and snatched the whip, which he was holding in a slack hand just then, and I pulled the pony round a little so that my hand with the whip in it was as far as possible from the servant on the tall horse.

"Give me that whip," he said between his teeth. I was going to say: Not unless you promise not to hit my pony again! but what good would a churl's promise be? So I simply said:

"I shan't!"

There then followed, right out in the open road, a most unseemly scuffle. He pulled his horse round and made a grab for the whip, but I was ready and brought it down smartly on his wrist; he cursed and made another snatch, not this time at the whip, but at the top of my arm, which he seized and twisted. I was quite helpless then, and the only way to break his hold was to slip out of the saddle and stand in the road; even so I dangled for a moment, held by his hand, before my weight carried me to the ground.

I was by this time thoroughly frightened; dismounting so hastily and carelessly had rubbed my sore bottom, and my arm had had a cruel twist, so I started to yell. I stood there, holding the whip behind me, my back pressed to Browny's heaving side, and I yelled as if I were being murdered.

"Give me that whip and get back on that pony," the servant said. I yelled louder. He was in a rather awkward position; he could lift me back onto the pony, but to do that he must himself dismount, and when he did, I thought—some part of me quite calm for all the fright and the pain and the yelling—I would strike his horse, hard, so that it galloped off, and while he chased it I would jump back on Browny and ride in the other direction.

The road was far from being deserted. Two old women were herding along a great gaggle of geese and looked at us with interest, not untinged with amusement, but they were too busy with their charges to stop and ask questions. A man with a panniered donkey, waiting for the geese to pass the place where the horse and the pony narrowed the road, did speak.

"Whassa matter? Hurt yersel'?"

"Mind your own business," said the Astallon man, so fiercely that the man with the donkey quailed, smacked his beast with the flat of his hand, and passed on.

"My Lady will hear about this," the servant said to me.

"Aye, from *me!*" I said, and was straightway frightened again at the thought of some great lady listening to both our tales and believing *him*. So I yelled some more. But I kept my eye on the man and saw that he was going to dismount. I got ready, but just then along came some horsemen, riding fast. The first one cried:

"Make way, make way!" and the Astallon man, instead of dismounting, pulled in a little to the side of the road. The gentleman rode past, his companion followed, but he looked at us, the third gentleman passed. Then the second rider wheeled round and rode back. He was about the age of, and not unlike, my Uncle Godfrey.

"What is all this to-do?"

I said, "Oh, sir, please, please help me."

The Astallon man slipped from the saddle and put his hand to his forelock and began to speak rapidly . . . a sore task . . . sent to conduct the little lady . . . no will for the journey. . . .

I ran forward and took hold of the gentleman's foot in the stirrup.

"It isn't true. It's all lies. I was going willingly till he hit Browny."

The gentleman said, "If you would speak one at a time, I might make some sense of it." He leaned forward a little and studied the badge. "Astallon of Beauclaire?"

"That's right, sir. And sent to conduct . . ."

"Ladies first," said the gentleman. "Now, why do you stand here and make a noise like a hound in full cry?"

I told him in as few words as possible. "You can see I speak the truth," I said, and I pointed to the welts that had already risen on Browny's smooth rump.

"All right. Now you be quiet for a moment. You, tell me, was there any particular urgency about this journey?"

"I was told to make it with all possible speed, sir."

"All possible speed. Well, your master would know that so small a child would not be mounted on a saddle horse. All possible speed for that pony would be . . . let me see . . . three days. I shall pass close by Beauclaire, I'll turn aside and say that if you arrive earlier you have overdriven both pony and rider and should be beaten."

He turned to me with a smile and said, "A pleasant journey and a safe arrival, demoiselle. Would you like me to take that whip?"

I said, "Oh, I do thank you. Thank you. What is your name?"

"My name? Why, what is my name to you?"

"I shall mention it in my prayers every night as long as I live."

He laughed. "Then I shall be greatly in your debt. But I hope you will outlive all memory of me by fifty years. My name is John Fitz Arle. And what is yours?"

"Maude Reed."

"I wish you well. As for you, fellow, mind what I said."

(I put his name into my prayers that night, and I kept it there, for years and years, by rote and habit, long after I had forgotten what he looked like and everything about him, except that he had stood by me in a moment of great need.)

So I had won, but victory has its price. At inns one's accommodation and food depends very largely upon one's servant and his care for one's comfort. Jack had seen that I slept and ate well in Colchester, Chelmsford, and Brentwood. Now anything would do.

What I didn't know was that in all great establishments all the servants are forever trying to make their duties profitable. My escort had been given money for the journey. If he could have shortened it by a night—even if Browny had ended broken-winded —the price of a night's lodging for us and our mounts would have gone into his own pocket. This form of cheating was rife at Beauclaire, as it must be, I suppose, in any establishment too large to be sharply looked to by one person. Even over the candles my Lord Astallon was swindled by his house steward, whose duty it was to see that new candles were placed in every sconce and stand every evening. The short ends were one of his perquisites, and, since hundreds of candles were used every day, they would have amounted to something. But he was not content. The new candles were put in place and they were lighted; then some minion of the steward's would run around, replacing them by the stubs of another evening. So the cry, "Bring fresh candles," was constantly to be heard, together with complaints that candles these days lasted only half the time that they were wont to do.

Even taking three days for the journey, thanks to my behaviour, I think the man made some small profit for himself. I do not think that my Uncle Godfrey, nor my cousin Astallon, would have wished me to lie in the common sleeping room with tinkers and drovers; or to dine on boiled goose-grass root three days in succession. Fortunately, as my homesickness and misery grew, my appetite lessened. And as the appetite lessens so do the spirits. It was a very miserable, quiet little girl who got stiffly down from her pony's back, and saw him led away and thought: There goes my last friend.

The servant indicated that I was to follow him, so on foot we went through another archway and into a court with a well in its centre. An old man was drawing up water in a bucket and tipping it into a barrel which fitted into a frame with two wheels and shafts; a donkey stood between the shafts and a boy stood by the donkey's head. This vast household used so much water that the old man worked at the well and the barrel made journeys to and fro, all day long.

One side of this court was enclosed by a wing of the house itself, and here was an entry, a deep, dark porch with an iron-studded door set within it. As a sign of his displeasure with me the servant halted by this door, instead of taking me in and handing me over.

"In there," he said, and walked away.

I stepped into the porch, feeling smaller than I had ever done in my life, knowing how dwarfs feel in a world fitted to ordinary people. I stood for a moment, gathering my breath and my courage, then I pulled off my glove, and, making a fist, knocked on the door. It was, I soon saw, a very thick door, and plenty of noise was being made on its farther side. Nobody answered my knock. I beat on the door again and, when it stayed closed, turned the great iron handle and pushed.

Immediately inside the door was a kind of small room, the door behind me forming one wall of it, the other three made of finely

carved screening through which I could see. Our solar at the Old
Vine was reckoned to be a wonderful apartment, unmatched in the
whole of Baildon, but this room was three times as large and half
as high again. Yet it seemed full, for the young ladies within were
all wearing wide-spreading dresses and enormous headdresses. Four
of them sat in a group, with a piece of embroidery spread over
their laps, each stitching away at her own portion, and talking and
laughing as they worked. One sat alone on a window seat, playing
a lute, very softly and sweetly. Some others, at the end farthest from
the hearth, stood at a table, throwing dice and making loud ex-
clamatory noises; and three stood quite near the door, divided from
me by the lacy woodwork of the screen.

I stood in the enclosure, like something in a cage, and looked
about, then I pushed against each side in turn, and the left side
proved to be a swing door. I walked into the room and went near
to the three young ladies who were talking. One was telling some
tale, making gestures as she did so.

". . . so I said, 'Oh, *is* that so? Then what about the evening of
Holy Cross Day?' Could you have seen her face?"

One of the listeners said, "Oh, Ella, we swore never to mention
that!"

"I was so much provoked. But listen! She then said, 'That is
what comes of lending one's cloak!' And she tossed her head and
turned. . . . God have mercy, where did *you* spring from?"

Tossing her head and imitating the turn, she had come face to
face with me.

"I came by the door."

"And what do you want?"

"I've come to live here. My uncle arranged it."

"Who is your uncle?"

"Sir Godfrey Blanchfleur."

"Oh. Well, I don't think he is here now."

Perhaps she would have shown more concern, but one of the
other girls tugged at her sleeve.

"Ella, go on! I must skip in just one minute. Lend her cloak,
why, she wouldn't lend a pin!"

There was nothing to be hoped for from them, so I went farther
into the room and from shyness approached the lady who sat alone,
rather than another group.

All I had time to see, or wit to notice then, was that she was pretty, with a beautiful pale unblemished skin and hair so fair that it was almost silver.

I planted myself in front of her and said all in one shaky gulping sentence, "My name is Maude Reed and my Uncle Sir Godfrey Blanchfleur invited me here, and now he is gone and I don't know what to do and I want to go to the privy very badly indeed!"

"Poor poppet!" she said, and laid the lute aside, jumped up and took my hand and hurried me through a doorway, into a passage, up some steps, down some steps, into another passage and so into a room where stood a row of big square boxes covered with black velvet. She threw open the lid of one of them and showed a gleaming copper pot, sunk in the black velvet of the inner frame.

"There you are," she said cheerfully.

Urgent as my need was, I waited for her to go. I was unused to the ways of the great. At home there was a privy, with a screen of bushes around it, and there was, of course, the night-pot under the bed in case of need, but I had not—at least since I could remember —used either with anyone watching.

While I stood, almost weeping with indecision, the door opened, and one of the young ladies who had been dicing hurried in. I knew her by her violet-coloured dress. She threw up her skirt and took the stool next to the one opened for me.

"Holy Virgin," she said, "that onion broth! It goes through me like a purge."

Encouraged, I sat down and did what I wanted.

My friend, so pale and slender, looking so far removed from such gross human needs, lifted her sleeve and held it before her nose.

"Catherine, what a stink! Little one, have you done?"

She took up a bell which stood on the ledge of a niche like an unglazed window set in one of the inner walls, and rang it vigorously.

"Now," she said, "if anyone knows about you, it will be Dame Margaret and I think she is in the Still Room. We'll find her. So you are Blanchfleur's niece; yes, you have his eyes."

In the passage we met an old woman carrying a bucket and a jar of sudsy water; she stood aside to let us pass. When the passage widened the young lady took my hand, asked me to tell her my name again, asked how old I was, was I homesick? Yes, so had she been, she said, when she first came to Beauclaire, but that soon passed; in the Children's Dorter there were several boys and girls, some about my age, and I should enjoy playing with them; and Dame Margery, who governed us, was not too strict, it was said.

I made bold to ask her her name.

"Melusine." It was one I had never heard before, and I repeated it to make sure I had it right.

"Yes, Melusine. I was named for a fairy lady in a French romance."

"You could be one," I said. "I thought just now . . ." But I could not tell her the thought I had had in the Stool Room.

"What did you think?"

"That you are beautiful."

She laughed.

"You have the Blanchfleur tongue, too."

But she sounded pleased.

When we had walked for what seemed to me a long, long way, she stopped and opened a door. It smelt as though the lid had been taken off a spice box. Behind the door was a smallish, cosy room, lined with shelves and cupboards, all the shelves full of jars and bottles and boxes. At a solid table in the middle of the room sat a stout, elderly woman with a plain linen head-piece, moving her hands about in a wooden trough, full of some dry-looking, sweet-smelling mixture. Ranged along the table were many bowls, some of silver, some of pottery, pewter, and wood.

"What have we here?" she asked, looking up.

"We have Maude Reed, who has come to live here."

"Why, yes, of course. They were warned at the entrance that she would arrive today or tomorrow, and should be taken to Dame Margery. What has happened?"

"She came to the Well Yard door, and Dame Margery has taken all the children blackberrying, or so I thought."

"You thought right—so tomorrow I shall be busy with the cordials. And this not off my hands yet! Very well, very well. They will be back very soon, it's nearly dark. She can stay with me."

Melusine smiled and left me. Dame Margaret asked if I were at ease, and if I needed to eat now or could wait until supper.

I said I could wait. So, having tossed the mixture again, she said I could help her to dish it out into the bowls.

It was just the kind of task most useful at the moment; it kept me busy and made me feel a little less lost and unwanted. When she saw that I was careful and neat-handed, she left it all to me.

She took a cup and poured some dark rosy-red liquid into it and sat down, leisurely sipping. Between sips she asked me questions. At one point she snapped a finger and thumb and said:

"But of course. Your mother was Anne Blanchfleur. I remember her well." She looked at me with a new, close interest, up and down, noting my very shoes.

"Reed, you said? And your father is a wool merchant."

"No. My father is dead. My grandfather is a wool merchant, the biggest between London and Lincoln."

She made a little noise as though clearing her throat.

"Family ties are strong, for all that. Lucky for you, you are like your mother—in appearance, I mean."

"I'm not. My mother is very pretty, and I have red hair."

"It runs in this family. My Lord Astallon is red as a fox. As for prettiness, one day you may be pretty too if you learn not to glower."

The door opened, and another plain linen head-piece poked around its edge.

"Ha, Margaret! There is no linen, nor towels laid out for the Merlin Chamber, and my Lord Ashford just arriving."

"God be my judge!" cried Dame Margaret, jumping up. "It was tomorrow. I swear my Lady said tomorrow . . ." She trotted out of the room.

In the moment or so that the door had stood half open, the scent of roasted meat had come in and mingled with the spicy air of the room. I realised that I was, if not actually hungry, very empty. All through the journey my stomach had been full of misery, and the food at the inns, for the last three days, had been very unappetizing. Scratching up the last of the mixture of rose petals and lavender and bergamot heads out of the wooden trough and into the bowls, I began to think about supper. And that made me think of the Old Vine, of the bustle and chatter as the weavers and pack-whackers and smiths came trooping into the dining hall, my grandfather, quiet but kindly, taking his place at the end table, Mother beside him and Walter next to her. My place empty . . .

Here, at least, I was alone and could snivel a little; so I did, folding my arms on the table's edge and leaning my face on them. I snivelled until one of the candles went out. The Still Room was on the inner side of the house, with only one small window which looked out on a narrow court, so the candles had been lighted there early. Now one, and then another, guttered away. And I was afraid of the dark. Walter was too; but somehow he had managed to make his fear known, and when one day I confessed to Mother an equal dread of darkness she had said, "Copy cat! Just because Walter has this whim, so must you." So after that I had made light of it, sheltering behind Walter's need to have a light through all the hours of darkness. Now I was alone in a strange room, and where there had been six candles there were now four, and two were failing.

I went over and opened the door. The passage outside was quite brightly lighted. I walked along it, following my nose, which would, I thought, lead me to the food, the scent of which was now powerful. Soon the passage divided, one arm of it, narrow and dimly lighted, ran off to the left, the other, wider, very bright, led towards a set of stairs. I went that way, and at the stair head found myself in a room which was as much bigger than the one by the Well Yard door as that was compared with the solar at the Old Vine.

It was so magnificent, so unlike anything I had ever seen before, that for a moment I could forget that I was homesick, alone, hungry, and forgotten, and just stood staring. Every inch of the walls was covered with tapestry. At home we had one, and that was reckoned a marvel; here one joined onto the next, all the way round the great room. Ours at home was a scene from the Bible, Adam and Eve in the Garden of Eden, their nakedness screened by flowers and bushes, Eve offering Adam the fatal apple and the Serpent, coiled about a tree trunk and wearing a human face, watching the triumph of his wiliness. The tapestries in the Long Gallery at Beauclaire were pictures of stories which I had never heard; there was a knight on a great horse driving a lance into the body of a thing all covered with scales like a fish, but with a thick solid tail and claws like a bird and a head more like that of a horse than anything else. The knight wore a red cross on a white background on his breastplate. Every one of the woven pictures was concerned with knights. In one a knight lay on the ground, sorely wounded to judge by the blood that oozed over his shoulder from under the edge of his gorget, but he was blowing a great horn, and his enemies made a ring about him, waving their swords, aiming their pikes, while far off, on a distant hill, a gathering of knights seemed to be waiting and listening.

I walked all the way round, looking at the pictures and wishing that there were someone with me who could tell me the stories about them.

At the far end there was another high doorway, and I went through it and found myself in a smaller room, all hung with rose-pink draperies; and beyond that was another passage. There were many doors in it, and I opened them, one by one. Most of them opened onto darkness, and one, just opposite a candle sconce on the passage wall, gave me a fright, for it was full of suits of armour on their stands, and looked, at first glance, like men. That room smelt of the oil used on the harness, and of the vinegar which was mixed with the wood ash for polishing the metal.

By this time I could not even smell the food and knew I was lost. But just as I knew this I opened the door and found myself in the room into which, a lifetime ago, I had walked. There was the screen about the door, the table at which the ladies had diced, the piece of embroidery, and, on the window seat, Melusine's lute, just as she had flung it down. The candles were burning low here, too, but there were so many of them that the light still served. I walked over to the window seat and stood there, thinking that this was her place, and she was the only one who had been kind to me. I touched a string of the lute and it gave a little tunable twang.

There was a lute at home; it hung by a silk ribbon from a peg in the solar, and I had always wanted to handle it; but it had belonged to my father and was sacred. One day, however, Mother had reached it down and put it into my hands. "There you are," she said, "see what you can do."

All I could do, to start with, was to make a discordant noise. She sat and watched me, which was not helpful. I had, however, just begun to work it out, that when I touched this string such and such a sound came forth and when I touched this, another . . . and in a moment I felt sure I should have made a less distasteful noise when she jumped up, snatched the lute from me, and hung it back on its peg, saying:

"You have no art."

Now, left alone with a lute, I would have tried all the strings again and endeavoured to remember what I had learned in that one brief handling; but, as I reached the window seat where Melusine's lute lay, I could look out of the window and saw that the wall which ran out at right angles to the Well Yard Room was pierced with windows, all aglow, and as I looked a door opened and a man came out, holding something in his hand which he raised to his mouth and bit upon. So I went through the screen and out by the door and across the Well Yard and in through that opened door.

I was at the lowest end of the dining hall, from which all but a few servants and a tableful of pages had gone. At the other end was a low platform, with a table running across it, from side to side of the hall, and that table was edged with crimson velvet, heavily embroidered, a little like an altar cloth. Another vast table ran the whole length of the hall, and at the lower end there were others, set near the wall. Broken meats, half-eaten trenchers of bread soaked in gravy, spilled ale, gnawed bones, and apple cores littered the boards. Some men, each with a bucket, were going around sweeping everything from the tables, and behind each man came a boy with a filthy cloth which he drove—swish—across each surface as it was cleared.

The pages were eating heartily and talking and laughing at the same time. One looked up and saw me, nudged his neighbour, who looked and nudged his. They all stared but not one did more, and though some of the servants eyed me they said nothing. I walked along by the long central table, looking for something to eat. When I found it—it was a pigeon, all that was left of a dishful, to judge by the bones scattered round—I sat down, pulled the dish towards me, and began to eat. It was in that worst state, no longer hot, yet not quite cold, and I should have liked some bread with it; however, it took the edge from my hunger. As I ate I watched the clearing being done and thought how much more carefully we did things at the Old Vine, where the bones were collected separately and put onto the dung-heap where they softened down into manure, and all the soft waste went into the swill pail for the pigs. Nor would my mother, or for that matter Old Nancy, have allowed such filthy cloths as the boys were using anywhere within reach of our tables.

I crammed the last piece into my mouth just as the clearing man reached the place where I sat. I then walked down the hall again and out into the Well Yard and into the room where the ladies had been, hoping to find Melusine. There was no one there and the candles were almost dead.

I have known sharper grief, deeper misery, but never a feeling of more complete wretchedness, of being alone in a hostile world. Dame Margaret had spoken of my having been expected by the main entry; if I only knew where that was, I thought, I might find someone who would know me and tell me where to go. The idea of still being alone and lost when all the lights were dead and darkness everywhere filled me with panic.

Often, during the next few days, I looked back on my first evening at Beauclaire and thought how contradictory was its way of life. I truly believe that a homeless person, provided he or she were decently dressed, could have moved about in the house, eaten in the hall, slept in a corner, and gone unchallenged for a week, a month, maybe forever. Everyone would assume that the stranger belonged to some other department, or to some visitor's train. Yet, side by side with this, was the equally true fact that, once you *were* claimed and recognised and made part of the establishment, you could never for a moment get out of the place. There was somewhere where you must be, someone you must be with, something you must be doing from the moment you left your bed until you went back to it.

The household, which to me just then seemed so dreadfully disorganised, was, in fact, very closely and highly organised. All my misery was the result of having been sent to the wrong doorway.

Not daring to stay longer in the empty darkening room, I opened a door, found myself in a passage, and could hear some music and the sound of someone singing. The sounds seemed to come from the top of a flight of steps, so I climbed them and opened the door at the top and knew at once that I had solved one problem; I was no longer alone. The room was crowded with ladies and gentlemen, some ladies seated on benches and chairs with gentlemen around them, but most standing in groups. The music came from the other end of the apartment, and most of them were facing it, so had their backs to me.

I went in, like a pup looking for its master, hoping to find either Melusine or Dame Margaret. Here again, as I moved about people looked at me with a mild curiosity, but nobody asked *why* I was there. I was halfway up the room, at a point from which I could catch glimpses of the lute-player, and of a man with a harp and a boy with a wooden frame, the top bar hung with little bells, arranged in order of size, the smallest like a thimble, the largest as big as a cup, when I saw Melusine standing with a very fine young gentleman.

I had been moving diffidently, but at the sight of her I flung myself forward and took her hand.

"What!" she said. "You again. You should be abed."

"I know." I began to blurt out my woes, how Dame Margaret had left me and nobody had called me to supper and how I had been lost.

Faces began to turn in our direction; somebody said, "Hush!" The music ended with a loud sweep of the player's fingers across all the strings, and in the vibrating silence immediately following a sweet, high, languid voice called:

"What *is* all this ado?"

Holding me by the hand, Melusine led me towards where a lady sat on a bench with high, incurved ends, all gilded. The lady did look, indeed, like a statue of gold; her dress was yellow and so was her hair, and she wore it uncovered, pulled back from a high white forehead, and held in a net of gold, set with yellow stones where the strands crossed. Her face was like a statue's, too, carved into an expression of faintly shocked surprise, due to her eyebrows being shaved off and then painted on again, a full inch above their natural place.

Melusine let my hand fall and stepped back a pace and said in a stiff way, "Madam, this is Maude Reed."

"Maude Reed," she repeated the name, just as I had hours ago repeated Melusine's. She turned her head towards a man who stood behind the gilded bench. I remembered Dame Margaret's remark about the red hair. His was very red, quite different from mine. He leaned over and whispered in the lady's ear.

"Of course," she said, and turning back to me gave me a smile and said, "You are welcome."

I knew what to do and I meant to do it, to make her the best curtsey I had ever made, holding my skirt clear on each side and letting my head dip just at the right moment. And I did.

But the truth was that one of my reasons for misery and wanting to find Melusine was that I needed, once again, to visit the Stool Room; and my inside didn't know that I was making my duty to my mother's kin, Lord and Lady Astallon of Beauclaire, it thought I was attending to its needs. I felt the warm wetness run free, scouring my saddle-chafed thighs.

Forever disgraced, I thought, rising with the shamed blood scorching in my face. I cannot stay here. Tomorrow I must go home. And here they will remember me forever—Maude Reed the girl who made a curtsey and made water at the same time.

There was the little puddle; the moment I moved it would be seen by all, and, though I knew that I must move and that it would be seen, something made me try to defer the evil moment. I was like a person on his way to the tooth-puller's booth, lingering by every other booth that he passed.

"Madam," I said, "my mother sent you her loving greetings and her deep gratitude for taking me into your household."

"Your mother," she said, and again turned her head. My Lord again leaned forward and whispered into her ear.

"Your mother has trained you very prettily," said my Lady, turning back to me. "Now . . . You will join the Children's Dorter and be governed by Dame Margery, and I trust you will learn well."

Ignorant as I was, I recognised the tone of dismissal. But I still stood, guarding my shameful secret.

My Lord saved me. He made a sign to the musicians, who broke at once into a merry tune; and a slim young man with red cheeks came from behind the bench and bowed and extended his hand and said:

"Madam, I beg you, dance with me."

She smiled and stood up; and, since she could neither walk through me nor over me, I was bound to step aside.

Now, I thought, they will all see.

But her skirts were long and full and edged with fur. When she had passed there was nothing left to show that I had misbehaved myself. After a moment Melusine came to me and said, "I will take you to Dame Margery."

The young gentleman who had stood by her said, "When did you turn nursemaid? May I be your next charge?"

She said, "You do not expect to reach second childhood so soon, surely?"

Outside another door, which we reached after a long walk, Melusine halted, put her arm around me, and kissed me.

"Our paths may not cross again for many a long day," she said. "I hope you'll be happy."

I clung to her for a moment; then she put me gently away, and once we were inside the room, face to face with a dignified, solemn-looking lady, her manner was formal again.

"This is Maude Reed, Dame Margery," she said. "By some mistake she came in by the wrong door."

III

The Children's Dorter at Beauclaire was really an establishment on its own. The actual Dorter was the chamber in which we all slept, boys and girls together, but separated by screens down the centre of the room; when people spoke of the Children's Dorter, however, they meant also the big room in which we worked and played, and took all our meals except the midday dinner, and very occasionally our supper.

There were eight of us at the time when I joined the Dorter; my Astallon cousins had two children of their own, a boy of nine, named Ralph, a girl of six, Constance. There was another girl of eight who bore about the same relationship to them as I did myself, she was a Fortescue—sent, after the fashion of the time, to be schooled in the house of a cousin, while, in her own home, other girls and boys were being trained; her name was Alison. There were two brothers, aged nine and seven, Henry and William Rancon, whose father had died by my cousin Astallon's side in the French Wars lately ended; and there was an eleven-year-old girl named Helen Beaufort, who was a relative—some believed an illegitimate daughter—of the great Cardinal. There was also a girl named Madge FitzHerbert who was a true half-wit; she understood very little, spoke indistinctly, and had protruding brown eyes which did not see very well. I never knew her to manage to thread her needle. She was there because her own mother was dead and her father, when he remarried, did not wish his new wife to see what manner of child he had bred already. He had some position at Court and was in high favour, especially with the Duke of Gloucester, the King's uncle. My cousins had accepted Madge as an inmate of their Children's Dorter in return for some favour which her father was able to do for them. My Lady Astallon had ambitions and was always craving to live in London and take what she called her "proper place in the world," but her husband preferred to stay at Beauclaire, with only short visits to his other estates, to attend to the management of his affairs and mind no will but his own. I've heard him say that the Duke of Gloucester was "riding for a fall," that when the tree fell the ivy fell too, and that for himself he would sooner rule on his own acres than be just one voice on the Privy Council of the King.

Our days were strictly ordered, but by no means tedious. We girls learned to sew and to embroider; not to spin, spinning was at that time out of fashion for the gently reared and the distaffs lay idle in a corner. We learned to dance, and to play various games without showing chagrin when we lost, or pleasure when we won. Self-control was a virtue highly rated by Dame Margery; she never, for example, minded how much, how often, or how viciously we quarrelled but we were not allowed to smack one another, or scream, or cry. The boys, when they fell out, were allowed to use violence on one another, but not in the house.

"Into the yard and settle it," Dame Margery would say; and the one who came back defeated had scant sympathy.

"You'll take harder knocks, if you live."

The boys, when they were ten years old, were removed from her care altogether—"And I want no one saying, when you get amongst men, that I have brought you up soft."

We girls, though treated differently, were disciplined too. We must learn to stand still, perfectly upright, without fidgeting or sighing for long stretches of time on end; we must always eat, without any sign of distaste, anything put before us. We must learn to govern even the workings of our bowels.

"Bless you, child," Dame Margery once said to Helen Beaufort, "in a few years' time, when you wait upon some great lady and are tiring her hair, will you drop the pins and cry, 'I must to stool!'? You will *not*. Go stand in that corner, place your hands on your head, and await my permission to go."

Unlikely as it sounds, impossible as it seemed to us at the time, her methods did work; bowels and bladders learned that they were not masters to be pandered to, but servants to be obedient.

In many ways we were fortunate in our mistress; she was a countrywoman, who after some years in London had come back to the place that she loved, and she liked nothing better than to take us out, riding or afoot, naming us the wildflowers or the birds, warning us which berries were poisonous, letting us share, in a manner unusual in most households, the seasonal activities of the manor. On the day of my arrival the children had all been blackberrying; later we gathered mushrooms and hazelnuts. When the summer came, we were allowed—the girls demurely sunbonneted—to toss hay in the meadows, play amongst the stooks in the harvest fields. Once she took us all into the woods, carrying food with us, and let us make a fire and cook, tinker fashion. The meat was bitter with smoke on the outside and red raw within, but somehow it tasted different, and better than a dish similarly spoiled would have seemed eaten indoors.

My appreciation of our Dame did not come all at once. My first weeks at Beauclaire were very wretched. I made mistakes and was punished, I lost myself several times. When the boys teased me I fell into a rage, when Alison and Helen tried—as they did at first—to show themselves superior to me, I wept. So much that we did seemed to me useless, false, and hypocritical, and there was so much else that I did not understand.

This wool-merchant business, for example. Alison and Helen seemed to hold it against me that my grandfather was a wool merchant. At least here Helen, who was the older, always gave the lead and Alison followed her.

Once I cried, "And what's wrong with being a wool merchant?" and in fury took up the scissors and slashed into Helen's embroidery. Dame Margery punished me, and I yelled that it was not fair, I hadn't started the dispute.

"And do you expect fairness in this world, Maude? If so, you are going to be very sorely disappointed. Better learn now. Go stand in the corner and place your hands on top of your head."

I could learn, that was one blessing. I wasn't like poor Madge who could make the same mistake three times in one day. Next time Helen twitted me about the wool business I stayed calm. I didn't even look at her, I looked at the wall straight ahead and I said:

"My *father* was in the wool business too. And when I was born he did not call me his *niece!*"

Now for that I should have been whipped. But no! Dame Margery, a little later, said, "I am glad to see that you are learning to stand up for yourself in proper fashion."

Proper fashion, for young ladies, meant lashing out with hurtful words, not slashing with scissors.

Not long after that I performed, out of cowardice, an act of bravado which gave the boys a good opinion of me.

Every fine day, after the midday dinner, unless Dame Margery had something planned for us, we were allowed to go and play in what was called the Low Garden. In days long past, when Beau-claire consisted of the castle only, this garden had been the pleasance where, in times of peace, at least, the ladies could take the air. Since then new and better gardens had been made near the new house, but they were for the pleasure of grown-up people who did not wish to be disturbed by children's games. The Low Garden was now somewhat neglected, its grass tufty, its bushes overgrown, the walls surrounding it tumbled in some places. There was one stretch of wall, still quite sound, however, and one day the boys took a ladder into the garden, climbed by its help to the top of the wall and there strutted about like young cockerels, jeer-ing at us girls who, they claimed, couldn't do what they were doing. They then began a game of taking turns to run the length of the wall and back.

My head for heights had never been put to the test, and I couldn't see why William, a month or so younger than I was, could do some-thing which I could not, so in the end I called that it was now my turn; and I climbed the ladder and stood on the wall, which was about twelve inches wide at the top, and which, on the garden side, dropped ten feet, and on the outer side twice as much. The moment I stood on the wall and looked down I realised the truth of their jeers, this was something no girl could do, or should attempt. I also knew that to stand there, teetering, was the worst thing I could do; only speed could save me. Trying not to look at or think about the drop on either side, I walked briskly to the end of the stretch of wall where it ran into the side of a solid square tower. I turned and pressed my back against the blessed solidity of that tower and knew that I should never have the courage to leave it and set out on the return journey. My head was already spinning and my knees had turned to melted wax. So I did the only thing there was to do; crying, "I'll wager you daren't do *this!*" I jumped down into the garden. A sharp sickening pain stabbed through my ankle, but Dame Margery's exhortations of self-control bore fruit; I did not cry out, nor did I hobble, though my ankle remained swollen and painful for many days, and will even now, in wet weather, pain me.

Henry Rancon took up the challenge, climbed the wall, ran along, and jumped as I had done. William said he couldn't jump because he would jar a tooth that was already giving him trouble, and Ralph Astallon said it was time we went back to the house.

After that, however, whenever they wanted a fourth for any game they chose me rather than Helen, who was older and stronger.

So, bit by bit, I worked myself into place at Beauclaire, and before I had thoroughly recovered from my homesickness Christmas was drawing near. I expected to go home for Christmas, and I cherished a hope of being allowed to stay there. After all, one of the reasons for sending me away had been that it wouldn't be fair for Walter to go and for me to remain, and Walter had remained; and another reason was that I should learn, and I had taken care to learn all I could.

Advent came; the first Sunday in Advent, and then the second, and nothing was said about my going back to Baildon for Christmas. It seemed to me that it might be one of those things overlooked or gone awry—like my arrival—so during that week I said to Dame Margery:

"Madam, I am supposed to go home for Christmas."

"Are you indeed?"

"No one has spoken of any arrangements yet."

"Heaven bless you, child, have patience. Your home is . . . how far away?"

"Five days' ride."

"Then there is plenty of time."

Another Sunday came; and I reminded my Dame, and she said, "Maybe I should make inquiries."

She must have done so, for next day, at dinner in the hall, my Lady Astallon sent for me and when I stood close said, "This notion about going home for Christmas. What put that into your little head?"

I asked myself, what? When there was talk of Walter going to the Choir School and of me going to Clevely, there had been mention of being home for Christmas; but he was now at home and I was here. It was I, bidding Jack farewell at Brentwood, who had said, "Home for Christmas."

"It was understood, madam," I said in a weak voice.

"Not by me. And not I think by your uncle. In any case, travel at this time of the year is undesirable; the inns so uncomfortable and the likelihood of being snowbound . . ."

She waved an elegant hand in dismissal, and I now knew better than to argue.

Next day, on my way out of the Hall after dinner, I was stopped by my Uncle Godfrey. He had, on and off, paid me some attention, for which I was very grateful. He had returned to Beauclaire four or five days after my arrival and had at once sought me out and asked how I fared. Now he said:

"This going back to Baildon for Christmas, Maude, would be very silly. Christmas here is kept in such style. People come from London to share in the festivities."

"But I expected to go home."

"There you are mistaken. Your mother was clear on that point. You stay here until you are twelve."

"And not go home at all?"

"Running to and fro," he said, "is vastly expensive and bothersome and unsettling. And all to what purpose?"

"I want to see my mother and Walter and my grandfather."

Something changed in his face, so that for a moment I feared that I had offended him. Then he took a lock of my hair between his fingers and twisted it, saying slowly, "You know, child, sooner or later you have to learn to do without people. It's best to learn young."

"But why? If it is a question of expense I still have the broad gold piece my grandfather gave me."

"You'd only make it harder for yourself. . . ."

Where the words or the thought came from, I do not know, but I heard myself saying, "My mother doesn't want me at home, does she?"

"She knows that you will do better here. And so, for that matter, do I. Who else looks to go home?"

"Alison, Alison Fortescue."

"Does she so? Well, for your ear alone, in that house Christmas is so meanly celebrated I'll wager she'll wish she'd stayed here. Many's the Christmas I've spent there and, believe me, even the plums in the pudding are counted out, one by one."

I wanted to shout that it was no matter to me whether there was one plum in the pudding or a thousand. Most of all I wanted to go and cry somewhere, alone, by myself. But the truth was that at Beauclaire there was no place to cry alone; once you were part of it you lived a public life, where every sigh or frown or tear was observed and remarked. At this moment, because my uncle had stopped me on my way out of the Hall, there were Constance and Helen, Alison and Madge waiting for me.

I walked slowly to join them, thinking that when I had said that Mother didn't want me home my uncle had not denied it. I remembered then what I had forgotten, the face she had worn as she watched me ride away. Something within me hardened. I thought: Well, if she does not want me, I don't want her. It wasn't true at first, but thinking it over and over made it become true. I still yearned for the smallness and friendliness of the Old Vine, for the kitchen where I was welcomed and given gingerbread men, for the yard full of men like Jack who would call me "Little Mistress" one minute and "Maude" the next. But, over that Christmastime, I began to be weaned.

That I had not been expected to go home was made very clear by the arrival, two days before Christmas, of gifts for me. From my grandfather—or so I imagined—another broad gold piece, from my mother a blue velvet hood, lined and bordered with fur. With these gifts was a square of parchment, bordered all down the left side with leaves and berries painted in green and red, and with words written in the remaining space. The letters were very black, except for a few which were gaily coloured.

I held it out to Dame Margery and learned, to my surprise, that she could not read. But she knew what it was.

"It is a Christmas Piece, to bring you good wishes. Carry it down to the Well Yard Room. Most like one of the young ladies can spell it out for you. If not, you must ask the Chaplain."

I was delighted to have a chance to go where I might see Melusine, for whom I still entertained a passion of gratitude and admiration. There was, rightly, a firm barrier fixed between the Children's Dorter and the Well Yard Room and the Ladies' Dorter, and I seldom saw her except at a distance. That morning I found her and she read me out what Walter had written. It said:

> On this, the Birthday of Our Blessed
> Lord, I send Greetings to my Dear
> Sister and wish you Joy and God's
> Blessing on you, from your Brother
> Walter Reed.

Melusine read it for me three times, so that I could get it by heart. Then she asked how old was Walter, and when I told her that he was just my age she said, "He must be a clever scholar. It is nicely written and very even."

The Christmas Piece, bringing home almost as much as Walter to mind, made me homesick again. The pretty furred hood seemed a mockery, and when I returned to the Children's Dorter I gave it to Madge FitzHerbert, who had received no gifts at all.

The Christmas Piece I carried about with me all through the Twelve Days—which were kept, as my uncle had promised, with every possible gaiety.

While I was showing it to my Uncle Godfrey I said, "I would dearly like to read and write, too."

"You would *what?*"

I said it again.

"Then you must consult with Dame Margery."

"She cannot read. I had to ask the Lady Melusine to tell me the words."

"She has learning? Perhaps she could teach you. As I said, consult with your Dame."

Dame Margery showed more sympathy with my desire than I had dared to expect.

"You are to be a religious," she said thoughtfully, "and some learning might serve to advance you. I will speak to my Lady."

The answer, when it came, was typical of Beauclaire where the most prodigal extravagance ran side by side with sparing economy over trivial things. It seemed a pity for Melusine to waste her time teaching one child to read; who else would like to learn? Everyone else showed the utmost horror for the notion; I went round, pleading with one after another, even poor Madge. I argued that writing might be the one thing she *could* do, how could she know till she had tried. But she just giggled. In the end it was Henry Rancon, the least likely of all, who came to my aid. I thought of a good argument to use on him.

"At Easter you will move out of the Children's Dorter," I said, "and all your life will be changed. So you would have only a few lessons, and meanwhile I would do anything you asked. I would be your liege man."

Henry was always wanting somebody to be his faithful, unquestioning servant, and neither of the other boys was obliging.

"All right," he said. "I'll have lessons till Easter. Now you kneel down and put your hands between mine and swear to be my faithful liege and obey my every command."

That I did most gladly; and though Dame Margery said, "Won-

ders will never cease," when Henry professed his desire to learn to
read and write, by Candlemas the lessons were arranged.

Tucked away in that same long passage where the suits of armour
occupied a whole room, there was a small room in which some
earlier Lord Astallon had gathered several books; there was a table,
too, and a bench, and a slab of wood out of which sprouted three
horns. One held the ink, the other the quills, and the third the
sand for drying anything which was needed too hastily to permit
the ink to dry of itself.

And here, on three afternoons of the week, in the space between
our playtime and supper, Henry and I and Melusine met. On the
first day, when I thanked her, most eagerly, for agreeing to teach
us, she said:

"The saddle is on the other horse, Maude. To escape, even for
an hour, from the everlasting chatter and bickering; to get out of
that carp pond delights me."

Another time she said that it should be a law that every woman
who was not a busy housewife should learn to read.

"If they could find stories in books, they would be less ready to
make up tales about those they live amongst. And they would learn
that their own small joys and troubles do not fill up the world."

I learned fast, partly because I wanted to and partly to please
Melusine. Henry was content to learn how to write his name. Page
after page he filled with "Henry Rancon. Henry Rancon," then "Sir
Henry Rancon," or "Henry Rancon, Knight." He just lived for the
moment when he should be a knight; he had the same feeling for
my Uncle Godfrey—who was reckoned one of the best knights in
England—as I had for Melusine; and I think one thing which resigned him to the tedium of the lessons was that, every now and
then, and always unexpectedly, my uncle would look into the Book
Room to see what progress I was making. My uncle, unlike most of
his kind, spoke of learning with respect, and told Henry he was
lucky to be taught.

"I never had the chance," he said. "At your age I was never in one
place long enough."

"I could teach you now, Sir Godfrey," Melusine said.

"I am an old dog, too old for new tricks. But there are old tricks
that I could teach *you!*"

"Of that I have no doubt," she said, and laughed.

IV

It was towards the end of that February month that Henry made one of his demands upon me, in keeping with my vow. There had been some days of continuing snow, during which our afternoon playtime had been spent indoors, where tedium had led to squabbling and squabbling to punishment. Rheumy colds had afflicted us, too, and my cousin Ralph was still abed on one side of the screen, and Helen and Madge abed on the other side. Our Dame had her hands full and her temper was short.

On this day, however, the sun shone and the snow was melting fast, and as we came out of the Hall Henry said, "Come and play Hare and Hounds in the Maze."

The Maze at Beauclaire was a singular oddity. It was part of the old Low Garden, at least it formed one of its boundaries, but it was said to be older than the garden, older even than the castle. It was an intricate puzzle of narrow paths, crossing and turning back on themselves, bordered by clipped yew hedges as tall as a mounted man. In its very centre stood a block of black stone on a mound of grey ones. There was a story that in the very faraway past, when the people who lived in England were heathen, that stone was worshipped.

I had only penetrated deep into the Maze on one occasion; very soon after my arrival at Beauclaire, Helen Beaufort had mentioned, in Dame Margery's hearing, something about the Maze being the haunt of evil spirits, and Dame Margery had said:

"Rubbish. It is just a puzzle, laid out in the days when people could not walk far from the castle walls for fear of enemies, so they made the longest walk, and the most interesting, on the smallest possible space." And to prove that she believed what she said she had taken the lot of us, on a sunny autumn afternoon, and we had gone in and lost ourselves, and run this way and that, and shouted, and laughed and in the end come breathless to the black stone in the centre, and Dame Margery had said:

"You see. You have all lost your breath and wearied your legs as though you had run a mile. It is simply an exercise ground."

"Then what is the stone, madam?" Helen Beaufort asked.

"To mark the centre, so that people could know that they had arrived."

"It's a Rune Stone," Helen said in the stubborn way which she had mastered; not rude or ill-tempered, just a flat, unshakable way of stating something.

"And what might that mean?" Dame Margery asked.

"I don't know. I heard it spoken of as a Rune Stone."

"Meaning a marker, like a milestone," said Dame Margery. "Now, all take different paths and let's see who can be out first."

That night, in the Children's Dorter, after the light was out, Helen said to me, "A Rune Stone is not a marker, say what she may. Before I came to Beauclaire I lived at Greenwich and one was found there, and the priest had it hacked to pieces; he said it was evil."

There was no need for Dame Margery to tell us girls not to play in the Maze, we avoided it; but the boys often played a game of Hare and Hounds there, and certainly seemed to suffer no harm.

On this afternoon I said, "Oh, Henry, it's so cold and so sloppy underfoot."

"Running will warm you, and you can put on your thick shoes. Besides . . . you promised."

That was true, so I said meekly, "Can I be a Hound?" Hounds could run in company, the Hare must go alone.

"You are a Hound; with William. It is my turn to be Hare."

"I'll get my cloak and my thick shoes."

"We'll wait for you by the Maze," he said.

Alison and Constance were waiting for me, and as we went up the stairs I said, "I am going to play Hare and Hounds with William and Henry in the Maze. You come too."

"God's teeth," said Alison, who was fond of using grown-up expressions, "on a day like this? A cold thaw. I thank you, no!"

When we reached our room I went and stood before our Dame and said, "I am going to play with Henry and William."

I hoped that she, like Alison, might think a cold thaw a bad thing to brave. And that would let me out. But she only said that the fresh air would do me good, so long as I kept moving. So I fetched my cloak and looked for my thick shoes, and they had been taken away to be greased. So the bell must be rung and by the time it had been answered and the servant had been despatched for them, and had brought them, the brightness of the day had gone. In the Maze, I thought, it would soon be dusk.

However, I was sworn. So I ran out and joined the boys, who were waiting impatiently.

The rules were that the Hare started first, while the Hounds stood still and counted the fingers of both hands twice over. The Hare, as he ran, also counted twenty and when he had done cried, "Hee, hee, hee, you can't catch me!"

The Hounds then replied, "Woof, woof, woof."

Henry ran into the Maze and presently made his call. William and I ran in, crying, "Woof." It was already—for me, unpleasantly— nearly dusk between the high hedges, so I stayed close to William; at one place where two paths met he said:

"You take one, I'll go the other way." But William was not, even in pretence, my liege lord, so I let him run along his path and then I followed. At intervals Henry made the Hare call, and we responded. Henry's voice seemed to come from a different direction each time.

Presently William, as he ran, drew away from me. I tried to keep up, and when I couldn't, gasped out a shameless, breathless appeal.

"Wait for me."

He threw back over his shoulder, "We're not supposed to stay together; it spoils the game."

At the next turn I found that I had lost him, one path went left, one right, and so far as I could see along either he was not there. This was the moment that I had dreaded ever since Henry had issued his command. I stopped running and stood still. I needn't play any more; I could always say that I had tried to find them and failed. Had I had any sense at all, I thought, I should have fallen behind and turned back minutes ago, before I was far into the Maze.

Just before I turned I heard Henry's call far away to the left, and William's answering cry, to the right it seemed. To show that I hadn't given up too easily I cried, "Woof, woof, woof," too, but there was something about the sound of my voice that I didn't like, it sounded lost and frightened, less like a hound than a little bleating lamb.

I turned rightabout and began to walk, hoping that by going in that direction and keeping on long enough I must emerge at the entry. As I walked, I could hear Henry and William calling and counter-calling; once Henry sounded close at hand, and I hoped the next turn would reveal him. It did not. Nor the entry. And the dusk was deepening every second. To be alone in the Maze in the dark would be as bad as being in the Long Gallery at midnight on the sixth of November, when a long-dead Anne Astallon, whose husband had killed her in a fit of rage, was said to walk, weeping and wringing her hands.

I stood still and shouted, with all my strength, "Henry! Henry." There was no answer, and I thought, of course, he wouldn't answer, he'd think I was cheating in the game. One call though—if he heard it, he was bound to answer, being my liege lord, as I his man.

"À moi, Rancon! Aide! Aide!"

When that brought no response I knew I was out of earshot. I began to whimper and run any way, without trying to stick to one direction, and presently I found myself at the intersection of four paths and there was the big black stone.

I crossed myself and said, "God between me and all harm." I remembered what Dame Margery had said and tried to believe that it was placed there only to mark the centre; but Helen's words were much more powerful. It was still just light enough for me to see the chisel marks on the stone, deep in places, in others worn almost smooth.

I was extremely frightened, but with just sense enough left to know that what I feared was being alone in the dark, and that at such a place and such an hour even the most homely thing—a porridge bowl—could seem sinister. I didn't even know what "Rune" meant, so what happened next was not due to my imagination.

First I went to back away, into the mouth of the path by which I had come; and I found that I couldn't move. It was like one of those horrid nightmares when something pursues you and your feet are too heavy to run. My eyes were fixed on the stone, and I stood as fixed as it was. Then, in it, just level with my eyes, a light appeared, as though a small window had opened, with candles in the room within. The golden glow was faint at first, but it strengthened as I stared; and then out of the lighted square a face looked at me.

I did not, at that time, know what a cardinal looked like, the nearest I had been to one was when I listened to speculations about Helen's paternity, so I did not know what I was seeing. It was the face of the man that held my attention, not from any remarkable feature, but because his eyes, dark under heavy brows, looked straight at me in a very compelling, forceful way, as though he were using his will to beat mine down. I had no glimmer of a notion what he wanted of me, but I knew that whatever it was it was important to me; I knew also that I must not give in. As I thought that the face disappeared, the square glowed faintly for a moment and was gone.

By this time I was beyond fright. I knew I was about to die. I couldn't draw breath. It was as though an iron hand were clenched round my throat. Fighting against it, just to pull in breath once more took all my strength and I was failing, just about to die when the most beautiful sound in all the world reached my ears; a human voice, calling in its homely Sussex speech:

"Stay right where you be, little lady. I'm coming for ye."

The iron hand fell away, and I drew in breath with the sound of a cloth being ripped. I began to shake all over.

"Could ye give us a call for a bit of a guide?"

I tried, but my tongue was dry flannel between my chattering teeth.

"Now, now," the voice said, a trifle crossly, "'tis no use pretending, or hiding from me. The game's over now. You give us a shout!"

I tried and had just enough breath to make a small mew, like a kitten.

"Hi there! Can ye hear me?"

I managed to cry, "Hi!" and then, at the next try, "I'm by the stone."

"Stand still then."

In no time at all he was with me, a little bent gnome of a man, carrying a lantern. He put my fear—I was shaking still—down to the fact that I had been lost.

"That need never worrit you. We watch. We count 'em in and we count 'em out. Come on, now follow me."

As we walked he told me that once, long ago, when his own father was "just a little gaffer," some young people had gone into the Maze during the Christmas revels, and all come out but a young lady who was not missed until next day, and was dead when found.

"I should have died, too, if you hadn't found me."

"Oh no! 'Tisn't freezing tonight. Yon was a hard frost."

"I should have died of fear."

"There's naught to be feart of. There's two of us, and one is always on the watch."

"I didn't know that."

"No. We don't make much of ourselves. People don't like to think they're overlooked."

I don't think I was any more pious than the next child. I performed my duties and observed the Holy Days of Obligation and the fast days, but I seldom thought about religion. Now, however, I thought: That is like God, watching our comings and goings, Himself unseen but ready to help in time of need.

From that thought it was only a short step to be wondering whether the face I had seen in the Rune Stone was not really a heavenly vision and that what the man had been trying to convey to me was not to be frightened. The French girl, Jehan the Maid, had put visions and voices from Heaven in the forefront of everyone's mind. And *she*, I remembered, had been burned for a witch.

Dame Margery, who had not, I think, noticed my absence because she was so busy with the three sick children, scolded me for giving her needless anxiety, and set me yards of hemming to do for a punishment. William and Henry said I had spoiled the game, they thought I had given up too soon. I said to Henry, "I gave you the Cry of Extremity and you did not aid me, that cancels all vows."

I never mentioned my vision to anyone; and perhaps for that reason thought about it the more. Walter and I were born on St. Joseph's Day, and I thought it possible that the face I had seen had been of the Saint. After that I had a special devotion to St. Joseph, and when, around Eastertide, a seller of statues and medallions came round I broke into one of my gold pieces and bought a medallion of St. Joseph and fastened it to one of the cords of my velvet purse.

V

When the next Christmas came round I did not expect to go home and felt no sorrow about it. The love which I had felt for my mother was now firmly fixed upon Melusine, who was just as pretty, and just as sweet-scented, and who never pushed me away. When Henry moved, with my cousin Ralph, out of the Children's Dorter at Easter, he gave up his lessons, as I had known he would, but, as was the way at Beauclaire, a custom once established went on and on, and it would not surprise me if, in that house, one lady went on opening the Book Room and spending three evenings in it every week, with or without a pupil until the Wars of the Roses brought all those great houses to ruin.

For ruined they are, I have lived to see things change, and those great rambling houses where three hundred people would sit down to supper every evening, where any traveller of noble rank was welcomed like a brother, where everyone above the rank of knight had his own cook, and bloody battles—sometimes fatal—would be waged in the kitchens over who should use this hearth, this spit, they are gone. The Wars between the Red Rose of Lancaster and the White Rose of York are blamed for the change, but I sometimes think they were bound to end, those great establishments, out of their own unwieldiness and waste. And perhaps because, under all the glitter and splendour, there was something rotten, something that made human beings of small account, and wealth of too much.

Helen Beaufort was older than I, and had already left the Children's Dorter and joined the Ladies'. This had two results for me. Although Helen welcomed the change and thought herself greatly superior to me now, she was lonely at first, and would seize opportunities to talk and tell me bits of gossip which I should not otherwise have heard. And, with her going, I became the eldest in the Dorter, entrusted with certain duties and responsibilities, and allowed, in return, certain small privileges. The one I valued most was to be allowed now and then, to go and read in the Book Room after supper. Whenever I had that permission, I would tell Melusine and sometimes she would say that if she could slip away, too, she would come and join me.

One evening she *had* managed it and we were sitting close together on the bench, both reading from the same book, which was what I liked to do because it gave an excuse to press close to her. The writing of the book was poor and difficult to read, but the story was so interesting that we read on, taking turns to read a piece.

All at once the door flew open, and when we looked up, startled, it was to see Ella and two other young ladies with expressions of smiling mischief slowly changing to astonishment on their faces.

One of them, Millibrand, said, "Holy Mother of God! It *is* true. She *reads*."

Melusine said, "What did you think I was doing?" Her voice was cool, but her face was red-hot.

"We couldn't believe it," Phillipa said, gazing round the small room. "There is a Welsh minstrel in the Long Gallery. To miss him, in order to brood over a book that smells of mould . . ." She turned up her eyes, begging Heaven to witness the unlikelihood.

"To miss him, in order to spy on me seems even poorer exchange," Melusine said.

"Ah, but . . ." Ella began. Millibrand pulled her by the arm.

"We are missing the music. Come along."

They ran away, laughing and rustling their dresses.

I got up and closed the door which they had left open. As I sat down again, Melusine put her arm around me and gave me a quick hug.

"My good angel!" she said.

"Why?"

"Oh . . . well, if you had not been here they would have dragged me off with them."

Now that I was learning something which I enjoyed, and seeing so much of Melusine, and had lost all trace of homesickness, I was happy at Beauclaire, and my eleventh birthday, bringing with it the thought that the coming summer would be my last, saddened me. I began wondering whether it would be possible for me to stay and in the end join the ladies in the Well Yard Room, instead of being uprooted again and going to Clevely. It was plain to me that I wasn't wanted at home, and so long as I stayed away I couldn't see that it mattered to anyone but me where I was. Walter and I had now become competitive about our writing and sent letters to one another twice or three times a year; I would write to him, I thought, early in the summer, perhaps at Whitsun, and ask him to ask Mother if I might remain at Beauclaire. Walter was to me, now, hardly a memory; I had changed so much in these three years, I knew he must have, too; he had become somebody whose writing remained much neater and more stylish than mine, try how I would.

With the summer, life at Beauclaire always became very gay; besides the big Tournament, regularly held on St. Barnabas' Day, there were several smaller ones, and there were many unplanned entertainments, too; wandering players would come and perform their mysteries, jugglers their tricks, sword-swallowers and fire-eaters their seeming miracles. Most of these delights we children were allowed to share, increasingly so as we grew older. There had at one time been talk of two young children coming into the Dorter, but Dame Margery had argued against it; Constance was now "getting off her hands," she said, and she herself too old to start all over again. So in that summer of my eleventh year, when even Constance could stay up late without yawning or falling asleep where she sat, we had more fun than ever before.

One day in June—I remember that the garlands and banners from our Tournament were still up—there was a bear-baiting. We children took our places, at the back of the Ladies' Stand. I saw Helen Beaufort sit with the grownups, and reminded myself that I had not yet written that letter to Walter. It again seemed unfair, and unnecessary, that next year I should go to Clevely, and should have borne all Dame Margery's training for nothing.

I'd watched bear-baiting before and never been squeamish about it, but on this evening something happened to me. I stopped being Maude Reed, a spectator up in the stands, and entered into the feelings of the bear. I may be wrong, but I think learning to read had had an effect on me. When you read you must get out of your own skin and into the skin of the people you are reading about, that is the only way to enjoy it.

They'd cut the bear's nose, both to make him savage and to let the dogs smell blood to make them savage, and I began by having a pain in my nose; then, as the fight went on, pains went all over me, particularly low down in my body where I had never had a pain before, and between my thighs. I sighed and shifted about on the seat, and Dame Margery looked at me reprovingly.

It was a remarkably good bear; dog after dog it dealt with. Now and again, when a dog was clawed or crushed or bitten, my feelings went that way for a moment or two, but in the main I was with the bear, I was the bear.

Everybody became excited. The ladies, who must in all circumstances remain well behaved, smiled and clapped their hands and made little murmuring or squeaking sounds; the gentlemen were more noisy, wagering money on whether a dog would "score" or not, a "score" meaning a bite which held while one could count up to five; they shouted, and laughed, and yelled the counts aloud and groaned when a dog they had backed was shaken off too soon.

Presently, even from where we sat we could smell the blood.

Then somebody called, "Try two dogs at once." So they did and the bear dealt with them gallantly and cleverly.

The dogs—some were strays that had been collected and kept for such an occasion, or young hounds which had something wrong with them which made them of no value in their proper sphere—were let loose from one end of the Tourney Ground, and presently, from that end there was a cry.

"Only one dog left, my Lords and Ladies."

Then it'll soon be over, I thought; and despite all his wounds the bear will have won.

But somebody shouted, "Blind the bear!" and somebody else called for pepper.

After all that, to have pepper thrown in his eyes.

I knew then that I was going to be sick. I was surprised. The pain in my body hadn't been anything like the belly-ache which often ends in sickness. Nevertheless, I was going to be sick. I pressed my hands over my mouth and made for the stairs which led down from the stand. I was near them, and did not have to push past Dame Margery. I just blundered down and to the back of the stand and then I was sick.

I couldn't go back. Never willingly would I watch a bear-baiting again. I didn't much want to go into the house, either. It would be deserted. Some other entertainment was to follow the baiting, tumblers or mummers were to perform by torchlight. I'd walk about for a little while, I thought, and then, when the poor wretched bear had been taken away, and sand spread over the blood patches, creep back into my place.

From the Tourney Ground the nearest pleasant place for walking was the old Low Garden, so I went there, not minding being alone there, partly because being alone out-of-doors was never quite so uncomfortable to me as being alone within walls, and partly because somewhere, at the far end of the Low Garden, there was the Maze and nearby, keeping his watch, would be one of the old men. I didn't go near the Maze, though, I stayed on a path edged by ancient rosebushes, so long unclipped that they were almost wild again, but covered with a profusion of flowers, pale pink, striped with deeper colour, and very fragrant. In the mild evening air they shed their scent, and I breathed it in gladly after the reek of blood and terror in the Tourney Ground.

I walked up and down the path, and every time I turned I could see, at the other side of the overgrown garden, the tall blackish-green hedge which walled in the Maze; and one time, as I turned and looked that way, I saw two figures standing just inside the entry of it. At first my only feeling was of surprise because I had imagined that everybody was at the bear-baiting. As I looked, wondering who they were, and wondering also why they had avoided the entertainment, whether they had at one time been sickened, too, they moved together and so stood in a long embrace.

By this time, from my reading, from talks with Melusine, from gossiping with Helen, and from merely being alive and not stone-deaf, I had picked up all there was to know about the relationship between men and women. I knew exactly why this pair had been in the Maze rather than at the baiting, and I wondered whether they knew about the constant guard. Then I remembered that the old man had asked me to call out so that he could know my whereabouts, and thought with some relief that that showed that he could not see clean into the Maze, he could only watch the entry.

The man of this pair, whom I did not recognise, broke from the woman's arms and walked briskly away in a direction which would take him to the stable yard. The woman stood still for a moment or two and then took a path which would eventually meet, in a corner, the one upon which I stood. She had hardly taken four steps before I recognised her; it was Melusine. I knew by the way she walked. Recognition had been slow because she was wearing a new dress, scarlet, a colour she never wore, and a narrow, steeple head-dress instead of a wide, horned one.

My first impulse was to run and meet her, then I thought better of it. This had been a secret rendezvous, she might be displeased to know that it had been—at the end—overlooked. So instead of running to meet her where the paths joined, I drew back, and then, when she had passed, followed her. If she went into the house, then I could go into the house too. A little time in her company would be far more delightful to me than the best entertainment in the world.

At the end of the path she turned towards the house, not towards the Tourney Ground, and I followed her, keeping my distance all the time. I reached the Well Yard and was inside the deep porch when my Uncle Godfrey's voice hailed me.

"The baiting—is it over?"

I told him no, I had come in because I felt slightly unwell. He laid one of his hard hands against my neck, just under the ear, held it there a moment and said, "No fever."

He smiled and said he hoped I should feel better soon. That emboldened me to ask why he was not at the Tourney Ground and he said that he had been watching poultices applied to the leg of his destrier, Tristram, which had suffered a slight injury in the Tournament.

"Will he be better in time for the Dover Meeting?"

"It's to be hoped so," he said, and we parted. I was inside the Well Yard Room before my mind took notice of the fact that the man who had stood with Melusine just inside the Maze had worn a yellow doublet, and that my uncle was wearing that colour.

I knew by this time that my uncle was a knight without any land or other source of income, and that this was an unenviable thing to be. He had, more than once, tried to marry an heiress whose parents or guardians, in their turn, were looking out for a husband with money, and his efforts in this direction were now so bruited abroad that parents or guardians of heiresses looked at him a bit askance. That is what I mean when I say that the whole society of which Beauclaire was a sample was too much concerned with money. My Uncle Godfrey was handsome, kind, good-humoured, and acknowledged to be one of the best knights—some said the very best—in all the South of England. He was a man whom any girl could have been pleased and proud to marry, but he had no money, he could not be seriously considered. On the other hand, he was extremely popular with the ladies. In a strange, entirely false, stilted way it was the fashion, just then, for any married woman who was not positively repulsive in appearance to have a string of adorers who pretended to be in love with her. Perhaps pretended is a harsh word, some of them did, perhaps, cherish a hopeless passion; now and again perhaps a lady would slip from virtue, but it was rare; as a general rule the ladies wore their lovers and flaunted them as they wore and flaunted their jewels. Before a Tournament, for example, there was a competition amongst the ladies to count how many knights begged the honour of wearing their favours, just as fierce as the competition presently to be waged in the lists. There was a secret and very subtle game to be played with colours. A knight might ask a lady for a favour, a glove, a scarf, a sleeve to wear in the next event; he might be refused because her favour was already given; he would find out from her body servant what colour of gown she intended to wear, and then he would ride out on the day wearing somewhere about him that same colour. In this custom lay the origin of the ladies' hatred for having a gown the same colour as another's. There was another variation of the game, too. The ladies would go to great lengths and show much ingenuity in showing their preferences; my uncle's name being Blanchfleur, their task was easy, and at many a Meeting I have seen a dozen women wearing a white flower as a sign that they wished him well and had faith in his prowess. Officially my Uncle Godfrey "belonged" to my Lady Astallon, he was her kin by marriage, he was part of her husband's household, and she was very beautiful in the manner most admired just then, unreal, inhuman, with her shaved eyebrows and her hair plucked out all about her forehead to make her brow look high and the hairline as even as though it had been painted.

I thought of all this as I went into the Well Yard Room, and found it empty. I went on to the Stool Room, Melusine was not there, but she had been, just before me, I could smell her gillyflower-water fragrance through the faint, stored-up stink of the place. As I rang the bell I wondered had she gone into the Book Room. But when I reached the door it was locked. I turned back and, at the place where two passages joined, saw two old women; one had the bucket and jug of her occupation, the other carried a mug wrapped in a piece of flannel.

"Traipse, traipse, traipse," said the stool-emptier, bitterly, "all day long. And my feet as tender as the bird of your eye."

"But on the level," said the other. "Them stairs are my undoing. And I'll swear there's such a call for ginger, some of 'em must come round twice a month."

"Who is it this time?"

"The Lady Melusine. It ain't so long since ladies kept quiet about it, and danced the higher and laughed the louder so nobody should know, but *now!* No, we must lay abed and cosset our bellies with hot ginger twice a day."

"I'd swop with you."

"And after a week of the stairs you'd be glad to swop back."

I was close to them now, and I said, "I'm going up. Shall I take it?"

"Young ladies ain't allowed in the Ladies' Dorter."

"No one would know. I'd just put it in."

She looked at me with the suspicion of her kind; nobody ever did anything for nothing.

"Don't you go sipping at it. It's medicine, turn you black in the face if you drunk it without needing it."

But she handed it over.

I went upstairs slowly and carefully, pondering over why Melusine and my uncle must meet in secret. So far as I could see— quite apart from the fact that they were my two favourite people— they were well matched. Melusine was not a great heiress, she had a very modest dower, the freeholds of some properties in London, the rent of which was paid punctually four times a year and as punctually expended on new dresses or pieces of finery. Neither she nor my uncle was married, or betrothed to anyone else; her income, added to that he won in prize money, would keep them; she certainly wouldn't need a new dress if she lived to be a hundred.

I had reached the Ladies' Dorter, a room I had never, in all my time at Beauclaire, entered before. It was very large; the walls were painted and all the beds had hangings, some of plain silk, some embroidered with the family emblems of the owner. Great chests stood by the side and at the foot of each bed, and in the centre of the room was a table with several looking glasses on it. The room smelt of women, of musk, and violet and gillyflower and lavender, of linen fresh from the washing, of velvet, and under all of human flesh. My not-yet-settled stomach moved uneasily.

Melusine's bed was on the far side of the door; it had plain blue hangings. She had undressed and was lying flat with her bare arms exposed, her hands linked behind her head. She raised herself a little when I entered, and then, seeing me, sat up straight.

"Maude! What are you doing here? You know it is forbidden."

"Except for two old women we are alone in the house. So I brought your ginger."

"Why aren't you at the baiting?"

"I was sick."

"Poor sweet," she said, instantly sympathetic. "Look, you drink that posset. There's nothing more comforting to the stomach."

"I'm better now. It's for you."

The ends of her lips curved upwards in what was almost, but not quite a smile; it was a look I knew and generally accompanied some words of gentle mockery.

"It would be wasted on me. Drink it quickly and then run along. If you are found here . . ."

"Nobody will come yet. There is an entertainment by torchlight and it isn't nearly dark."

"Sit here and drink it then. Sit on the bed." She patted the place and then lay back, linking her hands behind her head again.

"Are you sure you don't want it?"

"That is one thing I am sure of." So I sat down and began to unwrap the flannel from the mug, saying, "The servant said that one sip would turn me black in the face."

"Why did she send you with it?" I explained that I had not been sent, I had offered to carry it.

She accepted—as I realised afterwards—this evidence of my devotion, plumbing its depths by the simple question, "How did you know it was for me?"

And I said, "She said so, besides I saw you come in."

"You saw me come in?" She was upright in the bed again. "Where have you been, Maude? *In the Low Garden?*"

I nodded.

"Then you saw us?"

I nodded again, stricken to think how I had given myself away.

She reached out and took hold of my arm; I could feel the heat of her hand through my sleeve.

"That's a secret. It must be kept, Maude, until the end of July. Do you understand? Will you promise?"

"Anything you said was a secret, Melusine, I would keep to myself, even on the rack."

"My poor dear child, you've never seen a rack! And it isn't *so* serious. Just till the end of July."

"And then you will be married?"

She nodded.

"Where will you live?"

"On his manor at Minsham."

I thought of that cold, bare hall, with the damp dew on the stone walls, the unrailed stairs, the bleak bedchambers above, and of that poor drooling old man, my Grandfather Blanchfleur.

"Oh no!" I said. "Couldn't you stay here?"

She said sharply, "No!" And then in an ordinary voice, "I forgot that you knew Minsham. Tell me about it."

I described it as well as I could. I also mentioned my grandfather. Melusine looked surprised and said she had never heard of him.

"He may be dead," I said. "I last saw him before I came here, and then he was almost dead."

"The house," she said, "it could be made comfortable—if money was spent on it?"

I pictured Minsham furnished with some of the comforts of the Old Vine, some of the elegance of Beauclaire.

"Oh yes."

"They'll soon be back," Melusine said, "you had better go. We'll talk tomorrow. And remember, this is between us."

I repeated the words which were traditional in the Children's Dorter for the making of any very special promise.

> "Else
> May my liver and lights die in me,
> May Old Scrat fly away with me."

Melusine laughed and said, "Oh, the memories that recalls! A most solemn oath."

I was in my bed and almost asleep when a thought jerked me wide awake again. If my Uncle Godfrey and Melusine were married and went to live at Minsham, perhaps I could go there too. That would be even better than staying at Beauclaire. Thanks be to St. Joseph, I thought, that I hadn't written my request to Walter. I wouldn't write now until the end of July when I could convey the news in any case, and, if I had persuaded Melusine to agree, beg to go to Minsham instead of to Clevely.

She was easily persuaded; she was, I think, genuinely fond of me, and as she said she would lack company, because my uncle would be away a great deal. I asked again couldn't she stay at Beauclaire, and I cannot remember whether it was then or another time that she told me what lay behind the secrecy and the need to leave Beauclaire once the truth was out. My Lady Astallon, Melusine said, would be furiously angry.

"But why? Uncle Godfrey is bound to get married some day."

"She sees no need for it. And if he did she would like to do the choosing for him, somebody he couldn't care for. You see . . ." She checked herself. "I shouldn't speak of such things to you, Maude. Here in this room I forget how young you are."

I would show her, I thought, that young as I was I fully understood the situation.

"He is her lover *in fact*? They bed together?"

"They *did*."

"Would she have minded his marrying Alys Courtney? There was talk of that, wasn't there?"

"Alys Courtney was very rich. That would have been understandable. She was plain, too. Our marriage will be a very different thing. He loves me, and that my Lady will find hard to accept."

"I see," I said; and I did, though not very clearly.

Another time when we were talking—for we now talked far more than we read in the Book Room—I asked her how long she and my Uncle Godfrey had been in love.

"He with me, or I with him? He with me only lately, a year maybe; I with him, oh, years, ever since I moved into the Well Yard Room. The first thing I noticed about you, poppet, was that your eyes were like his."

I remembered how she had said, "You have his eyes," and that simple statement which had pleased me when it was made, because it gave me a feeling of belonging somewhere, now hurt because I loved her and was afraid that all her kindness to me had been on account of that likeness and not for myself.

"A year, eh?" I said, fumbling about amongst the thoughts in my head. "Then how would you have felt had he married Alys Courtney?"

"How you harp on her! There was nothing in it. My Lady tried to match them, that is true. But Godfrey *loved* me and so nothing came of it."

That was not the way I had heard it; the failure of the match between my Uncle Godfrey and the Courtney heiress had been reported to me by Helen Beaufort, and she had said that he was willing, eager, the Courtney family reluctant. But then, Helen had a spiteful tongue and would gladly deal me a slap through my uncle. And Helen, naturally, did not know the truth.

In another of these most exciting conversations I learned why the end of July was so important.

"He'll come riding back from Dover with that great prize in his hand, and then the announcement will be made. In the Hall? Is that the way it will be? Oh, I hope I shall be there," I said.

"Hope that he wins the prize! It will be all that we shall have to live on until my rents come in at Michaelmas. I've been such an improvident, prodigal fool. On Lady Day I had the price of as good a destrier as ever wore harness, and I frittered it away on a new dress and a brooch to go with it, and a ring for *him*. How was I to know that Tristram would take a wound?"

"Tristram. What has the horse to do with it?"

Melusine made her right hand into a fist and ground it in the palm of her left hand.

"This waiting," she said. "He must joust at Dover, and he must win. And his horse is unsound. My Lady Astallon has promised to mount him—a Great Horse from Flanders—so well trained, they say, that if you mounted a sack of flour on him, with a lance fixed, he could unseat his man. Godfrey, with such a horse, could not fail."

"He won again here," I said, "and on Tristram, wounded as he was."

"He'll win at Dover; a silver cup filled with gold pieces."

We counted the days to the end of July. I wanted to write my letter to Walter, asking him to ask Mother if I could go and live at Minsham, but of course I must not do that yet, for to do so would betray the secret.

In our counting of the days we reached the place where we could say, "Only twenty days more."

VI

Earlier in the summer, in June when the people assembled for our St. Barnabas Tourney, some of them had brought rumours that this year the plague was worse than usual in London. Lord Astallon had seized upon this fact gleefully, and said in the Hall, loud enough to be heard from end to end of the High Table, "There you are! Was I not right to refuse Bowdegrave's invitation to spend the summer in his London house?"

Lady Astallon said discontentedly, "Your cousin Bowdegrave is now with the King at Windsor, which is full as healthful as this."

"I doubt it," said her husband.

And he was right. This year the plague reached Windsor, and amongst its victims were Madge FitzHerbert's father, his wife, and the child of their marriage, a boy of five years old. All in a moment Madge changed from being a half idiot, kept in the Children's Dorter because she was too stupid and ugly to be promoted to the Well Yard Room, into that most covetable piece of property—an heiress.

It was Helen Beaufort, who now knew everything—and who was quite pale and venomous with jealousy—who explained all this to me. Unmarried girls who had great fortunes were always taken into wardship by some man who administered their estates, and arranged a marriage for them, and out of both procedures made some pickings for himself. This was so well known and accepted a rule that the wardship of an heiress would be given away as a reward for service to the King.

"The King," said Helen, "is probably at this moment looking around to decide who shall have the privilege of being that ninny's guardian."

"My cousin Astallon should have it," I said. "She has lived under his roof all these years; as far as I can see nobody else has minded whether she had enough to eat or not, or anything to wear." It was a fact that any garment more than was strictly necessary which poor Madge possessed had been given to her by me, for I had passed on to her every thing my mother had sent me in the way of a present.

"Astallon," said Helen, "will never be thought of. He is not near the King, nor has he done him any service."

"Then it's very unfair."

"The whole thing is unfair," said Helen bitterly. "They'll probably marry her to an earl!"

"That couldn't happen. She still can't thread a needle, for all her riches," I said.

"If Astallon knew his business," said Helen in her most adult manner, and probably repeating something she had overheard, "he'd betroth her quickly to Ralph, or to Henry Rancon, and so keep control for himself."

Madge's new status, and her future, though a matter of interest to me, was not very near my heart, and as soon as Helen and I parted I half forgot about it, and went back to thinking about my own future, with Uncle Godfrey and Melusine at Minsham. However, on the evening of the next day I learned that Madge's future was very much my concern, and that Helen's gossiping prophecies had been wrong in only one respect. My cousin Astallon had taken the one way open to him to make use of Madge's fortune for the family good, but he hadn't chosen Ralph or Henry as a husband for the heiress; he had chosen his kinsman, Sir Godfrey Blanchfleur.

Before supper in the Great Hall, in full sight of the whole assembly, up stood the Beauclaire Chaplain, silly Madge, and my uncle, and the betrothal vows were made. Madge repeated her words in her thick flannelly voice, without any sign of understanding; my uncle pushed a ring on her finger and kissed her on the brow. And all over the Hall people got to their feet and raised their wine cups or their ale mugs and wished the happy couple well.

For a moment or two I was too stunned to think. When I did my first thought was a thoroughly selfish one. Now I should never go to Minsham! Immediately I thought of Melusine. If I was stunned and shocked, what, in God's name, was she feeling? I turned my head cautiously and looked along to where she sat. In my heart I saluted her. Men may win honour in battle and prizes and praise in tourneys, but women have their own kind of courage. You could never have guessed that the scene on the dais meant more to Melusine than to Ella or Phillipa or any other of the ladies. She was laughing and raising her cup.

All through the meal—and it was a festive one, with several extra dishes—Melusine's behaviour was so ordinary that in the end it deceived me. I thought to myself that this was just another trick—like getting the Great Horse of Flanders out of Lady Astallon. My uncle had gone through the act of betrothal in order to further some scheme of Lord Astallon's: now, if they sent from Windsor to take Madge into wardship, she need not go, she was betrothed. Then afterwards, when it was all forgotten, the betrothal could be annulled, and my uncle and Melusine be married after all.

That must be it, I thought; and Melusine knew. How else could she laugh and talk as though nothing had happened? I gripped onto this thought because it was the only comfort in my desolation, and soon I came to full belief and felt better.

However, next morning, in the Chapel, the Chaplain called the banns—for the second time, he said. And as soon as we were all back in the Children's Dorter my Lady Astallon came there, a thing rare in the extreme; she brought with her a sewing woman who carried a roll of rich tawny-coloured silk. Madge stood there like an ugly doll while the sewing woman measured her, and my Lady and Dame Margery conversed in voices too low for us to hear. Then the silk was spread out on the table and slashed into by the shears; the sewing woman treated the lovely stuff as though it were the coarsest, cheapest homespun. When the gown was cut out Lady Astallon said something that Alison and Constance and I *did* hear, all too clearly. We were to spend the day sewing the long seams of the skirt while the ladies in the Well Yard Room did the more skilled work on the bodice and the sewing woman managed the trickiest part of all, the long, falling sleeves. The wedding was going to be solemnised next day and the dress must be ready.

So it *was* going to happen.

Sewing was the worst occupation for me just then, since it left my whole mind free to brood over my misery, and Melusine's. Presently I thought: Nothing goes right for me! And all in a moment the tawny stuff and my needle and thread wavered and blurred; one tear, then another splashed onto the silk, making dark, star-shaped blotches. Dame Margery, who was watching, quickly thrust her plump white hand between me and the work and made the sign of the Cross.

"Tears on a wedding gown," she said in a shocked voice, "the worst possible luck, God and all the Saints guard against it! What ails *you*, Maude Reed, to behave so unseemly?"

I said the first thing that occurred to me.

"This is my morning for lessons; and I do not like to sew."

"And you dare show me this rebellious spirit, after I have governed you for three years? Shame on you," she said, and dealt me a clout on the ear. Her hand, for all its plump white velvet look, could deal a shrewd blow. "Get into the corner and put your hands on your head until you can control yourself."

She sat down in my place and began to stitch.

In the corner, gazing at the blank wall, I thought about Melusine. I had ceased crying, it is almost impossible to cry with your hands linked above your head; and presently I was able to say—without turning from the corner:

"Madam. I am now controlled."

"Then you may return to your work."

"The Lady Melusine," I said.

"What of her?"

"She will be awaiting me in the Book Room."

"I doubt that. She will be sewing too."

"She goes to the Book Room early. . . ."

"Then run along and tell her that you are sewing and she should be. And waste no time. You are to be back by the time I reach here." She measured off a tiny length of seam.

I held my skirt high and galloped in the most unseemly way to the Book Room, but it was locked. I thought she might have locked herself in, so I knocked on the door and called that it was I, Maude. There was no sound from within. I then turned and ran to the Well Yard Room, which was like running from the Old Vine into Baildon town; only two of the young ladies were there, sewing diligently on the tawny silk. One said that Melusine was in the Book Room, the other said she was in attendance upon Lady Astallon. Just as I was leaving three others, Ella amongst them, came rustling in and I asked them if they knew where Melusine was. Nobody knew; and I had already been away much longer than I had been given leave for; so I had no choice but to go back and sew on that hateful tawny silk. I looked forward to the dinner hour; somehow I would make an opportunity to speak to Melusine then, no matter what trouble I brought down on myself.

But Melusine was not in the Hall for dinner; several other young ladies were absent, Helen Beaufort amongst them. Word went round that my Lady had suddenly decided that she had nothing fit to wear for a wedding, and that they were sewing at full speed on a new, wonderful cloth-of-silver gown.

My Lady having decided to make the wedding properly festive (and from my talk with Melusine I could see that this was, to her, the most welcome match in the world), the Chapel was to be hung with wreaths, the symbol of unity. So first thing in the morning we were all sent out in search of flowers. We children were to confine our search to the Low Garden, which yielded very little, the first flood of flowers was over, the big daisies which grew in the long grass were withering, and the poppies which had taken their place were useless for wreaths as they shed their petals too easily. There were a few roses on the bushes and a few heads of blue bugloss and that was all. Then Alison said that she had seen, on the banks of the moat, a great bush of honeysuckle.

"Honeysuckle smells sweet, and it isn't prickly and it weaves well," she said.

So the four of us—Madge of course was indoors, being washed

and made ready—went off to find the bush. Alison had seen it when she went to the bear-baiting, and it certainly was a big, lush-growing bush but it was on the outer bank of the moat and to reach it our shortest way would be across the drawbridge, upon which we were expressly forbidden ever to set foot. William said:

"Who will know? And even if they did nothing would happen today. It's a *wedding!*"

Alison was in favour of venturing, because the bush was her find, and I didn't care one way or the other, and Constance always did what we did. So we ran across the bridge and set about the bush, pulling off great flowery strands, some of them a yard long. And I thought with what joy I should be gathering flowers and making the wreaths were Melusine to be the bride, and what a sorry mockery it was now.

Then we heard men's voices shouting from the inward end of the bridge, and looked up guiltily, thinking that they were calling us. But they were not. They were looking and pointing down into the water of the moat.

"One of them's dropped something," William said. "Look, they're bringing a rope and grapple. Here, you have these. . . ." He pushed all his flowers into my arms, and went scampering off to watch something he hoped would be exciting.

I laid the bundle of leaves and flowers that he had given me aside and went on, dully and methodically gathering more, until I heard Alison, just beside me, let out a kind of hissing breath. I looked at her and saw that she was staring bridgewards, so I looked that way and saw Melusine brought up from the water.

The hooks had taken her by the middle and she hung in a curve, very gracefully, almost as a girl might hang from a man's arm in a more than ordinarily roisterous dance. At one end of the curve hung her scarlet dress, at the other her silver-gilt hair, both a little darkened by the water and that was all; and as they pulled her up the water fell from her hair and from her skirts, in sparkling, sun-touched drops. The thought shot into my head and out again: Even so, she is lovely.

Then I began to cry. Clutching the latest-gathered sprays of honeysuckle and crying wildly, I ran back to the bridge and crossed it. By that time they had laid her flat on the grey stone pavement, and they tried to prevent me going near, but I pushed past and looked down on her. I noticed then, and later took comfort from

the fact, that she looked most peacefully happy; her eyes were closed
and her lips were almost, not quite, but almost smiling. My own
raucous, gasping sobs seemed an intrusion upon that peacefulness,
but I could not stop them.

One of the men took hold of me and told me in a rough, kind
voice not to distress myself. Alison came up beside me, and Constance; they stared, shocked but quiet.

"Come on now," one of the men said, "you must go in. Rightly
you shouldn't have been there, you know. What's your Dame about
this morning?"

Alison and Constance had gathered up all the flowers; they were
loaded. Alison said, "Come along, Maude, we still have the wreaths
to make, you know."

Across the bodice of Melusine's scarlet dress the green slimy
strands of water weed lay, soiling, out of place. I laid my strands
of honeysuckle over them, thinking: Wedding wreath! and sobbing
more and more noisily.

More and more people had come running; there was quite a
crowd. Alison said in my ear the most damning of all Dame Margery's rebukes, "Maude, you are making an exhibition of yourself!"

I knew that, but there was no help for it. I went on crying. One
of the men picked me up and carried me into the house.

Dame Margery was kind at first. She petted and patted me and
gave me something soothing to drink; then, when I continued to
cry, she lost patience, shook me, finally slapped me and forbade me
to attend the wedding. So I lay on my bed and wept for Melusine,
while silly Madge became my aunt-by-marriage.

I knew that crying was useless; all it did was make my head ache
more and more; I tried to stop, but I couldn't. Even when every
tear was squeezed out of me and I was as dry as sawdust inside, I
still went on making the hiccuping noise.

Dame Margery came back from the wedding feast, and, finding
me still crying, gave me another drink, a poppy-smelling one, which
sent me to sleep. But the moment I was awake I was crying again.

They began to treat me—perhaps rightly—as though I had gone
out of my wits. I was moved out of the Children's Dorter and
lodged in a small room alone. Dame Margery seemed most concerned because I could eat nothing; she was convinced that if I
would only *try*, I could do so. Once she seized my nose and held it
until, in order to draw breath, I was forced to open my mouth;

instantly she popped in a spoonful of something she had ready at hand. It was a dish of fresh raspberries sprinkled with crushed sugar which was a rare luxury, even at Beauclaire. For me that mouthful had the very taste of misery and I have never eaten raspberries again, nor indeed any sweet thing at all.

Finally, as though in desperation, they fetched the Chaplain to me.

Remembering that he had taken the betrothal vows and called the banns, and officiated at that farce of a marriage ceremony, I had nothing to say to *him*, and lay on the bed, with my face turned towards the wall, crying and hiccuping, my mind closed to his talk until he said:

"I am surprised. I was given to understand that there was an affection between you and Melusine Talboys."

"There was," I said, without realising that I was speaking at last. "She was my friend, the one person who was kind to me when I came here, frightened and alone."

"Then you owe her a debt which you should begin immediately to repay."

He now had my attention. I cried, "But she's dead, she's dead. I can never repay her now."

"Her body is dead. But her soul—and that surely was the source of her kindness to you—is still alive and more in need of help from you, from us all, than ever before. If you had seen her cast herself into the water, would you have stood in a safe place and wrung your hands and wept, or would you have tried to save her?"

"I *would* have saved her."

The arrogance of that remark he deplored with a small sigh and went on, "Her state of mind no one can know, therefore no one can say that she died finally impenitent; she *did* die unshriven and her last act on this earth was the sin of self-destruction. She will be long in Purgatory, I fear, poor child. But her time there could be shortened, and her way out of it eased, by *you*, by your faithful and unremitting prayers. The scales of God's justice are finely balanced, and against the sum of all her sins and her final awful wrongdoing, prayers inspired by love and gratitude would weigh heavy."

I gave a great gulp and said, "I will pray."

"Ah," he said, in a pouncing, triumphant voice, almost as though he had said, "I've *got* you!" "Ah, but are you in a state to pray effectively? This unrestrained grief—as though you were a heathen for whom physical death was the end of all things—this refusal to eat or sleep, as though you, too, were bent on self-destruction, do these make for a claim to God's ear?" He gave another small sigh. "You're very young. I will try to put it plainer. Suppose your friend Melusine had deeply offended Lady Astallon and was to be punished, quite rightly, but you wished to plead for some mitigation, would you, do you think, serve any purpose by rushing into the Bower, crying loudly, your clothes in disarray, your whole manner distraught? Answer me."

"No."

"Very well, then. If you believe, as you must believe, being a Christian, that Melusine is not that poor dead body, but a living and immortal soul, at this moment suffering the cleansing pains of Purgatory, you will get up from that bed, wash and tidy yourself, and eat some plain, nourishing dish. You may have small appetite for it, but our appetites should at all times be under our control. Tell yourself that you eat in order to gain strength because your strength is needed. When you have done these things, come into the Chapel. I shall be waiting for you there."

Later in my life, when I often heard priests discussed critically and designated "good" or "bad," I would remember the Chaplain at Beauclaire. He was, so far as anyone could judge from outward signs, a worldly man, he lived luxuriously, he did Lord Astallon's bidding quite unquestioningly (as in that hasty marriage between my uncle and silly Madge), he was fond of fine clothes, addicted to hunting, not in fact a "good" priest. But, and this I do believe, ordination to the priesthood does convey some power, some authority outside the layman's understanding. And those upon whom that power has been conferred carry it, as a man may carry a lantern. He may keep the horn clean and clear so that the light is always visible, or he may let it grow smoky and smeary so that you might not know that the light was there. It is there, however, and in a moment of emergency it can be produced. So now the Chaplain, without saying anything which was new to me, without even being persuasive in his talk, had altered everything. I no longer saw Melusine as they lifted her from the water, dripping and dead. I saw *her*, as alive and real as she had ever been, suffering the physical pain and the spiritual misery of Purgatory, but knowing that it was only for a season, hopeful, not lost, not despairing.

The effect of this was not only to assuage my sorrow; it altered my whole attitude towards life. I no longer wished to remain at Beauclaire, and as that summer passed into autumn, and the autumn into winter, I began more firmly every day to look forward to going to Clevely and joining the nuns. I made no hasty decision about becoming a nun myself; in that mood of religious mysticism which followed my talk with the Chaplain I doubted my own worthiness to make such a decision. When I thought of Clevely I thought of it as a quiet place, with no distractions, where I could spend hours on my knees praying for Melusine without seeming odd or making myself conspicuous. At the age of twelve, having seen only one of the world's many aspects, I was prepared to retire from it.

VII

I left Beauclaire soon after my twelfth birthday. With one exception nobody seemed sorry to see me go. Madge might have been, but she was gone already, making with my Uncle Godfrey a tour of all her estates and hereditaments. The exception to the general indifference was, most startlingly, Henry Rancon, to whom I had hardly spoken a word since he had left the Children's Dorter and become a page.

I had seen him, of course, in the Hall and about the courtyards and I had noticed, in an idle kind of way, that since leaving Dame Margery's rule his appearance had not improved. He was never very clean and he was often bruised, or scratched or scarred in some way. He'd grown very rapidly, too, and, however often he was given a new outfit of the Astallon green, his clothes seemed too small.

On my last afternoon at Beauclaire I was sorting out my possessions and packing what I had decided to take with me in the same little chest which I had brought from the Old Vine. I discarded whatever seemed to me, in my limited knowledge, to be unsuited to life in a nunnery. Nuns, I believed, were vowed to a life of poverty and non-possessiveness, and a girl who went to live with them would need very little.

The other children were in the Low Garden, it being a fine afternoon, and Dame Margery, having seen me employed, took a little nap and then went out to gossip with one of her cronies. When she returned she had Henry Rancon with her. She said, with one of her smiles which were secretive and sly and knowledgeable:

"Maude, Henry wishes to bid you Godspeed. He has remembered some of the mannerliness I beat into him, it seems."

I had been taught manners, too, so I said, "That is very kind."

We stood and looked at one another across the little chest and the pile of discarded clothes. He wore the Astallon green—velvet for pages and they were supposed to change from their uniform when they went to the stables or out for their exercises, but Henry plainly hadn't bothered; his velvet was rubbed and spotted and he stank of sweat, horse and human. His hair had just been roughly clubbed and should have been washed. He had a long scratch down one cheek and a large scab on his chin.

He said, in a grudging, aggrieved way, "I didn't know that you were leaving until just now, after dinner."

He spoke as though he should have been informed, and I almost said: What is that to you? But I remembered my manners and said, "I leave tomorrow."

"Back to Baildon?"

"Fancy you remembering that! Yes, Baildon, but not to stay. I'm going to the nuns at Clevely."

"To a nunnery?"

"Yes. I should have gone there in the first place, but they wouldn't have me until I was twelve."

"You're not going to be a nun?"

I said, and it was true, "I don't even know that myself. I should like to be, but . . ."

"Don't," he said. He looked over to where Dame Margery had seated herself in the window, and scowled fiercely. He tried to speak softly, but his voice had just broken and he had no note between a gruff growl and a squeak. "Soon I'll be a squire. With any sort of arms I do well, none better. I'll be a squire, and very soon a knight. Maude, don't, I beg you, decide on being a nun until I'm a knight." He said all this in a squeak and then suddenly dropped to a deep manly voice. "You can't be a nun yet, and in four years I swear I'll have my spurs if I have to break my neck to get them. And ever since we used to play together I've always thought . . ." He broke off and glared at Dame Margery again, his face going a dark, unbecoming crimson. "When I'm a knight, I want you for my lady, and you can't be that if you're a nun."

I laughed, for the first time since Melusine's death.

"If I decide not to be a nun, Henry, somebody else might have the same notion."

He said furiously, "But I asked you first!" He tugged at one of his dirty fingers and pulled off a ring; it was of some base metal—lead I should think, from the weight of it—with a zigzag pattern in blue enamel running round it. Even to make it fit his own finger he had been obliged to wad it with a twist of thread, now worn black and greasy.

"Here you are," he said, groping for my hand and pushing the ring on to my finger, "I've spoken for you and done it properly, ring and all. You can bear witness to that, Dame."

Dame Margery laughed.

"It's a bit one-sided, but it'll do for now. Unless Maude cares to say something." I could tell from the way she spoke that she thought it silly child's play, as I did myself. And then all at once it seemed pathetic that the awkward, blushing boy should be the only one to be serious; and I remembered that it was Henry who had offered to learn to read, so that I could have lessons. I said gently:

"I can't promise anything, Henry. But if you like, I'll keep the ring to remember you by."

"Do that," he said. "So then, good-by, Maude."

He pushed his head forward and kissed me. Most surprisingly the lips in his rough battered face were as smooth and soft as silk.

Interval

I

The gifts which Anne Reed had, in most cases, fashioned with her own hands and despatched to Maude at Beauclaire, and which had been passed on to Madge FitzHerbert, were not, in fact, such perfunctory and deceptive offerings as the girl imagined. Once Maude was out of sight, the pangs of memory and conscience eased, and Anne could think of, could speak of "my daughter" as any woman might.

When Maude's first letter arrived Anne said, with complacency to Martin, "Things have improved since my day; nobody bothered to teach us to write. And you will admit that she sounds happy."

(The letter had been written in the Book Room, with Melusine sitting nearby.)

It was presently possible for Anne to look back upon her own youth, and, with that selective memory common to all whom the years have damaged, to see those early days golden with sunshine, brightened by hope, lively with appreciation of any occasional joy. She was convinced that she, too, could have been happy at Beauclaire or any other of the places where she had sojourned so miserably, had she not been so wretchedly poor.

As the days went by she came to think of her daughter as a more fortunate version of herself, just as pretty and graceful, but well shod, elegantly clothed, moving against the background of the Long Gallery, the Great Hall, the Low Garden. One day, she assured herself, when she had persuaded Martin into the provision of a dowry, the elegant, eligible young man of good family for whom she herself had waited in vain would pay his court to Maude and all would be well.

Never once did she suspect that her attitude towards the child was that which most people, after the first burst of grief, held towards the dead. Gone away. In safekeeping. Happy now. Anne had never felt that way about her dead, and could not know that she had watched a little girl ride away on a brown pony with the finality with which other people see a coffin lowered into the earth. Anne's dead, Denys, her mother, Richard, were all her victims, to be thought of as little as possible, subjects of the occasional nightmare from which refuge must be sought in the wine cup.

She had Walter, whom she loved extravagantly, both for himself and for what she could see of Richard in him. Richard's dark hair and eyes, his delicate look, his skill with the lute. Even when, at an early age, Walter declared that he was never going to be a wool merchant, he was going to take his lute and wander the roads and play to admiring crowds, the statement roused in his mother much delight and little concern. Richard had cherished that dream, too. Walter was Richard's son. Upon that certainty she could rest, much of her guilt absolved. As a statement it was not to be taken seriously; he would know better when he was older.

Martin had found him a good tutor, a young man called Nicholas Freeman, who had been trained in the monks' school at Norwich and come very near taking his priest's orders, changed his mind, and worked for a time in the office of a leather merchant in Norwich.

At first Anne had attached little importance to him, minding only that he should teach Walter thoroughly and as gently as possible. Walter learned swiftly.

"It will help if I am a scrivener as well," he explained gravely. "I can play to please the people and myself, and then if any one wants a letter written or a copyright made, I can do it and so make sure of my bread."

To count he refused, absolutely; and when pressed twice ran away. He was soon recovered, a small boy carrying a lute was not difficult to trace and Martin's men knew the roads and were well mounted. He was beaten, sobbed tearlessly, worked himself into a fever and was cosseted, but still refused to learn to count.

"I know all I need to know. I am not going to be a wool merchant."

Nicholas Freeman, with time on his hands, began to take an active part in the business. Martin's lame leg grew stiffer as he aged and sometimes he found difficulty in mounting his horse. One morning Nicholas asked:

"Would you like me to go for you, sir?"

"You think there is no skill in fleece-buying? They'd sell you anything."

"My father has a sheep run. I helped him until I was nine. I know all the tricks."

"Go then. But bring back any maggoty polls and I'll knock their price off your wages."

The young man laughed.

"With the price of wool as it is, and my wages what they are, that would be to take a quart from a pint pot."

Anne thought that an impudent answer, but Martin laughed and said, "I've been doing that all my life, boy."

Little by little the young man worked his way into Martin's confidence, was allowed more responsibility, was moving, Anne felt, into the place that should be Walter's. On that eagerly awaited day when Walter should, as she termed it, "come to his senses" there would be Nicholas Freeman standing between him and his grandfather. Martin seemed to find him easy to talk to, and sometimes as they sat at table she would study them both. The young man wore, for a clerk, a very healthy look, as though his farmyard tan had survived the years in cloister and countinghouse; in a slightly saturnine way, he was handsome, with bright hazel eyes, brown hair, and excellent teeth. Beside him Martin's lined face looked old. Old, she would think, and he never spares himself. Suppose he died before Walter settled and knew anything of the business; we should depend upon this stranger, and he might cheat us, we are so ignorant.

Spurred by the fear of material loss, she began to take interest in the business, listening, asking questions, sometimes venturing a suggestion. Martin, after the initial surprise, took refuge behind the immemorial barrier, "Nothing for you to bother about, my dear," "You wouldn't understand if I did explain," and, "Leave all that to us."

With Nicholas she had no better luck; he was a vain young man and had from the first resented her manner towards him; he rebuffed her gleefully, saying, "Why not discuss this with Master Reed?" and once, "Master Reed engaged me and it is to him that I render account of my doings."

The years went by. The twins' twelfth birthday came. Walter showed no sign of change of heart, but so long as he was allowed to

go his own way he was amiable and inoffensive. When she thought
of Maude, Anne imagined her moving from the Children's Dorter
into the Well Yard Room at Beauclaire and taking her place with
the young ladies. Upon that thought Anne braced herself for the
tussle with Martin concerning the dowry. If he remained obdurate,
she had one other hope. Godfrey, now married to the FitzHerbert
heiress, was extremely wealthy; he might do something for Maude;
he should do, out of gratitude for what Anne had done for him,
long ago.

She had entirely forgotten that she had ever intended to send
Maude to the nunnery at Clevely. That had been a move in a secret
game, won at the moment when a little girl rode through the archway on a brown pony.

But Maude had remembered that she was to leave Beauclaire
when she was twelve; Dame Margery remembered it, too, and so
did Lady Astallon. And one lovely April morning, on that same
brown pony, now too small for her, Maude came riding home.

II

On a sunny morning, about a fortnight after Maude's return, Martin
Reed came down to breakfast with some of the pain lines eased
from his face. He flexed his lame leg two or three times as he sat
in his chair and said, with satisfaction, "This weather suits me. I
shall ride out to the Minsham run today."

Two years before, the whole of Suffolk had been ravaged by
sheep-tick fever, and in replenishing his flocks Martin had tried an
experiment. He had brought—with great expense and labour—
sheep from the Cotswolds, where, in the greater cold of the high
hillsides, the animals which flourished were the ones with particularly thick fleeces. He had been resigned to the possibility of the
sheep growing lighter wool once they were on pastures less exposed;
but that had not happened in their first year. He was anxious now
to see for himself what difference a second winter had made.

"Like to come with me, Maude?" he asked.

"Oh yes, I would," she said eagerly. Then doubt and uncertainty
clouded her face. Since the moment when the Chaplain at Beauclaire had given her a new aim in life, she had made some advances

of her own. Self-denial was good, as well as prayer; a thousand small sacrifices of comfort or pleasure might "count," if offered in the proper spirit against the pains which Melusine was suffering in Purgatory.

Perhaps, she thought, imagining the pleasure of riding out in the sunshine, she should retract that acceptance and go instead to church, kneel until she was dizzy, pray until she was tired. That would "count."

But her grandfather's face had brightened and he was already considering which horse she should ride. She hadn't the heart to withdraw. Presently, at Clevely, there would be time and opportunity to make everything right.

So they rode out together and for some time spoke little and of trivial things. He explained about the sheep from the hills. He said, in a disgruntled way, that he had last year asked Walter to ride out and see them and that Walter had said a sheep was a sheep and no more. Cuckoos were calling from every thicket and he described to her how, as a boy, bird's-nesting at Rede on a precious Good Friday holiday, he had seen a cuckoo throw a blackbird's egg from a nest and settle down to lay her own.

It was talk to interest any child, and over Maude's response there was the patina of Dame Margery's training—not enough to listen and be interested, one must *look* interested, give signs of pleasure, encourage the talker to go on. Unaware of this, Martin simply found his granddaughter most pleasingly responsive; he found himself telling her things that he had never told anyone, things he had once, long, long ago, planned to tell Stephen and Robin when they were old enough to listen to his tales.

Thinking of them, which he seldom did nowadays, made him feel very old. Sixty-six this year. Forty long years had passed since the priest at Rede had told a stalwart young man of twenty that half his life was already sped. A long life, and superficially dull, work and work and work again. Two great sorrows, some success, several disappointments. And now, towards the end of it, here he was, riding alongside his granddaughter and feeling, under natural affection, something more lively stir.

He broke the silence by saying abruptly, "You didn't mean what you said the other day about going to live with the nuns, did you?"

"Oh yes," she said, without any hesitation, "I meant it. I have to."

"What does that mean? Your mother? That was all some silly idea she got into her head when there was talk of sending Walter to school. She said it would be unfair to send him from home and keep you. But the nuns wouldn't have you then. So she wheedled me into letting you go to Beauclaire. Against my will, I may tell you. And now you're home, and if I have any say in the matter there'll you stay."

"I can't go without your permission. They ask five pounds a year for my keep. And I must take a bed and blankets, linen. But I should cost as much at home."

"Cost!" he said. "Cost. That is nothing to me. You stay home, Maude, and I'll show how little cost matters. I'll buy you a grey mare. I know where to go—a fellow at Flaxham breeds them and trains them to paces that suit a lady. They have manes and tails like floss silk. You shall have a grey mare, Maude, and silk dresses, and a gold ring, a ring with a blue stone to match your eyes."

She closed her eyes for a moment and prayed one of the simple, unorthodox prayers which had become almost a habit.

All this, God! You alone know how badly, at Beauclaire, I wanted a proper mount. The dresses, too, and a ring with a sapphire. I'll sacrifice them all for one hour of Melusine's sojourn in Purgatory. Please take it, God. It is mine to give. I could have it, and I refuse it.

She opened her eyes and said, "You are very kind. You help me more than you know. But I must go to Clevely."

"Why?"

It is his five pounds, she thought; his money pays for the bed, the blanket, and the linen. He has the right to know.

"It is all so sad. I'm afraid that if I speak of it, I shall cry."

"Your mother," he said, trying to be helpful. "You must mind this. Mothers tend to like their sons better than their daughters, and when the pair are twins it shows more. You mustn't mind her, Maude. Let her have Walter. You're my girl."

All this, God, too! Please count my grandfather's favour, which I am about to forgo, against one hour of Melusine's torment.

She said, "It has nothing to do with Mother. I know how she feels about me; and it must be very hard for a woman not to like her own daughter."

Dear God, that is tolerance. I learned that very hard, could that count too? Just a minute. Because it was *so* hard to learn. Please, of Thy mercy, just a minute.

"Then *why?*" Martin asked in a grating and impatient voice, "why do you say you *must* go and shut yourself away there. When I want you home."

A long and horrible story. Something which, in its entirety, she had never had to tell. The Chaplain had known the details.

"When I first arrived at Beauclaire," she began. And Martin tilted his head sideways, the better to listen. She told him everything. The story ran smoothly at first and then was broken, like a stream which in its course runs over rocks. When she came to the re-countal of Melusine's body being taken from the water, she leaned forward over the pommel of her saddle and wept, and Martin, speaking for the first time since the story started, said:

"There, there, say no more, I understand." And he saw himself with his head pressed against the cold, smoke-blackened stone of the buttress of the Abbey wall, and then, falling prone, nursed in the lap of Old Agnes. To love hard, he thought, that is in our blood. For that reason I struck through the red mist and hit my master; for the same reason I cherished that mountebank, Pert Tom, and Old Agnes. I paid it tribute when I brushed aside, as though it were a cobweb, the almost certain proof that Magda had witchcraft in her; and years later I pandered to Richard over the matter of his love for Anne Blanchfleur.

"But I must say more," Maude said, wiping her gloved hand across her face, "because how otherwise can you understand? The Chaplain . . ."

She told him of the interview with the Chaplain, of her restoration to life and hope, of the task which he had laid upon her.

Martin listened attentively, thinking at first, with deep irritation, that this was all the result of her going to Beauclaire, but presently his mood changed. He realised that when she spoke of Melusine she did so as one would speak of the living, that she had achieved what all Christians should, but rarely do, do, the power to look upon death as an incident, not as the end. He compared this with his own feeling in similar circumstances. Kate, Stephen, Robin, and then Richard, all, to him, irrevocably dead. And God non-existent. Brought face to face with a faith so simple and unquestioning, so urgent that this child was plainly prepared to govern her whole life according to its requirements, he felt a thrill of almost superstitious awe. Not for him to oppose her decision. At the same time something in him rose in protest. When he spoke he did so slowly and carefully.

"You don't feel that you could pray, and be self-denying and all the rest of it, equally well at home? Nobody would interfere."

She shook her head.

"You see, that would be doing what I want. All the end of the time at Beauclaire I did want to go to Clevely. But since I have been back . . . Days like this," she said, looking around at the fresh young green of trees and meadows, all aglimmer in sunshine. "No, I know what I should do; and I hope that you will give me permission."

"I'm sorry you stumbled upon heartbreak so young," he said. "I was older when the blow fell on me. And I had no faith. You have that comfort. And if you're set on Clevely, you must go. Promise me one thing though. Don't think that going there means that you must be a nun."

"Oh, I'm not nearly good enough for that."

He ignored that. "It'll be some time before you have to make such a decision; I may be dead by that time, so I'll say my say now. It means having no husband, Maude. That may not matter; in most cases I think wanting a husband is something that wears off after a time. But it means no child and that's a different thing. Women, unless there's something very queer about them"—he remembered Magda—"need children, live through them. I've seen a woman, aye and she was hungry too, give her share of a poor meal to a child who had gobbled down his own. There's all kinds of love, my dear, but none to touch that. I wouldn't wish you to forgo it. That poor drowned girl was friend to you, and if you feel she's in Purgatory and your praying and fasting for a couple of years'll help, I've nothing against that. You mustn't make a life job of it."

I'm a clumsy old fool, he told himself. Maybe I've gone and put the idea into her head. With a return to his gruff manner he said, "There's Minsham Old Hall. You want to see your Grandfather Blanchfleur?"

"Not today," she said, averting her eyes, so that she should not see the place about which she and Melusine had held those long, happy conversations, made so many plans. The memory revived her revulsion for money, money and the greed for it which had brought about the whole tragedy. And even her grandfather's kind offer of a grey mare with a mane like silk, of fine dresses and a gold ring—all to do with money. I will have none of it, she thought. Once again she thought kindly of Clevely, where she would be free of it all.

Part Five

NICHOLAS FREEMAN'S STORY

I

When Maude Reed came home to her grandfather's house in the April of 1447, she was just twelve years old, and I was twenty-three: a full quarter century too young, one would have supposed, to be attracted by a girl of her age. And age was not my only safe-guard; I am by nature unsentimental and cynical; I was at the time happily provided with a mistress who suited me; and I had already, in the most practical and cold-blooded manner, made up my mind to marry Maude in about four years' time whatever she was like, even if she were the spitting image of her mother, whom I disliked.

Martin Reed himself put the idea into my mind. He was one of the least communicative people I ever had to do with, but even he, when in particularly low spirits or provoked, would seek some relief in talk. Several times, when Walter had annoyed him, he would speak of Maude, saying that twins were tricky things and the girl had been born with all the sense: saying that since Walter refused to have anything to do with the business, the one hope for it was for Maude to marry some decent, steady man, capable of running it.

Why should not I be that man? I was already, in addition to teaching Walter all he would consent to learn, keeping the accounts, and being trusted, day by day, with more of the practical side. As far as Master Reed could know, I was as steady as Baildon Tower; decent, too, for I had learned by experience; my new mistress lived some distance away, and was safely married. Her husband was a game warden whose duties, most conveniently, took him abroad at a time when I was free of mine. In four years' time, I thought, I should be twenty-seven and ready to settle down; Maude would be sixteen, and, unless her grandfather and her mother changed their ways, she would have had little contact with men. The Reeds were singularly friendless people. In Baildon indeed Master Reed was hated, though farther afield he was held in respect as an honest man and just.

Not being a fool, I realised that my plan to marry my master's granddaughter was very vague and vulnerable. When I joined the household at the Old Vine, the child was placed with one of Mistress Reed's noble relatives. Mistress Reed was highly connected, and had married the woolmaster's son for money—by the cast of countenance she usually wore I judged that it had been a bad bargain, she had a very discontented look. She was mightily devoted to her son, and, I thought, to her daughter; she was always stitching away on some fine article of clothing to send to the girl at Beauclaire. And from a few words dropped here and there by Master Reed I gathered that the mother's ambition was that her daughter should marry back into the class to which she herself belonged. But there the matter of dower was paramount, and the old man was obstinate.

"I'm not laying out my good money as bait for some young popinjay," he told me once. "It wasn't by my wish that the girl ever left home. She was a merry little thing and I missed her sore."

I thought over that statement; Mistress Reed had had her way once; she might succeed again.

There was very little that I could do to influence events, so I did not worry. I made myself as indispensable to my master as I could, was civil to Mistress Reed and patient with Walter and lived comfortably for three years.

Then Maude Reed came home and I fell in love.

At the time it seemed unaccountable, even to me. Now that I am middle-aged and accustomed to wealth and power, I understand my young self better. I am a lover of, a collector of beautiful things, and to me for a thing to be beautiful it must have a touch of the exotic. Anything that is lovely and unusual either in workmanship or material is to me irresistible; the moment I see it it makes an immediate impact and appeal, and I am not easy until it is mine.

Maude was Walter's twin and I had expected her to be like him; it was hardly necessary to make allowance for the difference in sex, for Walter's looks were girlish; he had a slim, seemingly boneless body, soft dark hair, and large dark eyes with long lashes.

My first sight of Maude, therefore, gave me a surprise. I looked,

looked again, found myself unable to look away from her. And even now, after many years, I find it impossible to say exactly what it was that so charmed me. It was a face that *meant* something. Not pretty. Not young even. Already, at the age of twelve, her beauty was the beauty of the ageless, undamageable skull. It showed in her brow, in her cheekbones and jaw. Her eyes, which were very blue, were set back in hollows, and below the cheekbones her face was scooped out, too. Her nose was low between the eyes, and then jutted out, blunt-tipped and wide-nostrilled. The lips of her mouth were long and both flat and full, and on either side lines had already formed, lines of fortitude, or perhaps of humour, a little on the wry side. The hair which was revealed when she threw back her hood was a warm reddish brown, crisp and springy.

For the rest she was somewhat taller than Walter, and, though delicately made, not without bone; thin square shoulders, bony wrists, long, clear jointed fingers. No breasts yet; and as I stared, wondering at myself and seeking some reason for my interest and for feeling as I did, I suddenly bethought me of the carved and painted angels in the roof of the St. Mary Chapel in the Abbey. Her beauty, like theirs, was of angle and plane, not of curve, and, like theirs, it was sexless, and, despite what her grandfather had said about merriment, on the sombre side. I had always had a weakness for small, plump, smiling women.

She was noticeably ill-dressed in a gown that had been lengthened, not very skillfully, and was still too short, especially in the sleeves. Mistress Reed had every reason to start demanding where was this and that garment, recently despatched to Beauclaire. Maude said she had given the things away.

"In Heaven's name, *why?*"

"I had sufficient without them."

Mistress Reed gave her a look of intense exasperation and then asked, "What is that you have on your finger?"

"A ring," the girl said, clipping her other hand over the ornament protectively.

"Show me!"

She held out her hand unwillingly and withdrew it quickly. We had all seen the clumsy, ill-fashioned thing and the dark mark, like a bruise, which the base metal had left on her finger.

"Tawdry rubbish. I should have thought that after three years at Beauclaire you would have known better than to wear such trash. Where did you get it? At a fair?"

"It is a keepsake; from a friend."

Mistress Reed, through her delicate, high-bridged nose, gave a sort of snort, and said, "The things I sent you . . . good sound things, you gave away!"

"Yes," Maude said.

They stood eyeing one another like wrestlers, each of whom has once thrown the other, and who now hesitate to try another fall. I saw that I had been wrong in thinking Mistress Reed devoted to both her children; she had no fondness for her daughter. And as Maude stood there, very straight, defiant, and yet oddly vulnerable, I was conscious of a wish to take her part, to protect her. It was a feeling quite new to me. But, after all, we have, every one of us, a weak point. The most hardened blasphemer has one name he holds holy, and once, in Norwich, I heard a triple murderer on his way to the gallows call to someone in the crowd, "Look after my owd dog!" Maude Reed was my weak point, the place where ordinary rules no longer held. I began to love her at that moment; but there should be another word for it; there should be several words to cover the widely diverse feelings for which we can only use the one word "love." I loved myself; I loved my amiable, cuddlesome Bessie; I loved Maude. Three very different uses of the word.

Maude had been home only a few days before I had an opportunity to serve her, to please her, and to put myself into her favour. She chanced to say that Walter wrote a much better script than she did herself. It was at table, where generally I was content merely to look at her.

"Who taught you?" I asked.

"One of Lady Astallon's ladies." I saw her eyes change colour, the black centre expanding until the blue was a mere rim. I had noticed before that light-eyed people, however strictly they rule their expressions, betray themselves thus. "Her name was Melusine," she said, and looked down.

Now Melusine is an unusual name, the name of a character in a French romance. Just the name it seemed to me, to slip into the mind of a young girl who, for purposes of concealment, tells an unpremeditated lie. That could be thought over later. I said smoothly:

"Ladies seldom have the advantage of being taught by a cloister-trained clerk. My teacher was a famous penman. If you like, demoiselle, I can show you, in a very short time, how to better your script."

At my use of the word "demoiselle," Mistress Reed and Master Reed both looked at me, the former with surprise and a touch of approval, the latter with one eyebrow cocked sardonically. It was a term of courtesy, used only towards young ladies of high birth, and not one to slip easily from the tongue of a clerk.

"That would be very kind," Maude said gravely. Then she smiled and her whole face was transfigured.

Mistress Reed, who liked me very little, could not forbear saying to me, "I should have thought you had enough to do, without taking on any more."

And to Maude, "You would be better employed with your needle. You write as well as you will ever need to."

"Not if I go to Clevely," Maude said.

For the first time since she had entered the house her mother looked at her kindly, almost lovingly.

"You wish to go to Clevely?"

Before Maude could answer Martin Reed brought his hand down on the table in a smack which made the platters jump.

"We'll have no talk of that," he said. "You're only just home. There's a whole long summer ahead. You stay here, learn to write, read if you want to, be a bit of company about the place. There's Walter, always on the fidget. I want no more of it." As though fearing an argument, he jumped up and limped away.

"If you wish to go to Clevely you shall," Mistress Reed said, looking at Maude and then quickly away again in the way she had. "I shall support you."

"If you do you're mad," Walter said. "Shut in, doing the same things, seeing the same people day after day. I'd rather be dead."

"Nobody," said Mistress Reed, in the soft fond voice which she kept for her son, "is suggesting that you should go to Clevely, Walter. We're talking about Maude."

"I came home to go to Clevely," Maude said. "It was all arranged, long ago, wasn't it? When I was twelve, they said. I thought it was settled."

"Of course, of course," Mistress Reed said hastily. "There was just the likelihood of your preferring to stay at Beauclaire. So the final negotiations were never . . . But it will be all right, I am sure."

I saw then how those lines, so out of place on either side of a young mouth, had been made. The girl knew, as well as I did, that her mother wanted her out of the house. How far that knowledge had influenced her decision to go into a nunnery as a lay boarder— which was all she could be at her age—I did not know, but, with that curious extra sight which infatuation lends, I could see with painful clarity that upon this matter of going to Clevely she was in two minds; half of her mind welcomed the idea, the other half rejected it.

I rejected it absolutely. I knew very well that dozens of girls every year went into convents as lay boarders; it was the fashion for girls of good birth to go and spend some time in the company of nuns most of whom were well bred, educated, capable of inculcating good manners, a smattering of learning, and a shrewd business sense in their charges. Most of the girls emerged little or none the worse for their cloistered years; a few became novices. Of that few, half— invariably well dowered—went on and took vows. An ordinary girl, going as a lay boarder, would have a likelihood of, say, one in twenty of becoming a professed nun.

But I wanted Maude here, in the Old Vine, here with me, susceptible, malleable. There was something about her, a kind of otherworldliness that would make her very open to persuasion. I had been schooled by monks; I knew how insidious mere atmosphere could be. I knew also how greedy—not as individuals, but as a community—any professed religious body could be. Maude Reed's dower would be a tempting bait. Especially to Clevely, which was surely the poorest house in all England.

Walter had by this time given up even the pretence of taking lessons from me, so when, at the time arranged, Maude came to the schoolroom we were alone. I took a clean piece of parchment and across the top of it wrote the alphabet in small letters and in capitals.

"There it is," I said, "and the secret is to make each letter sharp and clear, with points rather than sprawling, circular strokes. And with the capitals be sparing, write as though ink were gold—it is with gold that the great penman wrote, you know—not to be wasted. You see, economy, economy, and clarity is the result. You try now."

She was twice as teachable as Walter, though about writing he had been eager and good. In no time at all she had mastered the better style. Presently, looking up, she said in a defensive way:

"You mustn't judge the teacher by the pupil, you know, Master Freeman. Melusine wrote *beautifully*."

Anxious to ingratiate myself, I said, "Of that I am sure." I then asked, as casually as I could, "You were fond of your teacher?"

For a moment I thought she was about to cry; but she set her mouth, deepening the lines each side of it, and merely nodded her head.

There sprang into my mind a complete and feasible theory. There had been a writing master at Beauclaire—I could see him, sly, meek, and ingratiating—and although he would not dare aspire to the affections of one of the highborn young ladies, the wool-master's granddaughter would be within his range. Something had happened, discovery, scandal perhaps, and so she had come home, a trifle broken-hearted and ready, with girlish impetuosity, to fling herself into a nunnery. Or again, he, in his cunning, might have suggested that, it being the safest place where a girl could wait a year or two. Was it his ring that she wore?

The coarse, cheap thing was prominent on her hand as she wrote, and presently I ventured to say, "I think your ring is very pretty."

With something of her grandfather's bluntness, she said, "Oh no. Nobody could think that! But I like it." Once again she put her other hand over it and held it fast. At the same time her mouth took on such a tender look that I detected, beneath that carved wooden-angel exterior, the possibility of great sensuousness. With a quickening of my own blood I thought: He kissed her when he gave her that trinket.

I bore him no ill-will; what has been done once is the more easily done again, even if it is falling in love with one's writing master. She was very young; he was far away and I was here on the spot.

Then I remembered that she was going to Clevely.

I let her write for a while; then I said, "You read as well as you write, I imagine."

"Tolerably well."

"It is a pity then that you will have small chance to practise either art at Clevely. It is a very poor house and the Ladies are few. They work in the fields and the dairy."

"How do you know that?"

"We buy their few poor polls of wool—or did, until they lost their sheep from the tick fever. I've seen the Ladies, their habits hitched up, working like hinds."

She said dreamily, "I like to read and write; therefore Clevely will be all the more suitable for my purpose."

"Your purpose?"

"Something I must do." As she spoke she reached out for the pen-rag and wiped the point of her quill clean; stood it in the stand; rose to her feet, and, after a few words of thanks to me for the lesson, walked away, very graceful and dignified.

I felt rebuffed, I tried to feel resentful, too, but the genuine feeling would not be evoked. For the first time in my life in connection with any female I was inclined to self-blame. I should not have dared presume, on so slight an acquaintance, to question her.

Master Reed continued obstinate about Clevely. Once, through a half-open door, I heard Mistress Reed ask, in a quiet, cutting tone, "Is it that you grudge the five pounds a year for her lodging?"

"You know better than that. I'm thinking of her happiness."

"It is her own choice."

"Of that I must make sure."

The weather warmed, and one day Maude and her grandfather went out together. When they returned he had somehow convinced himself that her desire to go to the nuns was genuine. I could see, by his glumness, that he had been convinced against his will; nevertheless, without further protest, the preparations for her leaving began to go forward.

I now began to be concerned, for the first time in my life, for another person's creature comfort. On my wool-buying visits to Clevely I had seen inside the house; the nuns had no Frater even, they ate at a table at one end of the kitchen, which had a floor made of trodden earth and walls of undressed stone, running with dampness. I had not seen the rest of their accommodation, but I imagined that it would be equally comfortless. For a professed nun, vowed to poverty and self-denial, such surroundings might be, ethically, more right than the ease and luxuries that some communities enjoyed; but I hated to think of Maude in such a place.

I was silly enough to make one last effort to dissuade her. It was not planned, would indeed have been impossible to plan, for since the writing lesson which had ended so abruptly there had been no chance and no reason for us to have speech in private.

On this evening, just after supper, I was in the office, doing an extra hour's work. The weather had changed again and for the time of year it was bitterly cold, with a driving rain and a howling wind. Even for the sake of Bessie's embraces I was not prepared to ride three miles out and back again on such a night.

The door opened and I looked up crossly, expecting to see Mistress Reed, who had the annoying habit of coming into the office now and again when she knew her father-in-law was not there. She'd turn things over and ask questions—some of them, I admit, shrewd ones; and sometimes she would make suggestions which I would ignore and then in my own good time present as my own.

It was not Mistress Reed, however, it was Maude, who, from the threshold, said, "I thought my grandfather was here."

"He's gone to bed. In weather like this his leg troubles him."

"We trouble him too. I could see that at supper. So I thought . . ."

It was true that at the table Walter had once more referred to the time when he would travel the roads, playing his lute. Mistress Reed's expression had changed from discontent to piteousness, and the old man had looked first at Walter, then at Maude, and heaved one of his tremendous sighs. Disappointed in both his grand-children.

I heard myself saying, without any of the respect or the desire to please that formerly I had used towards her, saying, in fact, quite roughly, "I'm sorry for your grandfather. Walter is past praying for; he was born with this bee in his bonnet. But the poor old man had hopes of you. Piety can be as selfish as anything else, and if you stayed at home and cheered your grandfather's last years Almighty God would probably count it more of a virtue than wearing your hands out in the Clevely dairy and your knees on the Chapel floor."

She looked at me with wide-eyed astonishment, as well she might. I was astonished at myself.

"I'm not trying to acquire virtue for *myself*. What made you think that?"

Master Reed, who had been in the office before supper, and who felt the cold, had lighted the fire; it had burned down now to a heap of ashes, fitfully glowing pink under a coating of grey. I had got to my feet when Maude opened the door; now I turned and threw two billets of dry wood onto the fire, and then, reaching past her, I closed the door.

"Come in and get warm, it's one of the last chances you'll have," I said, in that same brusque way. "I know what I'm talking about. I went to Clevely for their last lot of wool in the month of May, and Dame Clarice Gracey who acts as Treasuress still had chilblains to the elbow. *In May.* She had her sleeves rolled up while she weighed the wool."

Maude gave a little shudder, moved her hands together, twisting the ugly ring, and then moved towards the fire and sat down on the settle, holding her hands to the warmth.

"The worse it is, the better. Don't ask me why. There are some things that shouldn't be talked about. It makes them seem . . ." She paused. "It makes them seem less real, less important. Can you understand that? I have a reason for going to Clevely. I told it to my grandfather, because I thought he had the right to know, and because I wanted to speak of it . . . yes . . . there was that, too. And ever since," she turned her head from the fire at which she had been staring and looked into my face, "it hasn't seemed so real or so urgent. I've begun to wonder . . ." She paused again. "I believe that you could, if you wanted, talk a thing clean away, make it be nothing."

I had seated myself on the opposite settle, and now, leaning forward, I said, "Try. Tell me why you think you must go to Clevely. Maybe then you won't want to go."

"That is what I fear. Except that . . . there is this in it, the less I *want* to go the more it will count if I do."

"Count? Count against what? Come on," I said, "you can tell me. Another fortnight and the Bishop's hands laid on me and I should have been a priest, qualified to hear any confession and advise on any matter. Imagine that! So you see, you can tell me anything."

Like all women she went off at a tangent. They do it, not deliberately, or because they are incapable of sticking to one line of thought as any man who has been nagged can bear witness, they do it for the same reason that a partridge whose nest is in danger will go limping and flapping away, deluding the intruder into the hope that she can be taken by hand. It is a defensive measure.

"I did not know," Maude Reed said, "that you were almost a

priest. What stopped you?" She spoke as though I were a runaway horse, grabbed by the reins.

I could hardly tell her what was my chief reason—that I knew myself unable to live celibate and should tire of pretending to be; my other reason was enough.

"I'm a farmer's son, with no family and no wealth to count on. For me the ladder to promotion was set very steep and lacked several rungs. Besides, I preferred the life of a layman; a priest should have a vocation."

She nodded gravely, and her hair changed colour where the firelight caught it.

"I know. Something—just a little thing it was, too—happened to me and made me think there was something in the world, after all. But there is a long time before I have to decide about a vocation."

"You make such a mystery of it all," I said brusquely, "talking about a purpose and what will count and other vagaries. You're far too young to take life so seriously. I'll tell you what I think. . . ."

"Yes?" She looked straight into my eyes.

"I think that at Beauclaire you had a bad attack of puppy love and something went wrong with it, so you go jumping into a convent like a scalt cat. It's very silly."

"I'm not jumping into a convent. I'm only going to live at Clevely for a time, as anyone might do."

Quite a lively temper, too, I found myself noting with approval. And another defensive tactic.

"I'll hazard a further guess," I said recklessly, "your bit of heartbreak at Beauclaire was concerned with your writing teacher—the one you call Melusine."

Dear me, that brought a result for which I was not prepared. She gave me a wild look and half rose, and then dropped back, laid her arms on the side of the settle, put her head down and began to cry.

I've heard dozens of women cry, with cause and without, and the most I have ever felt was a mild pity if they had what I considered good reason to weep, a testy impatience if I thought otherwise. Maude's tears seemed to come from my throat, her sobs to rend my chest.

I went down on my knees by the settle and put my arm round her and began to talk rubbish, saying that I meant no harm, that a little sentimental attachment was nothing to cry about, that I would sooner lose my right hand—what things people say in the endeavour to be persuasive!—than cause her a moment's pain. I reverted to childishness and referred to myself by the name that no one had used since I went, a boy of nine, to the monks' school at Norwich.

"Tell Nick," I pleaded, "tell Nick all about it."

She did too! Melusine and Uncle Godfrey and Madge Fitz-Herbert and how everything depended on money, and what an awful world this was. I kept my arm round those thin little shoulders and held her steady, and pulled out my sleeve and wiped her face on it. I hated all the three that she talked about because they had hurt her. The wench who'd lifted her skirt before the ring was on her finger was dead and beyond ill wishes; I wished a pox on the other two; and on all at the great house who had let such a situation develop, not seen what was afoot, and then, after the end of it, let this child carry her grief all sealed away in loneliness.

Presently, when she had cried herself out, I asked, "This is what you told your grandfather?"

"Yes. But I must not cry. I promised not to cry about it any more."

"Who made you promise such a daft thing?"

"The Chaplain."

Pox on him, too, I thought; a few good crying bouts and the wound would have begun to heal. She actually said, in a sad way, "There, now I've told you and it seems even farther away."

"That is why miseries should be talked over, not bottled up."

I left her then and put another log on the fire and again sat down opposite.

"Now listen to me," I began. I raked through my mind for any scrap of comfort to offer her. Heresies I could have gone to the stake for poured from my lips. I told her that there wasn't a word of evidence of the existence of Purgatory in the Bible. That Christ never exhorted anybody to pray for the dead. That the descent into Hell mentioned in the Creed was a man-made myth. "On the Cross, to the dying thief, Christ said, 'Today you shall be with me in Paradise,' what could be plainer than that?"

My years of training for priesthood now served me, in reverse as it were; I was persuasive, logical, like a lawyer who can plead this side of a case or that, according to who hires his tongue.

The result was disappointing; she listened, but was not convinced. The point I thought most telling she countered with, "That man was only a thief; not a suicide."

"Your friend had been wronged," I said. And then I paused, remembering that I had wronged at least two women in precisely that same way, and never until this moment had a pang of conscience about it. "Nobody can judge in these matters. She may have been acting in a spirit of self-abnegation; if she was with child, and had a family who would have shared the disgrace. If you want to make a disputation about it, theft is forbidden in the Commandments, there is no mention of suicide there. And if you care to be strictly logical, Christ Himself was the outstanding suicide of all time; at any moment *He* could have called down an army of angels to rescue Him."

In my eagerness to comfort her I had gone too far, forgetting that I was talking to a child of twelve. I saw horror dawn and grow in her face and savoured the full irony of having done myself deep damage in her estimation, simply through pity. I stopped speaking.

She said, "Now I know where I have seen you before. It has bothered me, not being able to *quite* remember. In the Maze at Beauclaire."

"I never was there."

"Not you. Your image. In the Rune Stone."

It was my turn to stare. And it was my turn—I who have always been impatient of women who told long tales about their dreams, and sceptical of those who claimed to have had premonitions—to listen to the story of a supernatural experience, which had at least one redeeming feature of being comic. She described the man she had seen in her vision, and whom she claimed to be me, in full cardinal's wear! Maybe I had missed my mark after all.

"You were trying to convince me of something, just as you were just now. And I knew you were wrong, as I know it now. Though I am sure," she added with magnanimity, "you were trying to be kind. And I'm sorry to have made such a show of myself. The first thing we were supposed to learn at Beauclaire was self-control."

"Of which," I said, "as with many another thing, a certain amount is very good, and too much deadly poison. The one thing I wish for you—because it would mean happiness in the end—is that you shouldn't act hastily over this matter. It was a shock, and you've brooded over it in silence and the whole thing has grown out of all proportion. If you spent, say, just the one summer here, living an ordinary life and trying to keep your grandfather cheerful, I'm quite sure . . ."

She said, "You know what they say in Suffolk when temptation offers, 'Get you ahind me, Old Scrat!' I must say it to you." She smiled, with the tearmarks still damp on her face. "I know what I must do, and I am going to do it."

Master Reed could be stubborn, and Walter was obstinate past all reason, and she was of their blood. But there was something other than obstinacy, there was something almost piteous in her last words to me that evening.

"Besides, even if I wished to defer going it would be awkward; everything is prepared."

And that was true. Mistress Reed had brought her undoubted capacity for industry and organisation to bear upon getting Maude's clothes and household goods ready for Clevely with such effect that when, on St. Barnabas' Day, she left the Old Vine for the second time, two pack horses were needed to carry her gear.

II

I had never much cared for Mistress Reed, thinking her cold and proud, admirable only in her devotion to her children, and in that I was but half right. After seeing her with Maude I liked her less, and, because she had encouraged the girl to leave home, even hastened her going as far as possible, I began to detest her. Her punishment was on its way, however, and I sometimes wondered how far she had herself helped to fashion it. How could anyone account for Walter Reed, who was, of all the people I have ever known, the most peculiar?

His mother was ordinary enough; she had married beneath her, but when one compared the home from which she came with that to which she had come, that was understandable enough. She had never, I am certain, entertained a thought, or experienced an emotion uncommon to her kind. She preferred her son to her daughter, but then thousands of women do that, but conceal the fact, perhaps out of deference to their husbands, who usually have a fondness for their daughters and govern their sons strictly.

Walter's father, who had died young of the lung rot, was, by all accounts, ordinary, too. He was musical, and rather better educated than some merchant's sons, but everything that was remembered about him indicated that he had been industrious and businesslike and sensible.

Whence then Walter? How did two such ordinary human people ever breed that changeling child?

He cared for nothing but his music. He accepted his mother's adoration without the reciprocation of even the most tepid affection. He condescended to learn to read and write because those arts would, he thought, be useful to him when he was an itinerant musician. For music he had some talent; he could pick up the words of any song, however long it was, at one hearing, and from a fragment of a tune, hummed or whistled, he could reconstruct the whole. He also made good songs of his own. Mistress Reed up to a point encouraged him, often remarking that he had inherited his father's ability—that was how I learned that Richard Reed had been musical. Even when he talked of his future, although one could see that the thought of his leaving home cut her to the heart, she was curiously infirm of mind, saying oh there was a long time to go before he could think of that, saying when he was older he would have more sense, saying that his father had talked the same way and settled down to business in the end.

His grandfather's attitude towards the boy was equally uncertain; he was deeply disappointed, as any man who had built a great business out of nothing and then finds his heir scorns and repudiates it would be justified in being. But never once did he make an open protest or seem to realise that a child could be governed and controlled. In the first three years of my time at Baildon the harshest thing I ever heard him say to Walter about his wildcat plans was:

"All right, if you go, when the time comes, you go. Don't keep talking about it!" And even that order Walter disobeyed when he felt like it.

Twice in those three years Walter, after some row over his lessons, had run away and been brought back. Excused from learning to count—which in any case he was completely unable to do; he left home at last still counting on his fingers—he settled down until the summer which followed Maude's going to Clevely.

During that summer, in August, the height of the pilgrim season in Baildon, there was an incident, trivial but curious, which I remembered years after, when Walter's fate was decided.

He came in, on that warm, dusty evening, a little late for supper, his face flushed, his eyes fever-bright, and his whole manner that of one who moves in a trance. He sat down and, ignoring the food before him, told us that he had been playing his lute in the market place. Those who had listened had given him cakes and fruit and sweetmeats and a variety of small trinkets. He laid them out on the board; a little image of St. Christopher, a knife with a horn handle, a belt buckle, and a money pouch made of plaited straw.

"They had no money to spare," he said, "but those who had . . . Look!" He opened the pouch and spilled out six or seven shining farthings. "They liked it so much that they paid me! They paid me!" he said.

His grandfather looked at the coins as though they had been earned by blood, fraud, prostitution. Mistress Reed looked at them as though they were her death warrant. I simply stared, thinking: Well, if he can earn that much in an hour, he's cleverer than most; a good thatcher working from dawn to dusk earned a penny and a half in the day.

Mistress Reed spoke first. She said, "Of course they liked your playing, Walter. You play extremely well. I always said so. But you mustn't take all this," she pointed to the stuff on the table, "as proof that you can make a living playing the lute. You see, you are very young and rather small, so they think that it is *marvellous* that you should . . ."

"The Devil take your tongue," Walter cried. All the colour went out of his face, leaving it the colour that I had only seen before on a corpse. "That isn't true. They liked it, I tell you. No matter about me. When I sang of the death of Roland they wept. Great rough men. One man said, 'What magic is this? I have not shed a tear since my child died, and what is this Roland to me?' He said that with tears running down his face. And then you say it is because I am small."

He would have been weeping himself, had he been able, but he never could cry; he could sob and moan but I never saw him shed a tear.

His mother shrank back as though he had hit her across the face, but his grandfather leaned forward and said in a voice of controlled fury, "Never, in all my days, have I known a boy speak so insolently to his mother. She spoke for your good and she spoke the truth. So, in the market place a few fools praised you, and you come home calling on the Devil. You ask pardon this minute, or I'll give you what I should have years ago, a damned good hiding."

I watched, with great interest. When I first came to the Old Vine the boy's choosiness over what he would and would not learn had been attributed to my failure to manage him. Let them learn.

Walter looked defiantly at his grandfather, but the old man was not to be outfaced. Set in their myriad wrinkles, under the scowl-scarred brow, his grey eyes bore down, unflinching. Walter's stare flickered and wavered. He put out his hands and gathered all the things he had laid out for display, as though they were his defence and consolation. Across them he said:

"I ask your pardon, madam. But truly it was not because . . ."

"That will *do!*" Master Reed said.

There was a silence at the table, broken when Walter picked up his little silver coins and passed them lightly from hand to hand. Mistress Reed leaned forward and seemed to be about to speak, but though her lips moved and her throat jerked, no sound came. She lifted her cup and drank, set it down, and then, rather like a woman who has heard evil tidings, put her hand over her mouth and the lower part of her face. Her hands, I noticed for the first time, were like Maude's, very long and thin, the finger joints clearly marked.

I saw Master Reed give her a sidelong glance. I thought that this was where I, one of the company, yet not emotionally concerned, should make some tactful, impersonal remark which would smooth over the awkward moment. Before I could think of one Master Reed, in a casual way which contrasted sharply with his last manner of speech, said:

"It would serve you right, Walter, if nobody spoke to you for a week. But that would punish your mother more than you. You'd better ask her to say that she forgives you."

Walter said as meekly as possible, "Please forgive me, Mother."

Master Reed then seemed to be affected by madness. He hit the table with his hand and said more furiously than I had ever heard him speak even to a pack-whacker who had foundered two horses, "God's blood! Can't you just for once do what you're told?"

Mistress Reed again moved her lips and tried to protest, but the old man thundered on. "I said, *ask* her to say she forgives you. Do it, or I'll break your neck!"

By this time every eye in the dining hall was turned towards our table. Mistress Reed, ever mindful of formalities, moved a hand in a gesture very eloquent and graceful to draw Master Reed's attention to this fact. He shook his head like a horse tormented by flies and kept his eye on Walter, who, after a minute said:

"Mother, please say that you forgive me."

The words came from her like liquid from an upturned bottle. "I do, Walter, I do. I shouldn't have said what I did. Of course they liked your playing."

"Now mark this," Master Reed said, "when you lose your temper and say things like 'Devil take your tongue,' that is a plain invitation for the same ill wish to fall on you. You be mindful of what you say."

I admit that on the face of it it was no more than any man might say to any child, a mere paraphrase of the old adage about ill wishes coming home to roost: but the way he said it gave it weight and importance. It was almost as though he believed that Walter's angry words had affected his mother's speech; as though the grandfather believed that the boy had a power to ill-wish, and wanted to warn him, privily, against inflicting hurt.

Rubbish, I told myself, superstitious nonsense. The one power which Walter Reed possessed was that of making people think he played better than he did. In the main he was secretive about his music, shutting himself away in the solar and playing for hours alone. On those occasions when he would say, rather pompously, "Now I will play for you," I always reminded myself that I had been schooled at Norwich where the choir is famous, and had twice heard Blind Hob of Lincoln play for the Leather Merchants' Guild in that same city. But always, before the end, Walter would have me, and with all judgement suspended I would fall under the spell, too.

During the time immediately after Maude's departure, whenever I heard Walter play, I would ask myself whether both these children hadn't been born with a curious power to charm, Walter by his music, Maude by just being. Walter's charm ended when his lute was silent, but Maude's could survive her absence. I thought of her, not always sentimentally, sometimes critically, at almost every moment during the day when my mind was not actually engaged upon some immediate business. I would try to recall her face and succeed only partially, making a picture in my mind of a blur dominated by one overprominent feature, the way one does when someone tries to describe a person unknown. "He has a big nose," they say, and you see just a nose. So I would think in turn of her blue, deep-set eyes, the hollow in her cheek, the turn of her lip, or the way her hair grew. Then, at another, unexpected time, I could recall the whole of her, down to the nails on her fingers. I thought of her, at such times, much as a man on short commons would think of some favourite, flavoursome dish. I craved to see her, and when, one day early in December, Martin Reed said, "I take it Maude will come home for Christmas," I wanted to jump up and shake him by the hand, slap him on the back, give loud and obvious evidence of my approval.

"I take it Maude will come home for Christmas," he said.

Mistress Reed said in a doubtful voice, "I don't know about that. Nobody mentioned it. Would it be allowed?"

Forgetful of my place, I said, "Of course it would. Who could prevent it? She isn't a novice, or even a school child. She can come home when she wishes."

"So I should think," Master Reed said.

"I'm not so sure." Mistress Reed looked me in the eye and said, "You were schooled by monks; did you go home for Christmas?"

She'd heard me say—the cunning bitch—that I did not.

"My home was thirty miles from my school, madam; and in return for my lessons I sang in the Choir. I could not miss the Christmas Masses. The cases are hardly comparable." I almost added and it would have been true: Except that my brothers didn't want me home, any more than you want Maude.

"It shouldn't be too difficult to find out," Master Reed said in his dry way. "Nicholas can write a letter, which I will sign."

"But are you sure that it is wise to unsettle her so soon? . . ."

"Holy Virgin, you talk as though we wanted her there, Anne. She took this whim to go, but if she's outlived it there's nothing I'd like better than to unsettle her. Unsettle, that's fool's talk."

Mistress Reed said with cold dignity, "I'm remembering my own childhood, always on the move and longing for some settled place. That was all."

"Well, if you can't see the difference," he said angrily and snatched up his mug, drank from it, and set it down with a clang.

Later, in the office, he stamped about, bringing his good leg down heavily.

"I'm the customer, ain't I?" he demanded of me. "I pay five pounds a year for her to be there when I'd pay four times the amount to keep her at home. You can tell them that if you like. The whole thing was a mistake from beginning to end. She should never have gone to Beauclaire. Beware of women, my boy. You don't have to be in love with one for her to lead you by the nose and you don't notice till too late. Get your things and write. How do you address a prioress? You should know. Now I'll say what I want to say, and you wrap it up so she'll not think she's dealing with an ignorant old fellow."

My former visits to the nunnery had been made after the shearing season, when the sun was warm and the fields green; even then I had been struck by the dreariness of the place, set all alone, far from the highway behind a barrier of trees. The House and the Chapel were both shaped like haystacks built of dark, dressed flint, the least cheerful of all building materials. They were linked by a kind of cloister, begun in stone and finished in wood; some of the pillars indeed were simply tree trunks, stripped of their branches but retaining their bark. Immediately in front of the cloister was a little herb garden, at this season bleached and depleted, but as neat as a piece of embroidery. Everything at Clevely was as neat as it was bleak.

The only door in the House opened directly upon the kitchen, and there was no portress here. My old acquaintance, Dame Clarice, answered my knocking, told me that the Prioress was ill in her bed, and without ceremony opened the letter.

"This is for Maude to decide. You may ask her. Let me see, Tuesday. You'll find her in the dairy." She indicated a door immediately opposite the one at which we stood, and said, "At the end of the passage."

I stepped in, aware at once of the smell of a religious house. Ordinary people on their way home from church shake the incense odour off into the air; professed religious on their short cloistered walk carry it with them to mingle with the scent of boiled onions and stockfish and the porridge that burned very slightly in the pan. With this smell of my schooldays in my nose and my heart jumping because I was, in a moment, going to see Maude again, I walked along the cold dim passage, feeling suddenly young and unsure of myself.

I could hear, before I reached the dairy door, the sound of girlish chatter, once a merry laugh, mingled with the clatter of pans and the swish of a scrubbing brush. Perhaps she was happy here, I thought, and perversely took no joy in the thought.

There were three of them in the cold dairy, all wearing coarse sacking smocks over their clothes, wooden clogs on their feet, and linen hoods covering their hair. One was engaged in scrubbing the shelves, one, on her knees, was scrubbing the floor, the other was scouring a bucket. The three faces turned to me with looks of surprise, then the one who was kneeling scrambled to her feet and said, "Oh, Master Freeman, is anything wrong?"

Even as I assured her, I was thinking to myself: Name of God, yes! Wrong that she who had never been full-fleshed should have grown so much thinner; wrong that her hands should be so red and swollen, the nails broken short and grimed from the dirty water. I told her my errand, and for one unguarded moment pure pleasure lightened her face, only to go out again like a blown candle. She said in a wooden way:

"I thank my grandfather for so kind a thought; but I had best stay here."

"He is counting upon your presence. Would you ruin his Christmas, when in the course of nature he can have few more? Remember what I said to you about selfishness."

"And you remember what I said about Owd Scrat!"

I longed to pick her up in my arms and run with her, out of the place; to shake the obstinacy out of her. I could only use words, and I was choosing, out of my own hurt, the most wounding ones I could muster, when the bucket scourer came to my aid.

"Oh, Maude," she said, "please go home and bring us back some Christmas fare. Raisins," she said, in an ecstatic voice.

"Ham," said the other, and I swear that her teeth shone for a second like a hungry dog's. "Ham for me, Maude. Please. We'll do your work. You go home and bring us back some goodies."

"A fine impression we shall make upon Master Freeman," Maude said. "He'll think us entirely governed by our appetites."

I took note of the conventual "we." I said, "You see, demoiselle, at the cost of a very slight sacrifice of your own self-esteem, you could mightily please three people—these and your grandfather."

"Four," she said. "I should myself be pleased."

"Five then, for I also should be . . . delighted."

"I should have to ask leave."

"It is already given. Dame Clarice said that it was for you to decide."

"The words must have *choked* her," cried the girl who had asked for ham. She giggled and put her hand to her mouth.

"Not for twelve days, then. Four."

"Good Maude. Kind Maude. The sooner I shall have my raisins."

Maude made a gesture of impatience, and moved towards me and the door. We went out together, and she pulled the door closed and leaned against it.

"You must not misjudge," she said. "They are both orphans and have lived here for four years. We have enough to eat."

"That I beg leave to doubt. You've grown very thin."

"We eat with the nuns and they work far harder than we do."

"You and they, in there, are growing," I protested.

"Which we shouldn't do if we lacked sufficient nourishment."

"There's no arguing with you. Shall I fetch you on Christmas Eve?"

"If you have time to spare." She smiled at me, and I saw that her odd little face which so easily assumed an expression of melancholy could just as easily shape itself to merriment. Martin had mentioned that she was a merry, hoydenish little girl. I cursed once again the bad management, the ignorance, and false values that had brought her to *this*.

Yet there was no denying that six months at Clevely had done a good deal to lighten her misery of spirit. During those four days of Christmas when my eyes, whenever possible, were upon her, as though they could never look their fill, I noticed that the old haunted look of desperate unhappiness had gone, and been replaced by a serenity which had a beauty of its own. Life at Clevely might be harsh and comfortless—some of the things Maude let slip shocked even her mother—but it seemed to be spiritually satisfactory and I, watching every blown straw that betrayed the wind's direction, saw several ominous signs.

Mistress Reed, as before, grumbled about her daughter's clothing. Why was this one dress so much worn, had Maude donned it every day, and why, where were the others? She was little pleased to hear that Jill was wearing one and Avice the other. Even I, doting as I was, detected a certain priggishness in the way Maude said:

"At Clevely we have all things in common. Except shoes. Feet vary so much. But," she added as though in extenuation, "we share the clogs."

Mistress Reed said, with a tartness which I understood, "That calls up the three-legged race which children run."

Maude laughed. "So it does! I should have said that we wear any clogs which come to hand, or to foot."

I recalled how teachable she was; in six months she had mastered the art of Christian imperturbability, as one of my teachers had called it.

Then again, at the well-spread table, the question of convent food arose.

"When you go back," Master Reed said, "that is if you insist upon going back, I shall send some hams and salt beef, and good wheat flour."

Maude said, and, hate the word as any man of sense must, there is no other, *demurely*, "That would be very much appreciated. Dame Winifred Challis who often has sick poor people in the guest-room is mostly at her wit's end to find them tasty dishes."

"You mean you wouldn't eat what I sent?"

"Oh no. We all eat from the same dish. Even the Prioress."

"Going hungry is no virtue," Master Reed said. "Thousands of people live their whole lives without knowing the feel of a full belly. You're enjoying what you're eating now, aren't you?"

"Oh yes. Very much. But to eat like this every day would be gluttony."

How well I knew it, this prate about the deadly sins! It could have only two effects. Hearing it often enough the young must give in, accept that to enjoy a comfortable bed was sloth, to eat a good meal was gluttony, to think one independent thought was pride, and on and on, until in one day of ordinary living you could commit the whole seven, twice over. (Whoever named them did so cunningly. Murder, which comparatively few people are tempted to, is not among them, anger, which every man must feel, is.) The only other way for the young to take is plain rebellion, bouncing away in the other direction, as I myself had done. Was Maude capable of it? That only time could tell.

In the privacy of the office Master Reed loosed his complaints.

"I've worked very hard, and at times been ruthless to see my family secure and comfortable, now the one I care most for might as well be a scullion. Better. Scullions grow fat on the dripping." He scowled at me. "I always thought food was plentiful in such places. They hand it out. When I was first lamed I lived on what was given me at the Abbey Alms Gate."

"It varies," I said. "All religious are supposed to be vowed to poverty. Their interpretation of it varies, and some merely disregard it. I believe Clevely is genuinely poor. They never managed to replace their sheep and so lost what piteous income their wool brought in."

His scowl lifted.

"I'll give them some sheep. How many could they look after properly without unduly adding to their labours? Three dozen? Fifty?"

"They had eight, if I remember rightly, before. I don't know how much pasture they have."

"Ask when you take Maude back. I'll give them what they can take, of my good Cotswolds from Minsham. And I'll buy every handful of wool at top price. That should help them to feed those poor girls a bit better."

"It wouldn't benefit Maude in any way, sir. The sick poor might fatten. And you'd be putting the gyves on Maude tighter than ever. Once make Maude a supply line between you and Clevely, and next time you see her she'll be in novice garb. I know my monks, and nuns differ from them only in ways that have no effect on greed."

He said, "I think you're wrong, Nicholas. Oh, right about the persuasion, possibly, but wrong as to the result. My family is naturally perverse. I believe if they tried to coax her *into* a habit, she'd run home and turn Lollard."

"You say that because she resisted our persuasions." I saw one of his eyebrows twitch when I said "our." "Yes, I tried to talk her into waiting, at least. But we were arguing against something that she felt she should do; and we were only using words. They—if they do try to persuade her—will be arguing for what she feels she should do, and words will be the least of it. Inside every community there is an atmosphere, a kind of mental climate which is very difficult to withstand."

He gave one of his enormous sighs, and said, as he had once

said when Walter was under discussion, "People do what they must, I suppose. But in this case," he scowled as he sought for the words he needed, "I never can feel that this is something that was in Maude and must out. It's been brought on from outside. If you knew what drove her to religion, you'd understand what I mean.

"She told me the whole story once. And sorry hearing I found it. *One* person had been kind to her in her loneliness, so she fixed on her the whole affection of a young and tender heart. And then the only word of real comfort she was given came from a priest. The result was inevitable."

There was a pause and I thought he was finished with the subject, but he said, "I failed her, too, perhaps. I thought of my own griefs—over which by this time, God knows, the grass should have grown. I envied her the certainty of her faith. I said as much. And I was wrong."

"As to that," I said, "I answered her with no faith, only with logic. It was a waste of breath."

He gave me one of his sharp looks.

"You seem to have a . . ." I thought by the way his lips shaped that he was going to say "a fondness," he amended it, "an interest in the girl."

I said boldly, "I am very fond of her, sir. Who could help it? Her looks are charming, her mind is lively, and even her obstinacy shows a good spirit."

He was pleased; it showed in the softening of his harsh old face. Then his eyes narrowed, as though he were regarding a bale of wool, assessing its weight and value.

"Her mother," he said slowly, "is often somewhat harsh towards her. You notice that?"

"Too often. I am tempted at times to forget my place and speak up in defence."

"Ah," he said, as though some question had been asked—not in words—and answered in the same fashion. "And you are now how old?"

"Twenty-four."

"You know the business; you are trustworthy and healthy, as handsome as a man needs to be. And twenty-four. Are your affections or interests engaged elsewhere?"

I told him, no, which was near enough to the truth as mattered.

"Then I'll tell you, Nicholas; if I could wish one wish it would

be that in two years' time, or three, you and Maude would marry.
I could die easy then."

I muttered some deprecating words about time being young yet,
and being honoured by this proof of his confidence and liking.
Never again did the matter come into the open; but the words had
been said; and if justification of my action was needed, later on,
there it lay.

III

The next two years seem to me, when I look back, to have been as
long as any other ten in my life. At Master Reed's insistence Maude
came home at fairly frequent intervals, always for Christmas, for
the birthday she shared with Walter, and again, either in August
or September; between these visits time sagged and dragged.

I had always held that any man who suffered any avoidable trouble or pain was a fool, and after Maude had gone stubbornly back
after that first Christmas visit I made great efforts to rid myself
of my infatuation.

I tried a change of mistress. My Bessie was as cheerful and cuddlesome as ever and I was fond of her, but I had become increasingly aware of some lack in our relationship. It was a coupling of
the flesh only—a business with which I had always hitherto been
supremely content but which now seemed to fulfil only half my
needs. I had only just determined to do something about this when
an astonishing and unlooked-for piece of luck came my way. Mistress Reed's brother, Sir Godfrey Blanchfleur, he who was responsible for all the trouble that had sent Maude to Clevely, came down
to visit his mad, moribund old father at Minsham and was shocked
by the conditions in which he found him. It chanced that on one
of the manors he had gained by his marriage he had found some
distant relative of his wife's family, a widow with two young sons,
living on sufferance. He spent a little money on making Minsham
Old Hall weathertight and slightly more comfortable and installed
this lady, with three good servants, to rule the household.

Clemence Kentwoode, had she possessed the minimum of
money or property, or even been childless, would not have re-

mained a widow for a week; she was pretty, witty, and amorous. She had the smattering of learning, and the grace of manner common to her kind, and although, at first, the greater freedom and independence which life at Minsham offered pleased her, she was soon desperately lonely. For me it was an easy conquest, but as soon as the excitement of the advances, and the novelty of the affair had worn off, there I was, in no better case than before. Worse indeed, having proved the failure of any substitute, however delightful. I was still in love with a child, a sanctimonious, sentimental, stubborn child.

And then, suddenly it seemed, a child no more. It was the birthday visit when she and Walter were fourteen years of age. I went, as had now become customary, to escort her home on the afternoon of the twelfth of March, and the moment I saw her I noticed the change. The sexless, carved-angel look had vanished. Though the Clevely diet and her growth upwards had assured that no flesh should accumulate on her bones, from somewhere Nature had found material enough for little pointed breasts which pressed against the material of her plain grey bodice, pulling it taut. The child had become a woman, the joy-giver, the child-bearer.

For me that was a miserable holiday; she seemed to have turned shy, losing what frank and confident friendliness she had ever felt for me. Nor was I the only one to suffer. Master Reed had bought her, as a birthday present, a fine gold ring with an inset sapphire, a trinket both valuable and beautiful. At the sight of it she burst into tears in which my experienced ear detected unmistakable hysteria and, holding one hand over the ring she had brought from Beauclaire, sobbed out that at Clevely nobody was allowed to wear more than one ring.

Her grandfather, with what I considered admirable restraint, said, "Well, wear them turn and turn about, then!" She turned, and sobbing flung herself upon him, putting her hands about his neck and saying that he had always been so good to her and she did not wish to displease him. He patted her awkwardly, and said, rather as though soothing a frightened horse, "There there. There there. It's all right. Don't upset yourself. There there."

Mistress Reed, with a look of controlled loathing, said, "If this is cloister hysteria, we want none of it here."

And where, I wondered, in her restricted life had she heard of "cloister hysteria," that ease in the shedding of tears which, alongside its opposite, stoic fortitude, is reckoned a virtue by all those communities who must make virtues or sins out of every natural thing. Her words inevitably made me take Maude's part and I said:

"Sudden contrasts are very upsetting. At Clevely she has so little and here she has so much. I remember when I was at Norwich we were all, for some prank which no one would confess to, confined to Dorter and Frater for a week. Then we were let out, and in the grass a single daisy had flowered. We all wept at the sight of it as though we had received news of bereavement."

"That," Mistress Reed said with cold dignity, "is exactly what I mean. Cloister hysteria. We don't want it here."

Maude pulled herself free of her grandfather's patting hand.

"You mean you don't want *me* here. That is nothing new. You never did. I've known for years that the sight of me affronts you. Everything you've ever given me was a sop to your conscience. I know. And you need not worry about my bringing the cloister here. I shall not come here again. When I go back I shall begin my novitiate."

Martin Reed banged his hand on the table.

"Enough!" he said. "That's enough. In all my days I never heard such a to-do over nothing. You, my girl," he looked at Maude, "will never be a novice with my consent. Five good pounds a year I paid them for your keep, and never in all my dealings have I had worse value for money. That'll stop. Tell them that. If they take you in a veil, they take you bare. See how they like that. As for you," he swung round and faced Mistress Reed, "all the wench said was true. Out of the house, first to Beauclaire, then to the nunnery. Why, God alone knows." He reached out and snatched up the ring which had precipitated the scene, and tossed it towards me. "Take it," he said, "give it to your leman. She can sell it and buy one of her boys some bit of gear that'll set him on the road to knighthood." He spat out the word as though it were an obscenity and rushed on, "That's been the ruin of us all, pretensions, with nothing behind them, sacrificing decent sober hard-working people and silly little girls who love the first person to speak a kind word and fine gentlemen so fine they'll wed lunatics for the sake of their acres. . . ." He had, on the whole, been coherent up to that point, then he began to mutter and babble.

I jumped up and went to him and took him by the arm.

"Master Reed, you are unwell. Let me help you to your room."

His weight, greater than I had reckoned for, defied me. I said to Walter, who throughout the whole business had sat watching, detached and observant, "Give me a hand." He came forward unwillingly and took the old man's other arm. We got him to bed and sent for the doctor, who bled him and diagnosed a fit of the choleric humour. No meat, he said, and no wine for two days, and we were all to take care not to anger him; he advised, too, that during the two days of low diet the old man should remain in bed.

So next morning, speaking as usual, looking pale after his bleeding, Master Reed said, "Send Maude to me." My heart, which had been very low since those words about the novitiate, rose a little. He looked very pitiable, propped against his pillows, and she, I knew, was fond of him; maybe he could talk her round. But I found, when I went in search of her, that she had gone already, stealing out before breakfast and taking one of the yard boys with her to bring back her horse.

I began then to think seriously about my future. With Maude in a nunnery and Master Reed likely, according to the doctor, to fall down dead any time he was crossed, my prospects were not promising. It was too late now to begin insinuating myself into Mistress Reed's favour; in the event of my master's dying I should be out on my ear smartly.

Up to that time I had been completely honest in my dealings, which included handling considerable sums of money and negotiating even larger ones. But from that St. Joseph's Day I began to emulate the Unjust Steward in the Bible story, whom Our Lord Himself praised for his foresight rather than blamed for his dishonesty. I was very careful, never taking more in coin, or making as a false entry more than could, at a pinch, be regarded as a genuine mistake; and it was all the easier because after that birthday visit and Maude's running away my master began to decline, not only in body but in mind and spirit. He began to talk of Maude as though she were dead, and sometimes he would call her Kate, and then catch himself.

I said to him once, "You mustn't despair too soon. Every novice doesn't take vows by any means."

"Despair," he said. "It isn't that. It's acceptance. It all goes by rule and the rule laid down for me was that Walter the smith's son should never have anything."

Then he said, "Did I say Walter the smith's son? My memory plays tricks. I knew him as a boy. It's I who must lose all I gain."

"Oh, come," I said, "you've been very successful in business."

"Yes, I've got a good business." He said it as though he mocked himself and it.

When the time came round for the five pounds to be sent to Clevely he sent it meekly; and charged me to tell Maude that she had but to ask for anything more that she needed. That message I was not able to deliver since Maude was either not allowed or had herself chosen not to see me. Dame Clarice took the money and told me, kindly but firmly, that it was impossible for me to see Maude.

Before I got back to the highway I dismounted and lay in a field full of tall white marguerites. I threw myself from side to side, crushing the flowers, full of misery and self-pity and fury at my own folly. To have let romantic love get hold of me and wreck my happiness, fool, sick-minded fool! Gay Nicholas Freeman, over whom several women had cried, lying in a damp field, perilously near crying himself!

I resolved to throw off this weakness. Good-by to Maude Reed, I thought, when at last I rose up and brushed the grass and broken petals from my clothes. Being already halfway to Minsham, I would go on, and see Clemence and take full pleasure in the thing I had, instead of crying, like a baby, for what was out of reach.

IV

Halfway through the next month, July, any wrong which Mistress Reed had done her daughter, and through her Master Reed and me, was repaid tenfold.

Walter walked into the dining hall for the midday dinner carrying his lute and wearing his best clothes. His mother made some comment upon his attire, and he said, as casually as though he were announcing a visit to church or a nearby fair:

"I'm going to Walsingham. A party sets out this afternoon."

I knew, and so did his grandfather, that the hour had struck. Mistress Reed, ever blind to what she did not wish to see, spoke for a moment as though he were merely joining a pilgrimage. Did they go mounted or afoot? Were any of the party known to her by name?

His smooth, secret face took on for a moment the bony stubborn look that was his sister's.

"They're tumblers and jugglers, riffraff. We shall walk, from Walsingham to Lynn and then to Lincoln."

She could not be blind to that. She turned pale, and with trembling lips began to plead.

"Too young," she said. "You're too young, Walter. Wait just a year, one more year. I promise then that you shall go, if you want to, with my blessing."

"I'm as old as Maude, and she has chosen what she is to be."

"Girls are always older for their age. Besides, Maude is safe." She reached out and took him by the wrist. "Walter, I beg of you. The roads are full of dangers. Thieves," she said. "Cutthroats."

"The poor are safe enough. Thieves only set upon merchants with fat moneybags." He gave Master Reed a saucy, provocative glance.

"Don't be so sure," his grandfather retorted. "The only time I was set upon, beaten, and left for dead, I was in rags and hadn't a farthing to my name."

"There are plenty on the road who would kill you for your shoes," Mistress Reed said. She turned, still holding her son's wrist, and appealed to the old man. "Forbid it," she said. "You are head of the family and he is only a child. Forbid him to go."

He said harshly, "What would be the use?"

Walter jerked his wrist free.

"All this fuss," he said disgustedly. "It isn't even sudden. I've been saying for years what I would do. And now, I know, is the time."

As he said the last words he threw back his head, and the fine black hair that was smoothly clubbed about his skull shifted and stirred, as though, in that still place, a free wild wind blew on him.

"You must take some money," Master Reed said, "in case of sickness, or other ill-fortune. It must be sewn into the lining of your jerkin."

"You're encouraging him," said Mistress Reed, beginning to cry. "I see it . . . because I let Maude go, you . . . Walter . . . yes, I see. I'll fetch her home, I promise. Make Walter stay here and I'll persuade Maude."

Walter jumped up and grabbed his lute and looked ready to run.

"Wait," the old man said. "You must have the money and the names of honest men I know in many towns, who would help in case of trouble. I'd have done as much for her," he added inconsequently, "if I had known."

"Nor is that all," cried Mistress Reed, checking her tears. "Walter, wait. I never wholly believed—you see, your father talked the same way and he never . . . no matter now—I never believed you would go, or so soon. I would have done something about it. Don't waste your music on the greasy gaping crowd, Walter. Make something of it. Go to Beauclaire or Rivington, or to your Uncle Godfrey at Horsbury where you could be heard by those who could advance you. Music like yours should be played at Westminster or Windsor."

That was flattery. To do him justice, I will say that during the last months his playing had improved and the spell which he could cast on his hearers now had solid worth behind it. But Westminster and Windsor!

Walter said, "I would hate that way. To be taken up because this man was my cousin or that one my uncle. Not for me! When I go to Windsor or Westminster it will be as plain Walter Reed, the strolling player. *And I shall go by invitation.*"

Since the day when I heard the fourteen-year-old grandson of a wool merchant speak those words, I have mingled with the great; I have spoken with crowned kings and stood in the presence of St. Peter's anointed successor. I have never, anywhere at any time, heard anyone speak so arrogantly.

Mistress Reed, her last card thrown and the game lost, said in a dull voice, "Come, let me sew in your money."

"Wait," Walter said. He looked into the hall, where the weavers and yardmen and such pack-whackers as were home for dinner that day had their eyes and ears upon our table, even as they plied their knives and spoons. He climbed onto the bench where he had been sitting and took up his lute.

"I am going away for a little while," he said in the clear, confident voice of one already used to addressing a mob. "This is my farewell to you. It is called 'A Song at Parting.' I made it for this occasion."

He had based it on one of those old pagan tales which had managed to slip through the close net of censorship which the Church had tried to drop between the stories of the antique world and those of Christendom. In a light, pleasing voice, neither child's nor man's, he sang of the final leave-taking between Orpheus and Eurydice, when, he having broken the condition of her release from Hades, she must turn back into the shadow world.

I suppose everyone within hearing, the stolid Flemish weavers, the rough urchins who swept the stables, the brutal drivers of the pony teams, and the maids who came crowding into the doorway to the kitchen, had at some time known a parting from someone of whom they were fond. The song spoke direct to the memory. I sat there, thinking of Maude, that tender mouth never to be kissed, that slim, just nubile body doomed to sterile virginity. I felt my own eyes moisten. Mistress Reed broke down and put her face in her hands and sobbed without restraint. Everyone cried except Master Reed, who stared straight ahead of him, God knows at what ghosts.

Walter struck the last note; looked around with satisfaction and jumped down from the bench.

Perhaps his music had touched his own heart. He laid a hand on his mother's shoulder and said, "I'm not going for good. I shall be back one day."

Master Reed got heavily to his feet and said, "I'll go get the money. Show it to nobody, Walter, and don't speak of it. Keep it in case of need."

V

Walter's departure had two results. Martin Reed now began to speak openly of me as his successor.

"It'll be in your hands," he said, speaking of the business. "Even if Walter comes home when he tires of the road, he'll know nothing. I want my daughter-in-law kept in comfort so long as she lives and I've always helped keep her father who'll probably live to be a hundred. Then there's Maude's dower. And I hope you'll get a family of your own. So you'll need to keep busy."

The third time he spoke to me in this strain I said to him frankly, "Unless, sir, you make a will and state clearly that it is your wish for me to take charge of the business, all these plans will come to nothing. If you die intestate, Walter is your heir, and his mother on the spot will be his regent. Before you are in your grave—God forgive me for mentioning such a thing—I shall have a month's wage and my quittance."

I spoke the more surely because, since Walter's going, the relationship between Mistress Reed and myself had undergone a great change for the worse; and for a reason which no one would credit.

She had attempted to assuage her melancholy over the loss of her son in a way unusual to women; she took to drink. Openly, at the supper table, she would drink three or four cups of wine in place of her usual one; and secretly too. I've gone into the solar in an evening and found her there, her hands idle on a piece of embroidery or plain sewing, and the air reeking of brandewijn; I've seen the cup standing on the floor, half, but not quite, hidden by her skirts. I've passed her on the stairs, standing aside where they widened and turned to allow her to go by, and smelled the same pungent odour, and she just come from her bedroom, early in the day.

She was never noisy or truculent; indeed in her cups she became more agreeable; the lines of her face would lift and soften. One realised, for the first time that, if she married young as most girls do and quickened soon after, she could still be just short of thirty. My Clemence was thirty-two. Mistress Reed had always seemed at least ten years older. But drunken, she lost something of her stiff, cool, self-contained look.

One evening, when Walter had been gone a month, I came in late, from Minsham. I had no more reason for secrecy, for over the episode of the ring on that fatal birthday morning Master Reed had betrayed that he knew about my attachment. After that any errand of supervision of the Minsham sheep run, where the sheep from the Cotswolds still flourished and produced their overweight in wool, would be undertaken in the afternoon; then I would have supper with Clemence, make love, and ride home.

It was now four months since Maude had gone back to Clevely without even a good-by, and my defences were building up. As I rode home I had thought to myself that if I could persuade Martin Reed to put me upon a sure footing, either now, or by will, which would take care of the future, I might do far worse than marry Clemence. She had much the same background as Mistress Reed and would be a match for her, I thought. And though the two boys were imps straight from Hell—you could almost smell the brimstone on them—one thorough good beating apiece, which as their stepfather I should have the right to administer, would improve their manners if not their characters. I toyed with this thought, not enthusiastically, but rather with the resignation of someone making the most he could of the second best, all the way home, while on the warm night air the scent of honeysuckle and meadowsweet lay heavy.

I noticed as I came to the Old Vine that there was a light in the solar window. Mistress Reed, a bit drunken, had left the candles burning, I thought. When I'd stabled my horse I would go in and pinch them out.

When I re-entered the passage which ran clear through the house, the solar door was open and she was standing just inside. Her hair, which I had never before seen completely uncovered, hung loose to her shoulders, very curly and pretty, pale gold. She wore a blue velvet bedchamber robe, so ungirded that I could see her breasts. And they were pretty too. She was very drunk.

I was reminded of my first visit to a house of ill-fame. It stood in a narrow lane, just off Tombland, in Norwich; the girls had worn exactly that half-revealing, half-concealing garb, and that same air of deliberate welcome.

"You're very late," she said.

"Yes, I am. Would you like me to put out the candles for you?"

"No. Not yet. Come and talk to me for a little while." She put her hand on my arm and I went into the room with her. She moved towards the window, which stood wide on the garden. The lop-sided moon which had lighted me home hung like a lantern, and the sweet night air, the breath of flowers and green things growing came in to mingle with the sharp scent of the brandewijn.

"I'm so lonely," she said. "Years and years and years with nobody to talk to."

She sat down on the window seat and would have pulled me down beside her, but I stiffened myself, and her hand, as I resisted, slid down from my arm to my hand. She twisted her fingers so that for a moment they were twined with mine, and she looked at me with as plain an invitation as any woman ever gave any man.

I thought very rapidly; a dozen thoughts in a breath's space. Ha, I thought, and I had believed that it was too late to work my way in with her. And I thought how amusing to see the trollop who had lived behind that screen of whalebone and good breeding. And I thought: You are the one who sent Maude to Beauclaire and therefore to Clevely and I will have no truck with you. Other thoughts I had too, of how long she had lived widowed, of things Clemence had murmured in moments of joy, of how it was better to live out your time as a maid than to be widowed since what you had never had you did not miss. Almost I could be sorry for her. But not quite. Besides, I had just come from Clemence and there was no desire in me. So I pulled my fingers free and said:

"Madam, it is too late now for talk. I am for bed. I advise you to do the same."

She began to whimper, saying that she could not sleep; that once the brandewijn would assure her slumbers, but now no more.

"In the end there is nothing," she said. "Nothing left. Nothing at all."

I reached over her bowed head and closed the window and latched it. As I did so she half rose and pressed herself against me. I stepped back and said, "Madam, you are not quite yourself this evening. Come take my arm and I will help you upstairs." I left one candle burning and put out the rest.

Still whimpering, she said, "I *am* myself. Locked in, all alone with terrible things to remember." She looked at me with drunken cunning and with a change of tone said, "Ah, you would like to know, wouldn't you? And all I'll tell you is that God has taken away Walter, to punish me. So I'm all alone and even you won't be kind to me."

My surprise and mixed feelings had settled down now into simple disgust. I said briskly, "I am always civil to you, madam. Even now I am offering you my arm, and to light you upstairs."

She gave me a beaten look, but she put her hand in the crook of the arm I offered and moving unsteadily mounted the stairs. At the door of her own room she paused.

"They come and stand by the bed and look at me," she said in a complaining, confidential way. "They never did that before. I'm afraid." For a second I suspected that this was a cunning trick to get me into her bedchamber; but almost immediately her manner underwent another sudden change. "I shan't flinch," she said. "The blood of brave men runs in me. Let them do their worst."

She opened the door and marched in, as though meeting a challenge, and before I could give her the candle slammed the door in my face.

I went on to my bed thinking about Joseph and Potiphar's wife.

As a character I had never much admired him, but now I saw the story from his viewpoint. I only hoped that when she woke, sore-headed and sober in the morning, she would have forgotten the whole episode. But her manner betrayed her. She had never been markedly pleasant to me, now she became even less so, always speaking to me in a cold, contemptuous way and taking trouble to make wounding remarks. She told me that I was going bald very early, and another time said that I was getting fat, unbecoming in a young man; she even hinted that my hose could do with a wash. One would have thought that I was the one who had made an attempt to seduce her.

That was why I spoke frankly to Master Reed of the need to make his will; but like all unlearned and self-made fellows he regarded the making of a will as tantamount to signing his death warrant.

"Yes," he said, "I will see about that." And did nothing.

For a boy who had evinced so little affection for his family while he lived in its bosom, Walter wrote very regularly and at some length. I suspect that some, at least, of his letters were written to advertise his skill and in the hope of drawing custom. He had plainly become one of the great fellowship of the open road, and at various times his letters were delivered to the Old Vine by tinkers, minstrels, pilgrims, friars, and merchants. Once even a gay young knight, with two squires in his train and his jousting armour on a pack horse, came jingling along to hand in a letter which Walter had written at Nottingham Castle.

"The boy played with such skill," he explained, "that I invited him to come with me to Colchester, where I join my Lord Delahaye who has a lively appreciation of talent. The young knave made mock of my offer, but said that if I went to Colchester I could deliver a letter for him. It has added some miles to my journey, but no matter; I have seen the nest that hatched so sweet a throstle."

Master Reed and I had just finished supervising the loading of one of the pony trains, and were on our way into the house.

"If you would be pleased to dismount and enter, sir," Martin said, "you would be welcome to the best I have to offer."

"I thank you, but I am already delayed."

"Run find your mistress," Master Reed said to me; and to

the young knight, "One moment more, for charity. The boy's mother . . . it would ease her mind to speak with one who saw him so recently."

Mistress Reed came running out, and the knight doffed his feathered cap and answered with civility the questions she asked about how Walter looked, was he still well shod, and what kind of company he was in. He repeated the story of his offer to introduce Walter to Lord Delahaye, and Mistress Reed, already a little mazed with wine, drew herself up with great dignity and said:

"If Walter had wanted advancement in that way he could have gone to his cousin Astallon at Beauclaire."

The young knight said, "Madam, your son will never lack advancement. With his skill and effrontery he should go far."

If Walter's letters were to be believed, such offers, and some even more dazzling, were an everyday matter to him. His reply was always that to him confinement in a great house, even a palace, would be as irksome as in a small. He seemed more impressed by his smaller triumphs, "everybody wept," "some women came and kissed my hand," "a man gave me his last farthing."

Mistress Reed kept all the letters in a box of carved wood, spent hours brooding over them and fingering them, and constantly referred to them as proof that Walter was dutiful, that he remembered his home and family with affection and would most surely return.

Once when she said that, Master Reed said, mildly but with meaning, "We trust that he will. And it would be a pity if he found us in less good fettle than he left us."

That was the most pointed remark he ever made to her in my presence; but then, despite his lack of learning and his gruffness, he was not insensitive. Whether in private he remonstrated with her I do not know. To me, on one occasion, when her insobriety was such as no one could overlook, he said:

"Poor woman. She cannot face grief. When her mother died it was the same, and when Richard died. It is her refuge, as work has been mine." He thought for a second, sticking out his underlip. "At least she hurts nobody but herself," he said. "By my work I've ruined two men that I know of, and probably others."

I forgot Mistress Reed. I thought to myself: It is a bad sign when old men who have led successful lives begin to look back and reckon what damage they have done. It is a foreshadowing of the final reckoning which they are preparing to face.

Time went on; the seasons changed. My little secret hoard of coins grew, more swiftly as Martin Reed relaxed, bit by bit, the strictness of his supervision. Physical changes in those one sees several times every day escape one's observation; it was with surprise that one summer evening, coming suddenly upon Mistress Reed in the garden, with the level rays of the westering sun full upon her, I realised that she had grown fat and that puckers of loose skin hung like little bags beneath her eyes and under her jaw. She was drunk, as usual; and she was staring so fixedly at a place where the grass grew lush under an apple tree that I thought she had dropped something and was searching for it. She actually pressed one hand against the trunk of the tree for support, and, thus balancing, bent over and with her other hand touched the grass.

I was going straight past her, but she heard my step on the path and straightened up, and, squeezing her eyes against the light of the sun, said, as though we had been for some time in converse:

"That is the *one* thing that is sure and certain, the one thing you can count on. God punishes every sin."

"So we are taught," I agreed, and made to pass on.

"But we don't believe it. That is where we make our mistake. And then it is so subtle. The punishment never comes either from the direction, or in the form that you expect. Bear that in mind. You plant a sin like a grain of wheat and you think punishment will come up, a full ear of wheat. For that you are prepared. But it isn't wheat that comes up; it's a damask rose, and you pluck it, and the thorns tear your flesh and the scent of it is poison. I know what I'm saying."

"I have no doubt of that, madam. Would you like my arm to assist you into the house? Then I must ask you to excuse me."

I went on into the house, thinking that here we were with another year almost half gone, Midsummer Eve again. And Master Reed still with his will not made, my future still very insecure, and Clemence growing a little, a very little, but still noticeably cooler. It was fifteen months since Maude had gone back to begin her novitiate, and though I had done my best to shut her out of mind, more than once, in the very act with Clemence, I had suddenly thought of her and gone impotent. That had frightened me; and

Clemence, sympathetic the first time, had turned suspicious the second.

Leaving Mistress Reed, maudlin under the apple tree, I thought to myself: It hardly needs God to punish us; we somehow contrive to punish ourselves.

VI

The news about Walter took a long time to reach us. A letter written in the April of 1451 arrived from Gloucester in June. It said he was well, and about to set out for Winchester. After that there was silence.

We should hear at Christmas, Master Reed said; yes, Mistress Reed echoed, we should certainly hear at Christmas. But the season came and went without a word. Mistress Reed burrowed more securely into her refuge, and the old man said, whether to comfort himself or her, that the absence of news might be a good sign. Probably in the autumn, faced with the discomforts of another winter, Walter had turned his face for home and therefore did not think to write.

Then, on a blustery March evening, my master and I were in the office when a servant girl, white of face and wide of eye, ran in and said that there was a creature asking for Master Reed at the yard door.

"If you mean a beggar, say so," Martin said, and prepared to lever himself out of his chair.

"I'll go," I said, and jumped up.

"If it's a letter or a message from Walter, bring the bearer in. A spoken word tells twice as much," Master Reed called after me.

The servant girl ran straight back to the kitchen instead of hanging about, as their habit is, to catch a word out of which to make a long story.

When I reached the door I realised that her use of the word "creature" had a frightful accuracy. There are the natural deformities to which the eye becomes accustomed, the squints, harelips, hunchbacks, mutilations due to accident or battle. But there is another sort, inflicted by unscrupulous showmen upon infant children. They take them when their bones are soft and pliable and shape them, as a gardener shapes a tree that is to be espaliered. Then, if the unfortunate child survives—few do—they have something truly unusual, something out of nature, for a sight of which, in a dim-lighted booth, the sensation seekers will hand over their pence.

This was one such, a striking example of the devilish art. His left arm had been trained to grow behind his head, so that he had two arms, one long and one short on the same side, and his head appeared to grow from under his arm, like those of a strange people mentioned in some traveller's tale.

In his armpit his head lay sideways, so that to look up he must turn his eyes almost out of their sockets.

"Are you Master Martin Reed?" he asked. His voice was muted.

"I'll take you to him," I said, sickened beyond being able even to ask his business. With my back to him as he pattered after me towards the office I managed to ask, "Is it anything concerning Walter Reed?"

"Yes. Yes. Bad news that I hate to tell. But I promised."

Outside the office door, which I had closed behind me because the wind was raging through the house, I said, "Wait here a moment." I went in.

"It is about Walter," I said, as gently as I could, "and bad news, he says. And the bearer, sir, is one of those freaks that they show at fairs—a shocking sight."

He drew a deep breath which lifted and straightened his heavy bowed shoulders.

"Let's know the worst," he said.

I admitted the poor creature, but did not go in myself. I went and sat on the stairs, near enough to be within call, telling myself that this was, after all, the proper thing to do. I was *not* one of the family, intimately as I lived with them; nevertheless, knowing the real reason for not going into the office, I knew that I was a deserter. Still, I was here if I was wanted. And in a minute, no more, the office door opened and Master Reed, grey-faced but quite calm, came out, turned towards the kitchen, saw me, and stopped. He lifted a warning finger.

"Go and ask them to mull some ale," he said, almost in a whisper, "and bring it and some bread and meat to the office. Then go and bring down my sheepskin coat. The poor creature's starving and soaked to the skin."

The stout old cook and the two serving girls were in a huddle by the kitchen fire, sharing a horrified pleasure.

"Is it gone?" asked the girl who had answered the door.

"The master is asking for mulled ale and bread and meat, in the office; and look lively," I said.

"I ain't taking it in. Opening the door and seeing *that* stand there hev took ten years off my life already."

"Put the things outside the door of the office, then, and knock. And look sharp," I said.

As I went out of the kitchen I heard the girl say, "Use a crock we can smash, Kitty; if I'd to set my lips to cup *that'd* used, it'd turn my stomach."

I went and fetched the coat, and, not wishing to behave like a silly serving wench, went into the room, determined to conceal my aversion. The poor creature knelt, shivering, by the fire. Master Reed still sat at his table. I looked at him questioningly and he said:

"The boy's dead, Nicholas; in bad circumstances."

I mumbled that I was sorry, which was true, though my feeling was, in the main, pity for him.

He was a remarkable man; there is a great deal of talking—and some writing too—about the beauties of chivalry, of physical courage, hardihood in the face of danger, all of it very far removed in most people's estimation from an old wool merchant whose hand had never closed on a sword hilt; but that evening he was magnificent in his fortitude. He got up and took the coat from me and went over to the grotesque and said:

"Throw off your wet things and hug this about you. You'll soon be warm. Food and drink are coming." Then, as though resuming the conversation which my entry had interrupted, he said, "That kind of thing means a lot to women. She may well ask what infirmary. Can we answer?"

"There is a House of White Ladies nearby."

"We'll tell her that. The best of nursing, the kindest of attention. After all, the boy's father," he paused and swallowed, "was in his own bed, he had every care, and a physician, yet he died. She will believe, and feel that no one was to blame."

The serving girl tapped on the door. She had gone by the time I opened it. I took in the cup and the platter and carried them to the freak, who had wriggled out of his clothes and was wearing the coat as a cape. His own jerkin, I noticed, with a fresh little thrill of distaste, had been made for him; it had no sleeve on one side, two on the other. He snatched at the things I offered, taking the mug in the hand nearest his face, the platter in the other.

Watching his ravenous attack upon the food, Master Reed said, "There's plenty more. Ask if you want it." He then gave one of his great sighs and set himself in motion. "I must break this to his mother. She might insist on seeing you. You know what to say if she does."

"I know, master. Maybe I should've softened the tale for you. It never entered my head."

"No, for me the truth was best. And I thank you for bringing it."

He indicated with a jerk of his head that I was to look after the freak and went limping away. I pulled a chair into a position from which I could look straight ahead of me without seeing the man who was still stuffing his mouth like a man filling a sack in a hurry.

"What is the truth?" I asked.

"He died, alongside me in Winchester gaol. November, December, cruel cold it was, the walls running with water and puddles on the floor. He took a cold and then a cough and it killed him. Not but what that was a mercy in a way; he'd have burned, otherwise. They'd got upwards of twenty witnesses and that was too much to overlook even though he did have friends in high places, and the Bishop himself was inclined to give Walter the benefit of the doubt. He was so young, too, and had such a nice way with him, enough to make anybody wonder. But twenty witnesses and more. No, that was too much. And in broad daylight too."

"What had he done?" I asked; though I knew all but the details of the answer, for I remembered that summer evening, the hasty angry words, the grandfather's warning.

The man by the fire crammed his mouth and chewed loudly.

"Mind, I wasn't there. I was in the gaol then—for stealing—but never mind me. I only know what Walter said, and that wasn't much, till they took his lute away he used to spend his time playing, only afterwards, when he was sick and heartbroke did he talk. And of course when I was turned loose I heard the talk. They're talking about it still in Winchester; some feel a bit ill-done by to have missed the burning."

He chewed again and resumed his tale.

In Winchester there was always a fair on St. Luke's Day, and most often it was a summer day crept into autumn. "St. Luke's little summer" people called it. This year was no exception; the sun shone clear and bright. There was a man who sold medicine, guaranteed to cure anything from a winter cough to the stone, and he gathered his crowd about him by banging on a drum. Twice during the morning Walter's playing had stolen his crowd away before he had sold much, and about midday the man had approached Walter and protested. Walter had moved away, but the people had followed, and within an hour the medicine-seller had come to him again and suggested a partnership.

"They say—but of course afterwards people will say anything—they say he offered him a fourth share, Walter to play and gather the crowd and then break off in the middle of a tune and let the man cry his wares. And they say that then Walter went white with rage and said, 'Am I to play that you may gull fools? Devil take your pills and potions.' Fifty people claim to have heard him say that."

He broke the tale and I heard him chewing. I also heard, from the other side of the house, some wild, most lamentable crying. I pitied Master Reed from the bottom of my heart.

The story went on. Within five minutes, before in fact the medicine-seller could get back to his stall, a bullock, running amok from the nearby cattle market, crashed into it; became entangled; and stamping, rolling, tossing its head, smashed every pill to powder and broke to fragments the thing which had been the medicine-maker's greatest pride and treasure, a big flask of Venetian glass, half full of red liquid which he claimed to be the elixir of life—the other half had been, he said, poured into the pills.

"Well," the freak said in his soft voice, "that could have been accident, though they counted it uncanny that, except to that one stall, the beast did no damage and was easily taken. In itself that would never have damned him. But next day . . ."

Next day the medicine man, with nothing to sell and a damage to avenge, took his drum and followed Walter round, banging loudly and out of time, spoiling his music. At first only a few people, who cared neither one way nor the other found this amusing, but presently even those who wanted to hear the proper music gave way and found the situation rather comic, and laughed. Walter stopped playing. He took some coins from his pocket and threw them towards the man with the drum.

"Will that buy your silence?" he asked.

The man scooped up the money and said, "Aye"; then, as Walter began to play again, amended it to, "Aye, for two minutes," and banged on his drum. The crowd laughed. Walter said, and this was what twenty reliable people were prepared to swear to, "Then there's no help for it. Let your arm wither."

"And they say that it did. It fell limp and began to grow small. By evening it was dry and shrivelled as a twig. There it was, and no help for it. One day he was mixing medicine and banging his drum—the next helpless. And twenty people near enough to hear what the boy said. It was hopeless. The Church court had him first and they handed him over to the secular arm, and that meant the townspeople. And how they felt is shown by what happened to the bullock. They claimed that was no ordinary beast, but possessed of the Devil. They burned it alive, and those who hadn't tasted meat in six weeks or seven forbore to touch a shred of it, though it lay there, open to all."

How much to believe; how much to discount? I sat there and wondered.

At last I said, "The boy himself; did he think he was guilty?"

"How can I answer that? In the beginning I thought he was a thief, like me. In the end, when they'd taken away his lute and he was miserable and talked more, he said . . . Yes, once he said that to feel strongly enough was to have power. I do remember that. I remember because I said that it was not so, because I felt strongly the wish to be shaped like other people; and he said what was done was done. And then he said that he wished . . . No, he said, 'If I had the power they say I have, I'd wish one wish for myself, to be out of this, and free, in the open, with my lute in my hand.' And he had half of his wish, for presently he coughed and choked on the blood and died, and they did put his lute in the grave with him. Or so I am told."

He went on with his supper, and we sat in silence until Master Reed came in, looking like a man who had just been released from the rack. But his most immediate concern was to find a place for the deformed man to sleep. When that was settled and I ventured to offer a few words of sympathy, he looked at me steadily and said:

"Poor child. With such promise too. But the two things sprang from the same root. And I knew it. That made me less firm than

I should have been. Poor Walter." He sighed again. "Maude should be here," he said. "Her mother'll need her, and I need her. I've not been firm enough in the past, but over this I shall be firm. Maude must come home."

VII

From the way in which Mistress Reed had behaved since Walter's departure, and the wild cries with which she had received the news of his death, I expected the following days to be made hideous by the manifestations of her grief and by her efforts to escape it. I looked ahead and imagined that life at the Old Vine, never very cheerful of late, would become dreary in the extreme. For the first time I began to wonder whether there might not be something unlucky about the house itself, or about the family. I knew I was a long way from being the carefree, cheerful, philandering fellow who had come there to teach Walter his letters. However, I soon shrugged that thought aside as nonsense. I pitied Master Reed, and his daughter-in-law too, but Walter's death had not harmed me; my future indeed looked brighter and more certain. And, I thought to myself, although Walter was buried, far away in Winchester, there would surely be a Requiem Mass for him, and surely Maude would be bound to attend, and perhaps she would feel some pity for her grandfather and decide to come home and gladden his last years. It was a frail hope, but I clung to it.

I kept well away from the house all the morning, and at twelve o'clock went in for my dinner. The square family table was unoccupied. The men assembling at the long tables were quieter than usual, and the serving girls, running round with bowls of meaty broth, had an air of suppressed excitement. The news about Walter had spread, I thought. The door behind me, the one which led into the main part of the house, opened, and Master Reed, instead of entering, stood in the opening and beckoned me to join him.

"Come here," he said, and stumped away up the stairs and to the door of Mistress Reed's room. His face wore a strange expression, something only just short of pleasure as he opened the door and said, "What do you make of that?"

It was as though he were showing me something which, after

long labour, he had made, or, after long waiting, had at last achieved.

Mistress Reed sat on the edge of her bed, dressed as far as her petticoat; she held a comb in her hand and was slowly almost sensuously passing it through the length of her hair. She acknowledged our presence by the open door by turning her head; there was no interest, no recognition, no expression at all in her face. The lines which discontent, grief, and anxiety had graved had all been wiped away, leaving a blank placidity. It was the face of a half-finished statue whose maker has not yet decided whether it shall portray joy or sorrow.

Having once looked our way, she looked away again and resumed her slow combing. Master Reed gently closed the door and said, "She has been like that all morning. Pray God she stays so."

"Amen to that," I said. "Her father did."

"Aye. That's the way it takes them. He turned simple when his wife died." He pondered for a second. "It's not much of a life, but better than being crazed with grief; and easier for everybody else. I must set one of the wenches to mind her."

In one way Mistress Reed was more fortunate than her sire; if the materials were put in her lap, or by her side, she would stitch away, contentedly, for hours. She no longer made anything, just worked away on long hems and seams, or did embroidery stitches without any design or pattern. One of the serving girls, glad of the easy task, devoted all her time to her.

On the third or fourth day Master Reed said, "We need a girl to take Phyllis' place in the kitchen. And who has time to see to that? Not you. Not I. This house lacks a mistress. Maude should come home, now. She must come home."

"The question is, will she?"

"Properly tackled, I think so. For one thing a house without a mistress is as tempting to any woman worth her salt as a ship without a captain to a sailor. For another, it offers her a chance to do something that would *count*, as she calls it. To come home and look after the sick woman who, all these years, was never fair to her, is to return good for evil, surely. Yes, that'll appeal to Maude. I'll go to Clevely tomorrow."

It rained in the night, and though the morning was fine a biting wind blew and the heavy black clouds rushing across the sky threatened more rain or even snow. I was in the weaving shed, settling some petty dispute, when I looked through the wide window and saw Master Reed emerge from the house; so muffled in clothes as to be shapeless and wearing a woollen cap pulled over his ears and brow. Remembering how he had held close to the house all winter, and thinking of the inclement weather, I went down and said unwillingly, because I doubted the outcome of the errand and felt that if it failed he would blame me:

"Let me go, sir."

"No. You mean kindly, but you don't have enough authority. Today I'm going to have it out. My mind is made up, and when my mind is set I mostly get my way."

I realised, with a faint start of surprise, that that was true. Mild and quiet as he was, this whole great business with its many aspects ran smoothly under his absolute authority; only within doors, with his family, did anything displeasing to him continue for longer than it took for him to notice it. He had given in to Maude's whim, Walter's waywardness, Mistress Reed's insobriety, not from weakness, but from kindness of heart.

Well, I thought, all power go with you. I helped him into his saddle, and then stared at the evidence of his confidence in himself, another horse, saddled with Maude's own saddle, and wearing a leading rein was led out. Master Reed took the rein, said, "Come up, then," and they trotted out of the yard.

When I went in to dinner one of the maids was thumping about in Maude's room, making it ready.

And faith, we are told, can remove mountains.

While we were at dinner there was a short sharp shower; but immediately after, just as I was leaving the house, the sun came out. I stood for a moment beside a lilac bush which had thrust a branch over the garden fence; it shimmered with buds, wetly green. Somewhere in the depths of the garden a bird was singing with passionate joy and the golden light lay everywhere like a blessing. I was suddenly certain that Maude would come home that afternoon, and that everything would be well. Anticipation ran, with the tickling thrill of a finger touch, all the way from my thighs to my throat.

Half an hour later it was snowing lightly, and when, in the premature twilight, my master rode home, alone, he was furred all over with white, even his eyebrows bore their little load.

I had imagined, from the length of his absence, that Maude had packed her goods, and that the return journey had been made with laden slowness. But the led horse's saddle was empty except for the snow.

Master Reed replied to my unspoken comment, "I went on to Minsham and took a look at the sheep. Had to do something to settle my mind."

He dismounted stiffly, and, instead of pushing away my proffered arm, took it and leaned on it heavily.

"It's been a bad day, my boy. And a fine fool I made of myself, as you shall hear."

I had made a good fire in the office, and a pint of well-spiced ale in a pewter mug waited on the hearth. I'd had the poker in and out of the heart of the fire for the last two hours, and now I pushed it home again. By the time I had helped him to shuffle off his wrappings it was glowing red, and I plunged it into the ale.

"That'll warm you, sir," I said, handing him the steaming brew.

"It's cooling I need. Feel that if you doubt me." He reached out his free hand and touched mine. "You'll understand, if I can bring myself to tell you."

My curiosity was lively; but the hand he had laid on mine was unnaturally hot and I remembered what the doctor had said about the danger of his being upset. I said as soothingly as possible, "I can see for myself that you are disappointed. Beyond that you can tell me as much or as little as you like."

"That's right! Now you begin to talk to me as though I were a baby. That's all I need after the day I've had."

He sipped his ale and I saw the sweat break out on his forehead. He pulled at the neck of his jerkin, exposing his stringy throat. Another thought struck me.

"Mistress Maude . . . she is well, I hope."

"How can I know? I tell you I never even . . . But I'd best begin at the beginning."

Clevely had altered; he'd spotted the change as soon as the place came in sight. Upwards of fifty ewes gathered in a field for lambing, with a shepherd and a boy in charge; another man in the house-yard, and not a nun to be seen anywhere. And the old kitchen door was now fenced off and a new one made at the far end of the house, with a deep porch in front of it and a portress to answer the bell. He'd asked for the Prioress, which was mere courtesy, since everyone knew that she was now bedfast; but it was not our old friend Dame Clarice Gracey who came into the cold little room where he was bidden to wait; it was a new nun, young, not more than thirty, who said she was the Prioress, so favouritism must have been at work to set her so high at that age.

He explained the situation and asked to see Maude. The Prioress, in a manner as smooth as cream, commiserated with him on the loss of his grandson and the indisposition of his daughter-in-law, but said that it was impossible for him to see Maude.

"Nicholas," he said, leaning forward a little, "when she said that it was like being hit over the heart. I thought she'd taken the veil without a word to us and I might never set eyes on her again. Come to my senses just too late, I thought, and for the rest of her days the poor silly child will come and go, eat or fast, sit or stand according to the word of this highhanded, mim-voiced bitch. And that roused my blood. I said even a nun was allowed to see her grandfather; I said she could stand by and hear every word that was spoken: I told her they weren't an enclosed order and if she didn't let me see Maude I'd complain to the Bishop. She wouldn't be ruffled; she said Maude was still a novice, free to see me or anybody else she'd a mind to, but I couldn't talk to her today because she wasn't at Clevely."

He hadn't believed that. He thought the Prioress quick-witted enough to have guessed what he wanted of Maude; and he thought of his five pounds a year; and he thought that maybe the Prioress had already seen that Maude was in two minds about the matter. So he as good as called her a liar to her face and accused her of not daring to let him talk to his granddaughter.

"So then, Nicholas, she said, 'Daren't is a strange word to use to me. What have I to fear? That you remove her from this house? I assure you I could fill her place ten times over and with girls well dowered.' Dowered is a word I hate the sound of. Before she could toddle it was dower, dower, dower. Hearing the word then, on top of all else, maddened me. I said, 'Then, if you've nothing to fear, why daren't you let me see her?' And she said, 'If you suspect me of hiding her in this house, search it. It is unusual to make a man free of the house, but if it will set your mind at rest, you may have my permission to go anywhere and conduct your search.' And I thought to myself: There's been ample time for that woman at the door to carry warning and have the girl hidden somewhere. So I said, 'I thank you, madam. That I will do.' And I did."

He drained the mug and set it aside and began to twist his hands together. He had big hands, calloused and seamed with ingrained dirt which no amount of scouring would ever remove; but they were oddly skillful; he could splice a broken thread on a loom as neatly and delicately as any of the weavers who made the care of their hands an excuse for never handling a tool. Now he moved his hands as if he were trying to wrench out his fingers one by one.

"I went everywhere, not once only, twice, three times, turning back in my tracks in case they had Maude on the move. My boy, if she'd been the size of a bobbin I couldn't have missed her. Dorter, storeroom, chapel, cellar, everywhere. And it all so poor; I swear our bed in Squatters Row was softer and warmer than any in that house; and as for their storeroom, it was pitiable, braxy mutton and weevilly flour such as I wouldn't offer any seaman of mine to eat. And in the end, back I was in the little cold room and she waiting for me, saying, 'And now will you perhaps accuse me of spiriting the girl away?' Then she said she'd tell me what she would have at first if I had asked her. According to her, the singing at Clevely is an offence to the ear and an insult to God, so Maude and one other—the only ones that can carry a tune—are sent to Ramsey to learn better and come back and teach the rest."

"Enough to make any man angry," I said. "But why blame yourself? Your suspicion might have been correct. You acted rightly."

He moved one eyebrow.

"You think so? I felt all in the wrong. And I apologised. She took advantage of that. She talked about Clevely, all the improvements that must be made; how in the past it had not been a nunnery in the real sense of the word, just a place where women lived and worked together and went to Chapel when the milking was done or the butter made. She's going to alter all that; and her great need is money. Five pounds a year, she was good enough to say, was generous enough when Maude lodged there and worked to earn her keep, but since then, as I, a businessman should know, money had lost some value and the noble was worth but six shillings nowadays. She talked to me like a huckster. What did I propose to do for Maude when she took her vows? And there's Maude thinking that all the world outside has gone awry through love of money. And me, that always called a dower a bait for knaves. I'd have done better, Nicholas, to have sent her to Beauclaire with the promise of a dower on a tag about her neck. A knave would at least have seen that the bed he had to share was soft and warm."

"What did you promise?"

"Nothing. I'm not that much of a fool. I tell you, we bargained like a couple of stockfishmongers. I said I wanted Maude to come home and see the state her mother was in, and I wanted one last good talk. Then, I said, if I could be sure that her mind was made up and no hope for it, I'd give a dowry they'd talk about for years. And so I will, but I must be sure first. She said that was fair enough and Maude will come home as soon as she's back from Ramsey."

"When will that be?"

"Oh, that depends on the singing." His voice took on a sardonic note and then changed. "And she did say one other thing, whether to set much store by it or not, I don't know. She said the visit to Ramsey would do Maude good, aside from the music, to let her see a properly conducted house, because that was how Clevely would be in future and discipline must be accepted meekly. That sounded to me a bit . . . but there, they have such a way of wrapping things up, half the time they mean something other than you'd think."

He shuddered suddenly and held out his hands to the fire.

In the morning he woke with a cold, of which he made light; the Minsham shepherd, he said, had a much worse one the day before and was out in the snow making a lambing pen. Giving this as an excuse for not keeping to his bed, he sneezed through the day, saying after each bout of sneezing, "There, that cleared it." He went to bed early with hot brick to his feet and a basin of onion gruel inside him. He'd budged many a cold with such simple remedies.

This one refused to be budged. It resisted even the curative measure of a day in bed, and by the third day had settled on his chest. He drew his breath with a wheeze and a rattle, and spoke with a hoarse croak. But he held that it was nothing but a cold, he'd had many worse. A linseed poultice was what he needed; surely to goodness somebody in the kitchen could make a linseed plaster.

The cook made it; and also a concoction of honey, vinegar, horehound, and cinnamon, upon whose virtue she was prepared to stake her own.

I took upon myself the application of the poultices, since, with Phyllis minding Mistress Reed, they were shorthanded in the kitchen. When I put it on hot that evening for the last time and settled him for the night, he seemed easier, and still most resolutely cheerful. But his cough, a rattling, ineffective effort to clear the clogged rheum from his chest, kept me awake most of the night. Three times I made a fresh plaster, plied him with the mixture, warmed a cup of milk.

"I shall get the physician to you in the morning," I said. He made no protest. Surprised and a little frightened by this, I thought that perhaps I should fetch the priest, too.

I wished that that could have been done in a more casual, less ominous way. But the Old Vine was not a house where the priest was a visitor; we had nothing to do with Baildon, our parish was Flaxham St. Giles, and the church and the priest's house were three miles away. Sir Andrew, the priest there, was elderly. To send for him was to hint that things were in a bad way.

I might have spared myself these cogitations, for in the grey dawn of the fourth day, when my master roused from an uneasy, restless doze, he stared at me for a moment as though he did not recognise me and then said, his voice more hoarse and weak than ever:

"It's beat me, my boy. I want the priest. Make my confession and my will at the same time."

"Sir Andrew?"

"Yes. Send a good horse . . . pillion."

"I will. But you mustn't lose heart, you know. You've got a stubborn cold and you can't throw it off as you did when you were younger. I'll get the doctor to you, too."

He wheezed out something about a waste of time, and something I didn't quite catch, about a hawthorn tree. Then he coughed and hawked and spoke more clearly for a moment.

"You mustn't fret. I've had my day; and it's a long time since Kate went."

That name, as much as anything, convinced me that he was dying; dying men look back over their lives, they say, back to their very beginnings. And Kate, whoever she was, must have belonged to his youth; I had never heard anyone mention her, though in the yard there were one or two who claimed to remember his wife, "a queer body" who'd never settled down in Baildon, but gone to her own people and then come back to have her baby and died when it was born. Her name was not Kate, I'd heard it, once, I think, and it was outlandish.

The thought that Martin, my master, was about to die fell on my mind and clove it in halves, like an axe coming down on a billet of wood. On one side there was all concern for *my* future. He had no heir except a girl in a convent; I understood the business, he trusted me, and liked me. Surely I must be provided for. But he had spoken of giving Maude a dower which would be talked of for years; and if he thought he was dying it would matter very little to him whether she stayed at Clevely or not. Blood, when the test comes, is thicker than water, and I could well imagine him saying that it was all to go to Maude.

On the other side of my mind there was no material consideration at all. I just realised how much I held him in respect and esteem, how much, whatever happened, I should miss him, quiet, solid, and sensible. True I deceived him a little and robbed him a little, sometimes railed at him in my mind for being slow and stubborn and old-fashioned and fussy over details, but I knew his worth; and although his honesty had not made me honest, and his kindness had not made me kind, he had shown me a standard against which I myself, and any other man I ever met, would measure very small.

Having sent for the priest and the doctor and seen the work in the yard begun, I went in and carried up a new poultice and then a piece of clean parchment, the quill, and the inkhorn. I looked down at these and thought: Instruments of Fate. A few scratches one way or another and a whole future is settled and sealed. I was tempted to remind him that to leave a fortune to Maude would be to make sure that she stayed in Clevely for life. Without saying much he had limned that new Prioress for me; she would be capable of settling, in the way she wanted it, the shilly-shallying mind of any girl so richly dowered. When it came to the point, however, I found that the words would not be said. Instead of speaking I fluffed up his pillows, and then went and fetched my own to add to his, so that he was propped almost upright, and seemed to find relief so.

"You're very good to me," he croaked.

"I'll remind you of those words at Lady Day," I said lightly. I drew my wage then.

He saw the joke and smiled. But he said, "I've seen my last Lady Day."

A pang ran through me, for him, for myself, for all poor people who must, in the end, face the unknown dark. Kings, nobles, clerks, and swineherds, all laid level at last, the songs sung, the good meals eaten, the kisses forgotten and done with. A great hunger for life took me. I decided, all in a moment, that I wouldn't darken another day of my life by hankering for anything; if he doesn't leave me a farthing, I thought, I'll still be alive, and young, capable of enjoying myself.

The priest arrived, red-faced from his ride in the wind, carrying a bag of embroidered linen.

"I am sorry indeed to find you thus," he began. Master Reed dismissed me with a glance and I went out, closing the door.

The woman who cooked for us all caught me on my way out of the house. What, she asked plaintively, should she do about dinner, and supper moreover; it was four days since anybody had given her an order and she'd managed as best she could, with bits of this and that, but now she was at the end. With the mistress gone silly and the master taken to his bed, whom could she ask but me. "Thass all very sad, but when they come in, all them great hearty men, they ain't to be put off with sorrowful words and titbits."

That, I knew, would be the last thing that he would wish. His attitude towards food was extraordinary; very abstemious himself, he was always careful to see that his table was spread with good food and plentiful. Yet the waste of a crumb worried him. I had often noted this incongruity and concluded that he was a man who, in his time, had gone hungry and knew the value of food.

And now, once again, my severed mind bothered me. By the time dinner was on the table . . . Oh, let us not think of that! Dying can be a long business. They'll come in hungry; and this is one of the days in their lives, in my life; all of us being rushed along by uncheckable time towards the moment when food will concern, will please us no more.

"You say you've been on the makeshift," I said. "To put it even, what is the thing they like best?"

"Salt beef and dumplings." She was beautifully certain about that. "But that'll mean opening a new cask of beef. You say I am to do that?"

"Yes. Open a new . . ." I broke off, hearing overhead the imperative banging of the stick which I had placed by Master Reed's bedside so that he could summon attention.

"Cask," I said, "and plenty of dumplings." I took the stairs two at a time.

It was the priest who had done the banging. When I entered he stood there, the stick in his hand. He gave me a sidelong, curiously shamefaced look and then looked down at the carved knob of the stick.

"My hands," he said. "All knotted with old age and stiffness. It's as much as I can do to write my name nowadays."

And probably, I thought swiftly, as much as he could do at any time. In some places and in some circumstances very little learning was demanded of a man anxious to take orders. And that little, unpractised for thirty or forty years in a country parish, would shrivel to nothing.

Master Reed, coughing and hawking, said, "You do the scribing, Nicholas."

The priest threw me another look, faintly hostile. I knew how he felt; there was no real need, in his opinion, to have the will written down. Dozens of men every year disposed of their property by word of mouth—a nuncupative will as it was called—and when it came to the attesting of such unwritten testaments there was no word that carried so much weight as a priest's. I accuse Sir Andrew of nothing when I say that, had I not been there with my ready pen, he could have called two gaping oafs from kitchen or yard, listened to Martin Reed's wheezing expression of his last wishes, and later on very easily proved that on his deathbed the wool merchant had turned very pious and left most of his goods to Holy Church. That had been done a thousand times and would be again. The number of Chantries in the country, served by idle, self-indulgent priests who could not even remember the names of those for whom they were to sing Masses, and by whose bounty they lived, proves that.

In this case, here I was, seating myself sideways, awkwardly against the chest where I had set the writing things, leaving the table for the cloth, the wafer, and the wine of the ritual.

Master Reed, in a voice that sounded like an ungreased wheel in the distance, said, "First I want every man who's worked for me five years or more to have three shillings and fourpence; those less long, twenty pence."

Before I could set down a word the priest said, "A written will should be properly made. That is no way to begin. You commend your soul to Almighty God and then say that you are of good mind and memory."

"You can both see. I'm short of breath. We'll get the main things down. Trim it up afterwards." Master Reed signed to me to write, which I did hastily.

His habitual economy of words now served him well; the sentences, though barely audible, were brief and clear. Calling me his "faithful servant and good friend," he left me the premises, the goodwill, tools, and instruments which would enable me to carry on his business as wool merchant, weaver, and smith. His two ships and his flocks were not included in this bequest, but he left me twenty pounds in cash for immediate expenses. Out of the profits of the business I was to pay, each year, three pounds to Sir Godfrey Blanchfleur, the elder, and ten to Anne Reed, widow of Richard Reed deceased, so long as they should live.

It was easy enough to keep pace with his dictation because of his frequent pauses to cough and gather breath. Having written that I looked at him, hoping to convey my gratitude in a glance, but he was staring ahead, frowning. He drew a rattling breath and went on.

Everything else of which he was possessed, the house, his ships, his cash money, the sheep run at Minsham and the flocks; two house properties in Baildon Saltgate, the Great Field at Horringer, the freehold of the God Spare Mariners inn at Bywater, were to go to his dearly beloved granddaughter, Maude Reed. . . .

The name emerged in such an inconclusive way that for a second or two I was certain that he was going to add some conditional phrase. Holding the pen suspended, I looked at him again and as I did so a bout of coughing racked him. When it was done, he said: "That's all."

Slowly I placed the full stop which would hold Maude in the nunnery. There was a little silence, broken by the priest's rasping voice, saying with genuine horror, "Such a will a heathen might make. No mention of Holy Church, of alms or charity or so much as a Mass for your sinful soul. My son, I bid you think again. For your own sake."

"What do you want me to say?"

"I," Sir Andrew's voice conveyed his affront, "I want nothing, except to ease your passage through Purgatory and give you credit at the Last Judgement. You, Martin Reed, like the young man who came to Our Lord, are a man of great possessions. I would not have you, like him, go sorrowful away when all the reckoning is made. And of this will I say that a Saracen who had never taken the Body and Blood of Christ upon his tongue might leave it behind."

Master Reed had sunk a little farther back into his pile of pillows and half closed his eyes.

"Sir Andrew," I began, in an expostulatory voice.

"Be silent!" he said. "You were brought in to write and well you have done it. I have his soul to care for. Martin, for your own sake, make a gift to the Church, one of your many properties. One-third to buy Masses for your soul; one-third for the poor; and one-third to be used at the priest's discretion. At Flaxham we have no bell." He added the final words with a disarming simplicity.

"Then let it be the Minsham sheep run, that being nearest to you."

"I will see that the Masses are faithfully said."

I scratched the sheep run out of the list of properties that were to be Maude's, and thought how the Prioress would grudge it, could she but know. I added the bequest to those already written, with details of its disposal. Then a thought struck me.

"You have not named those who should execute your will, sir."

"You," he said, wearily. "And Sir Andrew, here, if he is willing."

"Right readily. And the bell, Martin, shall bear your name, with some reminder. 'Pray for the soul of Martin Reed, whenever you my tongue shall heed' or something like that."

"I thank you," Martin Reed said, but he looked at me as he spoke, and one of his eyebrows lifted as I had seen it do when Mistress Reed spoke with extra haughtiness, or Walter made some unusually extravagant statement. And I thought to myself: This is not the way he would have willed it on the afternoon when he came back from Clevely. I put the quill into the inkhorn and tipped it a little, so that a thin black stream ran from corner to corner of the written sheet.

"Now look what I have done," I said. "I am very sorry. The chest is awkward to write at. Shall I now make a fair copy?"

"Yes," said Sir Andrew firmly. "And in the rewriting make a proper beginning. Write, 'In the name of Almighty God, Amen.' And then go on, 'I, Martin Reed, being of good mind and memory, make my testament in this wise.' Can you bear that in mind? And first mention the gift to Flaxham Church, it will look better there than tagged on at the end."

I looked again at my master. Save for two small dusky red patches over the cheekbones, his face was the colour of a candle; his eyes were half closed.

"In all else, sir, this is as you wish?"

"Make a fair copy, Nicholas; while I make my peace with God."

I bent down and lifted one of his big, work-worn hands and put my lips to it. I fumbled in my mind for some words—not my own—with which to refute the priest's attitude, and found them, spoke them haltingly. " 'What more can a man do than love mercy, do justice, and walk humbly before his God?' That you have always done, and God will know His own, sir."

I picked up the writing things and went from the room as the priest settled his stole.

Downstairs in the office I rewrote the will in a neat clear script, setting it down as I had been bidden, until I came to the point where, leaving Maude's name hanging in the air, Master Reed had paused. There I wrote in what I genuinely believed he would himself have added at any other time: "on condition that she abandon all intention of becoming a nun." He had wanted Maude to come home and marry and have children; those few added words would give her the chance to do so at least.

Then I thought, nobody would make such a condition without providing against its non-acceptance. So I added that if Maude insisted upon becoming a professed religious all her portion was to go to Flaxham Church. It hurt me to dispose so lightly of such a fortune, but the priest had just shown me that, like many people who do not rely upon the written word, he had an excellent memory. That final sentence would blur his memory and stop his mouth. It also, in a curious way, cleared my conscience.

Two witnesses who had no interest in the will were needed. I fetched two men who were waiting in the forge. They made their crosses and I wrote their names below.

By midday Martin Reed was peacefully unconscious, and in that state he died, just before dawn on the following morning.

Interval

What he found so hard to stomach was that in the end he brought
about his own undoing; was punished for behaving well; sustained
a hurt which would last a lifetime simply because he had shown a
delicate consideration for another person's feelings and exercised
self-restraint.

That he had, perhaps, challenged Fate by being too certain,
somewhat arrogant, a trifle smug, never once occurred to him.

He had been right, surely, not to make an instant proposal of
marriage when Maude, at last, came back to the Old Vine. She had
suffered enough emotional strain, returning to Clevely, after three
days of hard travel, to learn that her grandfather was dead and
buried, and, while that grief was still raw, coming home to learn
of Walter's death and to be confronted by her idiot mother.

At Clevely the Prioress had lost no time in producing an aged
copy of the Bull Periculoso of Pope Boniface VIII.

"Here it is, clearly set down in black and white, in the vulgar
tongue for the benefit of the unlearned," she said. "A rule made
one hundred and fifty years ago, which has been disregarded by
the heads of many Houses with consequent disorder and ruin.
Read it."

It was a piece of stiff parchment which had been kept tightly
rolled for many years. Under the Prioress's white, well-kept hands
it opened a little and then tried to spring back into its roll.

"Take hold of it. It has no teeth! There. . . ."

Maude read a sentence about forbidding, on pain of excommuni-
cation, any nun or sister to go outside the bounds of a monastery.
She looked up with a puzzled frown. She and Dame Lucy had been
sent to Ramsey.

"There," said the Prioress, and the finger jabbed down upon the next sentence. "Read it aloud."

"Item," Maude read, "let no one be received as nun or sister until we have enquired more fully into the resources of the House."

"It could hardly be clearer," the cool voice said. "A convent is not, as so many people suppose, a refuge for the indigent. The terms of your grandfather's will ensure that if you stay here you will have nothing. Not even the miserable five pounds a year that has hitherto been paid, and which he as good as promised me should be increased. Old men in their dotage," she said savagely, "change their minds with every wind. And the Flaxham priest, naturally, had an eye to his own advantage."

Maude took her hands from the document, folded them in front of her in the approved manner, and stood silent. There was nothing to say. She knew, in her heart, that her grandfather, although he had allowed her to live at Clevely, had done so against his will; and that had she become a nun it would have been with his disapproval. She had often wondered, during the last year, whether he had not known her better than she knew herself; and since the installation of the new Prioress her uncertainty and lack of contentment had grown daily. Now, after the long and wearing indecision, the choice had been made for her.

"There is no need to tell you," the Prioress said, "that this is a House virtually without resources. What I brought to it is already spent and not half of what is needful is yet done. If, in the circumstances, I allowed you to stay here, I should act in direct disobedience to this Papal Bull, and should myself deserve to be removed."

She spoke as though she were repudiating some plea, refuting an argument. Maude wondered how often this scene would be reenacted; upon how many women who were sure of their vocation, and who perhaps had no resources, even sequestrated ones like her own, this Papal Bull would be used like an axe. For herself it did not matter. She drew a long breath, lifted her head and said clearly:

"Madam, I am not asking you to keep me."

She never guessed that a little humility at this point, a few tears, some pleading words would have persuaded the Prioress to disregard Boniface VIII's express command. She never guessed that she had been sent to Ramsey to make a study of the music, not because she had a better ear than most of the others but because the

Prioress hoped that the idea of improving the Clevely singing would forge another link, give her an aim and a purpose. Maude had taken less kindly than anyone except Dame Clarice, who was so old that she counted for little, to the new regime at Clevely, and Maude was, in fact, exactly the type of woman whom the Prioress wished to rule; educated, well connected on one side, at least, sensible, and rich.

Rich no longer. The Prioress's disappointment was commensurate with her hopes, which had ridden high after her interview with old Martin Reed; and since he was beyond her reproaches she expended her anger upon Maude.

"I don't *mind*," Maude told Nicholas in one of their many talks. "I wasn't sure; I don't think I ever was sure, and Grandfather knew it. I think that is why he made that condition. As a test. All the same," she frowned, and on her smooth white forehead the ghost of Martin's double horseshoe cicatrice appeared, "I was *shocked*. In the old days money never mattered at Clevely."

"Then it was," he said lightly, "the only place on earth where it did not; and now there is none. Money always matters."

"Not to Walter. He was the one person who never minded about it."

He was tempted to retort sharply that even so it was money, some infinitesimally small sum of it, that had led to Walter's premature death. But he had seen that same darkening of the eyes as had once accompanied any mention of Melusine, and, as on former occasions, all his impulse was to comfort and console. So he took her hand and told her gently that she must not grieve for Walter; Walter's life, short as it was, had held as much happiness as most people know in sixty years; he had always done exactly what he wanted, and nothing that he did not; he had loved nothing and nobody but his music, and that love had never failed him.

He could, even thus early, have gone on to speak of other forms of love, confessed his own. But he refrained.

Opportunities to step smoothly from the impersonal to the intimate abounded, seemed indeed to thrust themselves upon him. She spoke once, in an astonished way, of the fact that her grandfather had named no guardian.

"I expected to be somebody's ward, like poor Madge FitzHerbert," she said. "And when I left Clevely I made up my mind that nobody was going to marry me for my possessions."

He realised that the omission had been an oversight; in his hasty rewriting of the will the matter of Maude's age had never entered his mind. He could not now say what was true, that Martin, in the making of his will, had visualised her under the guardianship and management of the Prioress of Clevely.

"Your mother is still living," he pointed out, "and I am here to look after everything for you. You need no guardian. And the notion of being married for your money is an absurdity. You are no Madge FitzHerbert. You are beautiful."

Her face coloured and the pace of his heartbeat quickened. Now? Why not? So easy. You are beautiful and lovable and I love you; to marry you has been my one desire since the moment I saw you almost four years ago.

But he left it where it was. A compliment, accepted with a blush.

There had always been, at the core of his feeling for her, an element of the worshipful, novel to him in his experience of women, and therefore oddly enjoyable. There was also in his attitude something resembling that of the gourmet who, before setting about some particularly succulent dish, eyes it with pleasure, sniffs its savour with gloating. Some part of his restraint was also not far removed from fear. She was so innocently friendly; a word spoken too soon, some betraying gesture made before he had succeeded in endearing himself to her, might ruin all. He had come so far, waited so long, worked so cunningly, that in the end nothing but perfection would suffice.

He behaved—as he saw, looking back—in lunatic fashion. Not content with a dumb wooing, fetching and carrying, acting in all but the ultimate assertion of rights, like an elderly man with a lovely and capricious mistress, he went to other lengths. He broke with Clemence, promising her a pension of five pounds a year and bearing first her reproachful tears and then her vituperative anger with the utmost detachment, as though suddenly a wall of glass had reared itself between her and him. He rode home from Minsham whistling, and on the next day took himself into the confessional at St. Mary's Church, and, for some moderate penance and a contribution to the Poor Box, was absolved from all his sins of fornication.

Young men, on the eve of knighthood, made similar confessions, and washed themselves thoroughly and then kept vigil in churches all through the night. That thought occurred to him as he left the church, raising his eyes to the carved angels in the roof, the angels of whom Maude, at the age of twelve, had reminded him. A carving, once made, he thought, was finished, could never grow or change. *His* angel, while losing nothing that could deserve reverence, had developed all the qualities which would enable a man to say truly, "With my body I thee worship." It occurred to him that on the night before his marriage he would keep vigil in this church, under the angel roof.

So he stepped out into the greenish April dusk at almost the same moment as a young man, thoroughly washed, confessed, and absolved, went into the chapel of the Knights Hospitallers, at Dunwich, to keep his pre-knighting vigil.

The days lengthened; the trees shook out their young green; daisies and cowslips and lady's smocks gemmed the meadows. There had never been so sweet a spring as this one through which they rode, on her business, on his, or something which concerned them both. It was a matter for laughter that *his* pack ponies on their comings and goings must use *her* front door and trot through the very heart of *her* house. And his certainty that he had done right, that he had carried out both Martin's wish and Maude's was proved beyond all doubt on the day when Sir Andrew, riding a bony mule, came into the Old Vine and, with the air of doing Maude a favour, said that if she cared to return to Clevely and take vows she could. Flaxham Church, out of what would then fall into its hands, would endow her handsomely. The Prioress, upon whom he had called, was very anxious, he said, to have Maude back, providing her return was in accord with the Bull Periculoso. If she saw his real purpose, Maude gave no sign of such awareness, but thanked him heartily and said she had no wish to return to Clevely.

"There are other houses," he suggested.

"None where I am needed as I am here. I look after my mother."

He argued at some length, and then, finding her immovable, made a peevish complaint about the wording of the will.

"It was made hastily and badly."

"You were present at its making, Sir Andrew," Maude said mildly.

"Yes; and I said at the time that it was such a will as a heathen might make. And I had my mind set upon persuading your grandfather on another point, so that that condition slipped in without my noticing. Also I had a cold in my head and at such times I am a little hard of hearing. Of one thing I am *sure*, and that is that it was never your grandfather's intention to so make his will that you should renounce your vocation."

"I think it was his intention to prove to me that I had no vocation."

"Then why did you contemplate the religious life?"

She frowned thoughtfully.

"I was trying to run away from certain things in this world that I was unwilling to face."

"And have they changed?"

It was impossible to explain how the balance had been adjusted, Clevely, under the new regime, another lost illusion, and the Old Vine, free of her mother's dislike, no longer a place to flee from. She said simply, "The change has been in me."

Some hot and hasty words about the uncertainty of purpose, the halting faith, the self-indulgence of this new generation, formed in his mind, but stopped short behind his teeth. She was his parishioner, and a wealthy one; it would serve him ill to alienate her. He had already ordered the new bell; there was that much gained; and now, to test her attitude he said:

"I find that I made your grandfather a rash promise. I also was hasty that morning. The bell will cost more than I thought and I shall not be able to afford the engraving which was to remind all those who heard its voice to pray for his soul."

She said eagerly that she would pay for that.

When he left, disappointed in his main objective, he looked forward to a future rich in little extortions. She had not taken advantage of his offer, but he was sure that in her heart she had appreciated it. She was convent-schooled and would be amenable. He remembered a proverb, current amongst the homely members of his flock—there were more ways of catching a cony than by chasing it, shouting.

Nicholas Freeman decided to declare himself on May the third, which at the Old Vine had always been the date of a humble, rather curious little family festival, known as "Sparrowgrass Day."

At the end of the garden, beyond the rosebushes and the apple trees and the herb plot, was a bed of asparagus, twenty years old. Richard had brought the first crowns back from one of his trips to Flanders; they had spread and flourished to such an extent that each year, at the height of its bearing, the bed gave at least two cuttings of such plenty that every man and boy in the dining hall could have ten or twelve green spikes as a vegetable with his supper dish. Martin Reed had convinced himself that the plant had medicinal qualities, it cleansed the blood. Earlier in the season, when the first shoots were ready for cutting but not in such number that they would "go round," the asparagus presented a problem to a master of Martin Reed's nature; the square family table in the hall was always served with exactly the same food as any other. Luxuries were enjoyed later, in privacy. A cooked vegetable, however, could not be served after supper, casually from the livery cupboard; nor could the first, succulent green growth be wasted. So, for some years, in the last days of April, or the early ones of May, Martin and Richard, and later Anne and then the children, had observed Sparrowgrass Day, and had supper served at the table in the solar. Then someone had observed that it was on May the third that Martin had first approached Anne's father about her marrying Richard, and so the little feast day was fixed. Other delicacies, such as fresh fish hurried up from Bywater, were added to the table, and always jugs of good wine.

This year Nicholas intended to keep the festival and, because Maude's birthday had fallen during the days of mourning for her grandfather and gone unmarked, it could be a celebration of her birthday too. He had ridden into Colchester and bought her a present from the goldsmith's there. It was a reliquary pendant, hung on a thin gold chain. The pendant was a flat, slim oblong of gold which, upon pressure on a spring, opened into a triptych of pictures, beautifully worked in enamel, the centre picture showing the Crucifixion, the one to the left the Annunciation, and the one on the right Christ's Ascension. When closed it measured an inch and a half by two, and was a masterpiece of delicate workmanship. It had cost every penny of his filchings and three pounds of his cash legacy.

He planned it all to the last detail. Mistress Reed could go to bed and eat—in the disgustingly slovenly way she had lately developed—her dish of asparagus there. He and Maude would sit in the solar, at a table with a good linen cloth, set near the window to catch the evening light. There would certainly be, to start with at least, the sadness inseparable from any family anniversary after a bereavement, and he would exert himself to talk as entertainingly as possible. The servant would serve the asparagus, and then the fish, and go, leaving the sweetmeats on the cupboard. When they were alone he would remind Maude of her forgotten birthday and produce his gift. After it had been admired he would fix the chain about her neck, drop his hands to her shoulders, turn her towards him, and kiss her.

All this planning gave him the same half-incredulous pleasure as he had felt through the waiting time. He, Nick Freeman, whose approach to women had always been so forthright, setting a scene, preparing the very words he would say. It was amazing, but it was wonderful; he loved her, never having loved any woman before, therefore it must all be as different as he could make it.

The very day was exactly as he would have had it could he have ordered it as he had ordered the clothes he intended to wear that evening; a warm, fair day, full of the first scents of summer. The little pink monthly rose, always the first to come into bloom was covered with half-open buds; the lilacs were in heavy flower. A bowl of the roses, he thought, closely massed together in the centre of the table, between the silver candlesticks. Giving this order to the maid whom he had taken into his confidence, an odd thought occurred to him—it was almost as though he were a priest, arranging an altar! The thought provoked a smile, which still lingered in the corners of his mouth and in his eyes as he went on to have a word with Phyllis. Mistress Reed to be out of the solar and into bed by six o'clock.

Then, so that the whole thing might be a surprise to Maude, he sought her out with the suggestion that in the afternoon they should ride together. There was a clip of wool he wanted to inspect at Marly.

"I've never been there," Maude said.

"You turn off at Flaxham and ride alongside the river. It is a pretty ride, especially now, with the hawthorns coming into bud."

Before they left he took out his new clothes and laid them on the bed. Never in all his life had he had such clothes because always every garment he had bought, even for best, had ahead of it years of servile office wear. His new tunic and hose were garments for a young, prosperous merchant, garments that Maude's own father might have worn, a tawny yellow, slashed with buff, colours carefully chosen to enhance his dark good looks, and the easy cut of the tunic calculated to conceal the hint of threatening stoutness. He laid the pendant beside the clothes, ready to slip into his pouch when he changed.

They exchanged casual, unimportant remarks as they rode, until, in the distance, they could see the double arch of the ancient stone bridge, with its image perfectly reflected in the water below. On either bank of the river were the hawthorns covered with bright green leaves, just uncurling, and clusters of buds a little less white than the flowers into which presently they would break. Somewhere on the other side of the river a cuckoo called, and another answered.

Maude gave a great sigh which called her grandfather to Nicholas' mind.

"Beautiful!" she said. "So beautiful. And when I think how nearly I missed it all." The ecstatic note in her voice gave way to a kind of grating impatience. "Oh, I know that the summer will pass and the bloom will fade and the leaves will fall, whereas the spiritual things, the devotion and the duties and the joys go on, unchanging whatever the season . . . and when one is old. I *know* that. In my mind. But my heart was never convinced. It would not be. I prayed and prayed for some sign, for some proof that what I knew I should do was the thing that was right for me. And nothing happened. Then, when the sign came, it pointed the other way."

They had halted their horses who, after nuzzling one another, dropped their heads and strained towards the green grass.

"I warned you," he said. And she took that, not as a reproach, but as proof that he knew what she was talking about. That was what made him so delightful a companion; he did not need everything explained and underlined.

"I know. But when you are young what do you know about yourself? I mean . . . a dim-witted person might, for the best of reasons, wish to be a scholar, and try and try, and he would learn *something*; then one day he might be sent to feed pigs and realise that feeding pigs was what God meant him to do. You know why I went to Clevely; I told you. And for a long time it seemed right. Being cold and tired and hungry, salting the butter away in casks with the salt getting into the cracks of my hands was all helping, I thought. I offered my little sufferings so that Melusine . . . And

then, all at once it was no good for me any more. Nothing I did
was a gift; it was a tax, wrenched from me."

"I could see that," he said.

"There was one time when I was afraid I might go mad. Shall
I tell you what I thought? I thought that if this went on much
longer, I should begin to hate Melusine. I thought she should never
have done . . . never have got herself into such a situation in the
first place; or, having let it happen, she should have married one of
those silly young men who were always following her around.
Wasn't that shocking? The one person who had been kind to me.
The person who had taught me to read and write. To think such
shameful things."

"Thoughts walk in uninvited," he said.

She turned to him with a look of bright relief.

"That *is* true, isn't it? I was in the Chapel, at the end of a twenty-
four-hour fast. I was making a Novena. And that thought, as you
say, walked in. And after that it all seemed such a waste. But I went
on praying, and in the end there was a sign—the Bull Periculoso!"

"May Heaven reward Pope Boniface VIII," he said lightly. But
one day, or rather one night, one night very soon, when they lay
spent with loving, breathless with loving, when she had tasted to
the full all the joy she had so nearly missed, he would tell her to
whom she owed it. The story of how the long-dead Pope had had
a little help from a humble living clerk would be worth telling.

The thought of being in bed with her, of her hair spread loose
on the pillow, of the way he would handle and teach that virgin
innocence moved him so much that once again he was astonished.
He might have been a boy again, virgin himself, excited by the
prospect of his first experience in the art of love.

"I think we should move on," he said. "We mustn't be late for
supper. I have a surprise for you."

They rode towards the bridge, she trying to extract from him
some details about the surprise, he refusing to tell her, and both
finding cause for laughter in this simple business because they were
happy and it was a day for laughter.

How well, he thought, he had chosen his time. Her return to
the world had combined with the natural resiliency of youth to
enable her to throw off her sorrows. She was whole now, and happy,
and his for the taking.

Presently he had another notion, as farfetched as the earlier comparison of a supper table with an altar. They were already, he thought, like a married couple. The proposal, the acceptance, the ceremony would be nothing but formalities. The real bonds of affection and common interest and good companionship were already forged.

He looked back upon how he had come to Baildon, having been thrown out of the leather merchant's house in disgrace; upon how, before ever he had set eyes upon her, he had decided that to marry his master's granddaughter would be a desirable thing to do. How seldom in this life did one's desires and one's material advantages run alongside. How profoundly, how miraculously lucky he had been.

He fell silent and rode for some time indulging in those gloating, self-congratulatory thoughts which ignorant heathen everywhere and at all times have regarded as dangerous, likely to provoke the gods to jealousy and wrath.

The road by which he and Maude, at the end of their ride, approached the Old Vine, ran steeply downhill, and the road itself had been made, immemorial years ago, by heavily laden horses who, to ease the incline, had struggled not straight forward but from left to right and then from right to left. It had three sharp bends; and three times, riding downhill, one could catch, and then lose again, the sight of the house, the weaving sheds and stables, lying at the bottom of the slope, with, just beyond, the wall and south gate of Baildon.

On this afternoon, as the view came first into sight, they could see two horsemen ride through the gateway; both men, one riding a tall horse, the other a heavier animal which bore, beside its rider, a sizable bundle behind the saddle. They saw so much, and then the road turned and a clump of elms blocked out the view.

When they could next look down the riders had almost reached the house and were visible in some detail. The one on the tall horse was young, his tanned face dark against his straw-coloured hair; the other man was older, and the bundle behind him, by its awkward angular shapes and the fact that it was enclosed in a soft, yellowish bag of goatskin, could be identified as a suit of armour packed for transit. Two squires on their way to join their master. The view was obscured again.

The road ran out on to the level and made its last turn. The two riders had halted by the great door of the Old Vine. The younger was studying the house, looking it over, up and down, from side to side. Perhaps because he was conscious of the new clothes lying spread upon his bed, Nicholas observed, between one blink of the eyelid and the next, the shabbiness of the scuffed, rubbed, greasy leather jerkin worn by this young man. At the same time, not to be missed, was some indefinable hint of quality; in the way he sat in his saddle, in the turn of his head, as he looked the house over. This quality was oddly reflected in his mount; rawboned and rough-coated, it yet bore the stamp of breeding.

Nicholas looked at Maude and was about to say: It seems we have visitors; for the young man, making a sign with his hand which his companion interpreted as an order to wait where he was, turned his horse and rode into the great door of the house. There was no time to make the remark, for Maude brought her hand down in a slap on her horse's rump and it shot forward. Nicholas caught one glimpse of a face he had never seen before, transformed, almost idiotic with joyful surprise.

His own horse, without urging, hurried after its companion, and they clattered into the yard nose to tail.

The young man was in the act of dismounting, his eyes fixed on the back of the house in the same keen earnest scrutiny to which he had subjected the front.

He reached the ground and then, hearing the clatter of hoofs, turned about. Maude threw herself out of the saddle and cried, "Henry!" Her face was red as a rose from chin to brow and his turned even darker.

He said in a gruff, embarrassed way, "I told you I should come."

It was not what he had intended to say, nor the tone in which he had intended to speak. And just behind Maude a man, too old to be her twin brother, a neat good-looking man, was just dismounting.

Too full of sudden fear to mind his manners, he seized Maude's hands and pulled off both her gloves. Only one ring, and that the one which he had pushed onto that finger more than four years ago.

"You've worn it . . . all this time?"

She nodded, and laughed, and said, "It's still too big."

Satisfied, he remembered what, through four hard years, he had kept in mind, as part of his goal. Still holding her hand, he went on one knee and lifted her fingers to his lips.

"Sir Henry Rancon," he said, so thickly that he seemed about to choke, "now and forever at your service, demoiselle."

"Last time," she said, "it was the other way round. You remember? Stand up, Sir Henry, and let me look at you."

He had changed very little, except to grow; the shabby old jerkin was much too small. An old scar ran from one eyebrow to the edge of his badly cropped, dusty hair, and a newer one, hardly healed, showed just below the line of his jaw. She remembered the surprising softness of his lips and wondered . . . And was then aware that Nicholas had come to stand beside her. She turned to him, and, with a smile that haunted him to the end of his life, dealt him his mortal wound.

"This was the surprise! Oh, Master Freeman, how did you guess?" They had been on Christian name terms for at least a month.

Sometimes, during his almost meteoric rise to the upper ranks in the clerical hierarchy—for with money behind him, celibacy willingly embraced, and ruthless ambition as his motive power, nothing could stop him—he would ponder the irony of it all. Occasionally such musings ended with disconcerting thoughts about puppets and the strings they danced on, thoughts unsuitable in a churchman, tacitly dedicated to the theory of man's free will.

He suffered one such moment when, thirty years later, he was presented with his cardinal's hat. He recalled then, as though it had been something he had dreamed, Maude's story of the Rune Stone at Beauclaire. That was easily to be dismissed as girlish fancy. Less easy to ignore was the memory of old Martin Reed saying mildly, out of his garnered experience, "People do what they must."